DENTAL RADIOGRAPHY

Principles and Techniques

Fourth Edition

DENTAL RADIOGRAPHY

Principles and Techniques

Joen M. Iannucci, DDS, MS
Professor of Clinical Dentistry
The Ohio State University
College of Dentistry
Columbus, Ohio

Laura Jansen Howerton, RDH, MS
Instructor
Wake Technical Community College
Raleigh, North Carolina

ELSEVIER
SAUNDERS

3251 Riverport Lane
St. Louis, Missouri 63043

Dental Radiography Principles and Techniques   ISBN: 978-1-4377-1162-2

Copyright © 2012, 2006, 2000, 1996 by Saunders, an imprint of Elsevier Inc.

Notices

Previous editions copyrighted 2006, 2000, 1996

Library of Congress Cataloging-in-Publication Data

Iannucci, Joen M.
    Dental radiography : principles and techniques / Joen M. Iannucci, Laura Jansen Howerton. — 4th ed.
       p. ; cm.
    Includes bibliographical references and index.
    ISBN 978-1-4377-1162-2 (pbk.)
    1. Teeth—Radiography.   I. Howerton, Laura Jansen.   II. Title.
    [DNLM: 1. Radiography, Dental—methods.   WN 230]
    RK309.H36 2012
    617.6′07572—dc22

                                                                    2011005794

Acquisitions Editor: Kristin Hebberd
Developmental Editor: Joslyn Dumas
Publishing Services Manager: Catherine Jackson
Project Manager: Sara Alsup
Design Direction: Teresa McBryan
Cover Designer: Maggie Reid

Printed in the United States of America

Last digit is the print number: 9 8 7 6 5 4 3 2 1

Dedications

To my son, Michael —
To my dad, Angelo —
To my mom, Dolores —
thank you for your everlasting love,
your encouragement, and a life filled with laughter.

To each of my coworkers —
thank you for your brilliant creativity,
your support, and your extraordinary sense of humor.

To each of my students, past & present —
thank you for all you have taught me,
and for the true privilege of being a part of your life.

JMI

To my husband, Bruce, who inspires me every day of my life.

LJH

Reviewers

Roseann Bass, CDA
Dental Assistant Program Coordinator
Department of Extended Studies
Norwalk Community College
Norwalk, Connecticut

Terry L. Doty, RDH, MS
Assistant Professor
Department of Nursing and Allied Health
Baltimore City Community College
Baltimore, Maryland

J. Blake Perkins, DDS
CEO
Cascadia Dental Career Institute
Vancouver, Washington
Part-time Clinical Faculty
Department of Restorative Dentistry
Pacific University School of Dental Health Science
Hillsboro, Oregon

Sheri Lynn Sauer, CODA, CDA
Dental Assisting Instructor, Secondary
Department of Dental Assisting
Eastland Career and Technical Schools
Groveport, Ohio

Jane Helen Slach, CDA, RDA, BA
Professor
Department of Health Science
Kirkwood Community College
Cedar Rapids, Iowa

Lynne C. Weldon, CDA, RDH
Adjunct Professor
Department of Health Sciences/Dental Assisting
Northwest Florida State College
Niceville, Florida

April V. Williams, RDH, BHSA, MDH
Assistant Professor
Department of Dental Hygiene
University of Tennessee Health Science Center
Memphis, Tennessee

Preface

Welcome to the fourth edition of *Dental Radiography: Principles and Techniques*. As the title suggests, the purpose of this text is to present the basic principles of dental radiography, and provide detailed information about radiographic techniques. This text offers a reader-friendly format with a balance of theory and complete technical instruction to develop radiography skills. Our goal has always been to facilitate teaching and learning; the fourth edition continues the two purposes set forth by the previous edition.

ABOUT THIS EDITION

One of the strengths of this text is its organization. To facilitate learning, the fourth edition is divided into manageable parts for both the reader and instructor:

- Radiation Basics
- Equipment, Film, and Processing Basics
- Dental Radiographer Basics
- Technique Basics
- Digital Imaging Basics
- Normal Anatomy and Film Mounting Basics
- Image Interpretation Basics

Each chapter includes several features to aid in learning. A list of **objectives** and key terms to focus the reader on the important aspects of the material are presented at the beginning of every chapter. **Key terms** are highlighted in magenta and bold typeface as they are introduced in the text. A complete **glossary** of more than 600 terms is included at the end of the book. **Step-by-step procedures that provide students with everything they need to know are included in the technique chapters.** The material is organized in an instructionally engaging, sound way that ensures technique mastery and serves as a valuable reference tool. Each of the technique chapters include *Helpful Hints* that help students learn to recognize and prevent the most common pitfalls in the performance of that technique, and provides a checklist of items to guide both the novice, or the experienced practitioner. **Summary tables and boxes** are included throughout the text. These provide easy-to-read synopses of text discussions that support visual learners, and serve as useful review and study tools. **Quiz questions** are included at the end of each chapter to immediately test knowledge. **Answers and rationales** to the quiz questions are provided to instructors on the Evolve website.

NEW TO THIS EDITION

In this edition, you will find a new section entitled **Digital Imaging Basics** that addresses the advances made in Digital Imaging since the publication of the third edition. Chapter 25 – **Digital Radiography** has been completely updated with new illustrations and content. This section also includes a brand new chapter on **Three-Dimensional Digital Imaging** (Chapter 26). Chapter discussions are updated and expanded to provide additional information on all types of digital imaging and implants. One of the biggest additions to the fourth edition is the **TEACH Instructor's Resources**. For more information about this, see the section entitled: **About EVOLVE.**

The fourth edition is also presented in full color. This helps clearly delineate the various learning features, and engages the student in the content. Colored line drawings and positioning photos help modernize them, and improves the clarity in this highly visual subject area. New photos were added throughout the text regarding newer products and equipment. Additional radiographs illustrate periodontal conditions, and interpretation of common soft-tissue findings seen on intraoral films.

ABOUT EVOLVE

A companion Evolve website is available to students and instructors. The site offers a wide variety of additional learning tools and greatly enhances the text for both students and instructors. In addition, all of the content that was contained on the CD-ROM will now be on Evolve.

FOR THE STUDENT

Evolve Student Resources offers the following:
- **Self-Study Examination.** 200—multiple-choice questions are provided in an instant feedback format. This helps the student prepare for class, and reinforces what they've studied in the text.
- **Case Studies. Scenarios** similar to those found on the National Board Dental Hygiene (NBDH) examination, as well as clinical and radiographic patient data, is presented with challenging self-assessment questions. There is also a case scenario in each chapter followed by three to five questions.
- **Glossary Exercises.** Crossword puzzles by chapter or groups of related chapters created from the book's key terms and glossary.
- **Labeling Exercises.** Drag-and-drop labeling of equipment and positioning drawings and photographs.
- **Radiograph Identification Exercises.** Drag-and-drop labeling of radiographs.
- **WebLinks.** Links to relevant websites and information that supplement the content of the textbook and encourage further online research and fact-finding

FOR THE INSTRUCTOR

Evolve Instructor Resources offers the following:

- **TEACH Instructor Resource Manual.** Includes the following:
  - **TEACH Lesson Plans.** Detailed instruction by chapters and sections, with content mapping.
  - **TEACH PowerPoint Slides.** Slides of text and images separated by chapter.
  - **Test Bank in ExamView.** Approximately 1000 objective-style questions with accompanying rationales and page/section references for textbook remediation
  - **Answers to Textbook Quiz Questions and Student Self-Study Questions.** A mixture of fill-in-the-blank and short-answer questions for each chapter, with self-submission and instant feedback and grading.
- **Image Collection.** All the text's images available electronically for download into PowerPoint or other classroom lecture formats

FROM THE AUTHORS

Are there any tricks to learning dental radiography? Most definitely! Attend class. Stay awake. Pay attention. Ask questions. Read the book. Learn the material. Do not cram. Prepare for tests. Do not give up.

We hope that you will find the textbook and Evolve website to be the most comprehensive learning package available for dental radiography.

Joen M. Iannucci, DDS, MS
Laura Jansen Howerton, RDH, MS

Acknowledgements

We express our deepest appreciation to our families and friends for their unending support during preparation of this manuscript.

This textbook would not have been possible without the incredible work, commitment, and enthusiastic dedication of the team at Elsevier, which includes Kristin Hebberd, managing editor, Joslyn Dumas, developmental editor, and Sara Alsup, associate project manager.

We would also like to acknowledge the generosity and willingness of many dental manufacturing companies who loaned their permissions to display imaging equipment, with an enormous thanks to Jackie Raulerson, manger of media and public relations of DEXIS.

The authors would also like to thank the staff and dental offices of Drs. Timothy W. Godsey, and Liliana Gandini of Chapel Hill, NC, Drs. Robert Elliott and Julie Molina of Cary, NC, and Dr. W. Bruce Howerton, Jr., of Raleigh, NC, for all their contributions of sample images.

Joen M. Iannucci, DDS, MS
Laura Jansen Howerton, RDH, MS

Table of Contents

PART I   RADIATION BASICS

1   Radiation History, 2

DENTISTRY AND X-RADIATION, 2
　Basic Terminology, 2
　Importance of Dental Radiographs, 3
DISCOVERY OF X-RADIATION, 3
　Roentgen and the Discovery of X-rays, 3
　Earlier Experimentation, 4
PIONEERS IN DENTAL X-RADIATION, 4
HISTORY OF DENTAL X-RAY
　EQUIPMENT, 5
HISTORY OF DENTAL X-RAY FILM, 5
HISTORY OF DENTAL RADIOGRAPHIC
　TECHNIQUES, 6

2   Radiation Physics, 8

FUNDAMENTAL CONCEPTS, 9
　Atomic and Molecular Structure, 9
　Ionization, Radiation, and
　　Radioactivity, 11
　Ionizing Radiation, 12
X-RADIATION, 13
X-RAY MACHINE, 14
　Component Parts, 14
　X-ray Tube, 15
　X-ray Generating Apparatus, 16
PRODUCTION OF X-RADIATION, 17
　Production of Dental X-rays, 17
　Types of X-rays Produced, 18
　Definitions of X-radiation, 19
INTERACTIONS OF X-RADIATION, 19
　No Interaction, 20
　Absorption of Energy and Photoelectric
　　Effect, 20
　Compton Scatter, 20
　Coherent Scatter, 20

3   Radiation Characteristics, 26

X-RAY BEAM QUALITY, 27
　Voltage and Kilovoltage, 27
　Kilovoltage Peak, 27
　Density and Kilovoltage Peak, 27
　Contrast and Kilovoltage Peak, 28
　Exposure Time and Kilovoltage Peak, 29
X-RAY BEAM QUANTITY, 29
　Amperage and Milliamperage, 29
　Milliampere-Seconds, 29
　Density and Milliamperage, 30
　Exposure Time and Milliamperage, 30

X-RAY BEAM INTENSITY, 30
　Kilovoltage Peak, 30
　Milliamperage, 30
　Exposure Time, 30
　Distance, 30
　Inverse Square Law, 31
　Half-Value Layer, 32

4   Radiation Biology, 34

RADIATION INJURY, 35
　Mechanisms of Injury, 35
　Theories of Radiation Injury, 35
　Dose-Response Curve, 36
　Stochastic and Nonstochastic Radiation
　　Effects, 36
　Sequence of Radiation Injury, 37
　Determining Factors for Radiation Injury, 37
RADIATION EFFECTS, 37
　Short-term and Long-term Effects, 37
　Somatic and Genetic Effects, 37
　Radiation Effects on Cells, 38
　Radiation Effects on Tissues and Organs, 38
RADIATION MEASUREMENTS, 39
　Units of Measurement, 39
　Exposure Measurement, 39
　Dose Measurement, 40
　Dose Equivalent Measurement, 40
　Measurements Used in Dental Radiography, 40
RADIATION RISKS, 40
　Sources of Radiation Exposure, 40
　Risk and Risk Estimates, 41
　Dental Radiation and Exposure Risks, 41
　Patient Exposure and Dose, 41
　Risk Versus Benefit of Dental Radiographs, 42

5   Radiation Protection, 45

PATIENT PROTECTION, 46
　Before Exposure, 46
　During Exposure, 48
　After Exposure, 51
OPERATOR PROTECTION, 51
　Protection Guidelines, 51
　Radiation Monitoring, 52
RADIATION EXPOSURE GUIDELINES, 52
　Radiation Safety Legislation, 52
　Maximum Permissible Dose, 53
　Maximum Accumulated Dose, 53
　ALARA Concept, 53
RADIATION PROTECTION AND PATIENT
　EDUCATION, 53

PART II   EQUIPMENT, FILM, AND PROCESSING BASICS

6 Dental X-Ray Equipment, 57

DENTAL X-RAY MACHINES, 57
Performance Standards, 57
Types of Machines, 58
Component Parts, 58
DENTAL X-RAY FILM HOLDERS AND BEAM ALIGNMENT DEVICES, 59
Types of Film Holders, 59
Types of Beam Alignment Devices, 60

7 Dental X-Ray Film, 63

DENTAL X-RAY FILM COMPOSITION AND LATENT IMAGE, 64
Film Composition, 64
Latent Image Formation, 64
TYPES OF DENTAL X-RAY FILM, 65
Intraoral Film, 65
Extraoral Film, 68
Duplicating Film, 72
FILM STORAGE AND PROTECTION, 72

8 Dental X-Ray Image Characteristics, 76

DENTAL X-RAY IMAGE CHARACTERISTICS, 76
VISUAL CHARACTERISTICS, 77
Density, 77
Contrast, 78
GEOMETRIC CHARACTERISTICS, 80
Sharpness, 80
Magnification, 81
Distortion, 83

9 Dental X-Ray Film Processing, 86

FILM PROCESSING, 87
Film Processing Fundamentals, 87
MANUAL FILM PROCESSING, 88
Film Processing Steps, 88
Film Processing Solutions, 89
Equipment Requirements, 90
Equipment Accessories, 91
Step-by-Step Procedures, 92
Care and Maintenance, 94
AUTOMATIC FILM PROCESSING, 95
Film Processing Steps, 95
Equipment Requirements, 96
Step-by-Step Procedures, 97
Care and Maintenance, 97
THE DARKROOM, 97
Room Requirements, 97
Location and Size, 97
Lighting, 98
Miscellaneous Requirements, 98
Waste Management, 99

FILM DUPLICATION, 99
Equipment Requirements, 99
Step-by-Step Procedures, 99
PROCESSING PROBLEMS AND SOLUTIONS, 99
Time and Temperature, 100
Chemical Contamination, 103
Film Handling, 103
Lighting, 106

10 Quality Assurance in the Dental Office, 111

QUALITY CONTROL TESTS, 111
Equipment and Supplies, 112
Film Processing, 113
Digital Imaging, 116
QUALITY ADMINISTRATION PROCEDURES, 117
OPERATOR COMPETENCE, 117

PART III   DENTAL RADIOGRAPHER BASICS

11 Dental Radiographs and the Dental Radiographer, 121

DENTAL RADIOGRAPHS, 121
Importance of Dental Radiographs, 121
Uses of Dental Radiographs, 122
Benefits of Dental Radiographs, 122
Information Found on Dental Radiographs, 122
THE DENTAL RADIOGRAPHER, 122
Knowledge and Skill Requirements, 122
Duties and Responsibilities, 122
Professional Goals, 123

12 Patient Relations and the Dental Radiographer, 125

INTERPERSONAL SKILLS, 125
Communication Skills, 125
Facilitation Skills, 126
PATIENT RELATIONS, 127
First Impressions and Patient Relations, 127
Chairside Manner and Patient Relations, 127
Attitude and Patient Relations, 128

13 Patient Education and the Dental Radiographer, 130

IMPORTANCE OF PATIENT EDUCATION, 130
METHODS OF PATIENT EDUCATION, 131
COMMON QUESTIONS AND ANSWERS, 131
Necessity Questions, 131
Exposure Questions, 132
Safety Questions, 133
Digital Imaging Questions, 133
Miscellaneous Questions, 133

14 Legal Issues and the Dental Radiographer, 135

LEGAL ISSUES AND DENTAL RADIOGRAPHY, *135*
Federal and State Regulations, *135*
Licensure Requirements, *136*
LEGAL ISSUES AND THE DENTAL PATIENT, *136*
Risk Management, *136*
Malpractice Issues, *137*
Patient Records, *137*
Patients Who Refuse Dental Radiographs, *138*

15 Infection Control and the Dental Radiographer, 140

INFECTION CONTROL BASICS, *141*
Rationale for Infection Control, *141*
Infection Control Terminology, *141*
GUIDELINES FOR INFECTION CONTROL PRACTICES, *141*
Personal Protective Equipment, *142*
Hand Hygiene and Care of Hands, *142*
Sterilization or Disinfection of Instruments, *142*
Cleaning and Disinfection of Dental Unit and Environmental Surfaces, *143*
INFECTION CONTROL IN DENTAL RADIOGRAPHY, *143*
Infection Control Procedures Used Before Exposure, *143*
Infection Control Procedures Used During Exposure, *146*
Infection Control Procedures Used After Exposure, *146*
Infection Control Procedures Used for Processing, *146*

PART IV TECHNIQUE BASICS

16 Introduction to Radiographic Examinations, 152

INTRAORAL RADIOGRAPHIC EXAMINATION, *152*
Types of Intraoral Radiographic Examinations, *152*
Complete Mouth Radiographic Series/Full Mouth Series, *153*
Diagnostic Criteria for Intraoral Radiographs, *153*
EXTRAORAL RADIOGRAPHIC EXAMINATION, *153*
PRESCRIPTION OF DENTAL RADIOGRAPHS, *154*

17 Paralleling Technique, 155

BASIC CONCEPTS, *156*
Terminology, *156*
Principles of Paralleling Technique, *156*

Beam Alignment Devices, *157*
Receptors Used for Paralleling Technique, *158*
Rules for Paralleling Technique, *158*
STEP-BY-STEP PROCEDURES, *159*
Patient Preparation, *159*
Equipment Preparation, *159*
Exposure Sequence for Receptor Placements, *159*
Receptor Placement for Paralleling Technique, *163*
MODIFICATIONS IN PARALLELING TECHNIQUE, *164*
Shallow Palate, *173*
Bony Growths, *173*
Mandibular Premolar Region, *174*
ADVANTAGES AND DISADVANTAGES, *176*
Advantages of Paralleling Technique, *176*
Disadvantages of Paralleling Technique, *176*

18 Bisecting Technique, 180

BASIC CONCEPTS, *181*
Terminology, *181*
Principles of Bisecting Technique, *181*
Receptor Stabilization, *182*
Receptors Used in Bisecting Technique, *183*
Position-Indicating Device Angulation, *183*
Rules of Bisecting Technique, *185*
STEP-BY-STEP PROCEDURES, *185*
Patient Preparation, *186*
Equipment Preparation, *186*
Exposure Sequence for Receptor Placements, *187*
Receptor Placement for Bisecting Technique, *188*
ADVANTAGES AND DISADVANTAGES, *189*
Advantages of Bisecting Technique, *189*
Disadvantages of Bisecting Technique, *189*

19 Bite-Wing Technique, 210

BASIC CONCEPTS, *211*
Terminology, *211*
Principles of Bite-Wing Technique, *212*
Beam Alignment Device and Bite-Wing Tab, *212*
Bite-Wing Receptors, *213*
Position-Indicating Device Angulation, *213*
Rules of Bite-Wing Technique, *214*
STEP-BY-STEP PROCEDURES, *214*
Patient Preparation, *215*
Equipment Preparation, *215*
Exposure Sequence for Receptor Placements, *215*
Bitewing Receptor Placement, *216*
VERTICAL BITE-WINGS, *222*
BITE-WING TECHNIQUE MODIFICATIONS, *222*
Edentulous Spaces, *222*
Bony Growths, *223*

20 Exposure and Technique Errors, 226

RECEPTOR EXPOSURE ERRORS, 227
Exposure Problems, 227
Time and Exposure Factor Problems, 227
PERIAPICAL TECHNIQUE ERRORS, 228
Receptor Placement Problems, 228
Angulation Problems, 228
Position-Indicating Device Alignment
Problems, 229
BITE-WING TECHNIQUE ERRORS, 230
Receptor Placement Problems, 230
Angulation Problems, 231
Position-Indicating Device Alignment
Problems, 232
MISCELLANEOUS TECHNIQUE ERRORS, 233
Film Bending, 233
Film Creasing, 234
Phalangioma, 234
Double Exposure, 234
Movement, 234
Reversed Film, 235

21 Occlusal and Localization Techniques, 239

OCCLUSAL TECHNIQUE, 239
Basic Concepts, 239
Step-by-Step Procedures, 240
LOCALIZATION TECHNIQUES, 242
Basic Concepts, 242
Step-by-Step Procedures, 248

22 Panoramic Imaging, 256

BASIC CONCEPTS, 256
Purpose and Use, 257
Fundamentals, 257
Equipment, 259
STEP-BY-STEP PROCEDURES, 261
Equipment Preparation, 261
Patient Preparation, 261
Patient Positioning, 261
COMMON ERRORS, 262
Patient-Preparation Errors, 262
Patient-Positioning Errors, 262
ADVANTAGES AND DISADVANTAGES, 267
Advantages of Panoramic Imaging, 267
Disadvantages of Panoramic Imaging, 268

23 Extraoral Imaging, 274

BASIC CONCEPTS, 274
Purpose and Use, 275
Equipment, 275
STEP-BY-STEP PROCEDURES, 276
Equipment Preparation, 276
Patient Preparation, 276
Patient Positioning, 277
EXTRAORAL PROJECTION TECHNIQUES, 277
Lateral Jaw Imaging, 277
Skull Imaging, 277
Temporomandibular Joint Imaging, 282

24 Imaging of Patients with Special Needs, 290

PATIENTS WITH GAG REFLEX, 291
Patient Management, 291
Extreme Cases of Gag Reflex, 291
PATIENTS WITH DISABILITIES, 292
Physical Disabilities, 292
Developmental Disabilities, 292
PATIENTS WITH SPECIFIC DENTAL NEEDS, 293
Pediatric Patients, 293
Endodontic Patients, 295
Edentulous Patients, 296

PART V   DIGITAL IMAGING BASICS

25 Digital Imaging, 301

BASIC CONCEPTS, 302
Terminology, 302
Purpose and Use, 302
Fundamentals, 302
Radiation Exposure, 303
Equipment, 303
TYPES OF DIGITAL IMAGING, 305
Direct Digital Imaging, 306
Indirect Digital Imaging, 306
STEP-BY-STEP PROCEDURES, 307
Sensor Preparation, 307
Sensor Placement, 307
ADVANTAGES AND DISADVANTAGES, 307
Advantages of Digital Imaging, 307
Disadvantages of Digital Imaging, 309

26 Three-Dimensional Digital Imaging, 312

BASIC CONCEPTS, 312
Terminology, 313
Fundamentals, 313
Equipment, 314
Common Uses, 317
STEP-BY-STEP PROCEDURES, 319
Patient Preparation, 319
Patient Positioning, 319
ADVANTAGES AND DISADVANTAGES, 319
Advantages of Three-Dimensional Digital
Imaging, 319
Disadvantages of Three-Dimensional Digital
Imaging, 321

PART VI   NORMAL ANATOMY AND FILM MOUNTING BASICS

27 Normal Anatomy: Intraoral Images, 325

DEFINITIONS OF GENERAL TERMS, 326
Types of Bone, 326
Prominences of Bone, 326

Spaces and Depressions in Bone, *328*
Miscellaneous Terms, *328*
NORMAL ANATOMIC LANDMARKS, *328*
Bony Landmarks of the Maxilla, *328*
Bony Landmarks of the Mandible, *335*
NORMAL TOOTH ANATOMY, *340*
Tooth Structure, *340*
Supporting Structures, *340*

28 Film Mounting and Viewing, *345*
FILM MOUNTING, *345*
Basic Concepts, *346*
Normal Anatomy and Film Mounting, *348*
Film Mounting Methods, *348*
Step-by-Step Procedure, *349*
FILM VIEWING, *352*
Basic Concepts, *352*
Step-by-Step Procedure, *352*

29 Normal Anatomy: Panoramic Images, *357*
NORMAL ANATOMIC LANDMARKS, *358*
Bony Landmarks of Maxilla and Surrounding Structures, *358*
Bony Landmarks of Mandible and Surrounding Structures, *360*
AIR SPACE SEEN ON PANORAMIC IMAGES, *363*
SOFT TISSUE SEEN ON PANORAMIC IMAGES, *363*

PART VII IMAGE INTERPRETATION BASICS

30 Introduction to Image Interpretation, *369*
BASIC CONCEPTS, *369*
Interpretation Terminology, *369*
Importance of Interpretation, *369*
GUIDELINES, *370*
Who Interprets Images?, *370*
Interpretation versus Diagnosis, *370*
When and Where Are Images Interpreted?, *370*
Interpretation and Patient Education, *370*

31 Descriptive Terminology, *372*
DEFINITION AND USES, *372*
What Is Descriptive Terminology?, *372*
Why Use Descriptive Terminology?, *373*
Descriptive Terminology versus Diagnosis, *373*
REVIEW OF BASIC TERMS, *373*
Radiograph/Dental Image versus X-Ray, *373*
Radiolucent versus Radiopaque, *373*
Terms Used to Describe Radiolucent Lesions, *374*
Terms Used to Describe Radiopaque Lesions, *377*

32 Identification of Restorations, Dental Materials, and Foreign Objects, *383*
IDENTIFICATION OF RESTORATIONS, *384*
Amalgam Restorations, *384*
Gold Restorations, *385*
Stainless Steel and Chrome Crowns, *386*
Post and Core Restorations, *387*
Porcelain Restorations, *388*
Composite Restorations, *389*
Acrylic Restorations, *390*
IDENTIFICATION OF MATERIALS USED IN DENTISTRY, *390*
Materials Used in Restorative Dentistry, *390*
Materials Used in Endodontics, *391*
Materials Used in Prosthodontics, *391*
Materials Used in Orthodontics, *393*
Materials Used in Oral Surgery, *393*
IDENTIFICATION OF MISCELLANEOUS OBJECTS, *393*
Jewelry, *395*
Eyeglasses and Napkin Chain, *397*

33 Interpretation of Dental Caries, *402*
DESCRIPTION OF CARIES, *403*
DETECTION OF CARIES, *403*
Clinical Examination, *403*
Dental Image Examination, *403*
INTERPRETATION OF CARIES ON DENTAL IMAGES, *403*
Interpretation Tips, *404*
Factors Influencing Caries Interpretation, *404*
CLASSIFICATION OF CARIES ON DENTAL IMAGES, *404*
Interproximal Caries, *404*
Occlusal Caries, *406*
Buccal and Lingual Caries, *407*
Root Surface Caries, *407*
Recurrent Caries, *408*
Rampant Caries, *408*

34 Interpretation of Periodontal Disease, *412*
DESCRIPTION OF THE PERIODONTIUM, *412*
DESCRIPTION OF PERIODONTAL DISEASE, *413*
DETECTION OF PERIODONTAL DISEASE, *414*
Clinical Examination, *414*
Dental Image Examination, *414*
INTERPRETATION OF PERIODONTAL DISEASE ON DENTAL IMAGES, *415*
Bone Loss, *415*
Classification of Periodontal Disease, *416*
Predisposing Factors, *419*

35 Interpretation of Trauma, and Pulpal and Periapical Lesions, *426*
TRAUMA VIEWED ON DENTAL IMAGES, *426*
Fractures, *427*
Injuries, *427*

**RESORPTION VIEWED ON DENTAL
IMAGES,** *428*
    External Resorption, *429*
    Internal Resorption, *429*
**PULPAL LESIONS VIEWED ON DENTAL
IMAGES,** *429*
    Pulpal Sclerosis, *429*
    Pulpal Obliteration, *430*
    Pulp Stones, *430*

**PERIAPICAL LESIONS VIEWED ON DENTAL
IMAGES,** *430*
    Periapical Radiolucencies, *431*
    Periapical Radiopacities, *433*

Glossary, *437*

Index, *453*

part I

Radiation Basics

Chapter 1 Radiation History, 2
Chapter 2 Radiation Physics, 8
Chapter 3 Radiation Characteristics, 26
Chapter 4 Radiation Biology, 34
Chapter 5 Radiation Protection, 45

Radiation History

OUTLINE

DENTISTRY AND X-RADIATION
    Basic Terminology
    Importance of Dental Radiographs
DISCOVERY OF X-RADIATION
    Roentgen and the Discovery of X-Rays
    Earlier Experimentation

PIONEERS IN DENTAL X-RADIATION
HISTORY OF DENTAL X-RAY EQUIPMENT
HISTORY OF DENTAL X-RAY FILM
HISTORY OF DENTAL RADIOGRAPHIC TECHNIQUES

LEARNING OBJECTIVES

After completion of this chapter, the student will be able to do the following:

- Define the key words associated with radiation history
- Summarize the importance of dental radiographs
- List the uses of dental radiographs
- Summarize the discovery of x-radiation
- Recognize the pioneers in dental x-radiation and their contributions and discoveries
- List the highlights in the history of x-ray equipment and film
- List the highlights in the history of dental radiographic techniques

KEY TERMS

Cathode ray	Radiograph, dental	Radiology
Fluorescence	Radiographer, dental	Vacuum tube
Radiation	Radiography	X-radiation
Radiograph	Radiography, dental	X-ray

The dental radiographer cannot appreciate current x-ray technology without looking back to the discovery and history of x-radiation. A thorough knowledge of x-radiation begins with a study of its discovery, the pioneers in dental x-radiation, and the history of dental x-ray equipment, film, and radiographic techniques. In addition, before the dental radiographer can begin to understand x-radiation and its role in dentistry, an introduction to basic dental radiography terms and a discussion of the importance of dental radiographs are necessary. The purpose of this chapter is to introduce basic dental radiography terms, to detail the importance of dental radiographs, and to review the history of x-radiation.

DENTISTRY AND X-RADIATION

Basic Terminology

Before studying the importance of dental radiographs and the discovery and history of x-rays, the student must understand the following basic terms pertaining to dentistry and x-radiation:

Radiation: A form of energy carried by waves or a stream of particles

X-radiation: A high-energy radiation produced by the collision of a beam of electrons with a metal target in an x-ray tube

X-ray: A beam of energy that has the power to penetrate substances and record image shadows on photographic film or digital sensors

Radiology: The science or study of radiation as used in medicine; a branch of medical science that deals with the use of x-rays, radioactive substances, and other forms of radiant energy in the diagnosis and treatment of disease

Radiograph: A two-dimensional representation of a three-dimensional object. In practice, often called an "x-ray"; this is not correct. X-ray (also x ray) is a term that refers to a beam of energy

Dental radiograph: A photographic image produced on an image receptor by the passage of x-rays through teeth and related structures

Radiography: The art and science of making radiographs by the exposure of film to x-rays

Dental radiography: The production of radiographs of the teeth and adjacent structures by the exposure of an image receptor to x-rays

Dental radiographer: Any person who positions, exposes, and processes dental x-ray image receptors

Importance of Dental Radiographs

The dental radiographer must have a working knowledge of the value and uses of dental radiographs. Dental radiographs are a necessary component of comprehensive patient care. In dentistry, radiographs enable the dental professional to identify many conditions that may otherwise go undetected and to see conditions that cannot be identified clinically. An oral examination without dental radiographs limits the dental practitioner to what is seen clinically—the teeth and soft tissue. With the use of dental radiographs, the dental radiographer can obtain a wealth of information about the teeth and supporting bone.

Detection is one of the most important uses of dental radiographs (Box 1-1). Through the use of dental radiographs, the dental radiographer can detect disease. Many dental diseases and conditions produce no clinical signs or symptoms and are typically discovered only through the use of dental radiographs.

DISCOVERY OF X-RADIATION

Roentgen and the Discovery of X-rays

The history of dental radiography begins with the discovery of the x-ray. Wilhelm Conrad Roentgen (pronounced "ren-ken"), a Bavarian physicist, discovered the x-ray on November 8, 1895 (Figure 1-1). This monumental discovery revolutionized the diagnostic capabilities of the medical and dental professions and, as a result, forever changed the practice of medicine and dentistry.

Before the discovery of the x-ray, Roentgen had experimented with the production of cathode rays (streams of electrons). He used a vacuum tube, an electrical current, and special screens covered with a material that glowed (fluoresced) when exposed to radiation. He made the following observations about cathode rays:

- The rays appeared as streams of colored light passing from one end of the tube to the other.
- The rays did not travel far outside the tube.
- The rays caused fluorescent screens to glow.

While experimenting in a darkened laboratory with a vacuum tube, Roentgen noticed a faint green glow coming from a nearby table. He discovered that the mysterious glow, or "fluorescence," was coming from screens located several feet away from the tube. Roentgen observed that the distance

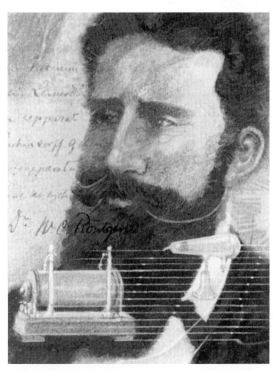

FIGURE 1-1 Roentgen, the father of x-rays, discovered the early potential of an x-ray beam in 1895. (Courtesy: Carestream Health Inc., Rochester, NY.)

BOX 1-1	Uses of Dental Radiographs

- To detect lesions, diseases, and conditions of the teeth and surrounding structures that cannot be identified clinically
- To confirm or classify suspected disease
- To localize lesions or foreign objects
- To provide information during dental procedures (e.g., root canal therapy, placement of dental implants)
- To evaluate growth and development
- To illustrate changes secondary to caries, periodontal disease, and trauma
- To document the condition of a patient at a specific point in time
- To aid in development of a clinical treatment plan

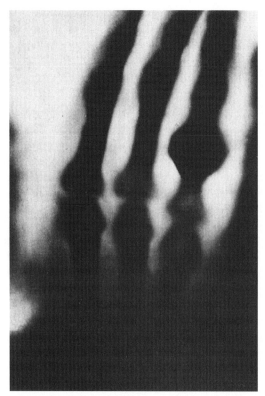

FIGURE 1-2 First radiograph of the human body, showing the hand of Roentgen's wife. (From Goaz PW, White SC: *Oral radiology and principles of interpretation*, ed 2, St Louis, 1987, Mosby.)

between the tube and the screens was much greater than the distance cathode rays could travel. He realized that something from the tube was striking the screens and causing the glow. Roentgen concluded that the fluorescence must be the result of some powerful "unknown" ray.

In the following weeks, Roentgen continued experimenting with these unknown rays. He replaced the fluorescent screens with a photographic plate. He demonstrated that shadowed images could be permanently recorded on the photographic plates by placing objects between the tube and the plate. Roentgen proceeded to make the first radiograph of the human body; he placed his wife's hand on a photographic plate and exposed it to the unknown rays for 15 minutes. When Roentgen developed the photographic plate, the outline of the bones in her hand could be seen (Figure 1-2).

Roentgen named his discovery x-rays, the "x" referring to the unknown nature and properties of such rays. (The symbol × is used in mathematics to represent the unknown.) He published a total of three scientific papers detailing the discovery, properties, and characteristics of x-rays. During his lifetime, Roentgen was awarded many honors and distinctions, including the first Nobel Prize ever awarded in physics.

Following the publication of Roentgen's papers, scientists throughout the world duplicated his discovery and produced additional information on x-rays. For many years after his discovery, x-rays were referred to as "roentgen rays," radiology was referred to as "roentgenology," and radiographs were known as "roentgenographs."

Earlier Experimentation

The primitive vacuum tube used by Roentgen in the discovery of x-rays represented the collective findings of many investigators. Before the discovery of x-rays in 1895, a number of European scientists had experimented with fluorescence in sealed glass tubes.

In 1838, a German glassblower named Heinrich Geissler built the first **vacuum tube**, a sealed glass tube from which most of the air had been evacuated. This original vacuum tube, known as the Geissler tube, was modified by a number of investigators and became known by their respective names (e.g., the *Hittorf-Crookes tube*, the *Lenard tube*).

Johann Wilhelm Hittorf, a German physicist, used the vacuum tube to study **fluorescence** (a glow that results when a fluorescent substance is struck by light, cathode rays, or x-rays). In 1870, he observed that the discharges emitted from the negative electrode of the tube traveled in straight lines, produced heat, and resulted in a greenish fluorescence. He called these discharges **cathode rays**. In the late 1870s, William Crookes, an English chemist, redesigned the vacuum tube and discovered that cathode rays were streams of charged particles. The tube used in Roentgen's experiments incorporated the best features of the Hittorf and Crookes designs and was known as the *Hittorf-Crookes tube* (Figure 1-3).

In 1894, Philip Lenard discovered that cathode rays could penetrate a thin window of aluminum foil built into the walls of the glass tubes and cause fluorescent screens to glow. He noticed that when the tube and screens were separated by at least 3.2 inches (8 cm), the screens would not fluoresce. It has been postulated that Lenard might have discovered the x-ray if he had used more sensitive fluorescent screens.

PIONEERS IN DENTAL X-RADIATION

After the discovery of x-rays in 1895, a number of pioneers helped shape the history of dental radiography. The development of dental radiography can be attributed to the research of hundreds of investigators and practitioners. Many of the early pioneers in dental radiography died from overexposure to radiation. At the time x-rays were discovered, nothing was known about the hidden dangers that resulted from using these penetrating rays.

Shortly after the announcement of the discovery of x-rays in 1895, a German dentist, Otto Walkhoff, made the first dental radiograph. He placed a glass photographic plate wrapped in black paper and rubber in his mouth and submitted himself to 25 minutes of x-ray exposure. In that same year, W.J. Morton, a New York physician, made the first dental radiograph in the United States using a skull. He also lectured on the usefulness of x-rays in dental practice and

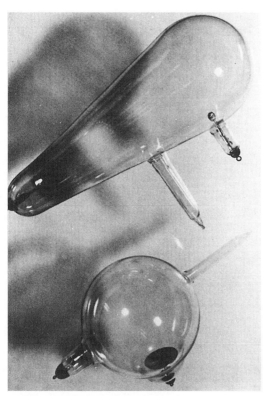

FIGURE 1-3 Hittorf-Crookes tubes used by Roentgen to discover x-rays. (From Goaz PW, White SC: *Oral radiology and principles of interpretation*, ed 2, St Louis, 1987, Mosby.)

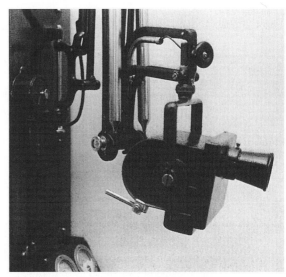

FIGURE 1-4 Victor CDX shockproof tube housing (1923). (From Goaz PW, White SC: *Oral radiology and principles of interpretation*, ed 2, St Louis, 1987, Mosby.)

made the first whole-body radiograph using a 3 × 6 ft sheet of film.

C. Edmund Kells, a New Orleans dentist, is credited with the first practical use of radiographs in dentistry in 1896. Kells exposed the first dental radiograph in the United States using a living person. During his many experiments, Kells exposed his hands to numerous x-rays every day for years. This overexposure to x-radiation caused the development of numerous cancers in his hands. Kells' dedication to the development of x-rays in dentistry ultimately cost him his fingers, later his hands, and then his arms.

Other pioneers in dental radiography include William H. Rollins, a Boston dentist who developed the first dental x-ray unit. While experimenting with radiation, Rollins suffered a burn to his hand. This initiated an interest in radiation protection and later the publication of the first paper on the dangers associated with radiation. Frank Van Woert, a dentist from New York City, was the first to use film in intraoral radiography. Howard Riley Raper, an Indiana University professor, established the first college course in radiography for dental students.

Table 1-1 lists highlights in the history of dental radiography. The development of dental radiography has moved forward from these early discoveries and continues to improve even today as new technologies become available.

HISTORY OF DENTAL X-RAY EQUIPMENT

In 1913, William D. Coolidge, an electrical engineer, developed the first hot-cathode x-ray tube, a high-vacuum tube that contained a tungsten filament. Coolidge's x-ray tube became the prototype for all modern x-ray tubes and revolutionized the generation of x-rays.

In 1923, a miniature version of the x-ray tube was placed inside the head of an x-ray machine and immersed in oil. This served as the precursor for all modern dental x-ray machines and was manufactured by the Victor X-Ray Corporation of Chicago (Figure 1-4). Later, in 1933, a new machine with improved features was introduced by General Electric. From that time on, the dental x-ray machine changed very little until a variable kilovoltage machine was introduced in 1957. Later, in 1966, a recessed long-beam tubehead was introduced.

HISTORY OF DENTAL X-RAY FILM

From 1896 to 1913, dental x-ray packets consisted of glass photographic plates or film cut into small pieces and handwrapped in black paper and rubber. The hand wrapping of intraoral dental x-ray packets was a time-consuming procedure. In 1913, the Eastman Kodak Company manufactured the first prewrapped intraoral films and consequently increased the acceptance and use of x-rays in dentistry. The first machine-made periapical film packets became available in 1920.

The films currently used in dental radiography are greatly improved compared with the films of the past. At present, fast film requires a very short exposure time, less than 2%

TABLE 1-1	Highlights in the History of Dental Radiography	
Year	**Event**	**Pioneer/Manufacturer**
1895	Discovery of x-rays	W.C. Roentgen
1896	First dental radiograph	O. Walkhoff
1896	First dental radiograph in United States (skull)	W.J. Morton
1896	First dental radiograph in United States (living patient)	C.E. Kells
1901	First paper on dangers of x-radiation	W.H. Rollins
1904	Introduction of bisecting technique	W.A. Price
1913	First dental text	H.R. Raper
1913	First prewrapped dental films	Eastman Kodak Company
1913	First x-ray tube	W.D. Coolidge
1920	First machine-made film packets	Eastman Kodak Company
1923	First dental x-ray machine	Victor X-Ray Corp, Chicago
1925	Introduction of bite-wing technique	H.R. Raper
1933	Concept of rotational panoramics proposed	
1947	Introduction of long-cone paralleling technique	F.G. Fitzgerald
1948	Introduction of panoramic radiography	
1955	Introduction of D-speed film	
1957	First variable-kilovoltage dental x-ray machine	General Electric
1978	Introduction of dental xeroradiography	
1981	Introduction of E-speed film	
1987	Introduction of intraoral digital radiography	
1998	Introduction of cone-beam computed tomography (CBCT) for dental use	
1999	Oral and maxillofacial radiology becomes a specialty in dentistry	
2000	Introduction of F-speed film	

than the initial exposure times used in 1920, which, in turn, reduces the patient's exposure to radiation.

HISTORY OF DENTAL RADIOGRAPHIC TECHNIQUES

The intraoral techniques used in dentistry include the bisecting technique, the paralleling technique, and the bite-wing technique. The dental practitioners who developed these radiographic techniques include Weston Price, a Cleveland dentist, who introduced the bisecting technique in 1904, and Howard Riley Raper, who redefined the original bisecting technique and introduced the bite-wing technique in 1925. Raper also wrote one of the first dental radiography textbooks in 1913.

The paralleling technique was first introduced by C. Edmund Kells in 1896 and then later, in 1920, used by Franklin W. McCormack in practical dental radiography. F. Gordon Fitzgerald, the "father of modern dental radiography," revived interest in the paralleling technique with the introduction of the long-cone paralleling technique in 1947.

The extraoral technique used most often in dentistry is panoramic radiography. In 1933, Hisatugu Numata of Japan was the first to expose a panoramic radiograph; however, the film was placed lingually to the teeth. Yrjo Paatero of Finland is considered to be the "father of panoramic radiography." He experimented with a slit beam of radiography, intensifying screens, and rotational techniques.

SUMMARY

- An x-ray is a beam of energy that has the power to penetrate substances and record image shadows on photographic film.
- A radiograph is a two-dimensional representation of a three-dimensional object.
- Radiography is the art and science of making radiographs by the exposure of image receptors to x-rays.
- A dental radiographer is any person who positions, exposes, and processes dental x-ray image receptors.
- Disease detection is one of the most important uses for dental radiographs.
- Wilhelm Conrad Roentgen discovered the x-ray in 1895.
- Following the discovery of the x-ray, numerous investigators contributed to advancements in dental radiography.

BIBLIOGRAPHY

Frommer HH, Savage-Stabulas JJ: Ionizing radiation and basic principles of x-ray generation. In *Radiology for the dental professional*, ed 9, St Louis, 2011, Mosby.

Haring JI, Lind LJ: The importance of dental radiographs and interpretation. In *Radiographic interpretation for the dental hygienist*, Philadelphia, 1993, Saunders.

Johnson ON, Thomson EM: History of dental radiography. In *Essentials of dental radiography for dental assistants and hygienists*, ed 8, Upper Saddle River, NJ, 2007, Pearson Education, Inc.

Langlais RP: *Exercises in oral radiology and interpretation*, ed 4, St Louis, 2004, Saunders.

Langland OE, Langlais RP: Early pioneers of oral and maxillofacial radiology, *Oral Surg Oral Med Oral Pathol* 80(5):496, 1995.

Langland OE, Langlais RP, Preece JW: Production of x-rays. In *Principles of dental imaging*, ed 2, Baltimore, MD, 2002, Lippincott Williams and Wilkins.

Miles DA, Van Dis ML, Williamson GF, Jensen CW: X-ray properties and the generation of x-rays. In *Radiographic imaging for the dental team*, ed 4, St Louis, 2009, Saunders.

White SC, Pharoah MJ: Radiation physics. In *Oral radiology: principles and interpretation*, ed 6, St Louis, 2009, Mosby.

White SC, Pharoah MJ: Radiation safety and protection. In *Oral radiology: principles and interpretation*, ed 6, St Louis, 2009, Mosby.

QUIZ QUESTIONS

MATCHING

For questions 1 to 9, match each term (a to i) with its corresponding definition.

a. Radiation
b. Radiograph
c. Radiograph, dental
d. Radiographer, dental
e. Radiography
f. Radiography, dental
g. Radiology
h. X-radiation
i. X-ray

____ 1. A photographic image produced on film by the passage of x-rays through teeth and related structures.

____ 2. A beam of energy that has the power to penetrate substances and record image shadows on photographic film.

____ 3. A form of energy carried by waves or a stream of particles.

____ 4. Any person who positions, exposes, and processes x-ray image receptors.

____ 5. The production of radiographs by the exposure of image receptors to x-rays.

____ 6. A high-energy radiation produced by the collision of a beam of electrons with a metal target in an x-ray tube.

____ 7. The science or study of radiation as used in medicine.

____ 8. The production of radiographs of the teeth and adjacent structures by the exposure of image receptors to x-rays.

____ 9. A two-dimensional representation of a three-dimensional object.

For questions 10 to 19, match the dental pioneers with their contributions (a to j).

a. Used paralleling technique in practical dental radiography
b. Discovered x-rays
c. Developed first x-ray tube
d. Introduced bisecting technique
e. Exposed first dental radiograph
f. Wrote first paper on the danger of x-radiation
g. Exposed first dental radiograph in United States (skull)
h. Introduced long-cone paralleling technique
i. Wrote first dental text; introduced bite-wing technique
j. Exposed first dental radiograph in United States (living patient)

____ 10. Coolidge
____ 11. Fitzgerald
____ 12. Kells
____ 13. McCormack
____ 14. Morton
____ 15. Price
____ 16. Raper
____ 17. Roentgen
____ 18. Rollins
____ 19. Walkhoff

ESSAY

20. Discuss the importance of dental radiographs.
21. Summarize the discovery of x-radiation.

chapter 2

Radiation Physics

OUTLINE

FUNDAMENTAL CONCEPTS
    Atomic and Molecular Structure
    Ionization, Radiation, and Radioactivity
    Ionizing Radiation
X-RADIATION
X-RAY MACHINE
    Component Parts
    X-Ray Tube
    X-Ray Generating Apparatus

PRODUCTION OF X-RADIATION
    Production of Dental X-Rays
    Types of X-Rays Produced
    Definitions of X-Radiation
INTERACTIONS OF X-RADIATION
    No Interaction
    Absorption of Energy and Photoelectric Effect
    Compton Scatter
    Coherent Scatter

LEARNING OBJECTIVES

After completion of this chapter, the student will be able to do the following:

- Define the key words associated with radiation physics
- Identify the structure of the atom
- Describe the process of ionization
- Discuss the difference between radiation and radioactivity
- List the two types of ionizing radiation and give examples of each
- List the characteristics of electromagnetic radiation
- List the properties of x-radiation
- Identify the component parts of the x-ray machine
- Label the parts of the dental x-ray tubehead and the dental x-ray tube
- Describe in detail how dental x-rays are produced
- List and describe the possible interactions of x-rays with matter

KEY TERMS

Absorption
Alpha particles
Aluminum disks
Amperage
Ampere (A)
Anode
Atom
Atom, neutral
Atomic number
Atomic weight
Autotransformer
Beta particles
Binding energy
Bremsstrahlung (braking radiation)
Cathode
Cathode ray
Circuit
Circuit, filament
Circuit, high-voltage
Coherent scatter
Compton electron
Compton scatter

Control panel
Copper stem
Current, alternating (AC)
Current, direct (DC)
Electrical current
Electricity
Electromagnetic spectrum
Electron
Electron volt (eV)
Electrostatic force
Element
Energy
Extension arm
Frequency
Insulating oil
Ion
Ion pair
Ionization
Kilo electron volt (keV)
Kilovolt (kV)
Kilovoltage peak (kVp)
Kinetic energy

Lead collimator
Leaded-glass housing
Mass number
Matter
Metal housing
Milliamperage (mA)
Milliampere (mA)
Molecule
Molybdenum cup
Nanometer
Neutron
Nucleon
Nucleus
Orbit
Periodic table of the elements
Photoelectric effect
Photon
Position-indicating device (PID)
Primary beam
Proton
Quanta
Radiation

Radiation, braking	Recoil electron	Tungsten filament
Radiation, characteristic	Rectification	Tungsten target
Radiation, electromagnetic	Scatter	Unmodified scatter
Radiation, general	Shell	Useful beam
Radiation, ionizing	Thermionic emission	Velocity
Radiation, particulate	Transformer	Volt (V)
Radiation, primary	Transformer, step-down	Voltage
Radiation, scatter	Transformer, step-up	Wavelength
Radiation, secondary	Tubehead	X-rays
Radioactivity	Tubehead seal	X-ray tube

To understand how x-rays are produced, the dental radiographer must understand the nature and interactions of atoms. A complete understanding of x-radiation includes an understanding of the fundamental concepts of atomic and molecular structure as well as a working knowledge of ionization, ionizing radiation, and the properties of x-rays. An understanding of the dental x-ray machine, x-ray tube, and circuitry is also necessary. The purpose of this chapter is to present the fundamental concepts of atomic and molecular structure, to define and characterize x-radiation, to provide an introduction to the x-ray machine, and to describe in detail how x-rays are produced. This chapter also includes a discussion of the interactions of x-radiation with matter.

FUNDAMENTAL CONCEPTS

Atomic and Molecular Structure

The world is composed of matter and energy. **Matter** is anything that occupies space and has mass; when matter is altered, **energy** results. The fundamental unit of matter is the **atom**. All matter is composed of atoms, or tiny invisible particles. An understanding of the structure of the atom is necessary before the dental radiographer can understand the production of x-rays.

Atomic Structure

The atom consists of two parts: (1) a central nucleus and (2) orbiting electrons (Figure 2-1). The identity of an atom is determined by the composition of its nucleus and the arrangement of its orbiting electrons. At present, 105 different atoms have been identified.

Nucleus. The **nucleus**, or dense core of the atom, is composed of particles known as protons and neutrons (also known as **nucleons**). **Protons** carry positive electrical charges, whereas **neutrons** carry no electrical charge. The nucleus of an atom occupies very little space; in fact, most of the atom is empty space. For example, if an atom were imagined to be the size of a football stadium, the nucleus would be the size of a football.

Atoms differ from one another on the basis of their nuclear composition. The number of protons and neutrons in the nucleus of an atom determines its **mass number** or **atomic weight**. The number of protons inside the nucleus equals the number of electrons outside the nucleus and determines the **atomic number** of the atom. Each atom has an atomic number, ranging from that of hydrogen, the simplest atom, which has an atomic number of 1, to that of hahnium, the most complex atom, which has an atomic number of 105. Atoms are arranged in the ascending order of atomic number on a chart known as the **periodic table of the elements** (Figure 2-2). **Elements** are substances made up of only one type of atom.

Electrons. **Electrons** are tiny, negatively charged particles that have very little mass; an electron weighs approximately 1/1800 as much as a proton or neutron. The arrangement of the electrons and neutrons in an atom resembles that of a miniature solar system. Just as the planets revolve around the sun, electrons travel around the nucleus in well-defined paths known as **orbits** or **shells**.

An atom contains a maximum of seven shells, each located at a specific distance from the nucleus and representing different energy levels. The shells are designated with the

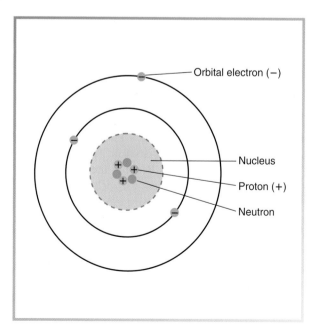

FIGURE 2-1 The atom consists of a central nucleus and orbiting electrons.

Orbital electron (−)
Nucleus
Proton (+)
Neutron

I A																	0
1 Hydrogen **H**	II A											III A	IV A	V A	VI A	VII A	**2** Helium **He**
3 Lithium **Li**	**4** Beryllium **Be**											**5** Boron **B**	**6** Carbon **C**	**7** Nitrogen **N**	**8** Oxygen **O**	**9** Fluorine **F**	**10** Neon **Ne**
11 Sodium **Na**	**12** Magnesium **Mg**	III B	IV B	V B	VI B	VII B		VIII		I B	II B	**13** Aluminum **Al**	**14** Silicon **Si**	**15** Phosphorous **P**	**16** Sulfur **S**	**17** Chlorine **Cl**	**18** Argon **Ar**
19 Potassium **K**	**20** Calcium **Ca**	**21** Scandium **Sc**	**22** Titanium **Ti**	**23** Vanadium **V**	**24** Chromium **Cr**	**25** Mangenese **Mn**	**26** Iron **Fe**	**27** Cobalt **Co**	**28** Nickel **Ni**	**29** Copper **Cu**	**30** Zinc **Zn**	**31** Gallium **Ga**	**32** Germanium **Ge**	**33** Arsenic **As**	**34** Selenium **Se**	**35** Bromine **Br**	**36** Krypton **Kr**
37 Rubidium **Rb**	**38** Strontium **Sr**	**39** Yttrium **Y**	**40** Zirconium **Zr**	**41** Niobium **Nb**	**42** Molybdenum **Mo**	**43** Technetium **Tc**	**44** Ruthenium **Ru**	**45** Rhodium **Rh**	**46** Palladium **Pd**	**47** Silver **Ag**	**48** Cadmium **Cd**	**49** Indium **In**	**50** Tin **Sn**	**51** Antimony **Sb**	**52** Tellurium **Te**	**53** Iodine **I**	**54** Xenon **Xe**
55 Cesium **Cs**	**56** Barium **Ba**	**57-71** Series of Lanthanide Elements	**72** Hafnium **Hf**	**73** Tantalum **Ta**	**74** Tungsten **W**	**75** Rhenium **Re**	**76** Osmium **Os**	**77** Iridium **Ir**	**78** Platinum **Pt**	**79** Gold **Au**	**80** Mercury **Hg**	**81** Thallium **Tl**	**82** Lead **Pb**	**83** Bismuth **Bi**	**84** Polonium **Po**	**85** Astatine **At**	**86** Radon **Rn**
87 Francium **Fr**	**88** Radium **Ra**	**89-103** Series of Actinide Elements	**104**	**105** Hahnium **Hn**													

Series of Lanthanide Elements

57 Lanthanum **La**	**58** Cerium **Ce**	**59** Praseo dymium **Pr**	**60** Neodymium **Nd**	**61** Promethium **Pm**	**62** Samarium **Sm**	**63** Europium **Eu**	**64** Gadolinium **Gd**	**65** Terbium **Tb**	**66** Dysprosium **Dy**	**67** Holium **Ho**	**68** Erbium **Er**	**69** Thulium **Tm**	**70** Ytterbium **Yb**	**71** Lutetium **Lu**

Series of Actinide Elements

89 Actinium **Ac**	**90** Thorium **Th**	**91** Protactinium **Pa**	**92** Uranium **U**	**93** Neptunium **Np**	**94** Plutonium **Pu**	**95** Americium **Am**	**96** Curium **Cm**	**97** Berkelium **Bk**	**98** Californium **Cf**	**99** Einsteinium **Es**	**100** Fermium **Fm**	**101** Mendelevium **Md**	**102** Nobelium **No**	**103** Lawrentium **Lr**

FIGURE 2-2 Periodic table of the elements.

letters K, L, M, N, O, P, and Q; the K shell is located closest to the nucleus and has the highest energy level (Figure 2-3). Each shell has a maximum number of electrons it can hold (Figure 2-4).

Electrons are maintained in their orbits by the **electrostatic force**, or attraction, between the positive nucleus and the negative electrons. This is known as the **binding energy**, or binding force, of an electron. The binding energy is determined by the distance between the nucleus and the orbiting electron and is different for each shell. The strongest binding energy is found closest to the nucleus in the K shell, whereas electrons located in the outer shells have a weak binding energy. The binding energies of orbital electrons are measured in **electron volts (eV)** or **kilo electron volts (keV)**. (One kilo electron volt equals 1000 electron volts.)

The energy required to remove an electron from its orbital shell must exceed the binding energy of the electron in that shell. A great amount of energy is required to remove an inner-shell electron, but electrons loosely held in the outer

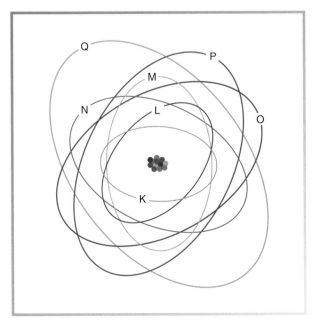

FIGURE 2-3 Orientation of electron orbits (shells) around the nucleus.

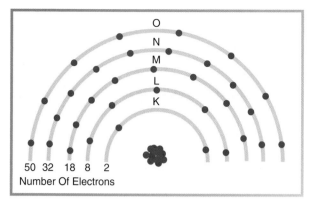

FIGURE 2-4 Maximum number of electrons that can exist in each shell of a tungsten atom. (Redrawn from Langlais RP: *Exercises in oral radiology and interpretation*, ed 4, St Louis, 2004, Saunders.)

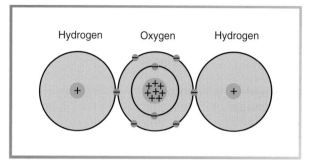

FIGURE 2-5 A molecule of water (H_2O) consists of two atoms of hydrogen connected to one atom of oxygen.

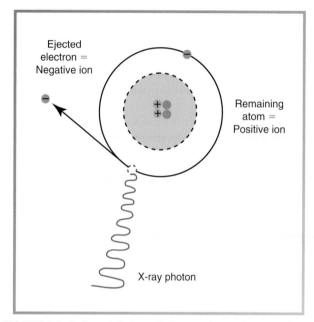

FIGURE 2-6 An ion pair is formed when an electron is removed from an atom; the atom is the positive ion, and the ejected electron is the negative ion.

shells can be affected by lesser energies. For example, in the tungsten atom, the binding energies are as follows:

70 keV	K-shell electrons
12 keV	L-shell electrons
3 keV	M-shell electrons

Note that the binding energy is greatest in the shell closest to the nucleus. To remove a K-shell electron from a tungsten atom, 70 keV (70,000 eV) of energy would be required, whereas only 3 keV (3000 eV) of energy would be necessary to remove an electron from the M shell.

Molecular Structure

Atoms are capable of combining with each other to form molecules. A molecule can be defined as two or more atoms joined by chemical bonds, or the smallest amount of a substance that possesses its characteristic properties. As with the atom, the molecule is also a tiny invisible particle. **Molecules** are formed in one of two ways: (1) by the transfer of electrons or (2) by the sharing of electrons between the outermost shells of atoms. An example of a simple molecule is water (H_2O); the symbol H_2 represents two atoms of hydrogen, and the symbol O represents one atom of oxygen (Figure 2-5).

Ionization, Radiation, and Radioactivity

The fundamental concepts of atomic and molecular structure just reviewed allow an understanding of ionization, radiation, and radioactivity. Before the dental radiographer can understand how x-rays are produced, a working knowledge of ionization and the difference between radiation and radioactivity is necessary.

Ionization

Atoms can exist in a neutral state or in an electrically unbalanced state. Normally, most atoms are neutral. A **neutral atom** contains an equal number of protons (positive charges) and electrons (negative charges). An atom with an incompletely filled outer shell is electrically unbalanced and attempts to capture an electron from an adjacent atom. If the atom gains an electron, it has more electrons than protons and neutrons and, therefore, a negative charge. Similarly, the atom that loses an electron has more protons and neutrons and thus has a positive charge. An atom that gains or loses an electron and becomes electrically unbalanced is known as an **ion**.

Ionization is the production of ions, or the process of converting an atom into ions. Ionization deals only with electrons and requires sufficient energy to overcome the electrostatic force that binds the electron to the nucleus. When an electron is removed from an atom in the ionization process, an **ion pair** results. The atom becomes the positive ion, and the ejected electron becomes the negative ion (Figure 2-6). This ion pair reacts with other ions until electrically stable, neutral atoms are formed.

TABLE 2-1	Particulate Radiations		
Particle	**Mass Units**	**Charge**	**Origin**
Alpha particle	4.003000	+2	Nucleus
Electron			
• Beta particle	0.000548	−1	Nucleus
• Cathode rays	0.000548	−1	X-ray tube
Protons	1.007597	+1	Nucleus
Neutrons	1.008986	0	Nucleus

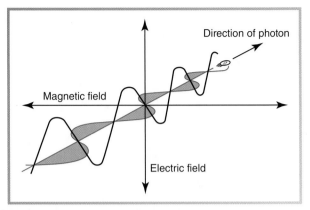

FIGURE 2-7 Oscillating electric and magnetic fields are characteristic of electromagnetic radiations.

Radiation and Radioactivity

Radiation, as defined in Chapter 1, is the emission and propagation of energy through space or a substance in the form of waves or particles. The terms radioactivity and radiation are sometimes confused; it is important to note that they do not have the same meaning.

Radioactivity can be defined as the process by which certain unstable atoms or elements undergo spontaneous disintegration, or decay, in an effort to attain a more balanced nuclear state. A substance is considered radioactive if it gives off energy in the form of particles or rays as a result of the disintegration of atomic nuclei.

In dentistry, radiation (specifically x-radiation) is used, not radioactivity.

Ionizing Radiation

Ionizing radiation can be defined as radiation that is capable of producing ions by removing or adding an electron to an atom. Ionizing radiation can be classified into two groups: (1) particulate radiation and (2) electromagnetic radiation.

Particulate Radiation

Particulate radiations are tiny particles of matter that possess mass and travel in straight lines and at high speeds. Particulate radiations transmit kinetic energy by means of their extremely fast-moving, small masses. Four types of particulate radiation are recognized (Table 2-1), as follows:

1. Electrons can be classified as beta particles or cathode rays. They differ in origin only.
   a. **Beta particles** are fast-moving electrons emitted from the nucleus of radioactive atoms.
   b. **Cathode rays** are streams of high-speed electrons that originate in an x-ray tube.
2. **Alpha particles** are emitted from the nuclei of heavy metals and exist as two protons and neutrons, without electrons.
3. Protons are accelerated particles, specifically hydrogen nuclei, with a mass of 1 and a charge of +1.
4. Neutrons are accelerated particles with a mass of 1 and no electrical charge.

Electromagnetic Radiation

Electromagnetic radiation can be defined as the propagation of wavelike energy (without mass) through space or matter.

The energy propagated is accompanied by oscillating electric and magnetic fields positioned at right angles to one another, thus the term electromagnetic (Figure 2-7).

Electromagnetic radiations are man made or occur naturally; examples include cosmic rays, gamma rays, x-rays, ultraviolet rays, visible light, infrared light, radar waves, microwaves, and radio waves. Electromagnetic radiations are arranged according to their energies in what is termed the **electromagnetic spectrum** (Figure 2-8). All energies of the electromagnetic spectrum share common characteristics (Box 2-1). Depending on their energy levels, electromagnetic radiations can be classified as ionizing or non-ionizing. In the electromagnetic spectrum, only high-energy radiations (cosmic rays, gamma rays, and x-rays) are capable of ionization.

Electromagnetic radiations are believed to move through space as both a particle and a wave; therefore two concepts, the particle concept and the wave concept, must be considered.

Particle Concept. The particle concept characterizes electromagnetic radiations as discrete bundles of energy called **photons**, or **quanta**. Photons are bundles of energy with no mass or weight that travel as waves at the speed of light and move through space in a straight line, "carrying the energy" of electromagnetic radiation.

Wave Concept. The wave concept characterizes electromagnetic radiations as waves and focuses on the properties of velocity, wavelength, and frequency, as follows:

- **Velocity** refers to the speed of the wave. All electromagnetic radiations travel as waves or a continuous sequence of crests at the speed of light (3×10^8 meters per second [186,000 miles per second]) in a vacuum.
- **Wavelength** can be defined as the distance between the crest of one wave and the crest of the next (Figure 2-9). Wavelength determines the energy and penetrating power of the radiation; the shorter the distance between the crests, the shorter is the wavelength and the higher is the energy and ability to penetrate matter. Wavelength is measured in **nanometers** (nm; 1×10^{-9} meters, or one

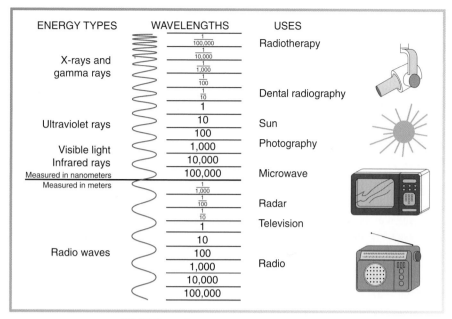

FIGURE 2-8 Electromagnetic energy spectrum.

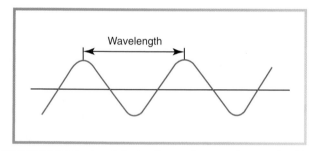

FIGURE 2-9 Wavelength is the distance between the crest (peak) of one wave and the crest of the next.

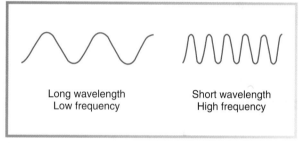

FIGURE 2-10 Frequency is the number of wavelengths that pass a given point in a certain amount of time. The shorter the wavelength, the higher the frequency will be, and vice versa.

BOX **2-1**	**Properties of Electromagnetic Radiations**

- Have no mass or weight
- Have no electrical charge
- Travel at the speed of light (3 × 186,000 miles/second; 108 meters/second)
- Travel as both a particle and a wave
- Propagate an electric field at right angles to path of travel
- Propagate a magnetic field at right angles to the electric field
- Have different measurable energies (frequencies and wavelengths)

billionth of a meter) for short waves and in meters (m) for longer waves.
- **Frequency** refers to the number of wavelengths that pass a given point in a certain amount of time (Figure 2-10). Frequency and wavelength are inversely related; if the

frequency of the wave is high, the wavelength will be short, and if the frequency is low, the wavelength will be long.

The amount of energy an electromagnetic radiation possesses depends on the wavelength and frequency.

Low-frequency electromagnetic radiations have a long wavelength and less energy. Conversely, high-frequency electromagnetic radiations have a short wavelength and more energy.

For example, communications media use the low-frequency, longer waves of the electromagnetic spectrum; the wavelength of a radio wave can be as long as 100 m, whereas the wavelength of a television wave is approximately 1 m. In contrast, diagnostic radiography uses the high-frequency, shorter waves in the electromagnetic spectrum; x-rays used in dentistry have a wavelength of 0.1 nm, or 0.00000000001 m.

X-RADIATION

X-radiation is a high-energy, ionizing electromagnetic radiation. As with all electromagnetic radiations, x-rays have the

BOX 2-2   Properties of X-Rays

- *Appearance:* X-rays are invisible and cannot be detected by any of the senses.
- *Mass:* X-rays have no mass or weight.
- *Charge:* X-rays have no charge.
- *Speed:* X-rays travel at the speed of light.
- *Wavelength:* X-rays travel in waves and have short wavelengths with a high frequency.
- *Path of travel:* X-rays travel in straight lines and can be deflected, or scattered.
- *Focusing capability:* X-rays cannot be focused to a point and always diverge from a point.
- *Penetrating power:* X-rays can penetrate liquids, solids, and gases. The composition of the substance determines whether x-rays penetrate or pass through, or are absorbed.
- *Absorption:* X-rays are absorbed by matter; the absorption depends on the atomic structure of matter and the wavelength of the x-ray.
- *Ionization capability:* X-rays interact with materials they penetrate and cause ionization.
- *Fluorescence capability:* X-rays can cause certain substances to fluoresce or emit radiation in longer wavelengths (e.g., visible light and ultraviolet light).
- *Effect on film:* X-rays can produce an image on photographic film.
- *Effect on living tissues:* X-rays cause biologic changes in living cells.

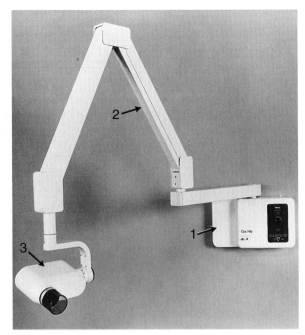

FIGURE 2-11 Three component parts of dental x-ray machine: **A,** control panel; **B,** extension arm; **C,** tubehead. (Courtesy Instrumentarium Dental, Inc. Milwaukee, WI.)

properties of both waves and particles. **X-rays** can be defined as weightless bundles of energy (photons) without an electrical charge that travel in waves with a specific frequency at the speed of light. X-ray photons interact with the materials they penetrate and cause ionization.

X-rays have certain unique properties or characteristics. It is important that the dental radiographer be familiar with the properties of x-rays (Box 2-2).

X-RAY MACHINE

X-rays are produced in the dental x-ray machine. For learning purposes, the dental x-ray machine can be divided into three study areas: (1) the component parts, (2) the x-ray tube, and (3) the x-ray generating apparatus.

Component Parts

The dental x-ray machine consists of three visible component parts: (1) control panel, (2) extension arm, and (3) tubehead (Figure 2-11).

Control Panel

The **control panel** of the dental x-ray machine contains an on-off switch and an indicator light, an exposure button and indicator light, and control devices (time, kilovoltage, and milliamperage selectors) to regulate the x-ray beam. The

control panel is plugged into an electrical outlet and appears as a panel or a cabinet mounted on the wall outside the dental operatory.

Extension Arm

The wall-mounted **extension arm** suspends the x-ray tubehead and houses the electrical wires that extend from the control panel to the tubehead. The extension arm allows for movement and positioning of the tubehead.

Tubehead

The x-ray **tubehead** is a tightly sealed, heavy metal housing that contains the x-ray tube that produces dental x-rays. The component parts of the tubehead include the following (Figure 2-12):

- **Metal housing,** or the metal body of the tubehead that surrounds the x-ray tube and transformers and is filled with oil—protects the x-ray tube and grounds the high-voltage components.
- **Insulating oil,** or the oil that surrounds the x-ray tube and transformers inside the tubehead—prevents overheating by absorbing the heat created by the production of x-rays.
- **Tubehead seal,** or the aluminum or leaded-glass covering of the tubehead that permits the exit of x-rays from the tubehead—seals the oil in the tubehead and acts as a filter to the x-ray beam.
- **X-ray tube,** or the heart of the x-ray generating system (discussed later) (Figure 2-13).
- **Transformer,** or a device that alters the voltage of incoming electricity (also discussed later).
- **Aluminum disks,** or sheets of 0.5-mm–thick aluminum placed in the path of the x-ray beam—filter out the non-

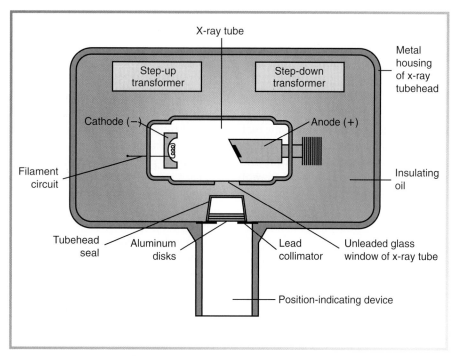

FIGURE 2-12 Diagram of dental x-ray tubehead.

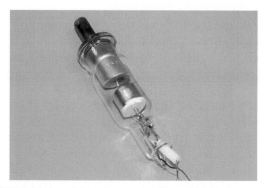

FIGURE 2-13 Actual dental x-ray tube. (From Bird DL, Robinson DS: *Modern dental assisting*, ed 10, St Louis, 2012, Saunders.)

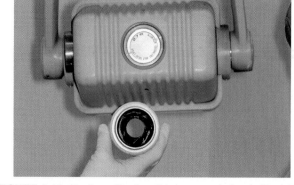

FIGURE 2-14 Aluminum filtration disk in x-ray tubehead. (From Bird DL, Robinson DS: *Modern dental assisting*, ed 10, St Louis, 2012, Saunders.)

penetrating, longer wavelength x-rays (Figure 2-14). Aluminum filtration is discussed in Chapter 5.

- **Lead collimator,** or a lead plate with a central hole that fits directly over the opening of the metal housing, where the x-rays exit—restricts the size of the x-ray beam (Figure 2-15). Collimation is also discussed in Chapter 5.
- **Position-indicating device (PID),** or open-ended, lead-lined cylinder that extends from the opening of the metal housing of the tubehead—aims and shapes the x-ray beam (Figure 2-16). The PID is sometimes referred to as the cone.

X-Ray Tube

The x-ray tube is the heart of the x-ray generating system; it is critical to the production of x-rays and warrants a separate discussion from the rest of the x-ray machine. The x-ray tube

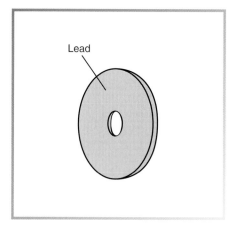

FIGURE 2-15 The lead collimator, or lead plate with a central opening, restricts the size of the x-ray beam.

is a glass vacuum tube from which all the air has been removed. The x-ray tube used in dentistry measures approximately several inches long by one inch in diameter. The component parts of the x-ray tube include a leaded-glass housing, negative cathode, and positive anode (Figure 2-17).

Leaded-Glass Housing

The **leaded-glass housing** is a leaded-glass vacuum tube that prevents x-rays from escaping in all directions. One central area of the leaded-glass tube has a "window" that permits the x-ray beam to exit the tube and directs the x-ray beam toward the aluminum disks, lead collimator, and PID.

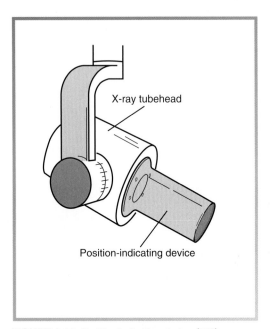

FIGURE 2-16 Position-indicating device (PID), or cone.

Cathode

The **cathode**, or negative electrode, consists of a tungsten wire filament in a cup-shaped holder made of molybdenum. The purpose of the cathode is to supply the electrons necessary to generate x-rays. In the x-ray tube, the electrons produced in the negative cathode are accelerated toward the positive anode. The cathode includes the following:

- The **tungsten filament**, or coiled wire made of tungsten, which produces electrons when heated.
- The **molybdenum cup**, which focuses the electrons into a narrow beam and directs the beam across the tube toward the tungsten target of the anode.

Anode

The **anode**, or positive electrode, consists of a wafer-thin tungsten plate embedded in a solid copper rod. The purpose of the anode is to convert electrons into x-ray photons. The anode includes the following:

- A **tungsten target**, or plate of tungsten, which serves as a focal spot and converts bombarding electrons into x-ray photons.
- The **copper stem**, which functions to dissipate the heat away from the tungsten target.

X-Ray Generating Apparatus

To understand how the x-ray tube functions and how x-rays are produced, the dental radiographer must understand electricity and electrical currents, electrical circuits, and transformers.

Electricity and Electrical Currents

Electricity is the energy that is used to make x-rays. Electrical energy consists of a flow of electrons through a conductor; this flow is known as the **electrical current**. The electrical current is termed **direct current (DC)** when the electrons

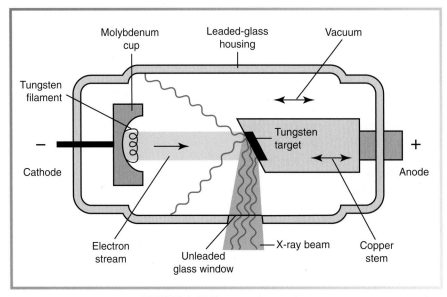

FIGURE 2-17 Diagram of x-ray tube.

flow in one direction through the conductor. The term **alternating current (AC)** describes an electrical current in which the electrons flow in two, opposite directions. **Rectification** is the conversion of AC to DC. The dental x-ray tube acts as a self-rectifier in that it changes AC into DC while producing x-rays. This ensures that the current is always flowing in the same direction, more specifically, from cathode to anode.

Generators on older machines produced an x-ray beam with a wavelike pattern, whereas newer constant-potential x-ray machines produce a homogeneous beam of consistent wavelengths during radiation exposure. Constant-potential machines also reduce patient exposure to radiation by 20%, an important consideration for patient protection.

Amperage is the measurement of the number of electrons moving through a conductor. Current is measured in **amperes (A)** or **milliamperes (mA)**. **Voltage** is the measurement of electrical force that causes electrons to move from a negative pole to a positive one. Voltage is measured in **volts (V)** or **kilovolts (kV)**.

In the production of x-rays, both the amperage and the voltage can be adjusted. In the x-ray tube, the amperage, or number of electrons passing through the cathode filament, can be increased or decreased by the **milliamperage (mA)** adjustment on the control panel of the x-ray machine. The voltage of the x-ray tube current, or the current passing from the cathode to the anode, is controlled by the **kilovoltage peak (kVp)** adjustment on the control panel.

Circuits

A **circuit** is a path of electrical current. Two electrical circuits are used in the production of x-rays: (1) a low-voltage, or filament, circuit and (2) a high-voltage circuit.

The **filament circuit** uses 3 to 5 volts, regulates the flow of electrical current to the filament of the x-ray tube, and is controlled by the milliampere settings. The **high-voltage circuit** uses 65,000 to 100,000 volts, provides the high voltage required to accelerate electrons and to generate x-rays in the x-ray tube, and is controlled by the kilovoltage settings.

Transformers

A transformer is a device that is used to either increase or decrease the voltage in an electrical circuit (Figure 2-18). Transformers alter the voltage of the incoming electrical current and then route the electrical energy to the x-ray tube. In the production of dental x-rays, three transformers are used to adjust the electrical circuits: (1) the step-down transformer, (2) the step-up transformer, and (3) the autotransformer.

A **step-down transformer** is used to decrease the voltage from the incoming 110- or 220-line voltage to the 3 to 5 volts used by the filament circuit. A step-down transformer has more wire coils in the primary coil than in the secondary coil (see Figure 2-18). The coil that receives the alternating electrical current is the primary, or input, coil; the secondary coil is the output coil. The electrical current that energizes the

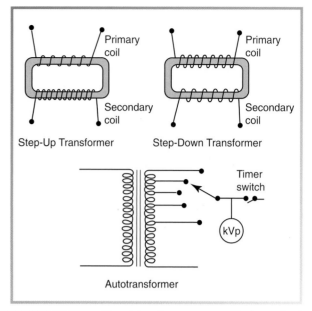

FIGURE 2-18 Three different transformers are used in the production of dental x-rays.

primary coil induces a current in the secondary coil. The high-voltage circuit uses both a step-up transformer and an autotransformer. A step-up transformer is used to increase the voltage from the incoming 110- or 220-line voltage to the 65,000 to 100,000 volts used by the high-voltage circuit. A **step-up transformer** has more wire coils in the secondary coil than in the primary coil (see Figure 2-18). An **autotransformer** serves as a voltage compensator that corrects for minor fluctuations in the current.

PRODUCTION OF X-RADIATION

Production of Dental X-Rays

With the component parts of the x-ray machine, the x-ray tube, and the x-ray generating apparatus reviewed, a discussion of the production of dental x-rays is now possible. Following is a step-by-step explanation of x-ray production (Figure 2-19):

1. Electricity from the wall outlet supplies the power to generate x-rays. When the x-ray machine is turned on, the electrical current enters the control panel through the cord plugged into the wall outlet. The current travels from the control panel to the tubehead through the electrical wires in the extension arm.
2. The current is directed to the filament circuit and step-down transformer in the tubehead. The transformer reduces the 110 or 220 entering-line voltage to 3 to 5 volts.
3. The filament circuit uses the 3 to 5 volts to heat the tungsten filament in the cathode portion of the x-ray tube. **Thermionic emission** occurs, defined as the release of electrons from the tungsten filament when the electrical current passes through it and heats the filament. The

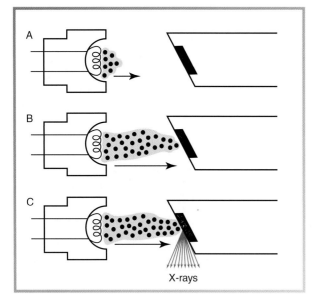

FIGURE 2-19 The production of dental x-rays occurs in the x-ray tube. **A**, When the filament circuit is activated, the filament heats up, and thermionic emission occurs. **B**, When the exposure button is activated, the electrons are accelerated from the cathode to the anode. **C**, The electrons strike the tungsten target, and their kinetic energy is converted to x-rays and heat.

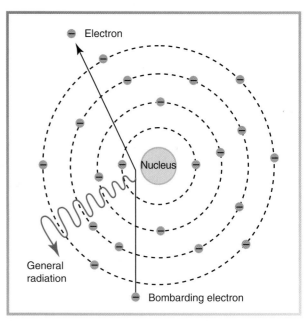

FIGURE 2-20 When an electron that passes close to the nucleus of a tungsten atom is slowed down, an x-ray photon of lower energy known as general (braking) radiation results.

outer-shell electrons of the tungsten atom acquire enough energy to move away from the filament surface, and an electron cloud forms around the filament. The electrons stay in an electron cloud until the high-voltage circuit is activated.

4. When the exposure button is pushed, the high-voltage circuit is activated. The electrons produced at the cathode are accelerated across the x-ray tube to the anode. The molybdenum cup in the cathode directs the electrons to the tungsten target in the anode.

5. The electrons travel from the cathode to the anode. When the electrons strike the tungsten target, their energy of motion (**kinetic energy**) is converted to x-ray energy and heat. Less than 1% of the energy is converted to x-rays; the remaining 99% is lost as heat.

6. The heat produced during the production of x-rays is carried away from the copper stem and absorbed by the insulating oil in the tubehead. The x-rays produced are emitted from the target in all directions; however, the leaded-glass housing prevents the x-rays from escaping from the x-ray tube. A small number of x-rays are able to exit from the x-ray tube through the unleaded glass window portion of the tube.

7. The x-rays travel through the unleaded glass window, the tubehead seal, and the aluminum disks. The aluminum disks remove or filter the longer wavelength x-rays from the beam.

8. Next, the size of the x-ray beam is restricted by the lead collimator. The x-ray beam then travels down the lead-lined PID and exits the tubehead at the opening of the PID.

Types of X-Rays Produced

Not all x-rays produced in the x-ray tube are the same; x-rays differ in energy and wavelength. The energy and wavelength of x-rays vary based on how the electrons interact with the tungsten atoms in the anode. The kinetic energy of the electrons is converted to x-ray photons through one of two mechanisms: (1) general (braking) radiation and (2) characteristic radiation.

General Radiation

Speeding electrons slow down because of their interactions with the tungsten target in the anode. Many electrons that interact with the tungsten atoms undergo not one but many interactions within the target. The radiation produced in this manner is known as **general radiation**, or **braking radiation** (**bremsstrahlung**). The term *braking* refers to the sudden stopping of high-speed electrons when they hit the tungsten target in the anode. Most x-rays are produced in this manner; approximately 70% of the x-ray energy produced at the anode can be classified as general radiation.

General (braking) radiation is produced when an electron hits the nucleus of a tungsten atom or when an electron passes very close to the nucleus of a tungsten atom (Figure 2-20). An electron rarely hits the nucleus of the tungsten atom. When it does, however, all its kinetic energy is converted into a high-energy x-ray photon. Instead of hitting the nucleus, most electrons just miss the nucleus of the tungsten atom. When the electron comes close to the nucleus, it is attracted to the nucleus and slows down. Consequently, an x-ray photon of lower energy results. The electron that misses the nucleus continues to penetrate many atoms, producing lower energy x-rays before it imparts all of its kinetic energy. As a result, general radiation consists of x-rays of many different energies and wavelengths.

Characteristic Radiation

Characteristic radiation is produced when a high-speed electron dislodges an inner-shell electron from the tungsten atom and causes ionization of that atom (Figure 2-21). Once the electron is dislodged, the remaining orbiting electrons are rearranged to fill the vacancy. This rearrangement produces a loss of energy that results in the production of an x-ray photon. The x-rays produced by this interaction are known as characteristic x-rays.

Characteristic radiation accounts for a very small part of x-rays produced in the dental x-ray machine. It occurs only at 70 kVp and above because the binding energy of the K-shell electron is approximately 70 keV.

Definitions of X-Radiation

Terms such as *primary*, *secondary*, and **scatter** are often used to describe x-radiation. Understanding the interactions of x-radiation with matter requires a working knowledge of these terms, as follows:

- **Primary radiation** refers to the penetrating x-ray beam that is produced at the target of the anode and that exits the tubehead. This x-ray beam is often referred to as the **primary beam**, or useful beam.
- **Secondary radiation** refers to x-radiation that is created when the primary beam interacts with matter. (In dental radiography, "matter" includes the soft tissues of the head, the bones of the skull, and the teeth.) Secondary radiation is less penetrating than primary radiation.
- **Scatter radiation** is a form of secondary radiation and is the result of an x-ray that has been deflected from its path by the interaction with matter. Scatter radiation is deflected in all directions by the patient's tissues and travels to all parts of the patient's body and to all areas of the dental operatory. Scatter radiation is detrimental to both the patient and the radiographer.

INTERACTIONS OF X-RADIATION

What happens after an x-ray exits the tubehead? When x-ray photons arrive at the patient with energies produced by the dental x-ray machine, one of the following events may occur:

- X-rays can pass through the patient without any interaction.
- X-ray photons can be completely absorbed by the patient.
- X-ray photons can be scattered (Figure 2-22).

A knowledge of atomic and molecular structure is required to understand such interactions and effects. At the atomic level, four possibilities can occur when an x-ray photon interacts with matter: (1) no interaction, (2) absorption or photoelectric effect, (3) Compton scatter, and (4) coherent scatter.

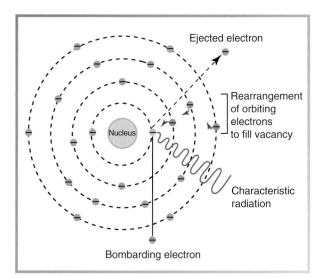

FIGURE 2-21 An electron that dislodges an inner-shell electron from the tungsten atom results in the rearrangement of the remaining orbiting electrons and the production of an x-ray photon known as *characteristic radiation.*

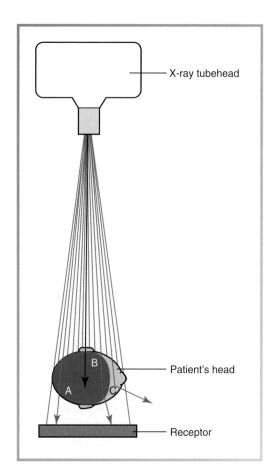

FIGURE 2-22 Three types of radiation interactions with the patient may occur. **A,** The x-ray photon may pass through the patient without interaction and reach the receptor. **B,** The x-ray photon may be absorbed by the patient. **C,** The x-ray photon may be scattered onto the receptor or away from the receptor.

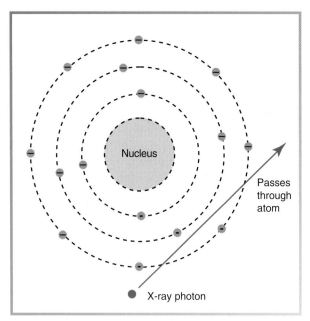

FIGURE 2-23 When an x-ray photon passes through an atom unchanged, no interaction has taken place.

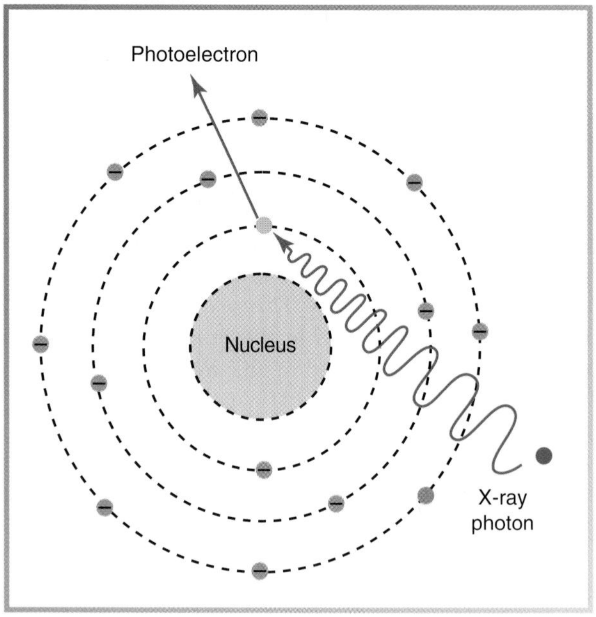

FIGURE 2-24 When an x-ray photon collides with an inner-shell electron, a photoelectric effect occurs: The photon is absorbed and ceases to exist, and a photoelectron with a negative charge is produced.

No Interaction

It is possible for an x-ray photon to pass through matter or the tissues of a patient without any interaction (Figure 2-23). The x-ray photon passes through the atom unchanged and leaves the atom unchanged. The x-ray photons that pass through a patient without interaction are responsible for producing densities and make dental radiography possible.

Absorption of Energy and Photoelectric Effect

It is possible for an x-ray photon to be completely absorbed within matter, or the tissues of a patient. **Absorption** refers to the total transfer of energy from the x-ray photon to the atoms of matter through which the x-ray beam passes. Absorption depends on the energy of the x-ray beam and the composition of the absorbing matter or tissues.

At the atomic level, absorption occurs as a result of the photoelectric effect. In the **photoelectric effect**, ionization takes place. An x-ray photon collides with a tightly bound, inner-shell electron and gives up all its energy to eject the electron from its orbit (Figure 2-24). The x-ray photon imparts all of its kinetic energy to the orbital electron, is absorbed, and ceases to exist. The ejected electron is termed a *photoelectron* and has a negative charge; it is readily absorbed by other atoms because it has very little penetrating power. The atom that remains has a positive charge. The photoelectric effect accounts for 30% of the interactions of matter with the dental x-ray beam.

Compton Scatter

It is possible for an x-ray photon to be deflected from its path during its passage through matter. The term *scatter* refers to

this type of radiation. At the atomic level, the Compton effect accounts for most of the scatter radiation.

In **Compton scatter**, ionization takes place. An x-ray photon collides with a loosely bound, outer-shell electron and gives up part of its energy to eject the electron from its orbit (Figure 2-25). The x-ray photon loses energy and continues in a different direction (scatters) at a lower energy level. The new, weaker x-ray photon interacts with other atoms until all its energy is gone. The ejected electron is termed a **Compton electron**, or **recoil electron**, and has a negative charge. The remaining atom is positively charged. Compton scatter accounts for 62% of the scatter that occurs in diagnostic radiography.

Coherent Scatter

Another type of scatter radiation that may take place when x-rays interact with matter is known as **coherent scatter**, or **unmodified scatter**. Coherent scatter involves an x-ray photon that has its path altered by matter (Figure 2-26). Coherent scatter occurs when a low-energy x-ray photon interacts with an outer-shell electron. No change in the atom occurs, and an x-ray photon of scattered radiation is produced. The x-ray photon is scattered in a different direction from that of the incident photon; no loss of energy and no ionization occur. Essentially, the x-ray photon is "unmodified" and simply undergoes a change in direction without a change in energy. Coherent scatter accounts for 8% of the interactions of matter with the dental x-ray beam.

SUMMARY

- An atom consists of a central nucleus composed of protons, neutrons, and orbiting electrons.

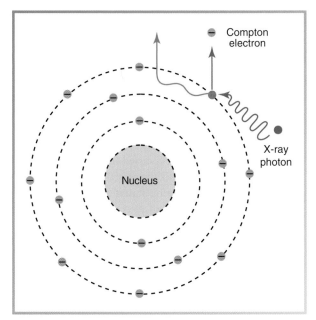

FIGURE 2-25 When an x-ray photon collides with an outer-shell electron and ejects the electron from its orbit, Compton scatter results: The photon is scattered in a different direction at a lower energy, and the ejected electron is referred to as a *Compton, or recoil, electron*.

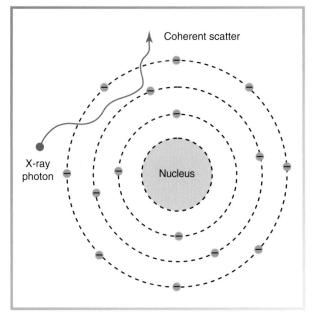

FIGURE 2-26 When an x-ray photon is scattered and no loss of energy occurs, the scatter is termed *coherent*.

- Most atoms exist in a neutral state and contain equal numbers of protons and neutrons.
- When unequal numbers of protons and electrons exist, the atom is electrically unbalanced and is termed an *ion*.
- The production of ions is termed *ionization*; an ion pair (a positive ion and a negative ion) is produced. The atom is the positive ion, and the ejected electron is the negative ion.
- Ionizing radiation is capable of producing ions and can be classified as *particulate* or *electromagnetic*.
- Electromagnetic radiations (e.g., x-rays) exhibit characteristics of both particles and waves and are arranged according to their energies.
- The energy of an electromagnetic radiation depends on wavelength and frequency.
- A low-energy radiation has a low frequency and a long wavelength; a high-energy radiation has a high frequency and a short wavelength.
- X-rays are weightless, neutral bundles of energy (photons) that travel in waves with a specific frequency at the speed of light.
- X-rays are generated in an x-ray tube located in the x-ray tubehead.
- The x-ray tube consists of a leaded-glass housing, a negative cathode, and a positive anode. Electrons are produced in the cathode and accelerated toward the anode; the anode converts the electrons into x-rays.
- After x-rays exit the tubehead, several interactions are possible: The x-rays may pass through the patient (no interaction), may be completely absorbed by the patient (photoelectric effect), or may be scattered (Compton scatter and coherent scatter).

BIBLIOGRAPHY

Frommer HH, Savage-Stabulas JJ: Ionizing radiation and basic principles of x-ray generation. In *Radiology for the dental professional*, ed 9, St. Louis, 2011, Mosby.

Johnson ON, Thomson EM: Characteristics and measurement of radiation. In *Essentials of dental radiography for dental assistants and hygienists*, ed 8, Upper Saddle River, NJ, 2007, Pearson Prentice Hall.

Johnson ON, Thomson EM: The dental x-ray machine: Components and functions. In *Essentials of dental radiography for dental assistants and hygienists*, ed 8, Upper Saddle River, NJ, 2007, Pearson Prentice Hall.

White SC, Pharoah MJ: Radiation physics. In *Oral radiology: principles and interpretation*, ed 6, St Louis, 2009, Mosby.

QUIZ QUESTIONS

MULTIPLE CHOICE

___ 1. Which of the following electrons has the greatest binding energy?
  a. N-shell electrons
  b. M-shell electrons
  c. L-shell electrons
  d. K-shell electrons

___ 2. What type of electrical charge does the electron carry?
  a. positive charge
  b. negative charge
  c. no charge
  d. positive or negative charge

___ **3.** Which term describes two or more atoms that are joined by chemical bonds?
  a. ion
  b. ion pair
  c. molecule
  d. proton

___ **4.** Which of the following describes ionization?
  a. atom without a nucleus
  b. atom that loses an electron
  c. atom with equal numbers of protons and electrons
  d. none of the above

___ **5.** Which term describes the process by which unstable atoms undergo spontaneous disintegration in an effort to attain a more balanced nuclear state?
  a. radiation
  b. radioactivity
  c. ionization
  d. ionizing radiation

___ **6.** Which of the following is *not* a type of particulate radiation?
  a. alpha particles
  b. beta particles
  c. protons
  d. nucleons

___ **7.** Which of the following is *not* a type of electromagnetic radiation?
  a. electrons
  b. radar waves
  c. microwaves
  d. x-rays

___ **8.** Which of the following statements is incorrect?
  a. Velocity is the speed of a wave.
  b. Wavelength is the distance between waves.
  c. Frequency is the number of wavelengths that pass a given point in a certain amount of time.
  d. Frequency and wavelength are inversely related.

___ **9.** Which of the following statements is incorrect?
  a. X-rays travel at the speed of sound.
  b. X-rays have no charge.
  c. X-rays cannot be focused to a point.
  d. X-rays cause ionization.

___ **10.** Which of the following statements is correct?
  a. X-rays are a form of electromagnetic radiation; visible light is not.
  b. X-rays have more energy than does visible light.
  c. X-rays have a longer wavelength than does visible light.
  d. X-rays travel more slowly than does visible light.

IDENTIFICATION

For questions 11 to 18, identify each of the labeled structures in Figure 2-27.
For questions 19 to 26, identify each of the labeled structures in Figure 2-28.

MULTIPLE CHOICE

___ **27.** Which of the following regulates the flow of electrical current to the filament of the x-ray tube?
  a. high-voltage circuit
  b. low-voltage circuit
  c. high-voltage transformer
  d. low-voltage transformer

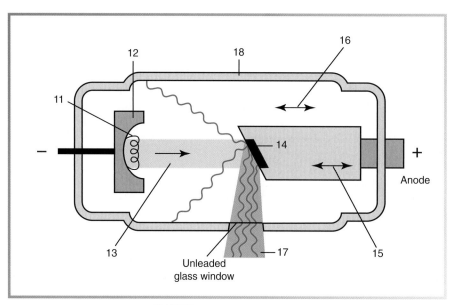

FIGURE 2-27 Dental x-ray tube.

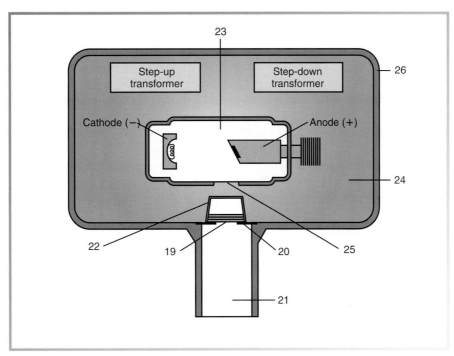

FIGURE 2-28 Dental x-ray tubehead.

___ **28.** Which of the following is used to increase the voltage in the high-voltage circuit?
  a. step-up transformer
  b. step-down transformer
  c. autotransformer
  d. step-up circuit

___ **29.** Which of the following does *not* occur when the high-voltage circuit is activated?
  a. The unit produces an audible and visible signal.
  b. Electrons produced at the cathode are accelerated across the tube to the anode.
  c. X-rays travel from the filament to the target.
  d. Heat is produced.

___ **30.** Which of the following is the location where x-rays are produced?
  a. positive cathode
  b. positive anode
  c. negative cathode
  d. negative anode

___ **31.** Which of the following is the location where thermionic emission occurs?
  a. positive cathode
  b. positive anode
  c. negative cathode
  d. negative anode

___ **32.** Which of the following accounts for 70% of all the x-ray energy produced at the anode?
  a. general radiation
  b. characteristic radiation
  c. Compton scatter
  d. coherent scatter

___ **33.** Which of the following occurs only at 70 kVp or higher and accounts for a very small part of the x-rays produced in the dental x-ray machine?
  a. general radiation
  b. characteristic radiation
  c. Compton scatter
  d. coherent scatter

___ **34.** Which of the following describes primary radiation?
  a. radiation that exits the tubehead
  b. radiation that is created when x-rays come in contact with matter
  c. radiation that has been deflected from its path by the interaction with matter
  d. none of the above

___ **35.** Which of the following describes scatter radiation?
  a. radiation that exits the tubehead
  b. radiation that is more penetrating than primary radiation
  c. radiation that has been deflected from its path by interaction with matter
  d. none of the above

___ **36.** Which of the following type of scatter occurs most often with dental x-rays?
  a. Compton
  b. coherent
  c. photoelectric
  d. none of the above

IDENTIFICATION

For questions 37 to 40, identify the x-radiation interaction with matter in Figures 2-29, 2-30, 2-31, and 2-32.

MULTIPLE CHOICE

For questions 41 to 44, refer to Figures 2-29, 2-30, 2-31, and 2-32.

____ 41. The interaction of x-radiation with matter illustrated in Figure 2-29 demonstrates:
  a. no scatter; no ionization
  b. no scatter; ionization
  c. scatter; no ionization
  d. scatter; ionization

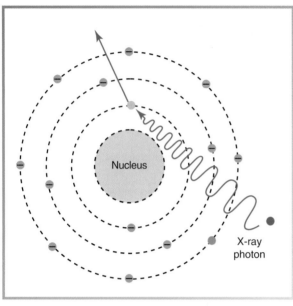

FIGURE 2-29

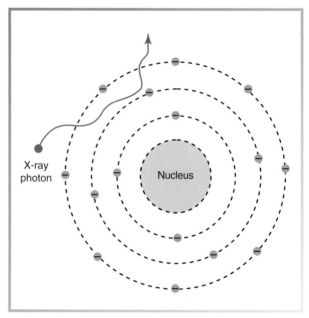

FIGURE 2-31

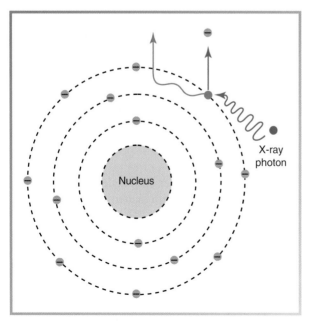

FIGURE 2-30

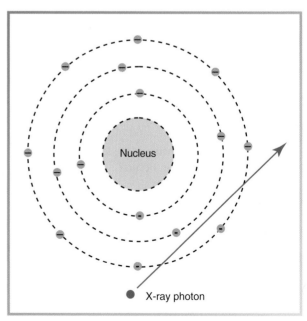

FIGURE 2-32

___ **42.** The interaction of x-radiation with matter illustrated in Figure 2-30 demonstrates:
   a. no scatter; no ionization
   b. no scatter; ionization
   c. scatter; no ionization
   d. scatter; ionization

___ **43.** The interaction of x-radiation with matter illustrated in Figure 2-31 demonstrates:
   a. no scatter; no ionization
   b. no scatter; ionization
   c. scatter; no ionization
   d. scatter; ionization

___ **44.** The interaction of x-radiation with matter illustrated in Figure 2-32 demonstrates:
   a. no scatter; no ionization
   b. no scatter; ionization
   c. scatter; no ionization
   d. scatter; ionization

chapter 3

Radiation Characteristics

OUTLINE

X-RAY BEAM QUALITY
    Voltage and Kilovoltage
    Kilovoltage Peak
    Density and Kilovoltage Peak
    Contrast and Kilovoltage Peak
    Exposure Time and Kilovoltage Peak
X-RAY BEAM QUANTITY
    Amperage and Milliamperage
    Milliampere-Seconds

    Density and Milliamperage
    Exposure Time and Milliamperage
X-RAY BEAM INTENSITY
    Kilovoltage Peak
    Milliamperage
    Exposure Time
    Distance
    Inverse Square Law
    Half-Value Layer

LEARNING OBJECTIVES

After completion of this chapter, the student will be able to do the following:

- Define the key words associated with radiation characteristics
- Describe the effect that the kilovoltage peak has on the quality of the x-ray beam
- Describe how milliamperage influences the quantity of the x-ray beam
- Identify the range of kilovoltage and milliamperage required for dental radiography
- Describe how increasing and decreasing exposure factors affect the density and contrast of the image

- State the rules governing kilovoltage, milliamperage, distance, and exposure time that are used when changing exposure variables
- Describe how kilovoltage, milliamperage, exposure time, and source-to-receptor distance influence the intensity of the x-ray beam
- Calculate an example of radiation intensity using the inverse square law
- Explain how the half-value layer determines the penetrating quality of the x-ray beam

KEY TERMS

Amperage	Intensity (of x-ray beam)	Milliampere-seconds (mAs)
Ampere (A)	Inverse square law	Polychromatic x-ray beam
Contrast	Kilovolt (kV)	Quality (of x-ray beam)
Density	Kilovoltage	Quantity (of x-ray beam)
Exposure time	Kilovoltage peak (kVp)	Volt (V)
Half-value layer (HVL)	Milliamperage	Voltage
Impulse	Milliampere (mA)	

Radiation characteristics include x-ray beam quality, quantity, and intensity. Variations in the character of the x-ray beam influence the quality of the resulting radiographs.

The dental radiographer must have a working knowledge of radiation characteristics. The purpose of this chapter is to (1) detail the concepts of x-ray beam quality and quantity, (2) define the concept of beam intensity, and (3) discuss how exposure factors influence these radiation characteristics.

Advances in dental radiographic equipment have produced control panels with predetermined settings for the various anatomic areas of the maxilla and mandible (Figure 3-1). On older radiographic units, the individual radiation characteristics of kilovoltage peak, milliamperage, and time could all be manually changed. On today's units, adjustments are not possible for milliamperage and kilovoltage peak. Although the modern equipment is easily understood and

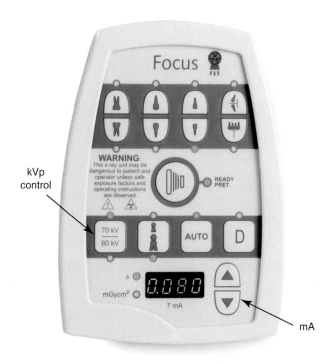

FIGURE 3-1 Kilovoltage peak (kVp) and milliamperage (mA) controls are located on the dental x-ray machine. (Courtesy Instrumentarium Dental, Inc. Milwaukee, WI.)

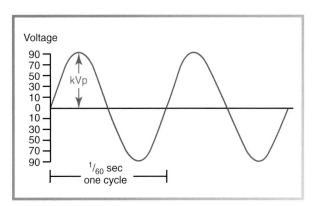

FIGURE 3-2 Kilovoltage peak (kVp) controls the quality of the x-ray beam and measures the peak voltage of the current.

convenient, the concepts of these three radiation characteristics must still be reviewed and understood.

X-RAY BEAM QUALITY

Wavelength determines the energy and penetrating power of radiation. X-rays with shorter wavelengths have more penetrating power, whereas those with longer wavelengths are less penetrating and more likely to be absorbed by matter. In dental radiography, the term **quality** is used to describe the mean energy or penetrating ability of the x-ray beam. The quality, or wavelength and energy of the x-ray beam, is controlled by kilovoltage.

Voltage and Kilovoltage

Voltage is a measurement of force that refers to the potential difference between two electrical charges. Inside the dental x-ray tubehead, voltage is the measurement of electrical force that causes electrons to move from the negative cathode to the positive anode. Voltage determines the speed of electrons that travel from cathode to anode. When voltage is increased, the speed of the electrons is increased. When the speed of the electrons is increased, the electrons strike the target with greater force and energy, resulting in a penetrating x-ray beam with a short wavelength.

Voltage is measured in volts or kilovolts. The **volt (V)** is the unit of measurement used to describe the potential that drives an electrical current through a circuit. Dental x-ray equipment requires the use of high voltages. Most radiographic units operate using kilovolts; 1 **kilovolt (kV)** is equal to 1000 volts.

Dental radiography requires the use of 65 to 100 kV. The use of less than 65 kV does not allow adequate penetration, whereas the use of more than 100 kV results in overpenetration.

Kilovoltage can be adjusted according to the individual diagnostic needs of patients. The use of 85 to 100 kV produces more penetrating dental x-rays with greater energy and shorter wavelengths, whereas the use of 65 to 75 kV produces less penetrating dental x-rays with less energy and longer wavelengths. A higher kilovoltage should be used when the area to be examined is dense or thick.

Kilovoltage Peak

On dental radiographic equipment that allows for the adjustment of individual radiation characteristics, kilovoltage is controlled by the kilovoltage peak adjustment dial on the x-ray control panel (Figure 3-2). **Kilovoltage peak (kVp)** can be defined as the maximum or peak voltage. The voltage meter on the control panel measures the x-ray tube voltage, which is actually the peak voltage of an alternating current (AC) (see Figure 3-3). This peak voltage is measured in kilovolts, and thus the term "kilovoltage peak" is used. For example, when 90 kVp is used to expose a receptor, the peak voltage of the tube current is 90,000 volts. As a result of varying kilovoltages occurring in the tube current, a **polychromatic x-ray beam**, or a beam that contains many different wavelengths of varying intensities, is produced.

The quality, or wavelength and energy of the x-ray beam, is controlled by the kilovoltage peak. The kilovoltage peak regulates the speed and energy of the electrons and determines the penetrating ability of the x-ray beam. Increasing the kilovoltage peak results in a higher energy x-ray beam with increased penetrating ability.

Density and Kilovoltage Peak

Density is the overall darkness or blackness of an image. An adjustment in kilovoltage peak results in a change in the density of a dental radiograph. When the kilovoltage peak is

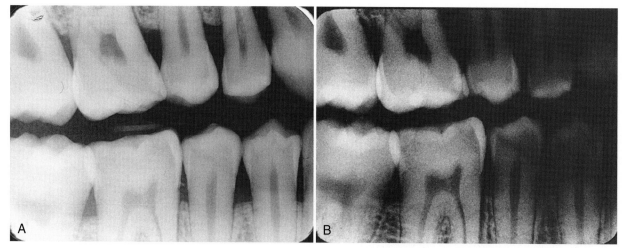

FIGURE 3-3 A, Diagnostic radiograph. **B,** Increase in kilovoltage results in an image that exhibits increased density; the image appears darker.

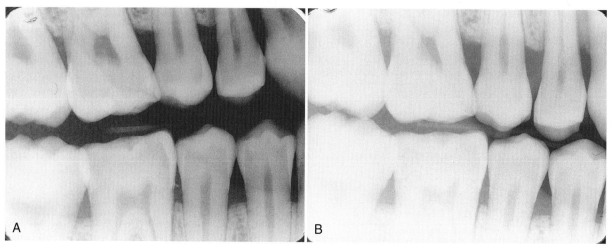

FIGURE 3-4 A, Diagnostic radiograph. **B,** Decrease in kilovoltage results in an image that exhibits decreased density; the image appears lighter.

increased while other exposure factors (milliamperage, exposure time) remain constant, the resultant image exhibits an increased density and appears darker (Figure 3-4A). If kilovoltage peak is decreased, the resultant image exhibits a decreased density and appears lighter (Figure 3-4B). Table 3-1 summarizes the effect of kilovoltage peak on density (also see Chapter 8).

Contrast and Kilovoltage Peak

Contrast refers to how sharply dark and light areas are differentiated or separated on an image. An adjustment in kilovoltage peak results in a change in the contrast of a dental radiograph. When low kilovoltage peak settings are used (65–70 kVp), a high-contrast image will result. An image with "high" contrast has many black areas and many white areas and few shades of gray (Figure 3-5). An image with high contrast is useful for the detection and progression of dental caries.

With high kilovoltage peak settings (690 kVp), low contrast results. An image with "low" contrast has many

TABLE 3-1	Effect of Kilovoltage Peak (kVp) on Image Density and Contrast		
Adjustment		**Density**	**Contrast**
↑ kVp		↑ (Darker)	Low
↓ kVp		↓ (Lighter)	High

↑, Increase; ↓, decrease.

shades of gray instead of black and white. An image with low contrast is useful for the detection of periodontal or periapical disease (Figure 3-6). Mounted radiographs that demonstrate low contrast and that are viewed properly on an illuminated surface with masked extraneous light are preferred in dental radiography.

A compromise between high contrast and low contrast is desirable. See Table 3-1 for a summary of the effect of kilovoltage peak on contrast (also see Chapter 8).

FIGURE 3-5 Image produced with lower kilovoltage exhibits high contrast; many light and dark areas are seen, as demonstrated by the use of the stepwedge.

FIGURE 3-6 Image produced with higher kilovoltage exhibits low contrast; many shades of gray are seen instead of black and white.

BOX 3-1 Kilovoltage Peak Rule

- When kilovoltage peak is increased by 15, exposure time should be decreased by half.
- When kilovoltage peak is decreased by 15, exposure time should be doubled.

Exposure Time and Kilovoltage Peak

Exposure time refers to the interval of time during which x-rays are produced. Exposure time is measured in **impulses** because x-rays are created in a series of bursts or pulses rather than in a continuous stream. One impulse occurs every 1/60 of a second; therefore, 60 impulses occur in 1 second.

To compensate for the penetrating power of the x-ray beam, an adjustment in exposure time is necessary when kilovoltage peak is increased (Box 3-1).

For example, a receptor is exposed using 90 kVp and 0.5 second. If the kilovoltage peak setting is decreased from 90 to 75, the exposure time must be increased from 0.5 to 1.0 second to maintain proper density and contrast.

X-RAY BEAM QUANTITY

Quantity of the x-ray beam refers to the number of x-rays produced in the dental x-ray unit.

Amperage and Milliamperage

Amperage determines the amount of electrons passing through the cathode filament. An increase in the number of electrons available to travel from the cathode to the anode results in production of an increased number of x-rays. The quantity of the x-rays produced is controlled by milliamperage.

The **ampere** (**A**) is the unit of measure used to describe the number of electrons, or current flowing through the cathode filament. The number of amperes needed to operate a dental x-ray unit is small; therefore, amperage is measured in milliamperes. One **milliampere** (**mA**) is equal to 1/1000 of an ampere. Some dental x-ray units have a fixed milliampere setting, whereas others have a milliampere adjustment on the control panel (see Figure 3-2). In dental radiography, the use of 7 to 15 mA is required; a setting above 15 mA is not recommended because of the resultant excessive heat production in the x-ray tube.

Milliamperage regulates the temperature of the cathode filament. A higher milliampere setting increases the temperature of the cathode filament and consequently increases the number of electrons produced. An increase in the number of electrons that strike the anode increases the number of x-rays emitted from the tube.

The quantity, or number of x-rays emitted from the tubehead, is controlled by milliamperage. Milliamperage controls the amperage of the filament current and the amount of electrons that pass through the filament. As the milliamperage is increased, more electrons pass through the filament, and more x-rays are produced. For example, if the milliamperage is increased from 5 to 10 mA, twice as many electrons travel from the cathode to the anode, and twice as many x-rays are produced.

Milliampere-Seconds

Both milliamperes and exposure time have a direct influence on the number of electrons produced by the cathode filament. The product of milliamperes and exposure time is termed **milliampere-seconds** (**mAs**), as follows:

$$\text{Milliamperes} \times \text{Exposure time (seconds)} = \text{Milliampere-seconds}$$

When milliamperage is increased, the exposure time must be decreased, and vice versa, if the density of the exposed radiograph is to remain the same.

EXAMPLE

Using 10 mA with an exposure time of 1.5 seconds would result in 15 mAs (10 mA × 1.5 seconds = 15 mAs). If the milliamperage is increased to 15, the time must be decreased to 1.0 second (15 mA × 1.0 second = 15 mAs).

Note that both these exposures result in the same number of milliampere-seconds, which produces the same density on a dental radiograph.

If a patient has difficulty holding still during the exposure, for example, the dental radiographer can increase the milliamperage and decrease the exposure time to compensate for the patient's movement.

Density and Milliamperage

Milliamperage, as with kilovoltage peak, has an effect on the density of a dental radiograph. An increase in milliamperage increases the overall density of the radiograph and results in a darker image. Conversely, a decrease in milliamperage decreases the overall density and results in a lighter image. Table 3-2 summarizes the effect of milliamperage on density.

Exposure Time and Milliamperage

Milliamperage and exposure time are inversely related. When altering milliamperage, the exposure time must be adjusted to maintain the diagnostic density of an image film. When milliamperage is increased, the exposure time must be decreased. When milliamperage is decreased, the exposure time must be increased.

Table 3-3 lists guidelines for adjusting kilovoltage peak, milliamperage, and exposure time.

X-RAY BEAM INTENSITY

Quality refers to the energy or penetrating ability of the x-ray beam; quantity refers to the number of x-ray photons in the beam. Quality and quantity are described together in a concept known as intensity. **Intensity** is defined as the product of the quantity (number of x-ray photons) and quality (energy of each photon) per unit of area per unit of time of exposure, as follows:

TABLE 3-2	Effect of Milliamperage (mA) on Image Density

Adjustment	Density
↑ mA	↑ (Darker)
↓ mA	↓ (Lighter)

↑, Increase; ↓, decrease.

TABLE 3-3	Guidelines for Adjusting Kilovoltage Peak (kVp), Milliamperage (mA), and Exposure Time

Adjustment	Exposure*
↑ kVp by 15	↓ Exposure time by 1/2
↓ kVp by 15	↑ Exposure time by 2
↑ mA	↓ Exposure time
↓ mA	↑ Exposure time

*Adjustment in exposure time needed to maintain diagnostic density of image.

$$\text{Intensity} = \frac{(\text{No. photons}) \times (\text{Energy of each photon})}{(\text{Area}) \times (\text{Exposure rate})}$$

Intensity of the x-ray beam is affected by a number of factors, including kilovoltage peak, milliamperage, exposure time, and distance.

Kilovoltage Peak

Kilovoltage peak regulates the penetrating power of the x-ray beam by controlling the speed of the electrons traveling between the cathode and the anode. Higher kilovoltage peak settings produce an x-ray beam with more energy and shorter wavelengths; higher kilovoltage levels increase the intensity of the x-ray beam.

Milliamperage

Milliamperage controls the penetrating power of the x-ray beam by controlling the number of electrons produced in the x-ray tube and the number of x-rays produced. Higher milliampere settings produce a beam with more energy, increasing the intensity of the x-ray beam.

Exposure Time

Exposure time, as with milliamperage, affects the number of x-rays produced. A longer exposure time produces more x-rays. An increase in exposure time produces a more intense x-ray beam.

Distance

The distance traveled by the x-ray beam affects the intensity of the beam. Distances that must be considered when exposing a dental radiograph include the following (Figure 3-7):
- *Target-surface distance:* The distance from the source of radiation to the patient's skin
- *Target-object distance:* The distance from the source of radiation to the tooth
- *Target-receptor distance:* The distance from the source of radiation to the receptor

The distance between the source of radiation and the receptor has a marked effect on the intensity of the x-ray

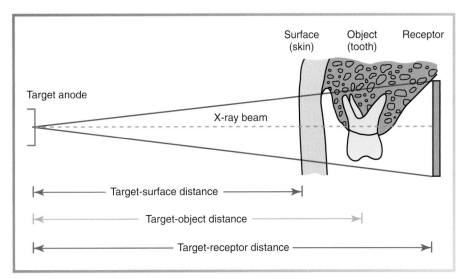

FIGURE 3-7 Distances to consider when exposing dental radiographs: target-surface, target-object, and target-receptor distance.

beam. As x-rays travel from their point of origin or away from the target anode, they diverge like waves of light and spread out to cover a larger surface area. As x-rays travel away from their source of origin, the intensity of the beam lessens. Unless a corresponding change is made in one of the other exposure factors (kilovoltage peak, milliamperage), the intensity of the x-ray beam is reduced as the distance increases.

The x-ray beam that exits from an 8-inch position-indicating device (PID) is more intense than one that exits from a 16-inch PID. The inverse square law is used to explain how distance affects the intensity of the x-ray beam.

Inverse Square Law

The **inverse square law** is stated as follows:

The intensity of radiation is inversely proportional to the square of the distance from the source of radiation.

"Inversely proportional" means that as one variable increases, the other decreases. When the source-to-receptor distance is increased, the intensity of the beam is decreased.

For example, when the PID length is changed from 8 to 16 inches, the source-to-receptor distance is doubled. According to the inverse square law, the resultant beam is one-fourth as intense (Figure 3-8). When the PID length is changed from 16 to 8 inches, the source-to-receptor distance is reduced by half. According to the inverse square law, the resultant beam is four times as intense.

The following mathematical formula is used to calculate the inverse square law.

$$\frac{\text{Original intensity}}{\text{New distance}^2} = \frac{\text{New intensity}}{\text{Original distance}^2}$$

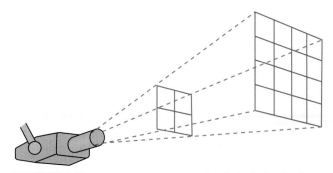

FIGURE 3-8 The inverse square law states that the intensity of radiation is inversely proportional to the square of the distance from the source. Note that as the source-to-receptor distance is doubled, the intensity of radiation is one fourth as intense. (Modified from White SC, Pharoah MJ: *Oral radiology principles and interpretation,* ed 5, St Louis, 2004, Mosby.)

EXAMPLE

If the PID length is changed from 8 inches to 16 inches, how does this increase in source-to-receptor distance affect the intensity of the beam?

$$\frac{1}{x} = \frac{16^2}{8^2}$$

$$\frac{1}{x} = \frac{256}{64}$$

$$\frac{1}{x} = \frac{4}{1}$$

$$x = \frac{1}{4}$$

This mathematical formula reveals that the intensity of the beam will be one fourth as intense if the source-to-receptor distance is changed from 8 to 16 inches (assuming that kilovoltage peak and milliamperage remain constant). In this example, the inverse square law reveals that doubling the distance from the source of radiation to the receptor (from an 8-inch to a 16-inch PID) results in a beam that is one fourth as intense. Remember: The intensity of the radiation is inversely proportional to the square of the distance.

Half-Value Layer

To reduce the intensity of the x-ray beam, aluminum filters are placed in the path of the beam inside the dental x-ray tubehead. Aluminum filters are used to remove the low-energy, less penetrating, longer-wavelength x-rays. Aluminum filters increase the mean penetrating capability of the x-ray beam while reducing the intensity. When placed in the path of the x-ray beam, the thickness of a specified material (e.g., aluminum) that reduces the intensity by half is termed the **half-value layer (HVL)**.

For example, if an x-ray beam has an HVL of 4 mm, a thickness of 4 mm of aluminum would be necessary to decrease its intensity by half. Measuring the HVL determines the penetrating quality of the beam. The higher the half-value layer, the more penetrating is the beam. (Filtration of the x-ray beam is discussed further in Chapter 5.)

SUMMARY

- Radiation characteristics include x-ray beam quality, quantity, and intensity.
- X-ray units may or may not have adjustable dials or buttons for kilovoltage peak, milliamperage, and time.
- *Quality* refers to the mean (average) energy or penetrating ability of the x-ray beam and is controlled by the kilovoltage peak.
- Increased kilovoltage peak produces x-rays with increased energy, shorter wavelength, and increased penetrating power; kilovoltage peak affects density and contrast.
- *Quantity* refers to the number of x-rays produced and is controlled by the milliamperage.
- Increased milliamperage produces an increased number of x-rays; milliamperage affects density.
- Exposure time also influences the number of x-rays produced.
- *Intensity* is the total energy contained in the x-ray beam in a specific area at a given time; intensity is affected by kilovoltage peak, milliamperage, exposure time, and distance.
- Increased kilovoltage peak, milliamperage, or exposure time results in increased intensity of the x-ray beam.
- Intensity of the x-ray beam is reduced with increased distance. The inverse square law is used to explain how distance affects the intensity of the x-ray beam.
- An aluminum filter is placed in the path of the x-ray beam to reduce the intensity and remove the low-energy x-rays from the beam.
- The thickness of aluminum placed in the path of the x-ray beam that reduces the intensity by half is termed the *half-value layer (HVL)*.

BIBLIOGRAPHY

Frommer HH, Savage-Stabulas JJ: Image formation. In *Radiology for the dental professional*, ed 9, St Louis, 2011, Mosby.

Frommer HH, Savage-Stabulas JJ: Image receptors. In *Radiology for the dental professional*, ed 9, St Louis, 2011, Mosby.

Frommer HH, Savage-Stabulas JJ: Ionizing radiation and basic principles of x-ray generation. In *Radiology for the dental professional*, ed 9, St Louis, 2011, Mosby.

Johnson ON, Thomson EM: The dental x-ray machine: components and functions. In *Essentials of dental radiography for dental assistants and hygienists*, ed 9, Upper Saddle River, NJ, 2007, Pearson Prentice Hall.

Johnson ON, Thomson EM: Producing quality radiographs. In *Essentials of dental radiography for dental assistants and hygienists*, ed 8, Upper Saddle River, NJ, 2007, Pearson Prentice Hall.

Miles DA, Van Dis ML, Williamson GF, Jensen CW: Image characteristics. In *Radiographic imaging for the dental team*, ed 4, St Louis, 2009 Saunders.

Miles DA, Van Dis ML, Williamson GF, Jensen CW: X-ray properties and the generation of x-rays. In *Radiographic imaging for the dental team*, ed 4, St Louis, 2009, Saunders.

White SC, Pharoah MJ: Radiation physics. In *Oral radiology: principles and interpretation*, ed 6, St Louis, 2009, Mosby.

QUIZ QUESTIONS

MULTIPLE CHOICE

____ 1. In dental radiography, the quality of the x-ray beam is controlled by:
   a. kilovoltage peak
   b. milliamperage
   c. exposure time
   d. source-to-receptor distance

____ 2. Identify the kilovoltage range for most dental x-ray machines:
   a. 50 to 60 kV
   b. 60 to 70 kV
   c. 65 to 100 kV
   d. greater than 100 kV

____ 3. A higher kilovoltage produces x-rays with:
   a. greater energy levels
   b. shorter wavelengths
   c. more penetrating ability
   d. all of the above

____ 4. Identify the unit of measurement used to describe the amount of electric current flowing through the x-ray tube:
   a. volt
   b. ampere
   c. kilovoltage peak
   d. force

___ 5. Radiation produced with high kilovoltage results in:
   a. short wavelengths
   b. long wavelengths
   c. less penetrating radiation
   d. lower energy levels

___ 6. In dental radiography, the quantity of radiation produced is controlled by:
   a. kilovoltage peak
   b. milliamperage
   c. exposure time
   d. both b and c

___ 7. Increasing milliamperage results in an increase in:
   a. temperature of the filament
   b. mean energy of the beam
   c. number of x-rays produced
   d. both a and c

___ 8. Identify the milliamperage range for dental radiography:
   a. 1 to 5 mA
   b. 4 to 10 mA
   c. 7 to 15 mA
   d. greater than 15 mA

___ 9. The overall blackness or darkness of an image is termed:
   a. contrast
   b. density
   c. overexposure
   d. polychromatic

___ 10. If kilovoltage is decreased with no other variations in exposure factors, the resultant image will:
   a. appear lighter
   b. appear darker
   c. remain the same
   d. either a or b

___ 11. Identify the term that describes how dark and light areas are differentiated on an image:
   a. contrast
   b. density
   c. intensity
   d. polychromatic

___ 12. A radiograph that has many light and dark areas with few shades of gray is said to have:
   a. high density
   b. low density
   c. high contrast
   d. low contrast

___ 13. The radiograph described in question 12 was produced with:
   a. low kilovoltage
   b. high kilovoltage
   c. low milliamperage
   d. high milliamperage

___ 14. Increasing milliamperage alone results in an image with:
   a. high contrast
   b. low contrast
   c. increased density
   d. decreased density

___ 15. A diagnostic image is produced using 90 kVp and 0.25 second. What exposure time is needed to produce the same image at 75 kVp?
   a. 0.50 second
   b. 0.75 second
   c. 1.00 second
   d. 1.25 second

___ 16. A diagnostic image is produced using 10 mA and 0.45 second. What exposure time is needed to produce the same image at 15 mA?
   a. 0.25 second
   b. 0.30 second
   c. 0.45 second
   d. 0.50 second

___ 17. The total energy contained in the x-ray beam in a specific area at a given time is termed:
   a. kilovoltage peak
   b. beam quality
   c. intensity
   d. milliampere-second

___ 18. Increasing which of these four exposure controls will increase the intensity of the x-ray beam: (1) kilovoltage, (2) milliamperage, (3) exposure time, (4) source-to-receptor distance?
   a. 1 and 2
   b. 2 and 3
   c. 1, 2, and 3
   d. 1, 2, 3, and 4

___ 19. The length of the position-indicating device is changed from 16 inches to 8 inches. The resultant intensity of the beam will be:
   a. four times as intense
   b. twice as intense
   c. half as intense
   d. one fourth as intense

___ 20. The half-value layer is the amount of:
   a. lead that restricts the diameter of the beam by half
   b. copper needed to cool the anode
   c. aluminum needed to reduce scatter radiation by half
   d. aluminum needed to reduce x-ray beam intensity by half

chapter 4

Radiation Biology

OUTLINE

RADIATION INJURY
Mechanisms of Injury
Theories of Radiation Injury
Dose–Response Curve
Stochastic and Nonstochastic Radiation Effects
Sequence of Radiation Injury
Determining Factors for Radiation Injury
RADIATION EFFECTS
Short-Term and Long-Term Effects
Somatic and Genetic Effects
Radiation Effects on Cells
Radiation Effects on Tissues and Organs

RADIATION MEASUREMENTS
Units of Measurement
Exposure Measurement
Dose Measurement
Dose Equivalent Measurement
Measurements Used in Dental Radiography
RADIATION RISKS
Sources of Radiation Exposure
Risk and Risk Estimates
Dental Radiation and Exposure Risks
Patient Exposure and Dose
Risk Versus Benefit of Dental Radiographs

LEARNING OBJECTIVES

After completion of this chapter, the student will be able to do the following:

- Define the key words associated with radiation injury
- Describe the mechanisms, theories, and sequence of radiation injury
- Define and discuss the dose–response curve and radiation injury
- List the determining factors for radiation injury
- Discuss the short-term and long-term effects as well as the somatic and genetic effects of radiation exposure
- Describe the effects of radiation exposure on cells, tissues, and organs

- Identify the relative sensitivity of a given tissue to x-radiation
- Define the units of measurement used in radiation exposure
- List common sources of radiation exposure
- Discuss risk and risk estimates for radiation exposure
- Discuss dental radiation and exposure risks
- Discuss the risk versus benefit of dental radiographs

KEY TERMS

Cell
Cell differentiation
Cell metabolism
Coulomb (C)
Critical organ
Cumulative effects
Direct theory
Dose
Dose, total
Dose equivalent
Dose rate
Dose–response curve
Exposure

Free radical
Genetic cells
Genetic effects
Gray (Gy)
Indirect theory
Injury, period of
Ionization
Latent period
Long-term effects
Mitotic activity
Nonstochastic effects
Quality factor (QF)
Radiation, background

Radiation absorbed dose (rad)
Radiation biology
Radioresistant
Radiosensitive
Recovery period
Risk
Roentgen (R)
Roentgen equivalent (in) man (rem)
Short-term effects
Sievert (Sv)
Somatic cells
Somatic effects
Stochastic effects

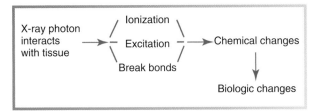

FIGURE 4-1 The x-ray photon interacts with tissues and results in ionization, excitation, or breaking of molecular bonds, all of which cause chemical changes that result in biologic damage.

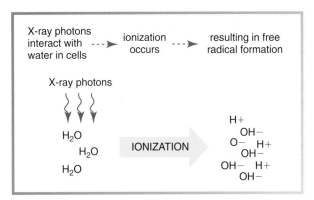

FIGURE 4-2 Examples of free radicals created when water is irradiated.

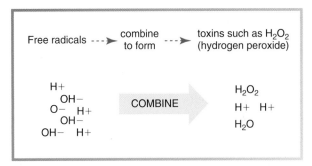

FIGURE 4-3 Free radicals can combine with each other to form toxins such as hydrogen peroxide.

All ionizing radiations are harmful and produce biologic changes in living tissues. The damaging biologic effects of x-radiation were first documented shortly after the discovery of x-rays. Since that time, information about the harmful effects of high-level exposure to x-radiation has increased on the basis of studies of atomic bomb survivors, workers exposed to radioactive materials, and patients undergoing radiation therapy. Although the amount of x-radiation used in dental radiography is small, biologic damage does occur.

The dental radiographer must have a working knowledge of **radiation biology**, the study of the effects of ionizing radiation on living tissue, to understand the harmful effects of x-radiation. The purpose of this chapter is to describe the mechanisms and theories of radiation injury, to define the basic concepts and effects of radiation exposure, to detail radiation measurements, and to discuss the risks of radiation exposure.

RADIATION INJURY

Mechanisms of Injury

In diagnostic radiography, not all x-rays pass through the patient and reach the dental x-ray film; some are absorbed by the patient's tissues. *Absorption,* as defined in Chapter 2, refers to the total transfer of energy from the x-ray photon to patient tissues. What happens when x-ray energy is absorbed by patient tissues? Chemical changes occur that result in biologic damage. Two specific mechanisms of radiation injury are possible: (1) ionization and (2) free radical formation.

Ionization

X-rays are a form of ionizing radiation; when x-rays strike patient tissues, ionization results. As described in Chapter 2, **ionization** is produced through the photoelectric effect or Compton scatter and results in the formation of a positive atom and a dislodged negative electron. The ejected high-speed electron is set into motion and interacts with other atoms within the absorbing tissues. The kinetic energy of such electrons results in further ionization, excitation, or breaking of molecular bonds, all of which cause chemical changes within the cell that result in biologic damage (Figure 4-1). Ionization may have little effect on cells if the chemical changes do not alter sensitive molecules, or such changes may have a profound effect on structures of great importance to cell function (e.g., DNA).

Free Radical Formation

X-radiation causes cell damage primarily through the formation of free radicals.* Free radical formation occurs when an x-ray photon ionizes water, the primary component of living cells. Ionization of water results in the production of hydrogen and hydroxyl free radicals (Figure 4-2). A **free radical** is an uncharged (neutral) atom or molecule that exists with a single, unpaired electron in its outermost shell. It is highly reactive and unstable; the lifetime of a free radical is approximately 10^{-10} seconds. To achieve stability, free radicals may (1) recombine without causing changes in the molecule, (2) combine with other free radicals and cause changes, or (3) combine with ordinary molecules to form a toxin (e.g., hydrogen peroxide [H_2O_2]) capable of producing widespread cellular changes (Figure 4-3).

Theories of Radiation Injury

Damage to living tissues caused by exposure to ionizing radiation may result from a direct hit and absorption of an

---

*A free radical with no charge is denoted by a dot following the chemical symbol (e.g., H·). A free radical with a charge is an ion.

x-ray photon within a cell or from the absorption of an x-ray photon by the water within a cell accompanied by free radical formation. Two theories are used to describe how radiation damages biologic tissues: (1) the direct theory and (2) the indirect theory.

Direct Theory

The **direct theory** of radiation injury suggests that cell damage results when ionizing radiation directly hits critical areas, or targets, within the cell. For example, if x-ray photons directly strike the deoxyribonucleic acid (DNA) of a cell, critical damage occurs, causing injury to the irradiated organism. Direct injuries from exposure to ionizing radiation occur infrequently; most x-ray photons pass through the cell and cause little or no damage.

Indirect Theory

The **indirect theory** of radiation injury suggests that x-ray photons are absorbed within the cell and cause the formation of toxins, which, in turn, damage the cell. For example, when x-ray photons are absorbed by the water within a cell, free radical formation results. The free radicals combine to form toxins (e.g., H_2O_2), which cause cellular dysfunction and biologic damage. An indirect injury results because the free radicals combine and form toxins, not because of a direct hit by x-ray photons. Indirect injuries from exposure to ionizing radiation occur frequently because of the high water content of cells. The chances of free radical formation and indirect injury are great because cells are 70% to 80% water.

Dose–Response Curve

If all ionizing radiations are harmful and produce biologic damage, what level of exposure is considered acceptable? To establish acceptable levels of radiation exposure, it is useful to plot the dose administered and the damage produced. With radiation exposure, a **dose–response curve** can be used to correlate the "response," or damage, of tissues with the "dose," or amount, of radiation received.

When dose and damage are plotted on a graph, a linear, nonthreshold relationship is seen. A linear relationship indicates that the response of the tissues is directly proportional to the dose. A nonthreshold relationship indicates that a threshold dose level for damage does not exist. A nonthreshold dose–response curve suggests that no matter how small the amount of radiation received, some biologic damage does occur (Figure 4-4). Consequently, there is no safe amount of radiation exposure. In dental radiography, as mentioned earlier, although the doses received by patients are low, damage does occur.

Most of the information used to produce dose–response curves for radiation exposure comes from studying the effects of large doses of radiation on populations, for example, atomic bomb survivors. In the low-dose range, however, minimal information has been documented; instead, the curve has been extrapolated from animal and cellular experiments.

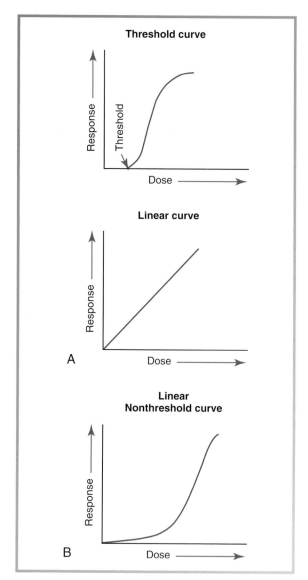

FIGURE 4-4 A, *Threshold curve:* This curve indicates that below a certain level (threshold), no response is seen. *Linear curve:* This curve indicates that response is proportional to dose. **B,** *Linear nonthreshold curve:* This dose–response curve indicates that a response is seen at any dose.

Stochastic and Nonstochastic Radiation Effects

Biologic effects from radiation can be classified as stochastic or nonstochastic. **Stochastic effects** occur as a direct function of dose. The probability of occurrence increases with increasing absorbed dose; however, the severity of effects does not depend on the magnitude of the absorbed dose. As in the case of nonthreshold radiation effects, stochastic effects do not have a dose threshold. Examples of stochastic effects include cancer (i.e., tumor) induction and genetic mutations.

Nonstochastic effects (deterministic effects) are somatic effects that have a threshold and that increase in severity with increasing absorbed dose. Examples of nonstochastic effects include erythema, loss of hair, cataract formation, and decreased fertility. Compared with stochastic effects, nonstochastic effects require larger radiation doses to cause serious impairment of health.

Sequence of Radiation Injury

Chemical reactions (e.g., ionization, free radical formation) that follow the absorption of radiation occur rapidly at the molecular level. However, varying amounts of time are required for these changes to alter cells and cellular functions. As a result, the observable effects of radiation are not visible immediately after exposure. Instead, following exposure, a latent period occurs. A **latent period** can be defined as the time that elapses between exposure to ionizing radiation and the appearance of observable clinical signs. The latent period may be short or long, depending on the total dose of radiation received and the amount of time, or rate, it took to receive the dose. The more radiation received and the faster the dose rate, the shorter is the latent period.

After the latent period, a **period of injury** occurs. A variety of cellular injuries may result, including cell death, changes in cell function, breaking or clumping of chromosomes, formation of giant cells, cessation of mitotic activity, and abnormal mitotic activity.

The last event in the sequence of radiation injury is the **recovery period**. Not all cellular radiation injuries are permanent. With each radiation exposure, cellular damage is followed by repair. Depending on a number of factors, cells can repair the damage caused by radiation. Most of the damage caused by low-level radiation is repaired within the cells of the body.

The effects of radiation exposure are additive, and unrepaired damage accumulates in the tissues. The **cumulative effects** of repeated radiation exposure can lead to health problems (e.g., cancer, cataract formation, birth defects). Table 4-1 lists disorders that may result from the cumulative effects of repeated radiation exposure on tissues and organs.

Determining Factors for Radiation Injury

In addition to understanding the mechanisms, theories, and sequence of radiation injury, it is important to recognize the factors that influence radiation injury. The factors used to determine the degree of radiation injury include the following:

TABLE 4-1	Tissue and Radiation Effect
Tissue or Organ	**Radiation Effect**
Bone marrow	Leukemia
Reproductive cells (ova, sperm)	Genetic mutations
Salivary gland	Carcinoma
Thyroid	Carcinoma
Skin	Carcinoma
Lens of eye	Cataracts

- *Total dose:* Quantity of radiation received, or the total amount of radiation energy absorbed. More damage occurs when tissues absorb large quantities of radiation.
- *Dose rate:* Rate at which exposure to radiation occurs and absorption takes place (dose rate = dose/time). More radiation damage takes place with high dose rates because a rapid delivery of radiation does not allow time for the cellular damage to be repaired.
- *Amount of tissue irradiated:* Areas of the body exposed to radiation. Total-body irradiation produces more adverse systemic effects than if small, localized areas of the body are exposed. An example of total-body irradiation is the exposure of a person to a nuclear energy disaster. Extensive radiation injury occurs when large areas of the body are exposed because of the damage to the blood-forming tissues.
- *Cell sensitivity:* More damage occurs in cells that are most sensitive to radiation, such as rapidly dividing cells and young cells (see later discussion).
- *Age:* Children are more susceptible to radiation damage than are adults.

RADIATION EFFECTS

Short-Term and Long-Term Effects

Radiation effects can be classified as either short-term or long-term effects. Following the latent period, effects that are seen within minutes, days, or weeks are termed **short-term effects**. Short-term effects are associated with large amounts of radiation absorbed in a short time (e.g., exposure to a nuclear accident or the atomic bomb). Acute radiation syndrome (ARS) is a short-term effect and includes nausea, vomiting, diarrhea, hair loss, and hemorrhage. Short-term effects are not applicable to dentistry.

Effects that appear after years, decades, or generations are termed **long-term effects**. Long-term effects are associated with small amounts of radiation absorbed repeatedly over a long period. Repeated low levels of radiation exposure are linked to the induction of cancer, birth abnormalities, and genetic defects.

Somatic and Genetic Effects

All the cells in the body can be classified as either somatic or genetic. **Somatic cells** are all the cells in the body except the reproductive cells. The reproductive cells (e.g., ova, sperm) are termed **genetic cells**. Depending on the type of cell injured by radiation, the biologic effects of radiation can be classified as somatic or genetic.

Somatic effects are seen in the person who has been irradiated. Radiation injuries that produce changes in somatic cells produce poor health in the irradiated individual. Major somatic effects of radiation exposure include the induction of cancer, leukemia, and cataracts. These changes, however, are not transmitted to future generations (Figure 4-5).

Genetic effects are not seen in the irradiated person but are passed on to future generations. Radiation injuries that produce changes in genetic cells do not affect the health of the exposed individual. Instead, the radiation-induced mutations affect the health of the offspring (see Figure 4-5). Genetic damage cannot be repaired.

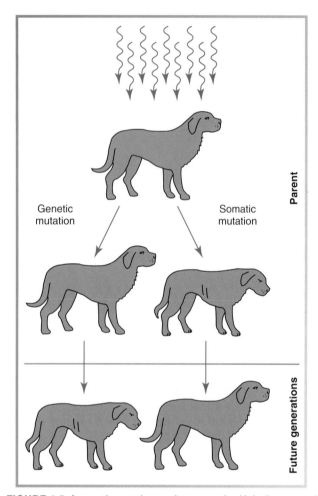

FIGURE 4-5 A somatic mutation produces poor health in the exposed animal but does not produce mutations in subsequent generations. In contrast, a genetic mutation does not affect the exposed animal but produces mutations in future generations.

(Figure labels: Genetic mutation, Somatic mutation, Parent, Future generations)

Radiation Effects on Cells

The **cell**, or basic structural unit of all living organisms, is composed of a central nucleus and surrounding cytoplasm. Ionizing radiation may affect the nucleus, the cytoplasm, or the entire cell. The cell nucleus is more sensitive to radiation than is the cytoplasm. Damage to the nucleus affects the chromosomes containing DNA and results in disruption of cell division, which, in turn, may lead to disruption of cell function or cell death.

Not all cells respond to radiation in the same manner. A cell that is sensitive to radiation is termed **radiosensitive**; one that is resistant is termed **radioresistant**. The response of a cell to radiation exposure is determined by the following:
- **Mitotic activity:** Cells that divide frequently or undergo many divisions over time are more sensitive to radiation.
- **Cell differentiation:** Cells that are immature or are not highly specialized are more sensitive to radiation.
- **Cell metabolism:** Cells that have a higher metabolism are more sensitive to radiation.

Cells that are radiosensitive include blood cells, immature reproductive cells, and young bone cells. The cell that is most sensitive to radiation is the small lymphocyte. Radioresistant cells include cells of bone, muscle, and nerve (Table 4-2).

Radiation Effects on Tissues and Organs

Cells are organized into the larger functioning units of tissues and organs. As with cells, tissues and organs vary in their sensitivity to radiation. Radiosensitive organs are composed of radiosensitive cells and include the lymphoid tissues, bone marrow, testes, and intestines. Examples of radioresistant tissues include the salivary glands, kidney, and liver.

In dentistry, some tissues and organs are designated as "critical" because they are exposed to more radiation than are others during radiographic procedures. A **critical organ** is an organ that, if damaged, diminishes the quality of a person's life. Critical organs exposed during dental radiographic procedures in the head and neck region include the following:
- Skin
- Thyroid gland
- Lens of the eye
- Bone marrow

TABLE 4-2	Tissue and Organ Sensitivity to Radiation
Radiosensitive Cells	**Radioresistant Cells**
Small lymphocyte (high sensitivity)	Muscle tissue (low sensitivity)
Bone marrow (high sensitivity)	Nerve tissue (low sensitivity)
Reproductive cells (high sensitivity)	Mature bone and cartilage (fairly low sensitivity)
Intestinal mucosa (high sensitivity)	Salivary gland (fairly low sensitivity)
Skin (fairly high sensitivity)	Thyroid gland (fairly low sensitivity)
Lens of eye (fairly high sensitivity)	Kidney (fairly low sensitivity)
Oral mucosa (fairly high sensitivity)	Liver (fairly low sensitivity)

TABLE 4-3	Units of Radiation Measurement	
Unit	**Definition**	**Conversion**
Traditional System		
Roentgen (R)	1 R = 87 erg/g	1 R = 2.58×10^{-4} C/kg
Radiation absorbed dose (rad)	1 rad = 100 erg/g	1 rad = 0.01 Gy
Roentgen equivalent (in) man (rem)	1 rem = rads × QF	1 rem = 0.01 Sv
SI system		
Coulombs per kilogram (C/kg)	–	1 C/kg = 3880 R
Gray (Gy)	1 Gy = 0.01 J/kg	1 Gy = 100 rads
Sievert (Sv)	1 Sv = Gy × QF	1 Sv = 100 rems

QF, quality factor; *J*, joule; *SI*, International System of Units.

RADIATION MEASUREMENTS

Units of Measurement

Radiation can be measured in the same manner as other physical concepts such as time, distance, and weight. Just as the unit of measurement for time is minutes, for distance miles or kilometers, and for weight pounds or kilograms, the International Commission on Radiation Units and Measurement (ICRU) has established special units for the measurement of radiation. Such units are used to define three quantities of radiation: (1) exposure, (2) dose, and (3) dose equivalent.

The dental radiographer must know radiation measurements to discuss exposure and dose concepts with the dental patient.

At present, two systems are used to define radiation measurements: (1) The older system is referred to as the *traditional system*, or *standard system*; and (2) the newer system is the metric equivalent known as the *SI system*, or *Système International de'Unités (International System of Units)*.

The traditional units of radiation measurement include the following:

- Roentgen (R)
- Radiation absorbed dose (rad)
- Roentgen equivalent (in) man (rem)

The SI units of radiation measurement include the following:

- Coulombs/kilogram (C/kg)
- Gray (Gy)
- Sievert (Sv)

This text uses both the traditional and SI units of measurement; the dental radiographer should be familiar with both systems and know how to convert measurements from one system to the other (Table 4-3). In addition, the dental radiographer must be familiar with a number of physics terms used in the definitions of both traditional and SI units of radiation measurement (Table 4-4).

TABLE 4-4	Radiation Measurement Terms
Term	**Definition**
Coulomb (C)	Unit of electrical charge; the quantity of electrical charge transferred by 1 ampere in 1 second.
Ampere (A)	Unit of electrical current strength; current yielded by 1 volt against 1 ohm of resistance.
Erg (erg)	Unit of energy equivalent to 1.0×10^{-7} joules or to 2.4×10^{-8} calories.
Joule (J)	SI unit of energy equivalent to the work done by the force of 1 newton acting over the distance of 1 meter.
Newton (N)	SI unit of force; the force that, when acting continuously on a mass of 1 kilogram, will impart to it an acceleration of 1 meter per second squared (m/sec^2).
Kilogram (kg)	Unit of mass equivalent to 1000 grams or 2.205 pounds.

Exposure Measurement

The term **exposure** refers to the measurement of ionization in air produced by x-rays. The traditional unit of exposure for x-rays is the **roentgen (R)**. The roentgen is a way of measuring radiation exposure by determining the amount of ionization that occurs in air. A definition follows:

Roentgen: *The quantity of x-radiation or gamma radiation that produces an electrical charge of 2.58×10^{-4} coulombs in a kilogram of air at standard temperature and pressure (STP) conditions.*

In measuring the roentgen, a known volume of air is irradiated. The interaction of x-ray photons with air molecules results in ionization, or the formation of ions. The ions (electrical charges) that are produced are collected and measured. One roentgen is equal to the amount of radiation that produces approximately two billion, or 2.08×10^9, ion pairs in one cubic centimeter (cc) of air.

The roentgen has limitations as a unit of measure. It measures the amount of energy that reaches the surface of an organism but does not describe the amount of radiation absorbed. The roentgen is essentially limited to measurements in air. By definition, it is only used for x-rays and gamma rays and does not include other types of radiation.

No SI unit for exposure that is equivalent to the roentgen exists. Instead, exposure is simply stated in coulombs per kilograms (C/kg). The **coulomb (C)** is a unit of electrical charge. The unit C/kg measures the number of electrical charges, or the number of ion pairs, in 1 kg of air. The conversions for roentgen and coulombs per kilogram can be expressed as follows:

$$1\,R = 2.58 \times 10^{-4}\,C/kg$$

$$1\,C/kg = 3.88 \times 10^3\,R$$

Dose Measurement

Dose can be defined as the amount of energy absorbed by a tissue. The **radiation absorbed dose**, or **rad**, is the traditional unit of dose. Unlike the roentgen, the rad is not restricted to air and can be applied to all forms of radiation. A definition follows:

Rad: *A special unit of absorbed dose that is equal to the deposition of 100 ergs of energy per gram of tissue (100 erg/g).*

Using SI units, 1 rad is equivalent to 0.01 joule per kilogram (0.01 J/kg). The SI unit equivalent to the rad is the **gray (Gy)**, or 1 J/kg. The conversions for rad and Gy can be expressed as follows:

$$1\,rad = 0.01\,Gy$$

$$1\,Gy = 100\,rads$$

Dose Equivalent Measurement

Different types of radiation have different effects on tissues. The **dose equivalent** measurement is used to compare the biologic effects of different types of radiation. The traditional unit of the dose equivalent is the **roentgen equivalent (in) man**, or **rem**. A definition follows:

Rem: *The product of absorbed dose (rads) and a quality factor specific for the type of radiation.*

To place the exposure effects of different types of radiation on a common scale, a **quality factor (QF)**, or dimensionless multiplier, is used. Each type of radiation has a specific QF based on different types of radiation producing different types of biologic damage. For example, the QF for x-rays is equal to 1.

The SI unit equivalent of the rem is the **sievert (Sv)**. Conversions for the rem and sievert can be expressed as follows:

$$1\,rem = 0.01\,Sv$$

$$1\,Sv = 100\,rems$$

Measurements Used in Dental Radiography

In dental radiography, the gray and sievert are equal, and the roentgen, rad, and rem are considered approximately equal. Smaller multiples of these radiation units are typically used in dentistry because of the small quantities of radiation used during radiographic procedures. The prefix "milli," meaning 1/1000 (e.g., millirad, or mrad), allows the dental radiographer to express small quantities of exposure, dose, and dose equivalent.

RADIATION RISKS

Sources of Radiation Exposure

To understand radiation risks, the dental radiographer must be familiar with the potential sources of radiation exposure. This knowledge can then be used to better understand the radiation risks associated with dentistry.

Humans are exposed daily to **background radiation**, a form of ionizing radiation that is ubiquitous in the environment. Naturally occurring background radiation includes cosmic radiation and terrestrial radiation. Cosmic radiation originates from the stars and the sun. A person's exposure to cosmic radiation depends on altitude: the higher the altitude, the greater is the exposure to cosmic radiation. Terrestrial radiation also occurs naturally and is emitted from radioactive materials present in the earth and air. Examples of terrestrial radiation include potassium-40 and uranium.

In the United States, the average dose of background radiation received by an individual ranges from 150 to 300 mrads (0.0015–0.003 Gy) per year. This exposure may vary according to geographic location. For example, geographic areas that contain more radioactive materials are associated with increased amounts of terrestrial radiation, whereas areas at higher elevations (e.g., Denver) are associated with increased amounts of cosmic radiation.

In addition to naturally occurring background radiation, modern technology has created artificial, or man-made, sources of radiation. Consumer products (e.g., luminous wristwatches, televisions), fallout from atomic weapons, weapons production, and the nuclear fuel cycle are all sources of radiation exposure.

Medical radiation, another source of radiation exposure, is the greatest contributor to artificial radiation exposure. Medical radiation includes medical radiographic procedures, dental radiography, fluoroscopy, nuclear medicine, and radiation therapy. Medical radiation exposure equals the average

TABLE 4-5	Radiation Sources and Exposure	
Radiation Source	**Whole Body (mrems/year)**	**Whole Body (Sv/year)**
Natural		
Radon	200.00	0.002
Cosmic	27.00	0.00027
Terrestrial	28.00	0.00028
Internal	39.00	0.00039
Artificial		
Medical or dental	53.00	0.00053
Consumer products	9.00	0.00009
Other		
Occupational	<1.00	<0.00001
Nuclear fuel cycle	<1.00	<0.00001
Fallout	<1.00	<0.00001

mrems, millirems; *Sv*, sieverts.

yearly dose from all other exposures combined and typically accounts for half of the total exposure received.

Table 4-5 summarizes the sources of low-level radiation.

Risk and Risk Estimates

A **risk** can be defined as the likelihood of adverse effects or death resulting from exposure to a hazard. In dental radiography, risk is the likelihood of an adverse effect, specifically cancer induction, occurring from exposure to ionizing radiation.

The potential risk of dental radiography inducing a fatal cancer in an individual has been estimated to be approximately 3 in 1 million. The risk of a person developing cancer spontaneously is much higher, or 3300 in 1 million. To keep the concept of risk in perspective, the risk of incurring a fatal cancer from dental radiographic procedures should be compared with commonplace risks. For example, a 1-in-1-million risk of a fatal outcome is associated with each of the following activities: riding 10 miles on a bike, 300 miles in an auto, or 1000 miles in an airplane; or smoking 1.4 cigarettes per day. These risk estimates suggest that death is more likely to occur from common activities than from dental radiographic procedures and that cancer is much more likely to be unrelated to radiation exposure. In other words, the risks from dental radiography are not significantly greater than the risks of other everyday activities in modern life.

Dental Radiation and Exposure Risks

To calculate the risk from dental radiographic procedures, doses to critical organs must be measured. As previously defined, a critical organ, if damaged, diminishes the quality of an individual's life. With dental radiographic procedures, the critical organs at risk include the thyroid gland and active bone marrow. The skin and eyes may also be considered critical organs.

Risk Elements

Thyroid Gland. Although the thyroid gland is not irradiated by the primary beam in dental radiographic procedures, thyroid radiation exposure does occur. An estimated dose of 6000 mrads (0.06 Gy) is necessary to produce cancer in the thyroid gland; such a large dose is not incurred in dental radiography. Instead, the average dose to the thyroid gland (rectangular collimation, D-speed film, long position-indicating device [PID], 20-film series) is 6 mrads (0.00006 Gy), or 1/1000 of the dose necessary to induce thyroid cancer.

Bone Marrow. The areas of the maxilla and mandible exposed during dental radiography account for a very small percentage of active bone marrow. The risk of cancer induction (leukemia) is directly associated with the amount of blood-producing tissues irradiated and the dose. Leukemia is induced most likely at doses of 5000 mrads (0.05 Gy) or more; a dose of such magnitude does not occur in dental radiography. The average bone marrow dose from periapical radiography is approximately 1 to 3 mrads (0.00001–0.00003 Gy) per film. Consequently, about 2000 to 5000 films would have to be exposed to induce leukemia.

Skin. A total of 250 rads (2.5 Gy) in a 14-day period causes erythema, or reddening, of the skin. To produce such changes, more than 500 dental films (F-speed film, exposure rate 0.7 R/second) in a 14-day period would have to be exposed. This is not a likely scenario in dental radiography.

Eyes. More than 200,000 mrads (2 Gy) are necessary to induce cataract formation (cloudiness of lens) in the eyes. Again, such high doses are not a consideration in dental radiography. Instead, the average surface dose to the cornea of the eye (D-speed film, long PID, 20-film series) is approximately 60 mrads (0.0006 Gy). In dental radiography, the chance of cataracts occurring is so unlikely that some scientists no longer consider the eyes a critical organ.

Patient Exposure and Dose

Dental patients must be protected from excess exposure to radiation. (Chapter 5 discusses patient protection in detail.) How much radiation exposure results from dental radiography? The amount of exposure varies, depending on the following:

- *Film speed*: Radiation exposure can be limited by using the fastest film available. The use of F-speed film instead of D-speed reduces the absorbed dose by 60%. Using F-speed film instead of E-speed reduces the absorbed dose by an additional 20%.
- *Collimation*: Radiation exposure can be limited by using rectangular collimation. The use of rectangular collimation instead of round collimation reduces the absorbed dose by 60% to 70%.
- *Technique*: Radiation exposure can be limited by increasing the source-to-film distance. The use of the long-cone paralleling technique and increased source-to-film distance reduces the skin dose.

TABLE 4-6	Absorbed Doses From Intraoral Radiographs

Film	Absorbed Dose (mrads)
Bite-Wing Examination	
F-speed, 4 films, 16-inch PID, round	15.6
F-speed, 4 films, 16-inch PID, rectangular	2.5
Full-Mouth Survey	
F-speed, 20 films, 16-inch PID, round	41.1
F-speed, 20 films, 16-inch PID, rectangular	12.9

mrads, millirads; *PID*, position-indicating device.

Exposure factors: Radiation exposure can be limited by using a higher kilovoltage peak. The use of higher kilovoltage peak reduces the skin dose.

Surface exposure, or the measure of the intensity of radiation at the patient's skin surface in coulombs per kilogram or roentgens, is typically used when referring to patient exposure. A single intraoral radiograph (D-speed film, 70 kVp, long PID) results in a mean surface exposure of 250 milliroentgens (mR). With F-speed film, a single intraoral radiograph results in a mean surface exposure of 100 mR.

The concept of absorbed dose may also be used when referring to patient exposure and dose. The absorbed dose from a 20-film series of dental radiographs (round collimation, F-speed film, long PID) is estimated to be 41 mrads (0.00041 Gy). If rectangular collimation is used, the absorbed dose decreases to approximately 13 mrads (0.00013 Gy) (Table 4-6).

Risk Versus Benefit of Dental Radiographs

X-radiation is harmful to living tissues. Because biologic damage results from x-ray exposure, dental radiographs should be prescribed for a patient only when the benefit of disease detection outweighs the risk of biologic damage. When dental radiographs are properly prescribed and exposed, the benefit of disease detection far outweighs the risk of damage from x-radiation (see Chapter 5).

SUMMARY

- All ionizing radiation is harmful and produces biologic changes in living tissue.
- Radiation injury results from ionization or free radical formation.
- A dose–response curve is used to demonstrate the response (damage) of tissues to the dose (amount) of radiation received.
- A threshold dose for damage does not exist, and the response of tissues is directly proportional to the dose received.
- Radiation injury follows a sequence of events: latent period, period of injury, and period of recovery.

- Radiation injury is affected by total dose, dose rate, amount of tissue irradiated, cell sensitivity, and patient's age.
- Short-term radiation effects occur when large amounts of radiation are absorbed in a short period; long-term radiation effects occur when small amounts of radiation are absorbed over a long time.
- Radiation effects are classified as somatic (seen in the irradiated person) or genetic (passed on to future generations).
- Cellular response to radiation depends on mitotic activity, cell differentiation, and cell metabolism.
- Radiosensitive cells include blood cells, immature reproductive cells, young bone cells, and epithelial cells. Radioresistant cells include the cells of bones, muscle, and nerve.
- Exposure is the measurement of ionization in air produced by x-rays; the units for exposure are the roentgen (R) and coulombs per kilogram (C/kg).
- Dose is the amount of energy absorbed by a tissue; the units for dose are the radiation absorbed dose (rad) and the gray (Gy).
- Dose equivalent measurement is used to compare the biologic effects of different types of radiation; the units for dose equivalent are the roentgen equivalent (in) man (rem) and the sievert (Sv).
- The risks of radiation exposure involved in dental radiography are not significantly greater than other everyday risks in life.
- The amount of exposure a patient receives from dental radiographs depends on the film speed, collimation, technique, and exposure factors used.
- Dental radiographs should be prescribed only for a patient when the benefit of disease detection outweighs the risk of damage from x-radiation.

BIBLIOGRAPHY

Bernstein DI, Clark SJ, Scheetz JP, Farman AG, Rosenson B: Perceived quality of radiographic images after rapid processing of D- and F-speed direct-exposure intraoral x-ray films, *Oral Surg Oral Med Oral Pathol Oral Radiol Endod* 96(4):486–491, 2003.

Frommer HH, Savage-Stabulas JJ: Biologic effects of radiation. In *Radiology for the dental professional*, ed 9, St Louis, 2011, Mosby.

Johnson ON, Thomson EM: Effects of radiation exposure. In *Essentials of dental radiography for dental assistants and hygienists*, ed 8, Upper Saddle River, NJ, 2007, Pearson Prentice Hall.

Miles DA, Van Dis ML, Williamson GF, Jensen CW: Radiation biology and protection. In *Radiographic imaging for the dental team*, ed 4, St Louis, 2009, Saunders.

White SC, Pharoah MJ: Radiation safety and protection. In *Oral radiology: principles and interpretation*, ed 6, St Louis, 2009, Mosby.

White SC, Pharoah MJ: Radiobiology. In *Oral radiology: principles and interpretation*, ed 6, St Louis, 2009, Mosby.

QUIZ QUESTIONS

MULTIPLE CHOICE

____ 1. The latent period in radiation biology is the time between:
   a. exposure of film and development
   b. subsequent doses of radiation
   c. cell rest and cell mitosis
   d. exposure to x-radiation and clinical symptoms
   e. none of the above

____ 2. A free radical:
   a. is an uncharged molecule
   b. has an unpaired electron in the outer shell
   c. is highly reactive and unstable
   d. combines with molecules to form toxins
   e. all of the above

____ 3. Direct radiation injury occurs when:
   a. x-ray photons hit critical targets within a cell
   b. x-ray photons pass through the cell
   c. x-ray photons are absorbed and form toxins
   d. free radicals combine to form toxins
   e. none of the above

____ 4. Indirect radiation injury occurs when:
   a. x-ray photons hit critical targets within a cell
   b. x-ray photons pass through the cell
   c. x-ray photons are absorbed and form toxins
   d. x-ray photons hit the DNA of a cell
   e. none of the above.

____ 5. Which of the following relationships describes the response of tissues to radiation?
   a. linear
   b. linear, threshold
   c. linear, nonthreshold
   d. nonlinear, nonthreshold
   e. none of the above

____ 6. Which of the following factors contributes to radiation injury?
   a. total dose
   b. dose rate
   c. cell sensitivity
   d. age
   e. all of the above

____ 7. Which of the following statements is correct?
   a. Short-term effects are seen with small amounts of radiation absorbed in a short period.
   b. Short-term effects are seen with small amounts of radiation absorbed in a long period.
   c. Long-term effects are seen with small amounts of radiation absorbed in a short period.
   d. Long-term effects are seen with small amounts of radiation absorbed in a long period.
   e. None of the above.

____ 8. Radiation injuries that are not seen in the person irradiated but that occur in future generations are termed:
   a. somatic effects
   b. genetic effects
   c. cumulative effects
   d. short-term effects
   e. long-term effects

____ 9. Which of the following is most susceptible to ionizing radiation?
   a. bone tissue
   b. small lymphocyte
   c. muscle tissue
   d. nerve tissue
   e. epithelial tissue

____ 10. The sensitivity of tissues to radiation is determined by:
   a. mitotic activity
   b. cell differentiation
   c. cell metabolism
   d. all of the above
   e. none of the above

____ 11. Which of the following is considered radioresistant?
   a. immature reproductive cells
   b. young bone cells
   c. mature bone cells
   d. epithelial cells
   e. none of the above

____ 12. An organ that, if damaged, diminishes the quality of an individual's life is termed a:
   a. critical organ
   b. somatic organ
   c. cumulative organ
   d. radioresistant organ
   e. none of the above

____ 13. The traditional unit for measuring x-ray exposure in air is termed:
   a. the gray
   b. coulombs per kilogram
   c. the rem
   d. the rad
   e. the roentgen

____ 14. Which of the following radiation units is determined by the quality factor (QF)?
   a. the roentgen
   b. the rad
   c. the rem
   d. the gray
   e. coulombs per kilogram

___ 15. The unit for measuring the absorption of x-rays is termed:
   a. the roentgen
   b. the rad
   c. the rem
   d. quality factor
   e. the sievert

___ 16. Which of the following conversions is correct?
   a. $1 R = 2.58 \times 10^{-4}$ C/kg
   b. 1 rad = 0.1 Gy
   c. 1 rem = 0.1 Sv
   d. 1 Gy = 10 rads
   e. 1 Sv = 10 rems

___ 17. Which of the following traditional units does not have an SI equivalent?
   a. the roentgen
   b. the rad
   c. the rem
   d. quality factor
   e. none of the above

___ 18. Which of the following is used only for x-rays?
   a. the sievert
   b. the gray
   c. the rem
   d. the rad
   e. the roentgen

___ 19. Which of the following conversions is correct?
   a. $1 R = 2.58 \times 10^{-4}$ C/kg
   b. 1 Gy = 100 rads
   c. 1 Sv = 100 rems
   d. 1 rem = rads × QF
   e. all of the above

___ 20. What is the average dose of background radiation received by an individual in the United States?
   a. 0 to 100 mrads (0–0.001 Gy)
   b. 50 to 100 mrads (0.0005–0.001 Gy)
   c. 150 to 300 mrads (0.0015–0.003 Gy)
   d. 200 to 500 mrads (0.002–0.005 Gy)
   e. 500 to 1000 mrads (0.005–0.01 Gy)

___ 21. What is the greatest contributor to artificial radiation exposure?
   a. radioactive materials
   b. medical radiation
   c. consumer products
   d. weapons production
   e. nuclear fuel cycle

___ 22. The amount of radiation exposure an individual receives varies depending on:
   a. film speed
   b. collimation
   c. technique
   d. exposure factors
   e. all of the above

___ 23. A single intraoral radiograph (D-speed film, 70 kVp, long PID) results in a mean surface exposure of:
   a. 50 mR
   b. 250 mR
   c. 500 mR
   d. 1 R
   e. 5 R

___ 24. What is the dose at which leukemia induction is most likely to occur?
   a. 500 mrads (0.005 Gy)
   b. 1000 mrads (0.01 Gy)
   c. 2000 mrads (0.02 Gy)
   d. 5000 mrads (0.05 Gy)
   e. none of the above

___ 25. Which of the following statements is incorrect?
   a. X-radiation is not harmful to living tissues.
   b. Dental radiographs benefit the patient.
   c. In dental radiography, the benefit of disease detection outweighs the risk of damage from radiation.
   d. Radiography should be prescribed only when the benefit outweighs the risk.
   e. Biologic damage results from x-ray exposure.

chapter 5

Radiation Protection

OUTLINE

PATIENT PROTECTION
    Before Exposure
    During Exposure
    After Exposure
OPERATOR PROTECTION
    Protection Guidelines
    Radiation Monitoring

RADIATION EXPOSURE GUIDELINES
    Radiation Safety Legislation
    Maximum Permissible Dose
    Maximum Accumulated Dose
    ALARA Concept
RADIATION PROTECTION AND PATIENT EDUCATION

LEARNING OBJECTIVES

After completion of this chapter, the student will be able to do the following:

- Define the key words associated with radiation protection
- Describe in detail the basics of patient protection before x-ray exposure
- Discuss the different types of filtration, and state the recommended total filtration for dental x-ray machines operating above and below 70 kVp
- Describe the collimator used in dental x-ray machines, and state the recommended diameter of the useful beam at the patient's skin
- List six ways to protect the patient from excessive radiation during x-ray exposure
- Describe the importance of receptor handling and processing after patient exposure to x-radiation

- Discuss operator protection in terms of adequate distance, shielding, and avoidance of the useful beam
- Describe personnel and equipment monitoring devices used to detect radiation
- Discuss radiation exposure guidelines, including radiation safety legislation, maximum permissible dose (MPD), maximum accumulated dose (MAD), and the ALARA concept
- Discuss with the dental patient what radiation protection steps will be used before, during, and after exposure to x-radiation

KEY TERMS

ALARA concept	Film, fast	Maximum permissible dose (MPD)
Beam alignment device	Filtration	Position-indicating device (PID)
Collimation	Filtration, added	Protective barrier
Collimator	Filtration, inherent	Radiation monitoring badge
Film, D-speed	Filtration, total	Radiation, leakage
Film, E-speed	Lead apron	Thyroid collar
Film, F-speed	Maximum accumulated dose (MAD)	

Many of the early pioneers in dental radiography suffered from the adverse effects of radiation. As discussed in Chapter 1, some of these pioneers lost their fingers, limbs, and, ultimately, lives to excessive doses of radiation. The hazards of radiation are now well documented, and radiation protection measures can be used to minimize radiation exposure to both the dental patient and the dental radiographer. The purpose of this chapter is to discuss patient protection before, during, and after exposure to x-rays; to detail operator protection methods; and to present radiation exposure and safety guidelines. In addition, this chapter includes a discussion of patient education about radiation protection.

PATIENT PROTECTION

X-radiation causes biologic changes in living cells and adversely affects all living tissues. With the use of proper patient protection techniques, the amount of x-radiation received by a dental patient can be minimized. Patient protection techniques can be used before, during, and after exposure to x-radiation.

Before Exposure

Patient protection measures can be used before any x-radiation exposure. Proper prescribing of dental radiographs and the use of equipment that complies with state and federal radiation guidelines can minimize the amount of x-radiation that a dental patient receives.

Prescribing Dental Radiographs

The first important step in limiting the amount of x-radiation received by a dental patient is the proper prescribing, or ordering, of dental radiographs. The person responsible for prescribing dental radiographs is the dentist. The dentist uses professional judgment to make decisions about the number, type, and frequency of dental radiographs.

Every patient's dental condition is different, and consequently, every patient should be evaluated for dental radiographs on an individual basis. A radiographic examination should never include a predetermined number of radiographs, nor should radiographs be taken at predetermined time intervals. For example, the dentist who prescribes a set number of radiographs (e.g., four bite-wings) at a set interval (e.g., every 6 months) for every patient is not taking the individual needs of the patient into consideration.

The American Dental Association (ADA), in conjunction with the U.S. Food and Drug Administration (FDA), has adopted guidelines for prescribing the number, type, and frequency of dental radiographic procedures. These guidelines summarize the recommendations that promote patient protection in diagnostic radiography (Table 5-1). For the latest information and changes on prescribing dental radiographs, visit www.ADA.org and www.FDA.gov.

Proper Equipment

Another important step in limiting the amount of x-radiation a dental patient receives is the use of proper equipment. The dental x-ray tubehead must be equipped with appropriate aluminum filters, lead collimator, and position-indicating device.

Filtration. Two types of **filtration** are used in the dental x-ray tubehead: inherent filtration and added filtration.

Inherent Filtration. **Inherent filtration** takes place when the primary beam passes through the glass window of the x-ray tube, the insulating oil, and the tubehead seal. The inherent filtration of the dental x-ray machine is approximately 0.5 to 1.0 millimeter (mm) of aluminum. Inherent filtration alone does not meet the standards

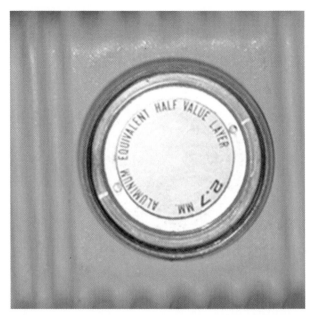

FIGURE 5-1 Aluminum discs are placed between the collimator and tubehead seal for added filtration. (From Bird DL, Robinson DS: *Modern dental assisting*, ed 10, St Louis, 2012, Saunders.)

regulated by state and federal laws. Therefore, added filtration is required.

Added Filtration. **Added filtration** refers to the placement of aluminum discs in the path of the x-ray beam between the collimator and the tubehead seal in the dental x-ray machine (Figure 5-1). Aluminum discs can be added to the tubehead in 0.5-mm increments. The purpose of the aluminum discs is to filter out the longer-wavelength, low-energy x-rays from the x-ray beam (Figure 5-2). The low-energy, longer wavelength x-rays are harmful to the patient and are not useful in diagnostic radiography. Filtration of the x-ray beam results in a higher energy and more penetrating useful beam.

Total Filtration. State and federal laws regulate the required thickness of **total filtration** (inherent plus added filtration). Dental x-ray machines operating at or below 70 kilovoltage peak (kVp) require a minimum total of 1.5 mm aluminum filtration, and machines operating above 70 kVp require a minimum total of 2.5 mm aluminum filtration.

Collimation. **Collimation** is used to restrict the size and shape of the x-ray beam and to reduce patient exposure. A **collimator**, or lead plate with a hole in the middle, is fitted directly over the opening of the machine housing where the x-ray beam exits the tubehead (Figure 5-3).

A collimator may have either a round or rectangular opening (Figure 5-4). A *rectangular* collimator restricts the size of the x-ray beam to an area slightly larger than a size 2 intraoral film and significantly reduces patient exposure. A *circular* collimator produces a cone-shaped beam that is 2.75 inches in diameter, considerably larger than a size 2 intraoral film (Figure 5-5A). Rectangular collimators may also be

TABLE 5-1 Guidelines for Prescribing Dental Radiographs*

Type of Encounter	Child With Primary Dentition (before eruption of first permanent tooth)	Child With Transitional Dentition (after eruption of first permanent tooth)	Adolescent With Permanent Dentition (before eruption of third molars)	Adult, Dentate or Partially Edentulous	Adult, Edentulous
New patient† being evaluated for dental development	Individualized radiographic exam consisting of selected periapical/occlusal views and/or posterior bite-wing images if proximal surfaces cannot be visualized or probed. Patients without evidence of disease and with open proximal contacts may not require radiographic exam at this time.	Individualized radiographic exam consisting of posterior bite-wing images with panoramic bite-wing images and selected periapical images	Individualized radiographic exam consisting of posterior bite-wing images with panoramic exam or posterior bite-wing images. Full-mouth intraoral radiographic exam is preferred when patient has clinical evidence of generalized dental disease or history of extensive dental treatment.	Individualized radiographic exam consisting of posterior bite-wing images with panoramic exam or posterior bite-wing images and selected periapical images	Individualized radiographic exam, based on clinical signs and symptoms
Recall patient† with clinical caries or at increased risk for caries‡	Posterior bite-wing exam at 6- to 12-month intervals if proximal surfaces cannot be examined visually or with probe			Posterior bite-wing exam at 6- to 18-month intervals	Not applicable
Recall patient† with no clinical caries and not at increased risk for caries‡	Posterior bite-wing exam at 12- to 24-month intervals if proximal surfaces cannot be examined visually or with probe		Posterior bite-wing exam at 18- to 36-month intervals	Posterior bite-wing exam at 24- to 36-month intervals	Not applicable
Recall patient† with periodontal disease	Clinical judgment as to need for and type of radiographic images for evaluation of periodontal disease. Imaging may consist of, but is not limited to, select bite-wing and/or periapical images of areas where periodontal disease (other than nonspecific gingivitis) can be identified.				Not applicable
Patients for monitoring of growth and development	Clinical judgment as to need for and type of radiographic images for evaluation and/or monitoring of dentofacial growth and development		As for child; Panoramic or periapical exam to assess developing third molars	Usually not indicated	
Patient with other circumstances§	Clinical judgment as to need for and type of radiographic images for evaluation and/or monitoring in these circumstances				

*The recommendations in this chart are subject to clinical judgment and may not apply to every patient. They are to be used by dentists only after reviewing the patient's health history and completing a clinical examination. Because every precaution should be taken to minimize radiation exposure, protective thyroid collars and aprons should be used whenever possible. This practice is strongly recommended for children, women of childbearing age, and pregnant women.

†Clinical situations for which radiography may be indicated include, but are not limited to, the following:
A. **Positive historical findings:** (1) previous periodontal or endodontic treatment, (2) history of pain or trauma, (3) familial history of dental anomalies, (4) postoperative evaluation of healing, (5) remineralization monitoring, or (6) presence of implants or evaluation for implant placement
B. **Positive clinical signs/symptoms:** (1) clinical evidence of periodontal disease, (2) large or deep restorations, (3) deep carious lesions, (4) malposed or clinically impacted teeth, (5) swelling, (6) evidence of dental/facial trauma, (7) mobility of teeth, (8) sinus tract ("fistula"), (9) clinically suspected sinus pathology, (10) growth abnormalities, (11) oral involvement in known or suspected systemic disease, (12) positive neurologic findings in head and neck, (13) evidence of foreign objects, (14) pain and/or dysfunction of temporomandibular joint, (15) facial asymmetry, (16) abutment teeth for fixed or removable partial prosthesis, (17) unexplained bleeding, (18) unexplained sensitivity of teeth, (20) unusual tooth morphology, calcification, or color, (21) unexplained absence of teeth, or (22) clinical erosion.

‡Factors increasing risk for caries may include, but are not limited to, the following: (1) high level of caries experience or demineralization, (2) history of recurrent caries, (3) high titers of cariogenic bacteria, (4) existing restoration(s) of poor quality, (5) poor oral hygiene, (6) inadequate fluoride exposure, (7) prolonged nursing (bottle or breast), (8) frequent high-sucrose content in diet, (9) poor dental health in family, (10) developmental or acquired enamel defects, (11) development of acquired disability, (12) xerostomia, (13) genetic abnormality of teeth, (14) many multisurface restorations, (15) chemotherapy and/or radiation therapy, (16) eating disorders, (17) drug/alcohol abuse, or (18) irregular dental care.

§Including, but not limited to, the following: (1) proposed or existing implants, (2) pathology, (3) restorative/endodontic needs, (4) treated periodontal disease, or (5) caries remineralization.
Modified from American Dental Association, US Food and Drug Administration: The selection of patients for dental radiographic examinations: www.ada.org; Accessed May 26, 2005.

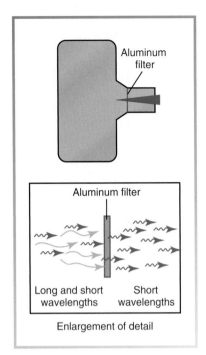

FIGURE 5-2 Aluminum discs are placed in the path of the beam to filter out the low-energy, longer-wavelength x-rays that are harmful to the patient.

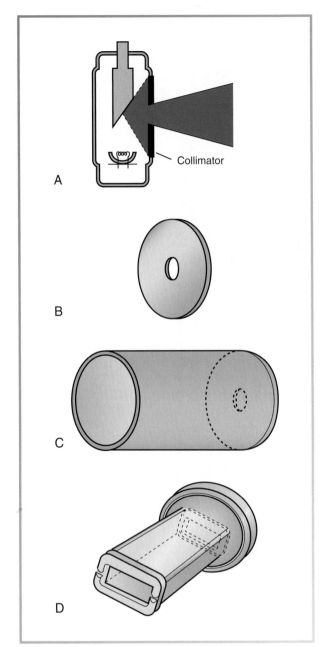

FIGURE 5-3 A, Collimation of an x-ray beam (*shown in color*) is achieved by restricting its useful size. **B,** Diaphragm collimator. **C,** Tubular collimator. **D,** Rectangular collimator. (From White SC, Pharoah MJ: *Oral radiology: principles and interpretation,* ed 5, St Louis, 2009, Mosby.)

added to the open end of a circular position-indicating device (PID) to reduce the amount of tissue being radiated (Figure 5-5B). When using a circular collimator, federal regulations require that the x-ray beam be collimated to a diameter of no more than 2.75 inches as it exits from the position-indicating device and reaches the skin of the patient (Figure 5-6).

Position-Indicating Device. The **position-indicating device (PID),** or *cone,* appears as an extension of the x-ray tubehead and is used to direct the x-ray beam. Three basic types of PIDs are currently used: (1) conical, (2) rectangular, and (3) round.

The *conical* PID appears as a closed, pointed plastic cone. When x-rays exit from the pointed cone, they penetrate the plastic and produce scatter radiation (Figure 5-7). To eliminate cone-produced scatter radiation, the conical PID is no longer used in dentistry. Open-ended, lead-lined rectangular or round PIDs limit the occurrence of scatter radiation (Figure 5-8).

Both *rectangular* and *round* PIDs are typically available in two lengths: short (8-inch) long (16-inch). The long PID is preferred because less divergence of the x-ray beam occurs (Figure 5-9).

Of the three types of PID, the rectangular type is most effective in reducing patient exposure.

During Exposure

Patient protection measures are used during x-ray exposure as well as before exposure. A thyroid collar, lead apron, fast film or digital imaging, and beam alignment devices are all used during x-ray exposure to limit the amount of radiation received by the patient. Proper selection of exposure factors and good technique further protect the patient from excessive exposure to x-radiation.

Thyroid Collar

The **thyroid collar** is a flexible lead shield that is placed securely around the patient's neck to protect the thyroid gland from scatter radiation (Figure 5-10). The lead prevents radiation from reaching the gland and protects the highly

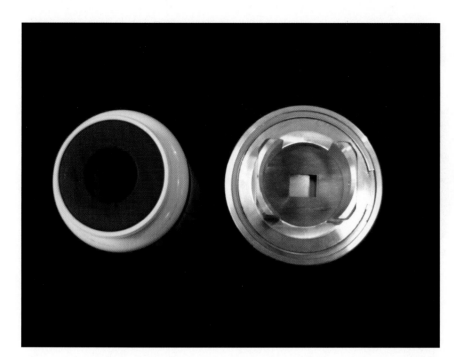

FIGURE 5-4 The hole in the collimator may be either round or rectangular in shape.

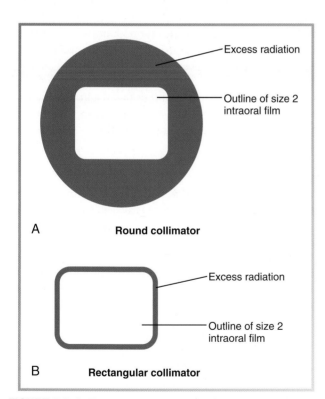

A   **Round collimator**

B   **Rectangular collimator**

FIGURE 5-5 A, The x-ray beam produced by a circular collimator is 2.75 inches in diameter, which is much larger than size 2 intraoral film. **B,** The x-ray beam produced by a rectangular collimator is only slightly larger than size 2 intraoral film.

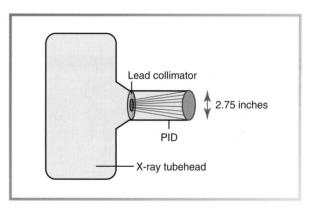

FIGURE 5-6 Federal regulations require that the diameter of a collimated x-ray beam be restricted to 2.75 inches at the patient's skin. *PID,* position-indicating device.

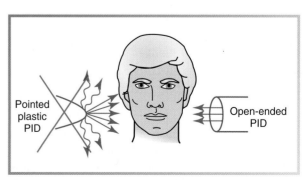

FIGURE 5-7 A plastic, pointed position-indicating device (PID) produces scatter radiation and is no longer used in dentistry.

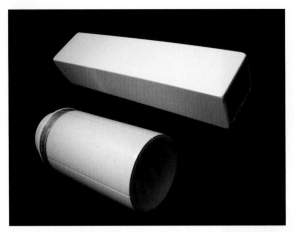

FIGURE 5-8 Open-ended, lead-lined round and rectangular position-indicating devices (PIDs).

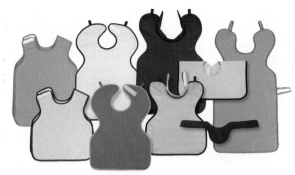

FIGURE 5-11 Examples of lead aprons. The thyroid collar may be attached to the lead apron or may be used as a separate shield. (Courtesy RINN Corporation, Elgin, IL.)

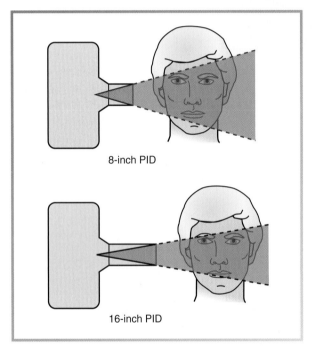

8-inch PID

16-inch PID

FIGURE 5-9 Compared with a short (8-inch) position-indicating device (PID), the longer (16-inch) PID is preferred because it produces less divergence of the x-ray beam.

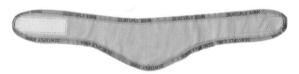

FIGURE 5-10 Thyroid collar. (From Bird DL, Robinson DS: *Modern dental assisting*, ed 10, St Louis, 2012, Saunders.)

radiosensitive tissues of the thyroid. The thyroid collar may exist as a separate shield or as part of the lead apron.

The thyroid gland is exposed to x-radiation during oral radiographic procedures because of its location. The use of the thyroid collar is recommended for all intraoral exposures.

However, use of the thyroid collar is not recommended with extraoral exposures because it obscures information and results in a nondiagnostic image.

Lead Apron

The **lead apron** is a flexible shield placed over the patient's chest and lap to protect the reproductive and blood-forming tissues from scatter radiation; the lead prevents the radiation from reaching these radiosensitive organs (Figure 5-11). Use of a lead apron is recommended for both intraoral and extraoral exposures. Many state laws mandate the use of a lead apron on all patients. Recently, lead-free aprons made of alloy sheeting have become available for use during intraoral or panoramic radiography. Without the weight of lead, these aprons weigh 30% less and are comfortable and easy to handle while providing the same protection as does the traditional lead apron.

Fast Film

Fast film is the most effective method of reducing a patient's exposure to x-radiation. Fast film is available for both intraoral and extraoral radiography. Currently, **F-speed film**, or *InSight*, is the fastest intraoral film available. Before the introduction of F-speed film, **E-speed film**, or *Ektaspeed*, was the fastest film available. F-speed film provides an additional 20% reduction in exposure over E-speed films (and 60% reduction in exposure from earlier **D-speed film**, or *Ultra-Speed*).

When compared with traditional film radiography, digital imaging requires less radiation exposure of the patient. The lowered absorbed dose is significant with regard to patient protection from excessive radiation. Digital imaging is discussed in detail in Chapter 25.

Beam Alignment Devices

Beam alignment devices are also effective in reducing a patient's exposure to x-radiation. A beam alignment device helps stabilize the receptor in the mouth and reduces the chances of movement (Figure 5-12).

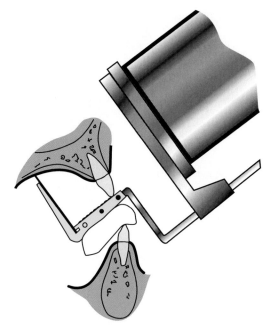

FIGURE 5-12 Beam alignment devices reduce the patient's exposure to radiation by stabilizing the receptor in the mouth. (Courtesy RINN Corporation, Elgin, IL.)

Exposure Factor Selection

Exposure factor selection also limits the amount of x-radiation exposure a patient receives. The dental radiographer can control the exposure factors by adjusting the kilovoltage peak, milliamperage, and time settings on the control panel of the dental x-ray machine. A setting of 70 to 90 kVp keeps patient exposure to a minimum. On some dental x-ray units, the kilovoltage peak and milliamperage settings are preset by the manufacturer and cannot be adjusted. (Chapter 3 discusses exposure factors and their effect on radiographs.)

Proper Technique

Proper technique helps ensure the diagnostic quality of images and reduce the amount of exposure a patient receives. Images that are nondiagnostic must be retaken; this results in additional exposure of the patient to radiation. *Retakes must be avoided at all times.*

To produce diagnostic images, the radiographer must have a thorough knowledge of the techniques most often used in dental radiography. Common approaches are the paralleling technique, bisecting technique, and bite-wing technique (see Chapters 17, 18 and 19, respectively). In addition to knowing how each receptor is exposed, an organized routine is important for the effective application of a technique.

After Exposure

The radiographer's role in limiting the amount of x-radiation received by a patient does not end during exposure. After the receptors have been exposed, they must be handled and processed. Meticulous handling and proper processing techniques are critical for the production of high-quality diagnostic images.

Proper Film/Sensor Handling

Proper film and/or sensor handling is necessary to produce diagnostic images and to limit patient exposure to x-radiation. From the time the receptors are exposed until they are processed or retrieved, careful handling is crucial. Artifacts caused by improper handling result in nondiagnostic images (see Chapter 9). A nondiagnostic image must be retaken, which exposes the patient to excessive radiation.

Proper Film Processing/Image Retrieval

Proper film processing (developing) and proper retrieval of digital images are also necessary to produce diagnostic images and to limit patient exposure to x-radiation. Improper film processing or image retrieval can render images nondiagnostic, thereby requiring retakes and needlessly exposing the patient to excessive x-radiation.

OPERATOR PROTECTION

The dental radiographer must use proper protection measures to avoid occupational exposure to x-radiation (e.g., primary radiation, leakage radiation, scatter radiation). The use of proper operator protection techniques can minimize the amount of radiation that a dental radiographer receives. Operator protection measures include following protection guidelines and using radiation-monitoring devices.

Protection Guidelines

The purpose of operator protection guidelines is to provide the dental radiographer with the basic safety information needed when working with x-radiation. Such guidelines are based on the following rule: *The dental radiographer must avoid the primary beam.* Operator protection guidelines include recommendations on distance, position, and shielding.

Distance Recommendations

One of the most effective ways for the operator to avoid the primary beam and limit x-radiation exposure is to maintain an adequate distance during exposure. The dental radiographer must stand at least 6 feet away from the x-ray tubehead during x-ray exposure. When maintaining this distance is not possible, a protective barrier must be used.

Position Recommendations

Another important way for the operator to avoid the primary beam is to maintain proper positioning during x-ray exposure. To avoid the primary beam, which travels in a straight line, the dental radiographer must position himself or herself perpendicular to the primary beam, or at a 90-degree to 135-degree angle to the beam (Figure 5-13).

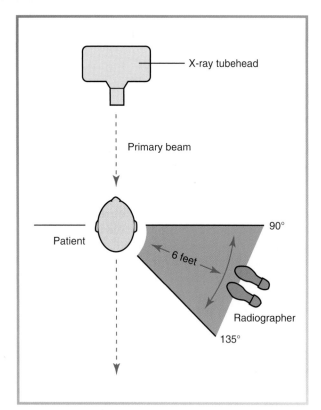

FIGURE 5-13 Operator protection guidelines suggest that the dental radiographer stand at an angle of 90 to 135 degrees to the primary beam.

Proper operator position also includes the following:
1. The dental radiographer must never hold a film in place for a patient during x-ray exposure.
2. The dental radiographer must never hold the tubehead during x-ray exposure.

Shielding Recommendations

Adequate shielding can greatly reduce the occupational exposure of the dental radiographer. **Protective barriers** that absorb the primary beam can be incorporated into the office design, thus protecting the operator from primary and scatter radiation. Whenever possible, the dental radiographer should stand behind a protective barrier, such as a wall, during x-ray exposure. Most dental offices incorporate adequate shielding in walls through the use of several thicknesses of common construction materials such as drywall.

Radiation Monitoring

Radiation monitoring can also be used to protect the dental radiographer and includes the monitoring of both equipment and personnel. The use of radiation monitoring can identify excessive occupational exposure.

Equipment Monitoring

Dental x-ray machines must be monitored for leakage radiation. **Leakage radiation** is any radiation, with the exception of the primary beam, that is emitted from the

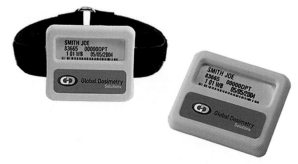

FIGURE 5-14 A radiation monitoring badge is used to measure the radiation exposure received by the dental radiographer. (From Bird DL, Robinson DS: *Modern dental assisting*, ed 10, St Louis, 2012, Saunders.)

dental tubehead. For example, if a dental x-ray tubehead has a faulty tubehead seal, leakage radiation results. Dental x-ray equipment can be monitored for leakage radiation through the use of a film device that can be obtained through the state health department or from the manufacturers of dental x-ray equipment.

Personnel Monitoring

The amount of x-radiation that reaches the body of the dental radiographer can be measured through the use of a personnel-monitoring device known as a **radiation monitoring badge**. A radiation monitoring badge can be obtained from a badge service company.

The radiation monitoring badge consists of a piece of radiographic film in a plastic holder (Figure 5-14). Each radiographer should have his or her own badge; the badge should be worn at waist level whenever the dental radiographer is exposing x-ray films or digital sensors. When badges are not worn, they should be stored in a radiation-safe area. A radiation monitoring badge should *never* be worn when the radiographer is undergoing x-ray exposure.

After the dental radiographer has worn the badge for a specified interval (e.g., 1 week, 1 month), the badge is returned to the service company. The company processes and evaluates the badge for exposure and then provides the dental office with an exposure report for each radiographer.

RADIATION EXPOSURE GUIDELINES

All x-radiation is harmful. Radiation exposure guidelines have therefore been established to protect the patient and operator from excessive exposure. These guidelines include radiation safety legislation and exposure limits for the general public and for persons who are occupationally exposed to radiation. Strict adherence to radiation exposure guidelines is mandatory for all dental radiographers.

Radiation Safety Legislation

Radiation safety legislation has been established at both state and federal levels to protect the patient, the operator, and the general public from radiation hazards. At the federal level, the Radiation Control for Health and Safety Act was enacted in 1968 to standardize the operation of x-ray equipment. Also, the federal Consumer-Patient Radiation Health and Safety Act was enacted in 1981 to address the issues of the education and certification of persons operating radiographic equipment.

Radiation legislation in the United States varies greatly from state to state; the dental radiographer must be familiar with the laws that apply to his or her workplace. For example, in some states, before a dental radiographer can expose patients to radiation, he or she must successfully complete a radiation safety examination.

Maximum Permissible Dose

Radiation protection standards dictate the maximum dose of radiation that an individual can receive. The **maximum permissible dose (MPD)** is defined by the National Council on Radiation Protection and Measurements (NCRP) as the maximum dose equivalent that a body is permitted to receive within a specific period. The MPD is the dose of radiation that the body can endure with little or no injury.

The NCRP published the complete set of basic recommendations specifying dose limits for exposure to ionizing radiation. This most recent report in 2003 states that the current MPD for occupationally exposed persons, or those who work with radiation (e.g., dental radiographers), is 5.0 rems/year (0.05 Sv/year). For nonoccupationally exposed persons, the current MPD is 0.1 rem/year (0.001 Sv/year). The MPD for an occupationally exposed pregnant woman is the same as that for a nonoccupationally exposed person, or 0.1 rem/year (0.001 Sv/year).

Maximum Accumulated Dose

Occupationally exposed workers must not exceed an accumulated lifetime radiation dose. This is referred to as the **maximum accumulated dose (MAD)**. MAD is determined by a formula based on the worker's age. To determine the MAD for an occupationally exposed person, the following formula is used:

$$MAD = (N - 18) \times 5 \text{ rems/year}$$

$$MAD = (N - 18) \times 0.05 \text{ Sv/year}$$

where N refers to the person's age in years. (Note that the number 18 refers to the minimum required age of a person who works with radiation.)

ALARA Concept

The **ALARA** (As Low As Reasonably Achievable) **concept** states that all exposure to radiation must be kept to a minimum. To provide protection to both patients and operators, every possible method of reducing exposure to radiation should be employed to minimize risk. The radiation protection measures detailed in this chapter can be used to minimize patient and operator exposure, thus keeping radiation exposure "as low as reasonably achievable."

RADIATION PROTECTION AND PATIENT EDUCATION

Patients often have questions about radiation exposure. The dental radiographer must be prepared to answer such questions and to educate the dental patient about radiation protection topics. Patient education about radiation protection may take the form of an informal conversation or printed literature.

The dental radiographer must be prepared to explain exactly how patients are protected before, during, and after x-ray exposure. An informal discussion can take place as the dental radiographer prepares the patient for x-ray exposure. For example, while placing the lead apron and thyroid collar on the patient, the dental radiographer can make the following comments:

- "Before we get started, let me tell you just how our office does all that is possible to protect you from unnecessary radiation."
- "Before we expose you to any x-rays, the dentist custom-orders your x-rays based on your individual needs. The x-ray equipment we use is frequently tested to ensure that state and federal radiation safety guidelines are met."
- "During x-ray exposure, we use a thyroid collar and a lead apron to protect your body from excessive radiation. We use the fastest film available and a device to hold the film so that your fingers are not exposed to radiation. We also use an effective technique so that we can avoid making mistakes that require further exposure."
- If using digital radiography: "Our office utilizes digital imaging procedures which reduce your exposure to radiation significantly when compared with traditional, film-based radiography."
- "Even after your dental x-ray films have been taken, we take steps to process the films carefully so that we don't have to take them again."
- "Hopefully, this quick review of radiation protection techniques has answered some of the questions you may have about dental x-rays. Do you have any other questions before we begin?"

In addition to such an informal discussion, printed handouts or pamphlets outlining the steps used to protect patients from excessive radiation can be provided to the patient. Pamphlets on radiation protection can be placed in the reception area or in the room where dental radiographs are taken.

SUMMARY

- Before x-ray exposure, proper prescribing of dental radiographs and proper use of radiographic equipment can minimize the amount of radiation that a patient receives.
- The dentist must prescribe radiographs on the basis of the individual needs of patients.

- In the x-ray tubehead, aluminum discs are used to filter out the longer-wavelength, low-energy x-rays from the x-ray beam.
- In the x-ray tubehead, a collimator (lead plate with a hole in the middle) is used to restrict the size and shape of the x-ray beam.
- A position-indicating device (PID) is used to direct the x-ray beam; the rectangular PID is most effective in reducing patient exposure to x-rays.
- A thyroid collar, a lead apron, fast film, digital imaging, and film-holding devices can be used during x-ray exposure to protect the patient from excessive exposure to radiation. Proper selection of exposure factors and good technique can also be used to protect the patient.
- After x-ray exposure, careful film/sensor handling, film-processing techniques, and image retrieval are critical for the production of diagnostic images.
- During x-ray exposure, the dental radiographer must always follow operator protection guidelines; he or she must avoid the primary beam (by maintaining an adequate distance) and use proper positioning and shielding.
- The dental radiographer must never hold a receptor or the tubehead in place for a patient during x-ray exposure.
- Radiation monitoring must include the monitoring of both equipment and personnel.
- Federal and state laws protect the patient, the operator, and the general public from radiation hazards.
- Exposure limits have been established for the general public and persons who work with radiation. The maximum permissible dose (MPD) for persons who work with radiation (e.g., dental radiographers) is 5.0 rems/year (0.05 Sv/year), and the MPD for persons who do not work with radiation is 0.1 rem/year (0.001 Sv/year).
- The ALARA (As Low As Reasonably Achievable) concept states that all exposure to radiation must be kept to a minimum.
- The dental radiographer must be prepared to explain to patients how they are protected before, during, and after x-ray exposure.

BIBLIOGRAPHY

Bernstein DI et al: Perceived quality of radiographic images after rapid processing of D- and F-speed direct-exposure intraoral x-ray films, *Oral Surg Oral Med Oral Pathol Oral Radiol Endod* 96(4):486–491, 2003.

Frommer HH, Savage-Stabulas JJ: Operator protection. In *Radiology for the dental professional*, ed 9, St Louis, 2011, Mosby.

Frommer HH, Savage-Stabulas JJ: Patient protection. In *Radiology for the dental professional*, ed 9, St Louis, 2011, Mosby.

Haring JI, Lind LJ: The importance of dental radiographs and interpretation. In *Radiographic interpretation for the dental hygienist*, Philadelphia, 1993, Saunders.

Johnson ON, Thomson EM: Patient relations and education. In *Essentials of dental radiography for dental assistants and hygienists*, ed 8, Pearson, 2007, Upper Saddle River, NJ.

Johnson ON, Thomson EM: Radiation protection. In *Essentials of dental radiography for dental assistants and hygienists*, ed 8, Pearson, 2007, Upper Saddle River, NJ.

Langland OE, Langlais RP, Preece JW: Radiologic health and protection. In *Principles of dental imaging*, ed 2, Baltimore, 2002, Lippincott Williams and Wilkins.

Miles DA, Van Dis ML, Jensen CW, Ferretti A: Intraoral radiographic technique. In *Radiographic imaging for the dental team*, ed 4, St Louis, 2009, Saunders.

Miles DA, Van Dis ML, Jensen CW, Ferretti A: Radiation biology and protection. In *Radiographic imaging for the dental team*, ed 4, St Louis, 2009, Saunders.

National Council on Radiation Protection and Measurements (NCRP): Limitation of exposure to ionizing radiation, NCRP Report No 116, 1993, NCRP.

White SC, Pharoah MJ: Health physics. In *Oral radiology: principles of interpretation*, ed 6, St Louis, 2009, Mosby.

USEFUL WEBSITES

American Dental Association (ADA)
www.ada.org/prof/resources/topics/radiography.asp
U.S. Food and Drug Administration (FDA):
www.fda.gov/Radiation-EmittingProducts/
RadiationEmittingProductsandProcedures

QUIZ QUESTIONS

TRUE OR FALSE

____ 1. Every patient should be evaluated individually for dental radiographs.

____ 2. The 8-inch PID is more effective than the 16-inch PID in reducing radiation exposure of the patient.

____ 3. Pointed cones should not be used because of increased scatter radiation.

____ 4. The thyroid collar must be worn for both intraoral and extraoral exposures.

____ 5. If necessary, the dental radiographer may hold a receptor in the patient's mouth to ensure a diagnostic image.

MULTIPLE CHOICE

____ 6. Which of the following describes the use of a filter in a dental x-ray tubehead?
  a. A filter reduces the size and shape of the beam.
  b. A filter removes low-energy x-rays.
  c. A filter removes the dose of radiation to the thyroid gland.
  d. A filter decreases the mean energy of the beam.

___ 7. Which of the following is not a component of inherent filtration?
   a. oil
   b. unleaded glass window
   c. a leaded cone
   d. tubehead seal

___ 8. Which of the following is the most effective method of reducing patient exposure to radiation?
   a. lead apron
   b. fast films
   c. round PID
   d. film-holding devices

___ 9. Which of the following position-indicating devices is most effective in reducing patient exposure?
   a. conical PID
   b. rectangular PID
   c. round PID
   d. all are equally effective in reducing patient exposure

___ 10. Which of the following devices restricts the size and shape of the x-ray beam?
   a. filter
   b. collimator
   c. barrier
   d. film badge

___ 11. Which of the following is used as a collimator?
   a. lead plate
   b. aluminum plate
   c. copper plate
   d. all of the above

___ 12. Which of the following describes the function of filtration?
   a. increases scatter radiation
   b. increases divergent rays
   c. increases long wavelengths
   d. reduces low-energy waves

___ 13. Which of the following is the recommended size of the beam at the patient's face?
   a. 2.75 inches
   b. 3.25 inches
   c. 3.50 inches
   d. 4.00 inches

___ 14. Which of the following terms describes the dose of radiation that the body can endure with little or no chance of injury?
   a. radiation limit
   b. maximum permissible dose
   c. occupationally exposed dose
   d. ALARA

___ 15. Which of the following is true of radiation monitoring badges?
   a. badges should be worn when the radiographer is undergoing x-ray exposure.
   b. badges can be shared between employees.
   c. badges should be worn at waist level when exposing x-ray receptors.
   d. All of the above are true.

FILL IN THE BLANK

16. Provide the requirements for proper filtration:
   a. Machines operating at 70 kVp or lower require _____ mm aluminum.
   b. Machines operating above 70 kVp require _____ mm aluminum.

17. State the angle that the dental radiographer should stand to the primary beam:_____ degrees.

18. State the formula for maximum accumulated dose:

_____

_____.

19. State the maximum permissible dose for occupationally exposed persons: _____ rems/year (_____ Sv/year).

20. State the maximum permissible dose for nonoccupationally exposed persons: _____ rem/year (_____ Sv/year).

part II

Equipment, Film, and Processing Basics

Chapter 6   Dental X-Ray Equipment, 57

Chapter 7   Dental X-Ray Film, 63

Chapter 8   Dental X-Ray Image Characteristics, 76

Chapter 9   Dental X-Ray Film Processing, 86

Chapter 10   Quality Assurance in the Dental Office, 111

Dental X-Ray Equipment

OUTLINE

DENTAL X-RAY MACHINES
    Performance Standards
    Types of Machines
    Component Parts

DENTAL X-RAY FILM HOLDERS AND BEAM ALIGNMENT
    DEVICES
    Types of Film Holders
    Types of Beam Alignment Devices

LEARNING OBJECTIVES

After completion of this chapter, the student will be able to do the following:

- Define the key words associated with dental x-ray equipment
- Discuss the regulation of dental x-ray machines at the federal, state, and local levels
- Recognize dental x-ray machines used for intraoral and extraoral films
- Identify the component parts of the dental x-ray machine
- Describe the purpose and use of dental x-ray film holders and devices
- Identify commonly used dental x-ray film holders and devices

KEY TERMS

Beam alignment device
Collimating device
Control devices
Control panel
Exposure button

Exposure light
Extension arm
Film, extraoral
Film, intraoral

Film holder
Indicator light
On-off switch
Tubehead

The dental radiographer must be familiar with dental x-ray equipment and dental x-ray film holders and beam alignment devices. With each passing year, digital imaging is becoming more prevalent and widely used. Because the majority of dental offices still use conventional radiography methods, the information presented in this section of the textbook is predominantly devoted to dental film and processing equipment. The purpose of this chapter is to introduce the dental radiographer to a variety of intraoral and extraoral dental x-ray machines, to detail the component parts of x-ray machines, and to describe the more common dental x-ray film holders and beam alignment devices.

DENTAL X-RAY MACHINES

A variety of intraoral and extraoral dental x-ray machines are available for diagnostic purposes. Dental x-ray machines vary in both design and operation. The dental radiographer must have a clear understanding of the operating procedures for the specific equipment that is used in the dental office to avoid improper exposure of patients and dental personnel.

Performance Standards

Before 1974, no federal standards existed for the manufacture of dental x-ray machines. All dental x-ray machines manufactured after 1974 must, however, meet specific federal guidelines regulating diagnostic equipment performance standards. The federal government regulates the manufacture and installation of dental x-ray equipment. State and local governments regulate how dental x-ray equipment is used and dictate codes that pertain to the use of x-radiation. Depending on state and local radiation safety codes, dental equipment must be inspected and monitored periodically. A fee is typically charged for such an inspection.

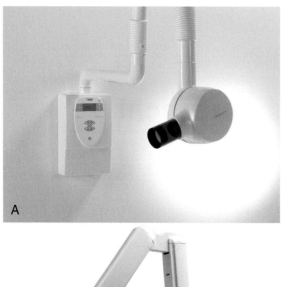

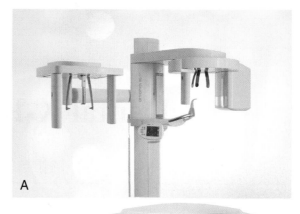

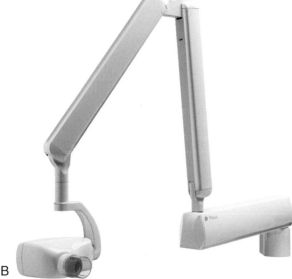

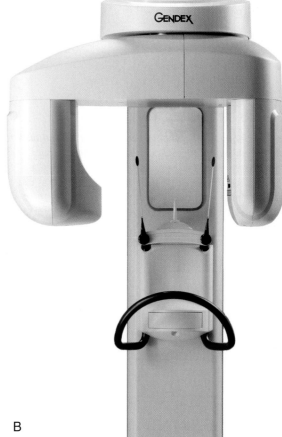

FIGURE 6-1 A, Heliodent intraoral x-ray machine (Sirona Dental Systems, LLC, Charlotte, NC). **B**, GX-770 intraoral x-ray machine. (Courtesy Instrumentarium Dental, Inc. Milwaukee, WI.)

FIGURE 6-2 A, Orthophos XGPlus extraoral x-ray machine. (Courtesy Sirona Dental Systems, LLC, Charlotte, NC). **B**, Orthoralix 8500 DDE extraoral machine. (Courtesy Gendex Dental Systems, Des Plaines, IL.)

Types of Machines

Dental x-ray machines may be used to expose **intraoral** receptors or **extraoral** receptors. Some machines are used only for intraoral exposures (Figure 6-1), whereas others are limited to extraoral exposures (Figure 6-2). A variety of dental x-ray machines are available from different manufacturers. (See Chapter 25 for examples of digital radiography units.)

Component Parts

As detailed in Chapter 2, the typical intraoral dental x-ray machine features three component parts: (1) tubehead, (2) extension arm, and (3) control panel.

Tubehead

The **tubehead,** or tube housing, contains the x-ray tube that produces dental x-rays (Figure 6-3). Extending from the tubehead opening is the position-indicating device (PID), or

cone. The PID may be circular or rectangular in shape and restricts the size of the x-ray beam.

Extension Arm

The **extension arm** suspends the x-ray tubehead, houses the electrical wires, and allows for movement and positioning of the tubehead.

Control Panel

The **control panel,** which allows the dental radiographer to regulate the x-ray beam, is plugged into an electrical outlet

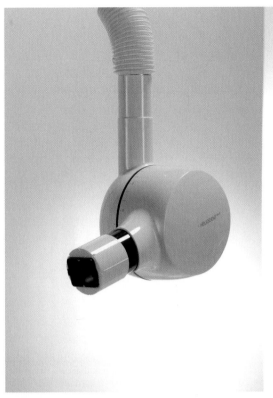

FIGURE 6-3 The tubehead of the Heliodent DS contains the x-ray tube. (Courtesy Sirona USA, Charlotte, NC.)

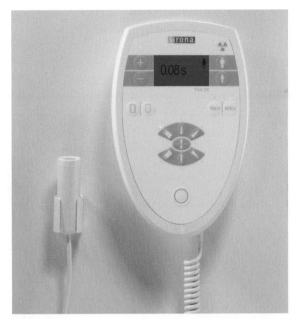

FIGURE 6-4 Heliodent DS control panel. (Courtesy Sirona USA, Charlotte, NC.)

and appears as a console or cabinet. A control panel may be mounted on a floor pedestal, a wall support, or a remote wall location outside the dental operatory. A single control panel may be used to operate more than one x-ray unit located in adjacent rooms. The control panel consists of (1) an on-off switch and indicator light, (2) an exposure button and exposure light, (3) a control device for time, and (4) with some units, control devices for kilovoltage peak and milliamperage (Figure 6-4).

On-Off Switch. The **on-off switch** must be placed in the "on" position to operate the dental x-ray equipment. An **indicator light** is illuminated when the equipment is turned on.

Exposure Button. The **exposure button** activates the machine to produce x-rays. The dental radiographer must firmly depress the exposure button until the preset exposure time is completed. As a visible sign that x-rays are being produced, an **exposure light** on the control panel is illuminated during x-ray exposure. In addition, a beep sounds during x-ray exposure as an audible signal that x-rays are being produced. The exposure light turns off and the beep stops when the x-ray exposure is completed.

Control Devices. The **control devices** that regulate the x-ray beam include the timer and the kilovoltage peak (kVp) and milliamperage (mA) selectors. The timer determines the length of exposure time in seconds or impulses. The kVp and mA selectors permit the dental radiographer to adjust and set

the correct kilovoltage peak and milliamperes. Some dental x-ray units have preset programmable settings for the various anatomic areas of the maxilla and the mandible or for different sizes of patients, thus eliminating the need to set the individual controls of kVp, mA, and time.

DENTAL X-RAY FILM HOLDERS AND BEAM ALIGNMENT DEVICES

A **film holder** is a device used to hold and align intraoral dental x-ray films in the mouth. Film holders eliminate the need for the patient to stabilize the film. With certain intraoral techniques (e.g., paralleling technique) the use of a film-holding device is required. Specific intraoral techniques and film-holding devices are discussed in Chapters 17, 18, and 19.

A **beam alignment device** is used to help the dental radiographer position the PID in relation to the tooth and the film. For use in conjunction with a beam alignment device, a **collimating device**, which is a metal plate with an opening, can be used to restrict the size of the beam.

Types of Film Holders

Intraoral film holders are commercially available from a number of manufacturers. The simplest film holder is a disposable Styrofoam bite-block with a backing plate and a slot for film retention; examples include XCP Bite-Block and Stabe Bite-Block (Rinn Corporation) (Figure 6-5). Molded-plastic devices that can be sterilized are also available, including EEZEE-Grip, formerly named Snap-A-Ray. EEZEE-Grip is a double-ended instrument that holds the film between two serrated plastic grips that can be locked in place (Figure 6-6).

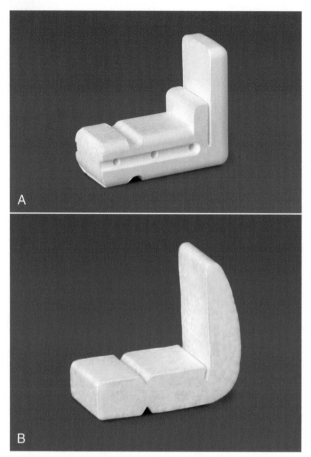

FIGURE 6-5 **A**, XCP Bite-Block. **B**, Stabe Bite-Block. (Courtesy Rinn Corporation, Elgin, IL.)

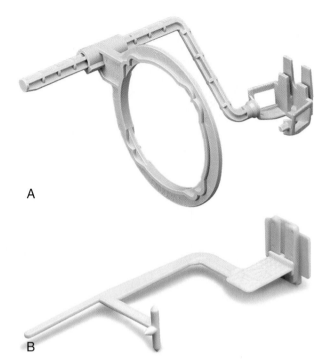

FIGURE 6-7 **A**, The EndoRay film holder is used during root canal procedures. It fits around rubber dam clamps and allows space for files to protrude from the tooth. **B**, The Uni-bite is a universal film holder that can be used with the bite-wing technique or the long-cone paralleling technique for film exposure. (Courtesy Rinn Corporation, Elgin, IL.)

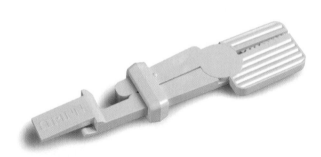

FIGURE 6-6 **Snap-A-Ray film holder.** The film can be positioned for anterior areas and most posterior areas. (Courtesy Dentsply Rinn, Elgin, IL.)

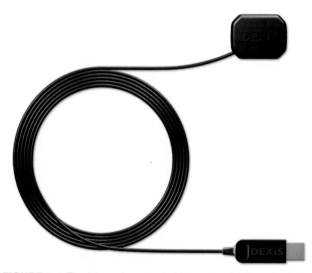

FIGURE 6-8 The intraoral sensor, held by a beam alignment device, allows the radiographer to use the paralleling technique for exposure. (Courtesy DEXIS LLC, Atlanta, GA.)

Other film-holding products include EndoRay and Uni-bite (Figure 6-7).

In digital radiography, a sensor is held in place by a bite-block attachment or by devices that aim the beam and sensor accurately. Beam alignment devices must be used to stabilize and secure the sensor (Figure 6-8).

Types of Beam Alignment Devices

Beam alignment devices and collimating devices, which are available from a number of manufacturers, are used to indicate the PID position in relation to the tooth and film. Metal beam alignment and collimating devices include the Precision film holders (Masel Orthodontics), which feature four metal collimating shields and film-holding devices that restrict the size of the x-ray beam to the size of the film (Figure 6-9).

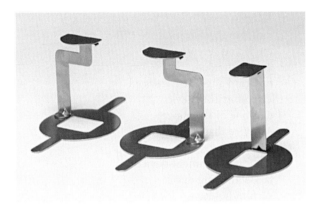

FIGURE 6-9 Precision film holders restrict the size of the x-ray beam to the size of the film. (Courtesy Masel Orthodontics.)

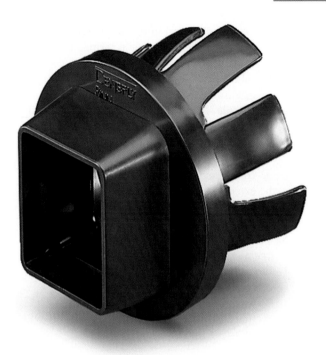

FIGURE 6-11 Rinn XCP Universal Collimator. (Courtesy Dentsply Rinn, Elgin, IL.)

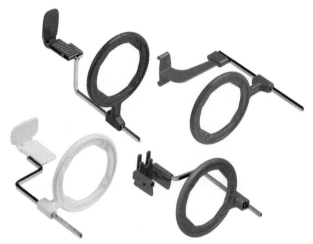

FIGURE 6-10 XCP instruments. The blue instruments are used in the anterior region, the yellow instruments are used in the posterior region, the red instruments are used in the bite-wing technique, and the torquoise instruments are used for endodontic procedures. (Courtesy Dentsply Rinn Corporation, Elgin, IL.)

SUMMARY

- The dental radiographer must be familiar with how x-ray equipment, film holders, and beam alignment devices are used in dentistry.
- The typical intraoral dental x-ray machine consists of three component parts: (1) tubehead, (2) extension arm, and (3) control panel.
- A film holder is used to stabilize an intraoral film.
- A beam alignment device helps the dental radiographer position the position-indicating device in relation to the tooth and the film.
- A collimating device is used with the beam alignment device to further restrict the size of the x-ray beam.

BIBLIOGRAPHY

Frommer HH, Savage-Stabulas JJ: Operator protection. In *Radiology for the dental professional*, ed 9, St Louis, 2011, Mosby.

Frommer HH, Savage-Stabulas JJ: Patient protection. In *Radiology for the dental professional*, ed 9, St Louis, 2011, Mosby.

Johnson ON, Thomson EM: The periapical examination. In *Essentials of dental radiography for dental assistants and hygienists*, ed 8, Pearson, 2007, Upper Saddle River, NJ.

The XCP and BAI beam alignment devices (Rinn) feature plastic bite-blocks, plastic aiming rings, and metal indicator arms (Figure 6-10). To reduce the amount of radiation a patient receives, a snap-on universal collimator can be added to the plastic XCP and BAI rings (Figure 6-11).

QUIZ QUESTIONS

MULTIPLE CHOICE

____ 1. No federal standards existed for dental x-ray machines manufactured before the year:
   a. 1954
   b. 1964
   c. 1974
   d. 1984

____ 2. Dental receptors placed inside the mouth are termed:
   a. intraoral
   b. extraoral
   c. occlusal
   d. all of the above

___ **3.** The component part of the dental x-ray machine that contains the x-ray tube is termed the:
   a. control panel
   b. tubehead
   c. extension arm
   d. console

___ **4.** The component part of the dental x-ray machine that allows movement and positioning of the tubehead is termed the:
   a. control panel
   b. extension arm
   c. console
   d. position-indicating device (PID)

___ **5.** The dental radiographer can regulate the x-ray beam (kilovoltage peak, milliamperage, time) through the use of the:
   a. control panel
   b. extension arm
   c. tubehead
   d. PID

___ **6.** An instrument that is used to help the dental radiographer position the PID in relation to the tooth and receptor is the:
   a. film holder
   b. beam alignment device
   c. collimating device
   d. none of the above

___ **7.** A device that is used to stabilize an intraoral receptor is a:
   a. beam alignment device
   b. collimating device
   c. film holder
   d. none of the above

___ **8.** A metal instrument that is used to restrict the size of the x-ray beam to the size of an intraoral receptor is the:
   a. collimating device
   b. film holder
   c. beam alignment device
   d. none of the above

chapter 7

Dental X-Ray Film

OUTLINE

DENTAL X-RAY FILM COMPOSITION AND LATENT IMAGE
    Film Composition
    Latent Image Formation
TYPES OF DENTAL X-RAY FILM

Intraoral Film
Extraoral Film
Duplicating Film
FILM STORAGE AND PROTECTION

LEARNING OBJECTIVES

After completion of this chapter, the student will be able to do the following:

- Define the key words associated with dental x-ray film
- Describe in detail film composition and latent image formation
- List and describe the different types of x-ray film used in dentistry
- Define intraoral film and describe intraoral film packaging
- Identify the types and sizes of intraoral film available
- Discuss film speed

- Discuss the differences between intraoral film and extraoral film
- Describe the difference between screen and nonscreen films
- Describe the use of intensifying screens and cassettes
- Describe duplicating film
- Discuss proper film storage and protection

KEY TERMS

Adhesive layer
Cassette
Film, bite-wing
Film, blue-sensitive
Film, cephalometric
Film, D-speed
Film, duplicating
Film, extraoral
Film, F-speed
Film, green-sensitive
Film, intraoral
Film, nonscreen
Film, occlusal
Film, panoramic
Film, periapical
Film, screen

Film, standard
Film, x-ray
Film base
Film emulsion
Film speed
Fluoresce
Gelatin
Halide
Identification dot
Image
Image receptor
Interproximal
Label side
Latent image
Latent image centers
Lead foil sheet

Outer package wrapping
Packet, film
Packet, one-film
Packet, two-film
Paper film wrapper
Phosphors
Protective layer
Radiograph, duplicate
Receptor
Screen, calcium tungstate
Screen, intensifying
Screen, rare earth
Sensitivity speck
Silver halide crystals
Tube side

The dental radiographer must have a working knowledge of the dental x-ray film. The film used in dental radiography is a type of photographic film that has been adapted for dental use. An image is produced on dental x-ray film when it is exposed to radiation that has passed through teeth and adjacent structures. To avoid film-related errors that result in increased patient exposure to x-radiation, the dental radiographer must understand the composition of the x-ray film and latent image formation. In addition, the dental radiographer must be familiar with the types of film used in dental radiography as well as film storage and protection.

The purpose of this chapter is to define film composition; to detail latent image formation; to describe the types of intraoral, extraoral, and duplicating film used in dental radiography; and to discuss film storage and protection.

DENTAL X-RAY FILM COMPOSITION AND LATENT IMAGE

In dental radiography, after the x-ray beam passes through teeth and adjacent structures, it reaches the x-ray film. The dental x-ray film serves as a recording medium, or **image receptor**; the term **image** refers to a picture or likeness of an object, and the term **receptor** refers to something that responds to a stimulus. Images are recorded on the dental x-ray film when the film is exposed to a stimulus—specifically, energy in the form of x-radiation or light. To understand how these images result, an understanding of film composition and latent image formation is necessary.

Film Composition

The x-ray film used in dentistry has four basic components: (1) a film base, (2) an adhesive layer, (3) film emulsion, and (4) a protective layer (Figure 7-1).

Film Base

The **film base** is a flexible piece of polyester plastic 0.2 mm in thickness that is constructed to withstand heat, moisture, and chemical exposure. The film base is transparent and exhibits a slight blue tint that is used to emphasize contrast and enhance image quality. The primary purpose of the film base is to provide a stable support for the delicate emulsion. The base also provides strength.

Adhesive Layer

The **adhesive layer** is a thin layer of adhesive material that covers both sides of the film base. The adhesive layer is added to the film base before the emulsion is applied and serves to attach the emulsion to the base.

Film Emulsion

The **film emulsion** is a coating attached to both sides of the film base by the adhesive layer to give the film greater sensitivity to x-radiation. The emulsion is a homogeneous mixture of gelatin and silver halide crystals.

Gelatin. The **gelatin** is used to suspend and evenly disperse millions of microscopic silver halide crystals over the film base. During film processing, the gelatin absorbs the processing solutions and allows the chemicals to react with the silver halide crystals.

Halide Crystals. A **halide** is a chemical compound that is sensitive to radiation or light. The halides used in dental x-ray film are made up of the element silver plus a halogen (bromine or iodine). Silver bromide (AgBr) and silver iodide (AgI) are two types of **silver halide crystals** found in the film emulsion; the typical emulsion is 80% to 99% silver bromide and 1% to 10% silver iodide. The silver halide crystals absorb radiation during x-ray exposure and store energy from the radiation (Figure 7-2).

Protective Layer

The **protective layer** is a thin, transparent coating placed over the emulsion. It serves to protect the emulsion surface from manipulation as well as mechanical and processing damage.

Latent Image Formation

Silver halide crystals absorb x-radiation during x-ray exposure and store the energy from the radiation. Depending on the density of the objects in the area exposed, silver halide crystals contain various levels of stored energy. For example, the silver halide crystals on the film that are positioned behind an amalgam restoration receive almost no radiation. Amalgam is dense and absorbs the x-ray energy. As a result, the silver halide crystals are not energized. In contrast, the

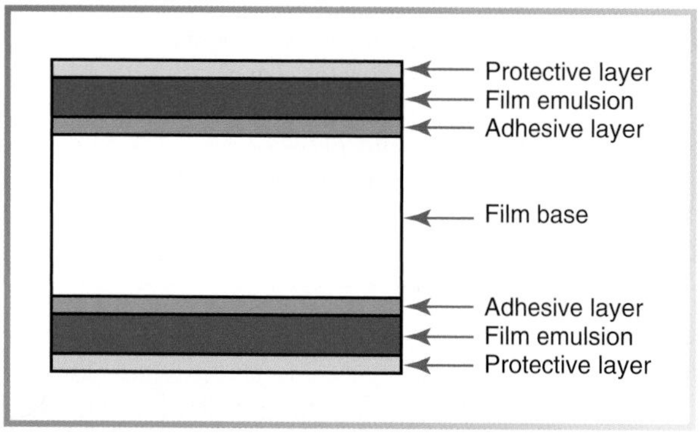

FIGURE 7-1 Schematic diagram showing construction of a typical dental x-ray film. The film emulsion is coated on both the top and the bottom surface of the polyethylene base; this allows for reduced exposure time and therefore a "faster" film. (From Miles DA, Van Dis ML, Razmus TF: *Basic principles of oral and maxillofacial radiology*, Philadelphia, 1992, Saunders.)

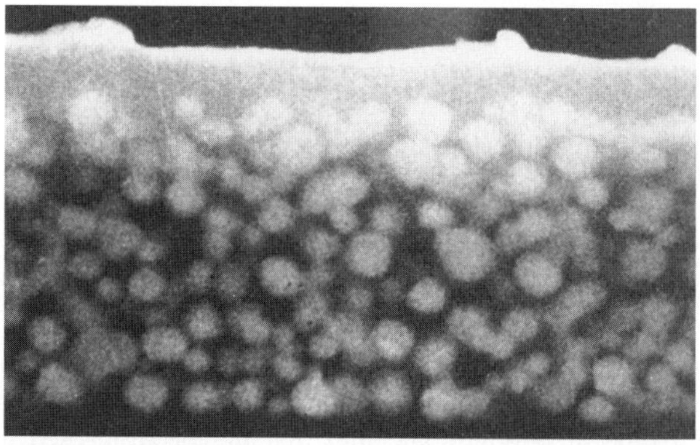

FIGURE 7-2 Scanning electron micrograph of unprocessed emulsion of Kodak Ultra-Speed dental x-ray film (magnification ×5000). Note white-appearing, unexposed silver bromide grains. (Courtesy Carestream Health, Inc., Rochester, NY.)

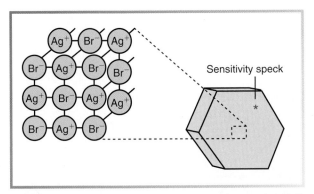

FIGURE 7-3 Each crystal in the radiographic emulsion consists of silver (Ag⁺) and primarily bromide (Br⁻) ions. Irregularities in the lattice structure form the sensitivity speck. (From Miles DA, Van Dis ML, Razmus TF: *Basic principles of oral and maxillofacial radiology*, Philadelphia, 1992, Saunders.)

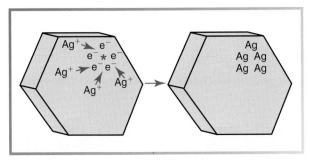

FIGURE 7-4 The sensitivity speck tends to attract free electrons (e⁻), which, in turn, attract positively charged silver ions (Ag). The aggregate of neutral silver atoms (Ag⁺) makes up the latent image center in the crystal. (From Bird DL, Robinson DS: *Modern dental assisting*, ed 9, Philadelphia, 2008, Saunders.)

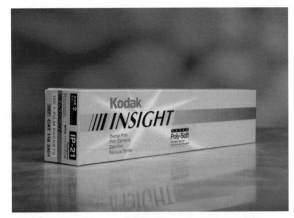

FIGURE 7-5 Intraoral film packets in a cardboard box that can be recycled. (Courtesy Carestream Health, Inc., Rochester, NY.)

silver halide crystals that correspond to air space (no density) receive more radiation and are highly energized.

The stored energy within the silver halide crystals forms a pattern and creates an invisible image within the emulsion on the exposed film. This pattern of stored energy on the exposed film cannot be seen and is referred to as a **latent image**. The latent image remains invisible within the emulsion until it undergoes chemical processing procedures. When the exposed film with latent image is processed, a visible image results (see Chapter 9).

How does the stored energy of the silver halide crystals result in a latent image? When the x-ray photons hit the surface of the film emulsion, some silver bromide crystals are exposed and energized, while other crystals are not exposed. The silver bromide crystals exposed to x-ray photons are ionized, and the silver and bromine atoms are separated. Irregularities in the lattice structure of the exposed crystal, known as **sensitivity specks**, attract the silver atoms (Figure 7-3). These aggregates of neutral silver atoms are known as **latent image centers** (Figure 7-4). Collectively, the crystals with aggregates of silver at the latent image centers become the latent image on the film.

TYPES OF DENTAL X-RAY FILM

Three types of x-ray film may be used in dental radiography: (1) intraoral film, (2) extraoral film, and (3) duplicating film.

Intraoral Film

An **intraoral film**, as defined in Chapter 6, is a film that is placed *inside* the mouth during x-ray exposure. An intraoral film is used to examine teeth and supporting structures.

Intraoral Film Packaging

Each intraoral film is packaged to protect it from light and moisture; the film and its surrounding packaging are referred to as a **film packet**. In dentistry, the terms "film packet" and "film" are often used interchangeably. Intraoral film packets are typically available in quantities of 25, 100, or 150 films per container. Film packets are packaged in convenient plastic trays or cardboard boxes that can be recycled (Figure 7-5). Boxes of intraoral film are labeled with the type of film, film speed, film size, number of films per individual packet, total number of films enclosed, and the film expiration date.

An intraoral x-ray film packet is made up of four separate items: (1) x-ray film, (2) paper film wrapper, (3) lead foil sheet, and (4) outer film wrapping (Figure 7-6).

X-Ray Film. The intraoral **x-ray film** is a double-emulsion film (emulsion on both sides). Double-emulsion film is used instead of single-emulsion film (emulsion on one side) because it requires less radiation exposure to produce an image. A film packet may contain one film (**one-film packet**) or two films (**two-film packet**). A two-film packet produces two identical radiographs with the same amount of exposure necessary to produce a single radiograph. The two-film packet is used when a duplicate record of a radiographic examination is needed (e.g., for insurance claims, patient referrals, etc.).

A small, raised bump known as the **identification dot** is located in one corner of the intraoral x-ray film (Figure 7-7). The raised bump is used to determine film orientation. After

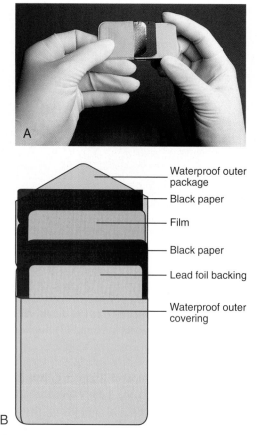

FIGURE 7-6 **A,** Back of an opened dental film packet. **B,** Diagram of A. (From Bird DL, Robinson DS: *Modern dental assisting*, ed 10, St Louis, 2012, Sounders.)

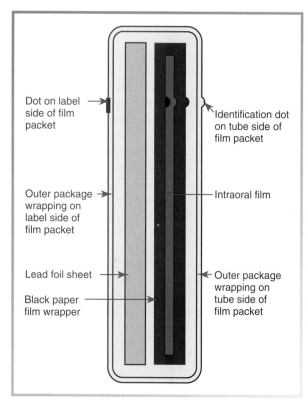

FIGURE 7-7 Labeled film packet.

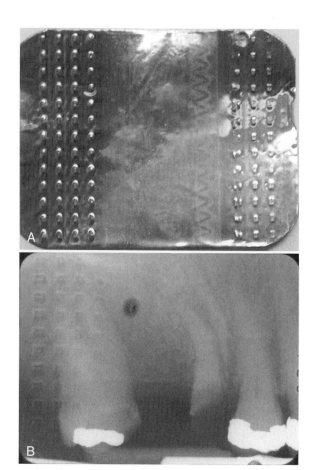

FIGURE 7-8 **A,** The lead foil insert in this packet has a raised diamond pattern across both ends. **B,** Radiograph showing the raised diamond pattern from the lead backing when the film is positioned backward in the mouth. (From Bird DL, Robinson DS: *Modern dental assisting*, ed 10, St Louis, 2012, Saunders.)

the film is processed, the raised identification dot is used to distinguish between the left and right sides of the patient. The dot is significant in film mounting and interpretation (see Chapter 27).

Paper Film Wrapper. The **paper film wrapper** within the film packet is a protective sheet that covers the film and shields the film from light.

Lead Foil Sheet. The **lead foil sheet** is a single piece of lead foil within the film packet that is located behind the film wrapped in protective paper. The thin lead foil sheet is positioned behind the film to shield the film from backscattered (secondary) radiation that results in film fog.

The manufacturer-placed embossed pattern on the lead foil sheet is visible on a processed radiograph if the film packet is inadvertently positioned in the mouth backward and then exposed (Figure 7-8).

Outer Package Wrapping. The **outer package wrapping** is a soft-vinyl or paper wrapper that hermetically seals the film packet, protective paper, and lead foil sheet. This outer wrapper serves to protect the film from exposure to light and saliva.

TABLE 7-1	Color Codes for Kodak Film Packets	
	PACKETS	
Film Type	**One-Film**	**Two-Film**
Ultra-Speed (D-Speed)	Mint	Gray
Insight (F-Speed)	Violet	Tan

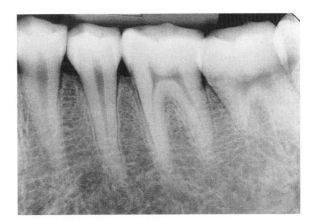

FIGURE 7-10 A periapical image. (Courtesy Carestream Health, Inc., Rochester, NY.)

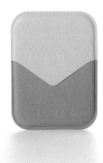

FIGURE 7-9 The label side of a film packet. (Courtesy, Carestream Health, Inc., Rochester, NY.)

The outer wrapper of the film packet has two sides: (1) the tube side and (2) the label side.

Tube Side. The **tube side** is solid white and has a raised bump in one corner that corresponds to the identification dot on the x-ray film. When placed in the mouth, the white side (tube side) of the film packet must face the teeth and the tubehead.

Label Side. The **label side** of the film packet has a flap used to open the film packet and remove the film before processing. The label side is color-coded to identify films outside of the plastic packaging container; color codes are used to distinguish one-film and two-film packets and film speeds (Table 7-1). When placed in the mouth, the color-coded side (label side) of the packet must face the tongue. It may be easier to remember that "the white side of the film faces the white teeth."

The following information is printed on the label side of the film packet (Figure 7-9):

- A circle or dot that corresponds with the raised identification dot on the film
- The statement "opposite side toward tube"
- The manufacturer's name
- The film speed
- The number of films enclosed

Intraoral Film Types

Three types of intraoral films are available: (1) periapical, (2) bite-wing, and (3) occlusal.

Periapical Film. The **periapical film** is used to examine the entire tooth (crown and root) and supporting bone (Figure 7-10). The term *periapical* is derived from the Greek root *peri*, meaning "around," and the Latin word *apex*,

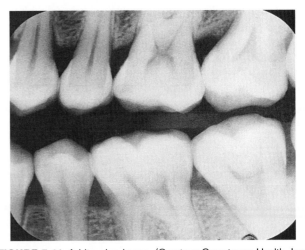

FIGURE 7-11 A bite-wing image. (Courtesy Carestream Health, Inc., Rochester, NY.)

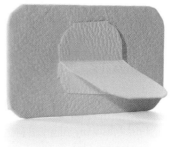

FIGURE 7-12 The bite-wing tab attached to the film. (Courtesy Carestream Health, Inc., Rochester, NY.)

referring to the terminal end of a tooth root. As the term suggests, this type of film shows the tip of the tooth root and surrounding structures as well as the crown.

Bite-Wing Film. The **bite-wing film** is used to examine the crowns of both maxillary and mandibular teeth on one film (Figure 7-11). The bite-wing film is particularly useful in examining **interproximal**, or adjacent, tooth surfaces. The bite-wing film has a "wing," or a tab, attached to the tube side of the film (Figure 7-12). The patient "bites" on the wing to

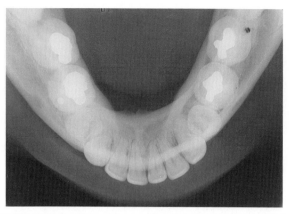

FIGURE 7-13 An occlusal image. (Courtesy Carestream Health, Inc., Rochester, NY.)

stabilize the film. Bite-wing films may be purchased with tabs attached to the film or may be constructed from a periapical film and bite-wing loop.

Occlusal Film. The **occlusal film** is used for examination of large areas of the maxilla or the mandible (Figure 7-13). The occlusal film is so named because the patient "occludes," or bites on, the entire film. The occlusal film is larger than periapical or bite-wing films.

Intraoral Film Sizes

The intraoral film is manufactured in five sizes to accommodate the varying mouth sizes of children, adolescents, and adults; the larger the number, the larger is the size of the film. Different sizes of film are used with periapical, bite-wing, and occlusal exposures (Figure 7-14).

Periapical Film. Three sizes (0, 1, and 2) of the periapical film are available.

- The *size 0* periapical film is the smallest intraoral film available and is used for very small children.
- The *size 1* periapical film is used primarily to examine the anterior teeth in adults.
- The *size 2* periapical film, also known as the **standard film**, is used to examine the anterior and posterior teeth in adults.

Bite-Wing Film. Three sizes (0, 2, and 3) of the bite-wing film are available. With the exception of the size 3 film, the size and shape of the bite-wing film are identical to the size and shape of the periapical film.

- The *size 0* bite-wing film is used to examine the posterior teeth in small children.
- The *size 2* bite-wing film is used to examine the posterior teeth in adults. This is the most frequently used bite-wing film.
- The *size 3* film is longer and narrower than the standard size 2 film and is used only for bite-wing images. This bite-wing film shows all the posterior teeth on one side of the arch in one radiograph.

Occlusal Film. The occlusal film is the largest intraoral film and is almost four times as large as a standard size 2 periapical film

- The *size 4* occlusal film is used to show large areas of the maxilla or the mandible.

Intraoral Film Speed

Film speed refers to the amount of radiation required to produce a radiograph of standard density. Film speed, or *sensitivity*, is determined by the following:

1. Size of the silver halide crystals
2. Thickness of the emulsion
3. Presence of special radiosensitive dyes

Film speed determines how much radiation and how much exposure time are necessary to produce an image on a film. For example, a fast film requires less radiation exposure because the film responds more quickly; a fast film responds more quickly because the silver halide crystals in the emulsion are larger. The larger the crystals, the faster is the film speed.

An alphabetical classification system is used to identify film speed. X-ray films are given speed ratings ranging from A speed (the slowest) to F speed (the fastest). Only the **D-speed film** and the **F-speed film** are used for intraoral radiography; the E-speed film has been discontinued by Kodak. The American Dental Association (ADA) and the American Academy of Oral and Maxillofacial Radiology (AAOMR) currently recommend the use of the F-speed film. The F-speed film requires 60% of the exposure time of the D-speed film and has comparable image contrast and resolution. Use of the F-speed film results in less radiation exposure of the patient. The F-speed film is a faster film than the D-speed film because of the larger crystals and the increased amount of silver bromide in the emulsion. Current F-speed films not only reduce radiation dose to the patient but also provide stable contrast characteristics under various processing conditions.

The speed of a film is clearly indicated on the label side of the intraoral film packet as well as on the outside of the film box or container.

Extraoral Film

An **extraoral film**, as described in Chapter 6, is placed *outside* the mouth during x-ray exposure. Extraoral films are used to examine large areas of the skull or jaws. Common extraoral films include panoramic and cephalometric films. A **panoramic film** shows a panoramic (wide) view of the maxilla and the mandible and surrounding structures on a single radiograph (Figure 7-15). A **cephalometric film** exhibits the bony and soft tissue areas of the facial profile (Figure 7-16).

Extraoral Film Packaging

Unlike intraoral films, extraoral films are designed for use outside the mouth and therefore are not enclosed in moisture-proof packets. Extraoral films used in dental radiography are available in 5 × 7–inch and 8 × 10–inch sizes as well as in the panoramic 5 × 12–inch and 6 × 12–inch sizes. Extraoral films are boxed in quantities of 50 or 100. Some manufacturers separate each piece with protective paper. Labels on the boxes of extraoral films contain information, including the type of film, film size, total number of films enclosed, and expiration date (Figure 7-17).

Extraoral Film Types

Two types of film may be used in extraoral radiography: (1) screen film and (2) nonscreen film.

Screen Film. The majority of extraoral films are screen films. A **screen film** is a film that requires the use of a screen for exposure (see later discussion). A screen film is placed between two special intensifying screens in a cassette (Figure 7-18). When the cassette is exposed to x-rays, the screens convert the x-ray energy into light, which, in turn, exposes the screen film. The screen film is sensitive to fluorescent light rather than to direct exposure to x-radiation.

Films used in a screen–film combination are sensitive to specific colors of fluorescent light. Some screen films are sensitive to blue light (Kodak X-Omat and Ektamat films), whereas others are sensitive to green light (Kodak Ortho and T-Mat films). **Blue-sensitive film** must be paired with screens that produce blue light, and **green-sensitive film** must be paired with screens that produce green light. Properly matched film–screen combinations are imperative to obtain high-quality images and to minimize exposure of the patient.

Nonscreen Film. A **nonscreen film** is an extraoral film that does not require the use of screens for exposure. A nonscreen extraoral film is exposed directly to x-rays; the emulsion is sensitive to direct x-ray exposure rather than to fluorescent light. A nonscreen extraoral film requires more exposure time than does a screen film and is not recommended for use in dental radiography.

Extraoral Film Equipment

In extraoral radiography, screen films are used in combination with two special equipment items: (1) intensifying screens and (2) cassettes.

Intensifying Screens. An **intensifying screen** is a device that transfers x-ray energy into visible light; the visible light, in turn, exposes the screen film. These screens intensify the effect of x-rays on the film. With the use of intensifying screens, less radiation is required to expose a screen film, and the patient is exposed to less radiation.

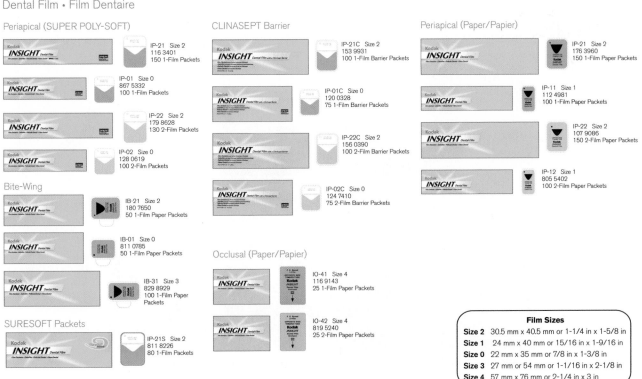

FIGURE 7-14 Film sizes for periapical, bite-wing, and occlusal films. (Courtesy Carestream Health, Inc., Rochester, NY.)

Continued

Kodak Ultra-speed
Dental Film • Film Dentaire

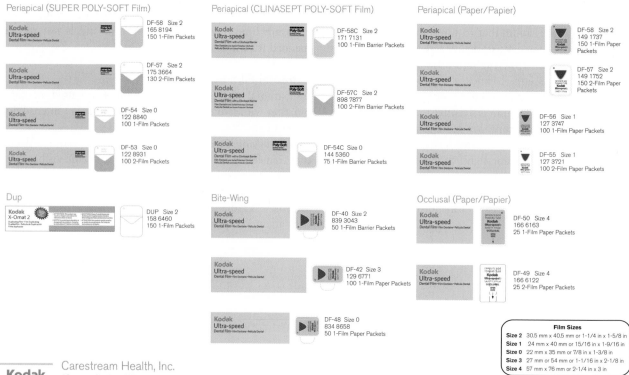

Periapical (SUPER POLY-SOFT Film)

Kodak Ultra-speed Dental Film • Film Dentaire • Pelicula Dental
Poly-Soft
DF-58 Size 2
165 8194
150 1-Film Packets

Kodak Ultra-speed Dental Film • Film Dentaire • Pelicula Dental
Poly-Soft
DF-57 Size 2
175 3664
130 2-Film Packets

Kodak Ultra-speed Dental Film • Film Dentaire • Pelicula Dental
Poly-Soft
DF-54 Size 0
122 8840
100 1-Film Packets

Kodak Ultra-speed Dental Film • Film Dentaire • Pelicula Dental
Poly-Soft
DF-53 Size 0
122 8931
100 2-Film Packets

Dup

Kodak X-Omat 2 Duplicating Film • Fine Duplicating • Du plaofilm • Pelicula de Duplicación Filme duplicateur
DUP Size 2
158 6460
150 1-Film Packets

Periapical (CLINASEPT POLY-SOFT Film)

Kodak Ultra-speed Dental Film with a Clinasept Barrier
Poly-Soft
DF-58C Size 2
171 7131
100 1-Film Barrier Packets

Kodak Ultra-speed Dental Film with a Clinasept Barrier
Poly-Soft
DF-57C Size 2
898 7877
100 2-Film Barrier Packets

Kodak Ultra-speed Dental Film with a Clinasept Barrier
Poly-Soft
DF-54C Size 0
144 5360
75 1-Film Barrier Packets

Bite-Wing

Kodak Ultra-speed Dental Film • Film Dentaire • Pelicula Dental
DF-40 Size 2
839 3043
50 1-Film Barrier Packets

Kodak Ultra-speed Dental Film • Film Dentaire • Pelicula Dental
DF-42 Size 3
129 6771
100 1-Film Paper Packets

Kodak Ultra-speed Dental Film • Film Dentaire • Pelicula Dental
DF-48 Size 0
834 8658
50 1-Film Paper Packets

Periapical (Paper/Papier)

Kodak Ultra-speed Dental Film • Film Dentaire • Pelicula Dental
DF-58 Size 2
149 1737
150 1-Film Paper Packets

Kodak Ultra-speed Dental Film • Film Dentaire • Pelicula Dental
DF-57 Size 2
149 1752
150 2-Film Paper Packets

Kodak Ultra-speed Dental Film • Film Dentaire • Pelicula Dental
DF-56 Size 1
127 3747
100 1-Film Paper Packets

Kodak Ultra-speed Dental Film • Film Dentaire • Pelicula Dental
DF-55 Size 1
127 3721
100 2-Film Paper Packets

Occlusal (Paper/Papier)

Kodak Ultra-speed Dental Film • Film Dentaire • Pelicula Dental
DF-50 Size 4
166 6163
25 1-Film Paper Packets

Kodak Ultra-speed Dental Film • Film Dentaire • Pelicula Dental
DF-49 Size 4
166 6122
25 2-Film Paper Packets

Film Sizes

Size 2	30.5 mm x 40.5 mm or 1-1/4 in x 1-5/8 in
Size 1	24 mm x 40 mm or 15/16 in x 1-9/16 in
Size 0	22 mm x 35 mm or 7/8 in x 1-3/8 in
Size 3	27 mm or 54 mm or 1-1/16 in x 2-1/8 in
Size 4	57 mm x 76 mm or 2-1/4 in x 3 in

Kodak Licensed Product   **Carestream Health, Inc.**
©Carestream Health, Inc. 2009.
Insight, SureSoft, Ultra-speed, Super Poly-Soft and Clinasept are trademarks of Carestream Health.
The Kodak trademark and trade dress are used under license from Kodak.

For more information / Pour plus d'informations, contactez nour via notre site : www.kodakdental.com

D6-53 859 3956
P/N 8H7447 2009-07-22

FIGURE 7-14, cont'd

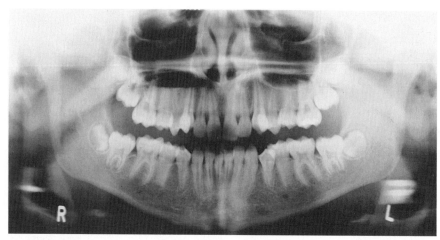

FIGURE 7-15 A panoramic image. (Courtesy Carestream Health, Inc., Rochester, NY.)

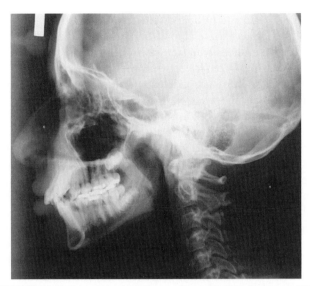

FIGURE 7-16 A cephalometric image. (From Bird DL, Robinson DS: *Modern dental assisting*, ed 10, St Louis, 2012, Saunders.)

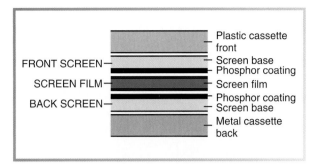

FIGURE 7-18 Inside cassette, the screen film is placed between two intensifying screens.

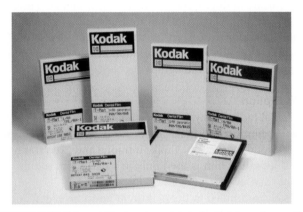

FIGURE 7-17 Extraoral film boxes are labeled with information on the type of film, film size, number of films enclosed, and expiration date. (Courtesy Carestream Health, Inc., Rochester, NY.)

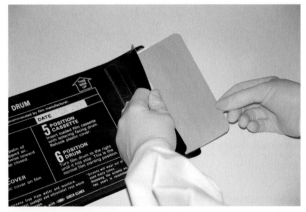

FIGURE 7-19 Cassette in open position, showing front and back intensifying screens and a piece of film. (From Bird DL, Robinson DS: *Modern dental assisting*, ed 10, St Louis, 2012, Saunders.)

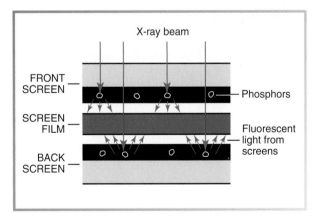

FIGURE 7-20 Phosphors in the intensifying screen emit visible light when hit by x-ray photons. Multiple visible light photons then strike and expose the film.

In extraoral radiography, a screen film is sandwiched between two intensifying screens of matching size and is secured in a cassette (Figure 7-19). An intensifying screen is a smooth plastic sheet coated with minute fluorescent crystals known as **phosphors**. When exposed to x-rays, the phosphors **fluoresce** and emit visible light in the blue or green spectrum; the emitted light then exposes the film (Figure 7-20). As discussed in Chapter 2, one of the properties of x-rays is that they cause certain materials (e.g., phosphors) to fluoresce.

Conventional **calcium tungstate screens** have phosphors that emit blue light. The newer **rare earth screens** have phosphors that are not commonly found in the earth (thus "rare earth") and emit green light. Rare earth intensifying screens are more efficient at converting x-rays into light than are calcium tungstate intensifying screens. As a result, rare earth screens require less x-ray exposure than do calcium tungstate screens and are considered faster. The use of rare earth screens means less exposure of the patient to x-radiation. Rare earth intensifying screens (Kodak Lanex Regular and Medium screens) are designed for use with green-sensitive films (Kodak Ortho and T-Mat films), whereas conventional screens (Kodak X-Omatic Regular screens) are used with blue-sensitive films (Kodak X-Omat and Ektamat films).

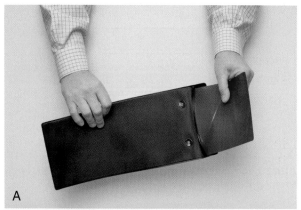

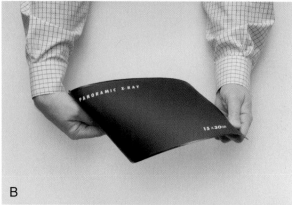

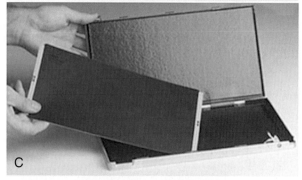

FIGURE 7-21 A and **B,** Close-up views of flexible 5 × 12–inch panoramic cassette. (Courtesy Instrumentarium Dental, Inc., Milwaukee, WI.) **C,** Rigid panoramic cassette.

Cassette. A **cassette** is a special device that is used to hold the extraoral film and the intensifying screens. Cassettes are available in a variety of sizes that correspond to film and screen sizes. A cassette may be flexible or rigid; most cassettes are rigid, although the panoramic cassette may be flexible (Figure 7-21).

A rigid cassette is more expensive but usually lasts longer than does a flexible cassette. A rigid cassette also better protects screens from damage. The film fits the rigid cassette exactly and cannot be loaded incorrectly. To load the flexible cassette properly, however, the film must be placed between the two screens and pushed to the end of the cassette.

Both rigid and flexible cassettes must be "light-tight" not only to protect the extraoral film from exposure but also to hold the intensifying screens in perfect contact with the extraoral film. Contact between the screen and the film is critical; lack of contact between screen and film results in loss of image sharpness.

A rigid cassette has a front cover and a back cover. The front cover is placed in such a way that it faces the tubehead and is usually constructed of plastic to permit the x-ray beam to pass through. The back cover is constructed of heavy metal and serves to reduce scatter radiation. Intensifying screens are installed inside the front and back covers of the cassette. The film is positioned between the two intensifying screens. Each screen exposes one side of the film.

The cassette must be marked to orient the finished radiograph; a metal letter "L" is attached to the front cover of the cassette to indicate the patient's left side, and a metal letter "R" indicates the patient's right side.

Duplicating Film

A **duplicate radiograph** is one that is identical to the original x-ray film. In dentistry, duplicate radiographs are used for patient referrals to specialists, for insurance claims, and as teaching aids. A special film, or duplicating film, is required to make a duplicate radiograph.

Description

In dental radiography, a **duplicating film** is a type of photographic film used to make an identical copy of an intraoral or extraoral radiograph. Unlike intraoral and extraoral films, the duplicating film is used only in a darkroom setting and is not exposed to x-rays.

When examined in the darkroom under safe light conditions, duplicating film has an emulsion on one side only. The emulsion side of the film appears dull, whereas the side without the emulsion appears shiny. The emulsion side of the film must contact the radiograph during the duplication process. (Chapter 9 describes the equipment necessary for film duplication and the duplication process.)

Packaging

Duplicating films are boxed in sets of 50 sheets and are available in three sizes: 5 × 12–inch, 6 × 12–inch, and 8 × 10–inch.

FILM STORAGE AND PROTECTION

Films are adversely affected by heat, humidity, and radiation. To prevent film fog (see Chapter 9), unexposed, unprocessed films must be kept in a cool, dry place. The optimum temperature for film storage ranges from 50° F to 70° F, and the optimum relative humidity level ranges from 30% to 50%. Films must be stored in areas that are adequately shielded from sources of radiation and should not be stored in areas where patients are exposed to x-radiation. Lead-lined or

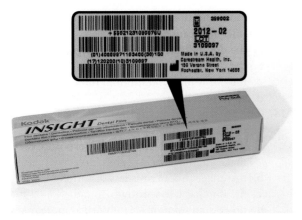

FIGURE 7-22 The expiration date is clearly labeled on the film package. (Courtesy Carestream Health, Inc., Rochester, NY.)

radiation-resistant film dispensers and storage boxes are ideal to prevent film fog.

All dental x-ray films have limited shelf life. Each box or container of films is clearly labeled with an expiration date (Figure 7-22). Films must be used before the labeled expiration date. The "first-in, first-out" rule of thumb should be applied to film use; the oldest films in stock should always be used before new films.

SUMMARY

- The dental x-ray film is an image receptor that has four basic components: (1) a film base, (2) an adhesive layer, (3) film emulsion, and (4) a protective layer.
- An image is recorded on the dental x-ray film when the film is exposed to x-radiation.
- The silver halide crystals in the film emulsion absorb the x-radiation during x-ray exposure and store the energy from the radiation. The stored energy forms an invisible pattern on the emulsion and is known as the latent image.
- When the exposed film with the latent image undergoes chemical processing, a visible image results.
- Three types of film are used in dental radiography: (1) intraoral film, (2) extraoral film, and (3) duplicating film.
- The intraoral film is placed inside the mouth and is then exposed; the extraoral film is placed outside the mouth and is then exposed; and the duplicating film is used to make a copy of a dental radiograph.

- An intraoral film packet is made up of four separate items: (1) x-ray film, (2) paper film wrapper, (3) lead foil sheet, and (4) outer package wrapping.
- Intraoral films are manufactured in five sizes (0, 1, 2, 3, 4); the larger the number, the larger is the size of the film.
- Intraoral films are available in two speeds: (1) D speed and (2) F speed. The F-speed film reduces patient exposure to radiation by 60% compared with the D speed film, with no loss of image contrast or quality.
- Extraoral films are typically screen films and require the use of intensifying screens and a cassette for exposure.
- Intensifying screens transform x-ray energy into visible light, which, in turn, exposes the screen film.
- The use of intensifying screens requires less radiation to expose a screen film and results in less radiation exposure of the patient.
- The duplicating film is a special type of photographic film used to make an identical copy of an intraoral or extraoral radiograph.
- The duplicating film is used in a darkroom setting and is not exposed to x-radiation.
- Films are adversely affected by heat, humidity, and radiation and must be stored away from sources of radiation at 50° to 70° F and with a relative humidity level of 30% to 50%.
- Dental films should always be used before the expiration date printed on the label.

BIBLIOGRAPHY

Frommer HH, Savage-Stabulas JJ: Image formation. In *Radiology for the dental professional*, ed 8, St Louis, 2005, Mosby.

Frommer HH, Savage-Stabulas JJ: Image receptors. In *Radiology for the dental professional*, ed 8, St Louis, 2005, Mosby.

Johnson ON, Thomson EM: Dental x-ray films. In *Essentials of dental radiography for dental assistants and hygienists*, ed 8, Pearson. Upper Saddle River, NJ, 2007.

Ludlow JB et al: Characteristics of Kodak Insight, an F-speed intraoral film, *Oral Surg Oral Med Oral Pathol Oral Radiol Endod* 91(1):120–129, 2001.

Miles DA, Van Dis ML, Jensen CW, Ferretti A: Film processing and quality assurance. In *Radiographic imaging for the dental team*, ed 4, St Louis, 2009, Saunders.

White SC, Pharoah MJ: X-ray film, intensifying screens, and grids. In *Oral radiology: Principles and interpretation*, ed 6, St Louis, 2009, Mosby.

QUIZ QUESTIONS

FILL IN THE BLANK

1. The component of an x-ray film described as "a thin transparent coating that is placed over the emulsion" is termed:

_____

2. The component of the x-ray film described as "a flexible piece of plastic that withstands heat, moisture, and chemical heat" is termed:

_____

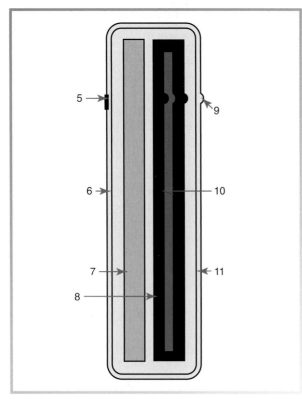

FIGURE 7-23

3. The chemical compounds that change when exposed to radiation or light are termed:

_____

_____

4. The invisible pattern of stored energy on the exposed film is termed:

_____

_____

IDENTIFICATION

For questions 5 to 11, identify the items indicated on the intraoral film packet illustrated in Figure 7-23.

MULTIPLE CHOICE

____ **12.** Dental x-ray film that is placed inside the mouth and used to examine the teeth and supporting structures is termed:
  a. duplicating film
  b. extraoral film
  c. intraoral film
  d. none of the above

____ **13.** The identification dot on the intraoral film is significant because:
  a. the dot indicates the patient's right or left side
  b. the dot determines film orientation
  c. the dot is important in film mounting
  d. all of the above

____ **14.** One advantage of a film with an emulsion coating on both sides (double-emulsion film) is that:
  a. the film requires less radiation exposure to make an image
  b. the image produced is less distorted
  c. the film has less sensitivity to radiation
  d. processing solutions are absorbed more easily

____ **15.** The purpose of a lead foil sheet in the film packet is:
  a. to protect the film from primary radiation
  b. to protect the film from saliva
  c. to protect the film from backscattered radiation
  d. to distinguish between the patient's right and left sides

____ **16.** Which of the following is not found on the label side of the film packet?
  a. film speed
  b. expiration date
  c. the phrase "opposite side toward tube"
  d. number of films enclosed

____ **17.** Which of the following film sizes is known as the standard film?
  Size 0
  Size 1
  Size 2
  Size 3

____ **18.** Which of the following is the largest intraoral film size?
  a. size 4
  b. size 3
  c. size 2
  d. size 1

____ **19.** The film characteristic that is "the amount of radiation needed to produce a radiograph of standard density" is:
  a. contrast
  b. speed
  c. image resolution
  d. size

____ **20.** The speed of a film is determined by the size of the silver halide crystals in the emulsion. Identify the true statement:
  a. The larger the crystals, the faster is the film speed.
  b. The larger the crystals, the slower is the film speed.
  c. The smaller the crystals, the faster is the film speed.
  d. None of the above is correct.

___ **21.** A film that is placed outside the mouth during x-ray exposure is termed a(n):
  a. extraoral film
  b. intraoral film
  c. duplicating film
  d. periapical film

___ **22.** A screen film is more sensitive to fluorescent light than to direct exposure to x-rays.
  a. True
  b. False

___ **23.** Nonscreen extraoral film is commonly used in extraoral radiography.
  a. True
  b. False

___ **24.** The device that transfers x-ray energy into visible light is termed a:
  a. cassette
  b. nonscreen film
  c. screen film
  d. intensifying screen

___ **25.** The intensifying screen that emits green light and must be used with green-sensitive film is a:
  a. calcium tungstate screen
  b. rare earth screen
  c. phosphor screen
  d. rare tungstate screen

___ **26.** The device used to hold the extraoral film and intensifying screens is termed a:
  a. screen holder
  b. film holder
  c. cassette
  d. any of the above

___ **27.** Which of the following statements is true?
  a. Cassettes are available in sizes that correspond to film and screen sizes.
  b. A flexible cassette is more expensive than is a rigid cassette.
  c. Film can be loaded incorrectly in the rigid cassette.
  d. Film cannot be loaded incorrectly in the flexible cassette.

___ **28.** Which of the following results if the intensifying screens are not in perfect contact with the screen film?
  a. The screen may be damaged.
  b. The film may be damaged.
  c. A loss of image sharpness occurs.
  d. None of the above.

___ **29.** Which of the following statements about the duplicating film is false?
  a. It is not exposed to x-rays.
  b. It is used in the darkroom.
  c. It may be placed intraorally or extraorally.
  d. It is used to make copies of radiographs.

___ **30.** Identify the ideal temperature and humidity levels for film storage:
  a. 50° F to 70° F; 30% to 50%
  b. 60° F to 80° F; 50% to 60%
  c. 70° F to 90° F; 60% to 70%
  d. below 50° F; 0% to 30%

chapter 8

Dental X-Ray Image Characteristics

OUTLINE

DENTAL X-RAY IMAGE CHARACTERISTICS
VISUAL CHARACTERISTICS
    Density
    Contrast

GEOMETRIC CHARACTERISTICS
    Sharpness
    Magnification
    Distortion

LEARNING OBJECTIVES

After completion of this chapter, the student will be able to do the following:

- Define the key words associated with dental x-ray image characteristics
- Differentiate between radiolucent and radiopaque areas on a dental radiograph
- Describe a diagnostic dental radiograph
- List the two visual characteristics of the radiographic image
- List the factors that influence density and contrast
- Discuss the difference between high contrast and low contrast
- Describe film contrast and subject contrast
- Describe the difference between short-scale contrast and long-scale contrast
- Identify images of high contrast, low contrast, no contrast, short-scale contrast, and long-scale contrast
- Describe a stepwedge
- List the three geometric characteristics of the radiographic image
- List the factors that influence sharpness, magnification, and distortion

KEY TERMS

Contrast	Distance, object–receptor	Operating kilovoltage peak
Contrast, high	Distance, target–receptor	Penumbra
Contrast, long-scale	Distortion	Radiograph, diagnostic
Contrast, low	Exposure factors	Radiolucent
Contrast, film	Exposure time	Radiopaque
Contrast, scale of	Focal spot	Sharpness
Contrast, short-scale	Magnification	Stepwedge
Contrast, subject	Milliamperage	Subject thickness
Density		

Dental x-ray image characteristics include both visual characteristics and geometric characteristics. A variety of factors affect the visual image characteristics of density and contrast as well as the geometric image characteristics of sharpness, magnification, and distortion.

The dental radiographer must have a working knowledge of dental x-ray image characteristics. The purpose of this chapter is to describe in detail the visual image characteristics of density and contrast; to define the geometric image characteristics of sharpness, magnification, and distortion; and to discuss how influencing factors alter these image characteristics.

DENTAL X-RAY IMAGE CHARACTERISTICS

A dental radiograph appears as a black-and-white image that includes varying shades of gray. When viewed on a light source, the darkest area of a radiograph appears black, and the lightest area appears white. Two terms are used to describe the black areas and the white areas on a dental radiograph, *radiolucent* and *radiopaque*, respectively.

- **Radiolucent** refers to that portion of a processed radiograph that is dark or black. A structure that appears radiolucent on a radiograph lacks density and permits the passage of the x-ray beam with little or no resistance. For example, air space freely permits the passage of dental x-rays and appears mostly radiolucent on a dental radiograph (Figure 8-1).
- **Radiopaque** refers to that portion of a processed radiograph that appears light or white. Radiopaque structures are dense and absorb or resist the passage of the x-ray beam. For example, structures that resist the passage of the x-ray beam include enamel, dentin, and bone and appear radiopaque on a dental radiograph (Figure 8-2).

The ideal dental radiograph is not too light and not too dark. The quality of a dental radiograph is determined by its image characteristics. The image characteristics of a dental radiograph include the visual characteristics of proper density and contrast as well as the geometric characteristics of sharpness with minimal magnification and distortion. The ideal dental radiograph is a diagnostic one. A **diagnostic radiograph** provides a great deal of information; the images exhibit proper density and contrast, have sharp outlines, and are of the same shape and size as the object radiographed.

VISUAL CHARACTERISTICS

Two visual characteristics of the radiographic image—density and contrast—directly influence the diagnostic quality of a dental radiograph.

Density

The overall blackness or darkness of a dental radiograph is termed **density**.

Description

When a dental radiograph is viewed against a light source, the relative transparency of areas on the radiograph depends on the distribution of black silver particles in the emulsion. Darker areas represent heavier deposits of black silver particles. Density is this degree of silver blackening.

Images of teeth and supporting structures must have enough density to be viewed on a light source; however, if the density of an image is too great, or the image appears too dark, images that cannot be visually separated from each other may result. A radiograph with the correct density enables the radiographer to view black areas (air spaces), white areas (enamel, dentin, and bone), and gray areas (soft tissue) (Figure 8-3).

Influencing Factors

A number of factors have a direct influence on the density of a dental radiograph. As discussed in Chapter 3, three

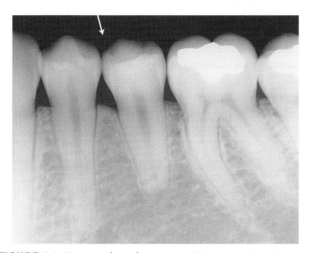

FIGURE 8-1 Air space (*arrow*) appears radiolucent, or dark, because the dental x-rays pass through freely.

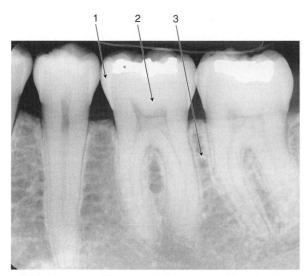

FIGURE 8-2 Dense structures, such as enamel (1), dentin (2), and bone (3), resist the passage of x-rays and appear radiopaque, or white.

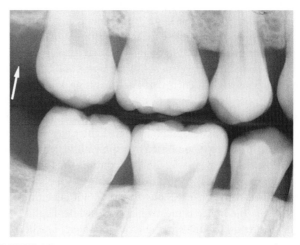

FIGURE 8-3 Note the grayish area behind the last molar teeth (*arrow*); this represents the gingival tissues.

TABLE 8-1	Visual Characteristics and Influencing Factors	
Visual Characteristic	Influencing Factors	Effect of Influencing Factors
Density	mA	↑ mA = ↑ density
		↓ mA = ↓ density
	kVp	↑ kVp = ↑ density
		↓ kVp = ↓ density
	Time	↑ Time = ↑ density
		↓ Time = ↓ density
	Subject thickness	↑ Thickness = ↓ density
		↓ Thickness = ↑ density
Contrast	kVp	↑ kVp = long-scale contrast; low contrast
		↓ kVp = short-scale contrast; high contrast

mA, milliamperage; *kVp*, kilovoltage peak; ↑, increased; ↓, decreased.

exposure factors control the density of a dental radiograph, as follows:

- Milliamperage (mA)
- Operating kilovoltage peak (kVp)
- Exposure time

Any increase in such exposure factors, separately or combined, increases the density of a dental radiograph. In addition, the thickness of the subject influences density (Table 8-1).

Milliamperage. Today, most modern dental x-ray machines do not allow for the adjustment of **milliamperage** (mA). In machines that do allow for adjustment, an increase in mA produces more x-rays that the receptor is exposed to and, as a result, increases density. If the milliamperage is increased, the density increases, and the radiograph appears darker. Conversely, if the milliamperage is decreased, the density decreases, and the radiograph appears lighter.

Operating Kilovoltage Peak. Today, many modern dental x-ray machines do not allow for the adjustment of **operating kilovoltage peak** (kVp). An increase in kVp increases density by increasing the average energy of the x-rays and by producing x-rays of higher energy. If the operating kilovoltage is increased, the density increases, and the radiograph appears darker. Conversely, if kilovoltage is decreased, the density decreases, and the radiograph appears lighter.

The kVp has been compared to a spray nozzle on a garden hose. Like the spray nozzle, the kVp controls the force of the emerging x-rays. Low kVp is like "opening up" the nozzle on a hose. The x-rays have less power and do not penetrate well. As a result, the image is mostly black and white. High kVp is like "closing down" the spray nozzle on a hose. The beam is highly penetrating and has high energy. As a result, many shades of gray are seen in the resultant image.

Although using a high kVp produces more x-rays, a linear relationship does not exist. For every increase of 15 kVp, a two-time increase in density occurs.

Exposure Time. Density is directly related to **exposure time**. An increase in exposure time increases density by increasing the total number of x-rays that reach the receptor surface. If the exposure time is increased, more x-rays reach the receptor, the density increases, and the radiograph appears dark. Conversely, if the exposure time is decreased, the density decreases, and the radiograph appears lighter.

The x-ray timer has been compared to a water faucet. It turns the flow of x-rays on or off. For example, if the faucet is open for a certain period, a specific amount of water will flow. If the faucet is opened for twice that amount of time, twice the amount of water will flow. The same is true with exposure time. If a receptor is exposed to x-radiation for a specific period, a specific amount of x-ray photons will come out of the machine. If the time is doubled, the amount of x-rays produced is doubled. The longer the exposure time, the more x-ray photons reach the receptor, expose it, and continue to darken the image.

Subject Thickness. Fewer x-rays reach the receptor in a patient with an increased amount of soft tissue or thick, dense bones. As a result, the image has less density and appears lighter. Adjustments in operating kVp, mA, or exposure time can be made to compensate for variations in the size of patients and **subject thickness**.

Contrast

The difference in the degrees of blackness (densities) between adjacent areas on a dental radiograph is termed **contrast**.

Description

The differences in the amount of light transmitted through adjacent areas of a dental radiograph can also be described as contrast. When viewed on a light source, a dental radiograph that has very dark areas and very light areas is said to have **high contrast**; the dark and light areas are strikingly different. A radiograph that does not have very dark and very light areas but instead has many shades of gray is said to have **low contrast**. In dental radiography, an image that is a compromise between low contrast and high contrast is preferred. The overall contrast of a dental radiograph is determined by the properties, or film contrast, and by the object radiographed, or subject contrast.

Film Contrast. **Film contrast** refers to the characteristics of the receptor that influence radiographic contrast. The characteristics that influence contrast include the inherent qualities of the film and film processing, and the qualities of the sensor. The inherent qualities of the film are under the control of the film manufacturer and cannot be changed by the dental radiographer. Film processing, however, is under the control of the dental radiographer. Development time or the temperature of the developer solution affects the contrast of a dental radiograph. An increase in development time or developer temperature results in a film with increased contrast.

Subject Contrast. **Subject contrast** refers to the characteristics of the subject that influence radiographic contrast. Subject contrast is determined by the thickness, density, and composition (atomic number) of the subject. Subject contrast can be altered by increasing or decreasing the kilovoltage. When a high operating kVp (0.90 kVp) is used, low subject contrast results, and many shades of gray are seen on the dental radiograph. Conversely, when a low operating kVp (65–70 kVp) is used, high subject contrast results, and areas of black and white are seen.

Influencing Factors

Only one exposure factor has a direct influence on the contrast of a dental radiograph. As discussed in Chapter 3, the operating kVp affects contrast.

Operating Kilovoltage Peak. Increasing the kilovoltage affects contrast by increasing the average energy of the x-rays and by producing higher energy x-rays. X-rays with higher energy are better able to penetrate tissue. As a result, more variations in tissue density are recorded on the receptor and appear as varying shades of gray. A higher kilovoltage produces an image with decreased or low contrast; the radiograph exhibits many shades of gray. Conversely, a lower kilovoltage produces an image with increased or high contrast; the radiograph has many black-and-white areas.

Table 8-1 summarizes the effects of kilovoltage on contrast. Figure 8-4 provides a series of dental radiographs showing the influence of kilovoltage on both density and contrast.

Scales of Contrast

The range of useful densities seen on a dental radiograph is termed the **scale of contrast**. In dental radiography, the terms **short-scale contrast** and **long-scale contrast** may be used to describe the appearance of a radiograph.

Short-Scale Contrast. A dental radiograph that shows only two densities, areas of black and areas of white, has a short contrast scale. A lower kilovoltage range results in a radiograph with a short-scale contrast; many areas of black and white, rather than shades of gray, are seen. A radiograph that exhibits a short contrast scale can also be described as having high contrast, in which the black and white areas are easily distinguished from each other (Table 8-2).

Long-Scale Contrast. A dental radiograph that exhibits many densities, or many shades of gray, has a long contrast scale. A higher kilovoltage range results in a radiograph with a long-scale contrast; many shades of gray, rather than areas of black and white, are present. A radiograph that exhibits a long contrast scale can also be described as having low contrast, in which areas of gray are not easily distinguished from each other (see Table 8-2).

Stepwedge. A device known as a **stepwedge** can be used to demonstrate short-scale contrast and long-scale contrast. A stepwedge consists of uniform-layered thicknesses of an

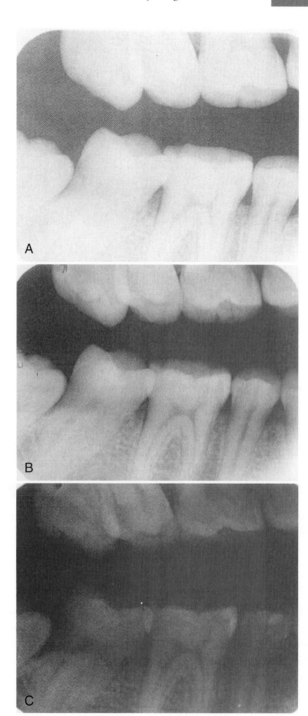

FIGURE 8-4 Exposure series showing the influence of operating kilovoltage peak (kVp). **A**, When kVp is low, the result is low density (the degree of blackness created by developed silver) and high contrast (the relative difference between the lightest and darkest elements in a radiograph). **B**, The optimal image is created when a proper balance between kVp and milliamperage (mA) is obtained. This image is considered optimal because it provides a full range of tones from white to black. **C**, When kVp is high, the result is very high density with very little contrast. (Courtesy Carestream Health, Inc., Rochester, NY.)

TABLE 8-2	The Effect of Kilovoltage on Contrast		
Kilovoltage	Contrast	Scale of Contrast	Example
High (>90 kVp)	Low	Long-scale	See Figure 8-16, *A*.
Low (<70 kVp)	High	Short-scale	See Figure 8-16, *B*.

kVp, kilovoltage peak.

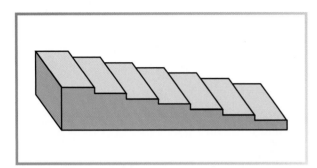

FIGURE 8-5 A stepwedge is made of uniform-layered thicknesses.

x-ray absorbing material, usually aluminum. The typical stepwedge is constructed of aluminum steps in 2-mm increments (Figure 8-5). When a stepwedge is placed on top of an image receptor and exposed to x-rays, the different steps absorb varying amounts of x-rays. As a result, different densities appear on the dental radiograph.

The use of a stepwedge to demonstrate corresponding densities and contrast scales is illustrated in Figure 8-6. The stepwedge can be used to monitor the qualities of the film, the film processing, and the sensor; quality control tests using the stepwedge are discussed in Chapter 10.

GEOMETRIC CHARACTERISTICS

Three geometric characteristics of the radiographic image—sharpness, magnification, and distortion—influence the diagnostic quality of a dental radiograph. These geometric characteristics must be minimized to produce an accurate radiographic image.

Sharpness

Sharpness (also known as *detail, resolution,* or *definition*) refers to the capability of the receptor to reproduce the distinct outlines of an object. In other words, sharpness refers to how well the smallest details of an object are reproduced on a dental radiograph.

Description

A certain lack of image sharpness, or unsharpness, is present in every dental image. The fuzzy, unclear area that surrounds a radiographic image is termed the penumbra (from the Latin *pene*, meaning "almost," and *umbra*, meaning "shadow"). **Penumbra** can be defined as the unsharpness, or blurring, of the edges of a radiographic image.

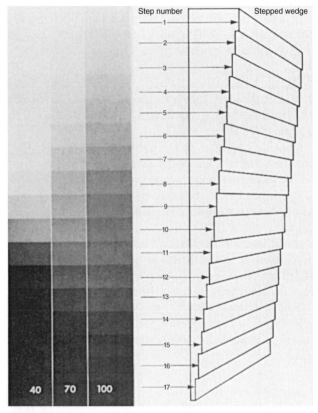

FIGURE 8-6 Radiographs taken at 40 kVp are predominantly black and white; that is, they have high contrast (a short-contrast scale). Those taken at 100 kVp show many shades of gray (a long-contrast scale). (From Miles DA, Van Dis ML, Jensen CW: *Radiographic imaging for the dental team,* ed 3, St Louis, 2009, Saunders.)

Influencing Factors

The sharpness of an image is influenced by the following three factors (Table 8-3):

- Focal spot size
- Film composition
- Movement

Focal Spot Size. As described in Chapter 2, the tungsten target of the anode serves as a **focal spot**; this small area converts bombarding electrons into x-ray photons. The focal spot concentrates the electrons and creates an enormous amount of heat. To limit the amount of heat produced and to prevent damage to the x-ray tube, the size of the focal spot is limited. The size of the focal spot ranges from 0.6 to 1.0 mm² and is determined by the manufacturer of the x-ray equipment; most manufacturers use the smallest focal spot area possible based on heat production restrictions.

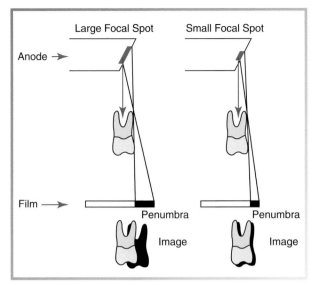

FIGURE 8-7 The smaller the focal spot area, the sharper the image appears; the larger the focal spot area, the greater is the amount of penumbra, and the greater is the loss of image sharpness.

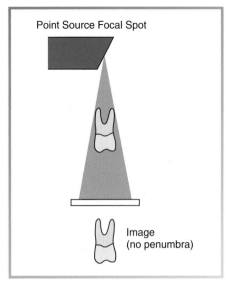

FIGURE 8-8 Theoretical "point source" of x-rays would produce a sharp image without penumbra.

TABLE **8-3**	Geometric Characteristics and Influencing Factors	
Geometric Characteristic	**Influencing Factors**	**Effects of Influencing Factors**
Sharpness	Focal spot size	↓ Focal spot size = ↑ sharpness
		↑ Focal spot size = ↓ sharpness
	Film composition	↓ Crystal size = ↑ sharpness
		↑ Crystal size = ↓ sharpness
	Movement	↓ Movement = ↑ sharpness
		↑ Movement = ↓ sharpness
Magnification	Target–receptor distance	↑ Target–receptor distance = ↓ magnification
		↓ Target–receptor distance = ↑ magnification
	Object–receptor distance	↑ Object–receptor distance = ↑ magnification
		↓ Object–receptor distance = ↓ magnification
Distortion	Object–receptor alignment	Object and receptor parallel = ↓ distortion
		Object and receptor not parallel = ↑ distortion
	X-ray beam angulation	Beam perpendicular to object and receptor = ↓ distortion
		Beam not perpendicular to object and receptor = ↑ distortion

↓, decreased; ↑, increased.

The smaller the focal spot area, the sharper the image appears; the larger the focal spot area, the greater is the loss of image sharpness (Figure 8-7). If x-rays were produced from one spot or a single "point source," no unsharpness would be present (Figure 8-8). However, a single point source of x-ray production is impossible because of the limited capacity of the x-ray tube.

Film Composition. The composition of the film emulsion influences sharpness. Sharpness is relative to the size of the crystals found in the film emulsion. The emulsion of faster film contains larger crystals that produce less image sharpness, whereas slower film contains smaller crystals that

produce more image sharpness. Unsharpness occurs because the larger crystals do not produce object outlines as well as smaller crystals do.

Movement. Movement influences image sharpness. A loss of image sharpness occurs if the tubehead, the receptor, or the patient moves during x-ray exposure (Figure 8-9). Even slight amounts of movement result in unsharpness (Figure 8-10).

Magnification

Image **magnification** refers to a radiographic image that appears larger than the actual size of the object it represents.

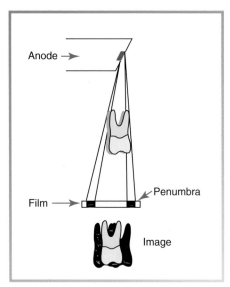

FIGURE 8-9 Diagram illustrating the influence of motion on image sharpness. Note that the image outline is blurred because of penumbra formation.

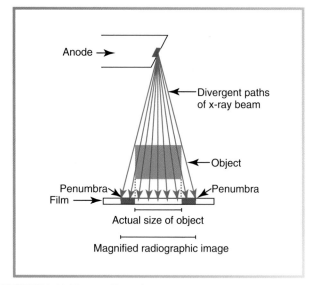

FIGURE 8-11 Diagram illustrating magnification as a result of the divergent paths of the x-ray beam.

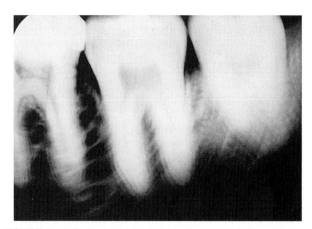

FIGURE 8-10 Radiograph of a patient who moved during x-ray exposure. Note the blurred image outline.

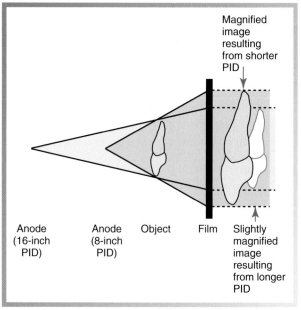

FIGURE 8-12 A longer position-indicating device (PID) (16 inches) and target–receptor distance results in less image magnification.

Description

Magnification, or enlargement of a radiographic image, results from the divergent paths of the x-ray beam. As you may recall from Chapter 2, x-rays travel in diverging straight lines as they radiate from the focal spot. Because of these diverging paths, some degree of image magnification is present in every dental radiograph (Figure 8-11).

Influencing Factors

The image magnification on a dental radiograph is influenced by the following (see Table 8-3):
- Target–receptor distance
- Object–receptor distance

Target-Receptor Distance. As defined in Chapter 3, the **target-receptor distance** (also known as the *source-to-receptor distance*) is the distance between the source of x-rays

(focal spot on the tungsten target) and the image receptor. The target–receptor distance is determined by the length of the position-indicating device (PID). When a longer PID is used, more parallel rays from the middle of the x-ray beam strike the object rather than the diverging x-rays from the periphery of the beam. As a result, a longer PID and target–receptor distance result in less image magnification, and a shorter PID and target–receptor distance result in more image magnification (Figure 8-12).

Object–Receptor Distance. The **object–receptor distance** is the distance between the object being radiographed (the

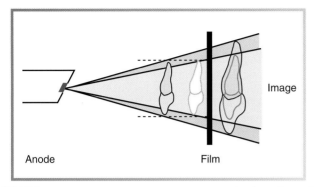

FIGURE 8-13 Object–receptor distance. Note that the closer the tooth is to the receptor, the less enlargement is seen on the image.

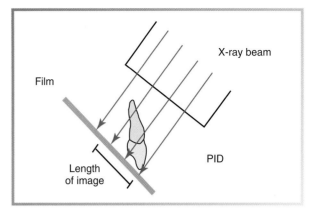

FIGURE 8-14 If the tooth and receptor are not parallel, an angular relationship is formed, and a distorted image results. In this example, the length of the tooth that appears on the image is shorter than the actual tooth.

tooth) and the image receptor. The tooth and the receptor should always be placed as close together as possible. The closer the tooth is to the receptor, the less is the enlargement of the image. A decrease in object–receptor distance results in a decrease in magnification, and an increase in object–receptor distance results in an increase in image magnification (Figure 8-13).

Distortion

Dimensional **distortion** of a radiographic image is a variation in the true size and shape of the object being radiographed. A distorted image does not have the same size and shape as the object being radiographed.

Description

A distorted image results from the unequal magnification of different parts of the same object. Distortion results from improper receptor alignment or beam angulation.

Influencing Factors

The dimensional distortion of a radiographic image is influenced by the following (see Table 8-3):
- Object–receptor alignment
- X-ray beam angulation

Object–Film Alignment. To minimize dimensional distortion, the object and receptor must be parallel to each other. If the object (tooth) and receptor are not parallel, an angular relationship results. An angular relationship produces a variation of distances between the tooth and the receptor that result in a distorted image. A distorted image may appear too long or too short (Figure 8-14). Such distortions are discussed in the later chapters on technique.

X-Ray Beam Angulation. To minimize dimensional distortion, the x-ray beam must be directed perpendicular to the tooth and the receptor. The central ray of the x-ray beam must be as nearly perpendicular to the tooth and receptor as possible to record the adjacent structures in their true spatial relationships (Figure 8-15).

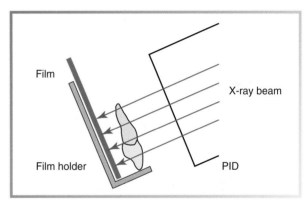

FIGURE 8-15 To limit distortion, the central ray of the x-ray beam must be perpendicular to the tooth and the receptor.

SUMMARY

- A number of factors influence the visual image characteristics of density and contrast as well as the geometric characteristics of sharpness, magnification, and distortion.
- Milliamperage, operating kilovoltage peak, and exposure time can be used to adjust the density of a dental radiograph. Subject thickness also influences the density of an image.
- Only the operating kilovoltage peak has a direct influence on contrast.
- A radiograph that exhibits areas of black and white is termed *high contrast* and is said to have a short contrast scale; a radiograph that exhibits many shades of gray is termed *low contrast* and is said to have a long contrast scale.
- A stepwedge can be used to demonstrate short-scale and long-scale contrast patterns.
- The factors that influence the geometric characteristics of sharpness, magnification, and distortion are reviewed in Table 8-3.
- To create a sharp image, the dental radiographer uses the smallest focal spot possible, chooses a film with small

crystals in the emulsion, and limits patient, tubehead, and image receptor movements.

- To limit image magnification, the longest target–receptor distance and the shortest object–receptor distance are used.
- To limit image distortion, the receptor and the tooth are positioned parallel to each other, and the x-ray beam is directed perpendicular to the tooth and the receptor.

BIBLIOGRAPHY

Frommer HH, Savage-Stabulas JJ: Image formation. In *Radiology for the dental professional*, ed 9, St Louis, 2011, Mosby.

Frommer HH, Savage-Stabulas JJ: Image receptors. In *Radiology for the dental professional*, ed 9, St Louis, 2011, Mosby.

Johnson ON, Thomson EM: Producing quality radiographs. In *Essentials of dental radiography for dental assistants and hygienists*, ed 8, Pearson, 2007, Upper Saddle River, NJ.

Miles DA, Van Dis ML, Jensen CW, Ferretti A: Image characteristics. In *Radiographic imaging for the dental team*, ed 4, St Louis, 2009, Saunders.

White SC, Pharoah MJ: X-ray film, intensifying screens, and grids. In *Oral radiology: principles and interpretation*, ed 6, St Louis, 2009, Mosby.

QUIZ QUESTIONS

MULTIPLE CHOICE

____ 1. The portion of a processed radiograph that appears dark or black is termed:
   a. dense
   b. radiolucent
   c. radiopaque
   d. transparent

____ 2. The portion of a processed radiograph that appears light or white is termed:
   a. radiolucent
   b. radiopaque
   c. dense
   d. high density

____ 3. Which of the following appears most radiolucent on a dental radiograph?
   a. bone
   b. enamel
   c. dentin
   d. air space

____ 4. An example of a radiopaque structure seen on dental x-rays is:
   a. bone
   b. enamel
   c. dentin
   d. all of the above

____ 5. The overall blackness or darkness of a dental radiograph is termed:
   a. density
   b. contrast
   c. subject thickness
   d. diagnostic quality

____ 6. Increasing the milliamperage (mA) will cause:
   a. an increase in density; the image appears darker
   b. an increase in density; the image appears lighter
   c. a decrease in density; the image appears darker
   d. a decrease in density; the image appears lighter

____ 7. Increasing the operating kilovoltage peak (kVp) will cause:
   a. an increase in density; the image appears darker
   b. an increase in density; the image appears lighter
   c. a decrease in density; the image appears darker
   d. a decrease in density; the image appears lighter

____ 8. Increasing the exposure time will cause:
   a. an increase in density; the image appears darker
   b. an increase in density; the image appears lighter
   c. a decrease in density; the image appears darker
   d. a decrease in density; the image appears lighter

____ 9. A dental patient has thick soft tissues and dense bones. To compensate for this increase in subject thickness and to provide an image of diagnostic density, the dental radiographer may:
   a. increase the exposure time
   b. increase the milliamperage
   c. increase the operating kilovoltage peak
   d. any of the above

____ 10. The difference in the degrees of blackness between adjacent areas on a dental radiograph is termed:
   a. density
   b. contrast
   c. subject thickness
   d. diagnostic quality

____ 11. When viewed on a light source, a dental radiograph that demonstrates many shades of gray is said to have:
   a. high contrast
   b. low contrast
   c. high density
   d. low density

____ 12. When viewed on a light source, a dental radiograph that demonstrates very dark areas and very light areas is said to have:
   a. high contrast
   b. low contrast
   c. high density
   d. low density

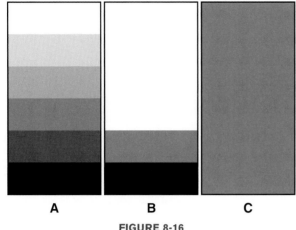

A   B   C

FIGURE 8-16

For questions 13 to 17, refer to Figure 8-16.

___ **13.** In Figure 8-16, which diagram exhibits high
  contrast?
  a. A
  b. B
  c. C

___ **14.** In Figure 8-16, which diagram exhibits low
  contrast?
  a. A
  b. B
  c. C

___ **15.** In Figure 8-16, which diagram exhibits long-scale
  contrast?
  a. A
  b. B
  c. C

___ **16.** In Figure 8-16, which diagram exhibits short-scale
  contrast?
  a. A
  b. B
  c. C

___ **17.** In Figure 8-16, which diagram exhibits no
  contrast?
  a. A
  b. B
  c. C

___ **18.** The one exposure factor that has a direct influence
  on the contrast of a dental radiograph is:
  a. operating kilovoltage peak
  b. milliamperage
  c. exposure time
  d. subject thickness

___ **19.** The type of contrast preferred in dental
  radiography is:
  a. low contrast
  b. long-scale contrast only
  c. short-scale contrast only
  d. a compromise between short-scale contrast and
    long-scale contrast

___ **20.** The stepwedge is used for all of the following
  except:
  a. to demonstrate short-scale and long-scale
    contrast
  b. to monitor quality control of film processing
  c. to increase the penetrating quality of the x-ray
    beam
  d. to demonstrate densities

___ **21.** The capability of the receptor to reproduce distinct
  outlines of an object is termed:
  a. sharpness
  b. magnification
  c. distortion
  d. diagnostic quality

___ **22.** The unsharpness or blurred edges seen on a
  radiographic image is termed:
  a. distortion
  b. umbra
  c. penumbra
  d. contrast

___ **23.** The geometric characteristic that refers to a
  radiographic image that appears larger than its
  actual size is termed:
  a. distortion
  b. detail
  c. definition
  d. magnification

___ **24.** A variation in the true size and shape of the object
  being radiographed is termed:
  a. magnification
  b. distortion
  c. sharpness
  d. resolution

FILL IN THE BLANK

For questions 25 to 35, fill in the blank with the words
increase or *decrease*.

25. Decrease focal spot size = _____ sharpness.
26. Increase crystal size = _____ sharpness.
27. Decrease crystal size = _____ sharpness.
28. Decrease movement = _____ sharpness.
29. Increase movement = _____ sharpness.
30. Increase target–receptor distance = _____
  magnification.
31. Increase object–receptor distance = _____
  magnification.
32. Decrease object–receptor distance = _____
  magnification.
33. Object and receptor are parallel = _____
  distortion.
34. Beam perpendicular to object and receptor =
  _____ distortion.
35. Beam not perpendicular to object and receptor =
  _____ distortion.

chapter 9

Dental X-Ray Film Processing

OUTLINE

FILM PROCESSING
    Film Processing Fundamentals
MANUAL FILM PROCESSING
    Film Processing Steps
    Film Processing Solutions
    Equipment Requirements
    Equipment Accessories
    Step-by-Step Procedures
    Care and Maintenance
AUTOMATIC FILM PROCESSING
    Film Processing Steps
    Equipment Requirements
    Step-by-Step Procedures
    Care and Maintenance

THE DARKROOM
    Room Requirements
    Location and Size
    Lighting
    Miscellaneous Requirements
    Waste Management
FILM DUPLICATION
    Equipment Requirements
    Step-by-Step Procedures
PROCESSING PROBLEMS AND SOLUTIONS
    Time and Temperature
    Chemical Contamination
    Film Handling
    Lighting

LEARNING OBJECTIVES

After completion of this chapter, the student will be able to do the following:

- Define the key words associated with processing of dental x-ray film
- Describe in detail how a latent image becomes a visible image
- List and discuss the five steps of manual film processing
- List and describe the four basic ingredients of the developer solution
- List and describe the four basic ingredients of the fixer solution
- Discuss the parts of the processing tank: insert tanks, master tank, and lid
- List and describe the equipment needed for manual film processing
- List and discuss the procedural steps for manual film processing
- Describe the care and maintenance of the processing solutions, equipment, and equipment accessories used in manual film processing
- Discuss the advantages of automatic film processing

- List and identify the component parts of the automatic film processor
- Describe the mechanism of automatic film processing
- List and discuss the four procedural steps for automatic film processing
- Describe the care and maintenance of the automatic film processor and automatic processing solutions
- Discuss the location, size, lighting, and equipment requirements necessary for the darkroom
- Discuss safelighting
- Discuss the equipment requirements and procedural steps for film duplication
- Describe film processing problems that result from time and temperature errors
- Describe film processing problems that result from chemical contamination errors
- Describe film processing problems that result from film handling errors
- Describe film processing problems that result from lighting errors

KEY TERMS

Accelerator	Air bubbles	Compartment, fixer
Acetic acid	Ammonium thiosulfate	Compartment, water
Acidifier	Compartment, developer	Darkroom

Darkroom plumbing
Darkroom storage space
Darkroom work space
Daylight loader
Developer cutoff
Developer solution
Developer spots
Developing agent
Development
Drying chamber
Elon
Film, cleaning
Film, duplicating
Film, fogged
Film, overdeveloped
Film, overlapped
Film, scratched
Film, underdeveloped
Film, yellow-brown
Film duplicator
Film feed slot
Film hangers
Film recovery slot
Fingernail artifact

Fingerprint artifact
Fixation
Fixer cutoff
Fixer solution
Fixer spots
Fixing agent
Hardening agent
Humidity level
Hydroquinone
Hypo
Latent image
Light-tight
Light leak
Oxidation
Potassium alum
Potassium bromide
Preservative
Processing, automatic
Processing, manual
Processor, automatic
Processor housing
Radiolucent
Radiopaque
Reduction

Reduction, selective
Replenisher
Replenisher pump
Replenisher solution
Restrainer
Reticulation of emulsion
Rinsing
Roller film transporter
Room lighting
Safelight filter
Safelighting
Sodium carbonate
Sodium sulfite
Sodium thiosulfate
Static electricity
Stirring paddle
Stirring rod
Sulfuric acid
Tank, insert
Tank, master
Tank, processing
Thermometer
Timer
Valve, mixing

To produce high-quality diagnostic dental radiographs, the dental x-ray film must be properly exposed and processed. Film processing procedures directly affect the quality of a dental radiograph. The dental radiographer must have a working knowledge of film processing procedures, problems, and solutions.

The purpose of this chapter is to detail film processing procedures, to discuss manual and automatic film processing, to describe darkroom requirements, and to explain film duplication procedures. In addition, this chapter discusses common processing problems and provides solutions.

FILM PROCESSING

Film processing refers to a series of steps that produce a visible permanent image on a dental radiograph. The purpose of film processing is twofold, as follows:

- To convert the latent (invisible) image on the film into a visible image
- To preserve the visible image so that it is permanent and does not disappear from the dental radiograph

Film Processing Fundamentals

As detailed in Chapter 7, the silver halide crystals in the film emulsion absorb x-radiation during x-ray exposure and store the energy from the radiation. The stored energy within the silver halide crystals forms a pattern and creates an invisible image within the emulsion on the exposed film. This pattern of stored energy on the exposed film cannot be seen and is referred to as the **latent image**. The latent image remains invisible within the film emulsion until it undergoes chemical processing procedures.

From Latent Image to Visible Image

How does the latent image become a visible image? Under special darkroom conditions, a chemical reaction takes place when a film with a latent image is immersed in a series of special chemical solutions. During processing, a chemical reaction occurs, and the halide portion of the *exposed, energized* silver halide crystal is removed; chemically, this is referred to as a **reduction**. Reduction of the exposed silver halide crystals results in precipitated black metallic silver.

During film processing, selective reduction of the exposed silver halide crystals occurs. **Selective reduction** refers to the reduction of the energized, exposed silver halide crystals into black metallic silver, while the *unenergized, unexposed* silver halide crystals are removed from the film. The latent image is made visible through processing procedures (Figure 9-1), as follows:

1. The film is placed in a chemical known as the **developer solution** for a specific amount of time and at a specific temperature. The developer distinguishes between the exposed and unexposed silver halide crystals. The developer initiates a chemical reaction that reduces the exposed silver halide crystals into black metallic silver and creates dark or black areas on a dental radiograph. At the same time, the unexposed silver halide crystals remain virtually unaffected by the developer.
2. Following the development process, the film is rinsed in water to remove any remaining developer solution.

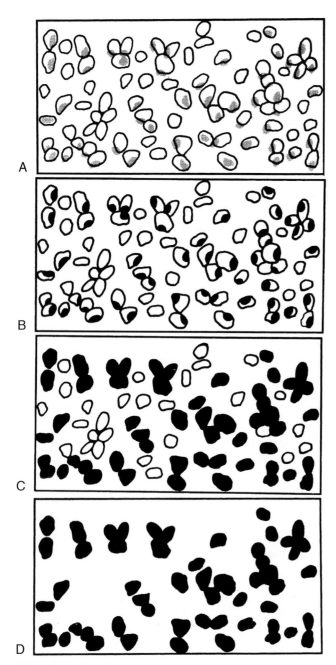

FIGURE 9-1 A, Schematic distribution of silver halide grains. The gray areas indicate a latent image produced by exposure. **B,** Partial development begins to produce metallic silver (*black*) in exposed grains. **C,** Development completed. **D,** Unexposed silver grains have been removed by fixation. (Courtesy Carestream Health, Inc., Rochester, NY.)

3. Next, the film is placed in a special chemical known as the **fixer solution** for a specific amount of time. The fixer solution removes the unexposed silver halide crystals and creates white or clear areas on the dental radiograph. Meanwhile, the black metallic silver is not removed and remains on the film. After the fixing process, the film is washed in water to remove any remaining traces of the chemical solutions and then dried.

The Visible Image

The visible image that results on a dental radiograph is made up of black, white, and gray areas. The black areas seen on a dental radiograph are created by deposits of black metallic silver. The amount of deposited black metallic silver seen on a dental radiograph varies depending on the structures being radiographed. The white areas on a dental radiograph result from the removal of the unexposed silver halide crystals. The amount of unexposed silver halide crystals removed depends on the structures being radiographed. As discussed in Chapter 8, structures that permit the passage of the x-ray beam appear black, or *radiolucent* (see Figure 8-1), as follows:

Radiolucent: A radiolucent structure is one that readily permits the passage of the x-ray beam and allows more x-rays to reach the film. If more x-rays reach the film, more silver halide crystals in the film emulsion are exposed and energized, thus resulting in increased deposits of black metallic silver. A radiograph with large deposits of black metallic silver appears black, or radiolucent.

As discussed in Chapter 8, structures that resist the passage of the x-ray beam appear white or *radiopaque* (see Figure 8-2), as follows:

Radiopaque: A radiopaque structure is one that resists the passage of the x-ray beam and restricts or limits the amount of x-rays that reach the film. If no x-rays reach the film, no silver halide crystals in the film emulsion are exposed, and no deposits of black metallic silver are seen. A radiograph with areas of unexposed silver halide crystals that have been removed during processing and with no black metallic silver deposits appears white, or radiopaque.

MANUAL FILM PROCESSING

Manual film processing (also known as *hand processing* or *tank processing*) is a simple method of developing, rinsing, fixing, and washing dental x-ray films. To process films manually, the dental radiographer must be knowledgeable about specific equipment requirements, step-by-step processing procedures, and care and maintenance of the equipment and supplies.

Film Processing Steps

Manual film processing consists of the following five steps:
1. Development
2. Rinsing
3. Fixing
4. Washing
5. Drying

Development

The first step in film processing is **development**. A chemical solution known as the developer is used in the development process. The purpose of the developer is to reduce the exposed, energized silver halide crystals chemically into black metallic silver. The developer solution softens the film emulsion during this process.

Rinsing

After development, a water bath is used to wash or rinse the film. **Rinsing** is necessary to remove the developer from the film and stop the development process.

Fixing

After rinsing, *fixing* takes place. A chemical solution known as the *fixer* is used in the fixing process. The purpose of the fixer is to remove the unexposed, unenergized silver halide crystals from the film emulsion. The fixer hardens the film emulsion during this process.

Washing

After **fixation**, a water bath is used to wash the film. A washing step is necessary to thoroughly remove all excess chemicals from the emulsion.

Drying

The final step in film processing is the drying of the films. Films may be air-dried at room temperature in a dust-free area or placed in a heated drying cabinet. Films must be completely dried before they can be handled for mounting and viewing.

Film Processing Solutions

Film processing solutions may be obtained in the following forms:

- Powder
- Ready-to-use liquid
- Liquid concentrate

Both the powder and the liquid concentrate forms must be mixed with distilled water. The liquid concentrate form is popular and is used in most dental offices; it is easy to mix and occupies little storage space (Figure 9-2). It is important to follow the manufacturer's recommendations for the preparation of such solutions.

Fresh chemicals produce the best radiographs. To maintain freshness, film processing solutions must be replenished daily and changed every 3 to 4 weeks; more frequent changing of solutions may be necessary when large numbers of films are processed. "Normal" use is defined as 30 intraoral films per day.

As described under Film Processing Steps, two special chemical solutions are necessary for film processing: developer and fixer.

Developer Solution

The developer solution contains four basic ingredients: (1) developing agent, (2) preservative, (3) accelerator, and (4) restrainer (Table 9-1).

Developing Agent. The **developing agent** (also known as the *reducing agent*) contains two chemicals, hydroquinone (paradihydroxybenzene) and Elon (monomethyl-para-aminophenol sulfate). The purpose of the developing agent is to reduce the exposed silver halide crystals chemically to black metallic silver.

Hydroquinone generates the black tones and the sharp contrast of the radiographic image. Hydroquinone is temperature sensitive; it is inactive below 60° F and very active above 80° F. Because this chemical is sensitive to temperature,

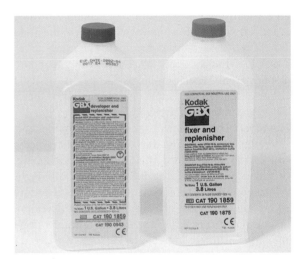

FIGURE 9-2 Liquid concentrates of developer and fixer. (From Bird DL, Robinson DS: *Modern dental assisting*, ed 10, St Louis, 2012, Saunders.)

TABLE **9-1**	Developer Composition	
Ingredient	**Chemical**	**Function**
Developing agent	Hydroquinone	Converts the exposed silver halide crystals to black metallic silver
		Slowly generates the black tones and contrast in the image
	Elon	Converts the exposed silver halide crystals to black metallic silver
		Quickly generates the gray tones in the image
Preservative	Sodium sulfite	Prevents rapid oxidation of the developing agents
Accelerator	Sodium carbonate	Activates the developer agents
		Provides the necessary alkaline environment for the developing agents
		Softens the gelatin of the film emulsion
Restrainer	Potassium bromide	Prevents the developer from developing the unexposed silver halide crystals

the temperature of the developing solution is critical. The optimal temperature for the developer solution is 68° F.

Elon, also known as *metol*, acts quickly to produce a visible radiographic image. Elon generates the many shades of gray seen on a dental radiograph. This chemical is not temperature sensitive. If hydroquinone and Elon were used individually and not in combination, Elon would produce a film that appeared gray with indistinct contrast, whereas hydroquinone would produce a film that appeared black and white. By using a combination of these chemicals, a film with black, white, and shades of gray is produced.

Preservative. The antioxidant **sodium sulfite** is the preservative used in the developer solution. The purpose of the **preservative** is to prevent the developer solution from oxidizing in the presence of air. The reducing agents hydroquinone and Elon are not stable in the presence of oxygen and readily absorb oxygen from the air. If these agents react with oxygen, the action of the developer solution is weakened. The preservative helps to prevent this weakening and to extend the useful life of hydroquinone and Elon.

Accelerator. The alkali **sodium carbonate** is used in the developer solution as an accelerator. The purpose of the **accelerator** (also called the *activator*) is to activate the developing agents. The developing agents are active only in an alkaline (high-pH) environment. For example, hydroquinone and Elon do not develop when used alone; the presence of an alkaline accelerator is required. The accelerator not only provides the necessary alkaline environment for the developing agents but also softens the gelatin of the film emulsion so that the developing agents can reach the silver halide crystals more effectively.

Restrainer. The restrainer used in the developing solution is **potassium bromide**. The purpose of the **restrainer** is to control the developer and to prevent it from developing the exposed and unexposed silver halide crystals. Although the restrainer stops the development of both exposed and unexposed crystals, it is most effective in stopping development of the unexposed crystals. As a result, the restrainer prevents the radiographic image from appearing fogged; a fogged film appears dull gray, lacks contrast, and is nondiagnostic.

Fixer Solution

The fixer solution contains four basic ingredients: (1) fixing agent, (2) preservative, (3) hardening agent, and (4) acidifier (Table 9-2).

Fixing Agent. The **fixing agent** (also known as the *clearing agent*) is made up of **sodium thiosulfate** or **ammonium thiosulfate** and is commonly called **hypo**. The purpose of the fixing agent is to remove or clear all unexposed and undeveloped silver halide crystals from the film emulsion. This chemical "clears" the film so that the black image produced by the developer becomes readily distinguished.

Preservative. The same preservative used in the developer solution, sodium sulfite, is also used in the fixer solution. The purpose of the preservative is to prevent the chemical deterioration of the fixing agent.

TABLE 9-2	**Fixer Composition**	
Ingredient	**Chemical**	**Function**
Fixing agent	Sodium thiosulfate; ammonium thiosulfate	Removes all the unexposed undeveloped silver halide crystals from the emulsion
Preservative	Sodium sulfite	Prevents the deterioration of the fixing agent
Hardening agent	Potassium alum	Shrinks and hardens the gelatin in the emulsion
Acidifier	Acetic acid; sulfuric acid	Neutralizes the alkaline developer and stops further development

Hardening Agent. The hardening agent used in the fixer solution is **potassium alum**. The purpose of the **hardening agent** is to harden and shrink the gelatin in the film emulsion after it has been softened by the accelerator in the developer solution.

Acidifier. The acidifier used in the fixer solution is **acetic acid** or **sulfuric acid**. The purpose of the **acidifier** is to neutralize the alkaline developer. Any unneutralized alkali may cause the unexposed crystals to continue to develop in the fixer. The acidifier also produces the necessary acidic environment required by the fixing agent.

Equipment Requirements

Dental x-ray film is processed in the darkroom using manual processing techniques or an automatic film processor. Special equipment is required for both manual film processing and automatic film processing.

Processing Tank

The essential piece of equipment required for **manual processing** is a **processing tank**. A processing tank is a container divided into compartments to hold the developer solution, water bath, and fixer solution. A processing tank has two insert tanks and one master tank (Figure 9-3), as follows:

- **Insert tanks.** Two removable 1-gallon insert tanks hold the developer and fixer solutions. Both are placed in the master tank. The developer solution is typically placed in the insert tank on the left, and the fixer solution is placed in the insert tank on the right. The water in the master tank separates the two insert tanks.
- **Master tank.** The master tank suspends both insert tanks and is filled with circulating water. The water surrounds both insert tanks. An overflow pipe is used to control the water level in the master tank.

Ideally, the processing tank should be constructed of stainless steel, which does not react with processing solutions and is easy to clean. The processing tank should be equipped

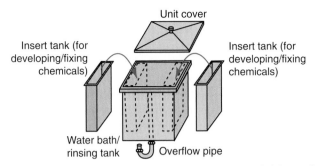

Unit cover

Insert tank (for developing/fixing chemicals)

Insert tank (for developing/fixing chemicals)

Water bath/ rinsing tank

Overflow pipe

FIGURE 9-3 Processing tanks showing developing and fixing tank inserts in bath of running water with overflow drain. (Modified from White SC, Pharoah MJ: *Oral radiology: principles and interpretation*, ed 6, St. Louis, 2009, Mosby.)

with a light-tight lid that is used to cover the solutions at all times. The cover protects the solutions from oxidation and evaporation, and during processing, it protects the developing films from exposure to light.

The temperatures of the developer and fixer solutions are controlled by the temperature of the circulating water in the master tank. A processing tank must be supplied with both hot and cold running water and a **mixing valve**. The water temperature is controlled through a mixing valve, which mixes the incoming hot and cold water (as in bathroom showers) to produce a water bath that maintains an optimum temperature of 68° F.

Equipment Accessories

In addition to a processing tank, a few accessory equipment items, including a thermometer, timer, and film hangers, are necessary for manual film processing.

Thermometer

A nonmercury **thermometer** is necessary for manual processing and is used to determine the temperature of the developer solution. A floating thermometer or one that is clipped to the side of the developer tank may be used (Figure 9-4). A thermometer containing metal or alcohol solution is recommended over one that contains mercury. Mercury is a toxic substance and spills must be handled according to Environmental Protection Agency (EPA) standards.

A thermometer must be placed directly in the developer solution and not in the water bath. Why? As previously stated, the temperature of the water in the master tank controls the temperature of the developer and fixer solutions in the insert tanks. The water in the master tank reaches the desired temperature almost as soon as it is turned on. The water, however, must circulate in the master tank for some time to equalize the temperatures of the processing solutions. Depending on the size of the insert tanks and the temperature of the solutions, the developer and fixer solutions may take up to 1 hour to reach the temperature of the water bath.

Using a thermometer, the developer temperature must be checked before processing. The optimum temperature for development is 68° F. Below 60° F, the chemicals work too

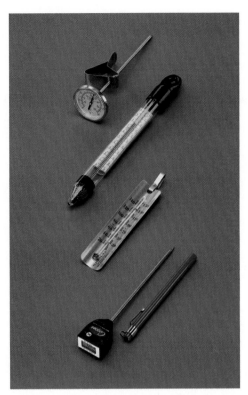

FIGURE 9-4 Examples of various thermometers used in manual film processing. (Courtesy Flow Dental, Deer Park, NY.)

slowly and result in underdevelopment. Over 80° F, the chemicals work too rapidly and produce film fog. The temperature of the developer determines development time. A time–temperature chart can be used to determine development time (Table 9-3). It is important to note that these temperatures refer to manual processing only. For automatic processor temperatures, refer to the section on automatic processing later in this chapter.

Timer

An accurate **timer** is also necessary for manual processing. X-ray film is processed in chemical solutions for specific intervals indicated by the manufacturer of the processing solutions. A timer is used to indicate such intervals (e.g., how long films have been placed in the developer solution, rinse water, fixer solution, and wash water). A timer is used to signal the radiographer that the films must be removed from the current processing solution. Development time depends on the temperature of the developer solution and must be adjusted based on time–temperature guidelines (see Table 9-3).

Film Hangers

Film hangers (also known as *film racks* or *processing hangers*) are necessary for manual processing. A film hanger is a device equipped with clips used to hold films during processing (Figure 9-5). Film hangers are made of stainless steel and include an identification tab or label. Film hangers are available in various sizes and can hold up to 20 intraoral films.

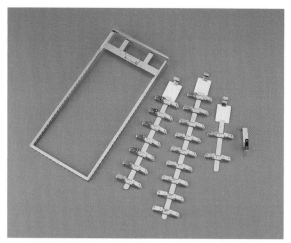

FIGURE 9-5 A variety of film hangers. (Courtesy Dentsply RINN Corporation, Elgin, IL.)

Miscellaneous Equipment

A **stirring rod** or **stirring paddle** is a necessary piece of equipment for manual processing. A stirring rod is used to agitate the developer and fixer solutions before processing. The stirring action mixes the chemicals and equalizes the temperature of the solutions. The stirring rod or paddle may be plastic or glass. Another useful item for manual processing is a *plastic apron*, which is used to protect clothing during the processing of films and the mixing of chemicals.

Step-by-Step Procedures

Before manual film processing, the exposed dental x-ray film and necessary equipment must be present in the darkroom. Specific infection control procedures that pertain to manual film processing are detailed in Chapter 15. For procedural steps, see Procedure 9-1.

PROCEDURE 9-1   Manual Film Processing

1. Identify the solutions.
   - Typically, the insert tank on the left is used for the developer, and the insert tank on the right is used for the fixer.
   - The fixer solution is easily identified by its vinegar-like odor.
2. Check the solution levels.
   - If the developer level is low, add fresh developer.
   - If the fixer level is low, add fresh fixer solution.
   - Never add water to raise the level of the solutions; it dilutes the strength of the chemicals.
3. Stir the solutions.
   - To avoid chemical contamination, use different paddles to stir the developer and the fixer.
   - Stirring the solutions mixes the chemicals and equalizes the temperature of the solutions.
4. Check the temperature.
   - Check the temperature of the developer solution.
   - The optimum temperature for the developer is between 68° F and 70° F; however, temperatures between 65° F and 75° F may be used.
   - If the temperature of the developer solution is outside this range, the circulating water temperature must be adjusted accordingly. Sufficient time must then be allowed for the developer to reach the correct temperature.
5. Label the hanger.
   - Label the film hanger with the name of the patient and the date of exposure.
6. Prepare the darkroom.
   - Close and lock the door of the darkroom.
   - Turn off the overhead white light, and turn on the safelights.

7. Unwrap the films.
   - For intraoral films, carefully unwrap each exposed film over a clean work surface (Figure 9-6, *A* to *C*), using proper infection control procedures (see Chapter 15).
   - Dispose of all film packet wrappings.
   - For extraoral films, carefully remove the film from the cassette.
   - Handle all films holding them on the edges only.
8. Load the hanger.
   - Clip each unwrapped film to the labeled film hanger, one film to a clip (Figure 9-6, *D*).
   - Verify that each film is securely attached by running a finger along the film edge.
   - Reattach any loose films.
9. Set the timer.
   - On the basis of the temperature of the developer solution and the manufacturer's instructions, set the timer.
   - A time–temperature chart is used to determine such time intervals (see Table 9-3).
   - If the optimal temperature of 68° F is used, the recommended development time is 4.5 to 5 minutes.
10. Immerse the films, and activate the timer.
    - Immerse the film hanger with films into the developer solution.
    - Films must not contact other films or the side of the processing tank during development.
    - Gently agitate the film hanger up and down several times to prevent air bubbles from clinging to the film.
    - Hang the film rack on the edge of the insert tank, and make certain that all films are immersed in the developer.
    - Activate the timer and cover the processing tank.

PROCEDURE **9-1**   **Manual Film Processing—cont'd**

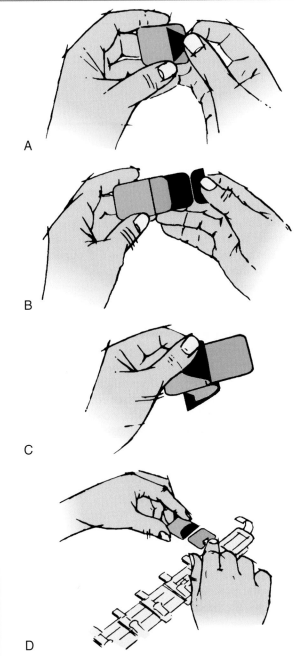

A

B

C

D

FIGURE 9-6 This figure illustrates uncontaminated films ready for processing. See Chapter 15, Figure 15-2, for removal of film barriers using proper infection control protocol. **A,** Pull the color-coded tab up and out to tear open the top of the packet. **B,** Pull on the black paper tab until about half of the black paper is out of the packet. **C,** Fold the black paper away from the film, put the clip on the film, and carefully remove the film from the packet. **D,** Clip film on hanger, one film to a clip. (Courtesy Carestream Health, Inc., Rochester, NY.)

11. Remove the films from the developer, and rinse them.
    • When the timer goes off, uncover the processing tank.
    • Remove the film hanger with films from the developer solution, and place it in the circulating water of the master tank.

• Agitate for 20 to 30 seconds.
• Remove and drain excess water for several seconds.

12. Determine the fix time.
    • On the basis of the development time, determine the fixation time and set the timer. A time–temperature chart is used to determine such time intervals (see Table 9-3).
    • Fixation time is approximately double the development time.

13. Immerse the films, and activate the timer.
    • Immerse the film hanger with films in the fixer solution.
    • Gently agitate it up and down several times.
    • Hang the film rack on the edge of the insert tank, and make certain that all films are immersed in the fixer.
    • Activate the timer and cover the processing tank.

14. Remove the films, and wash them.
    • When the timer goes off, uncover the processing tank, remove the film hanger with films from the fixer, and allow the excess fixer to drain back into the fixer tank.
    • Place the film hanger with films in the circulating water.
    • Allow the films to wash for a minimum of 20 minutes.

15. Dry the films.
    • Remove the film hanger with films from the wash water and gently shake off excess water.
    • Cover the processing tank.
    • To air-dry the films, suspend the film hanger with films from a rod or drying rack in a dust-free area over a drip pan.
    • If a heated drying cabinet is used, the temperature should not exceed 120° F.

16. Remove the films from the rack.
    • Remove the dry radiographs from the film hanger, and place them in an envelope labeled with the patient's name and date of exposure.
    • Outside the darkroom, use a viewbox to examine the radiographs, and place them in a labeled film mount.

17. Clean up.
    • After manual processing procedures have been completed, clean all processing equipment and work surfaces.
    • Make certain to clean hangers and clips after each use.
    • A clean darkroom is essential for the production of diagnostic radiographs.

TABLE 9-3	Processing Temperatures and Times			
Solution Temperature	Time in Developer (minutes)	Rinse Time (minutes)	Time in Fixer (minutes)	Wash Time (minutes)
65° F (18.5° C)	6.0	0.5	10–12	20
68° F (20.0° C)	5.0	0.5	10	20
70° F (21.0° C)	4.5	0.5	9–10	20
72° F (22.0° C)	4.0	0.5	8–9	20
75° F (24.0° C)	3.0	0.5	6–7	20
80° F (26.5° C)	2.5	0.5	5–6	20

Care and Maintenance

The processing solutions, equipment, and equipment accessories used in manual processing must be carefully maintained.

Processing Solutions

The manufacturer's instructions for the storage, mixing, and use of processing solutions must be carefully followed. Processing solutions deteriorate with exposure to air, continued use, and chemical contamination. Exhausted processing solutions result in nondiagnostic radiographs and therefore must be replaced. Processing solutions should be changed every 3 to 4 weeks; more frequent replacement of solutions may be necessary when large numbers of films are processed. Both the developer and the fixer solution should be changed at the same time. The processing solutions that require care and maintenance include the developer, fixer, and replenisher solutions.

Developer Solution. The developer solution becomes depleted from evaporation and the removal of small amounts from the tank on the film hanger and films. With time and use, the developer solution decreases not only in volume but in strength as well. A weakened or exhausted developer solution does not fully develop the latent image and produces a nondiagnostic radiograph with reduced density and contrast.

Six ounces of developer solution should be added to the developer tank at the beginning of each day. When the tank is holding its maximum capacity (e.g., 1 gallon), 6 ounces must be removed before adding the replenisher.

Fixer Solution. Fixer solution also decreases because of evaporation and the removal of small amounts from the tank on the film hanger and films. In addition, the fixer solution is diluted with water each time films are transferred from the rinse water to the fixer; this gradual dilution weakens the solution.

With time and use, the fixer solution decreases not only in volume but in strength as well. A full-strength fixer ensures adequate "clearing" of the film and hardening of the film emulsion. An exhausted or depleted fixer does not stop the chemical reaction sufficiently to maintain film clarity; the films will turn a yellow-brown color, transmit less light, and lose their diagnostic quality.

Three ounces of fixer solution should be added to the fixer tank at the beginning of each day. When the tank is holding its maximum capacity (e.g., 1 gallon), 3 ounces must be removed before adding the replenisher.

Replenisher Solutions. To maintain adequate freshness, strength, and solution levels, both the developer and the fixer solution must be replenished daily. A **replenisher** is a superconcentrated solution that is added to the processing solutions to compensate for the loss of volume and strength that results from oxidation. **Oxidation**, or the process that occurs when developer and fixer solutions combine with oxygen and lose strength, takes place when the processing solutions are exposed to air. A breakdown of the chemicals in the processing solutions results, shortening the length of time the solutions can be used to produce diagnostic radiographs. Replenishment maintains adequate concentrations of chemicals, which ensures uniform results between solution changes.

Processing Tank

The interaction between the mineral salts in water and the carbonate in the processing solutions produces deposits on the inside walls of the insert tanks. Such deposits contaminate the processing solutions. To produce diagnostic radiographs, the processing tank must be maintained in a clean state.

The master and insert tanks must be cleaned each time the solutions are changed. A commercial stainless steel tank cleaner or a solution of hydrochloric acid and water (1.5 ounces hydrochloric acid to 128 ounces of water) can be used to remove the mineral salts and carbonate deposits. Abrasive-type cleansers are not recommended for cleaning processing tanks; the cleansers may react unfavorably with the processing solutions. For procedural steps, see Procedure 9-2.

Miscellaneous Equipment

Cleanliness of manual processing equipment is essential. Film hangers and stirring paddles must be cleaned after each use. Both must be thoroughly cleaned, rinsed, and dried. The

PROCEDURE 9-2 **Cleaning the Processing Tank**

1. Drain the tanks.
   - Pull the drain plugs in the insert tanks and master tank.
   - Drain all liquid from each tank.
2. Clean and soak the tanks.
   - Pour cleaning solution into the master and insert tanks.
   - If the insert tanks are heavily coated with deposits, allow the tanks to soak for 30 minutes.
3. Scrub and rinse the tanks.
   - After soaking, use a brush to scrub all surfaces of the insert and master tanks as well as the tank cover.
   - Rinse thoroughly with water, wipe clean, and dry.
4. Add fresh solutions.
   - Pour fresh developer solution into the left insert tank and fresh fixer solution into the right insert tank.
   - Fill insert tanks until the solution level reaches the indicated fill line, about 1 inch from the top of the tank.
   - Fill the master tank with water.
5. Cover the tanks.
   - Place the lid on the processing tank.
   - The tank lid should be removed only when changing or adding solutions, when checking the developer temperature, or when processing films.

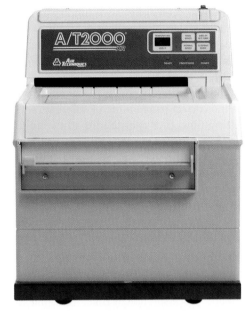

FIGURE 9-7 A typical automatic film processor used in the dental office. (Courtesy Air Techniques Inc., Melville, NY.)

plastic apron used to protect clothing should also be wiped clean after each use.

AUTOMATIC FILM PROCESSING

Automatic processing is another simple way of processing dental x-ray films.

Film Processing Steps

Automatic film processing consists of the following four steps:
   1. Development
   2. Fixing
   3. Washing
   4. Drying

The essential piece of equipment required for automatic processing is the automatic film processing machine, or **automatic processor**. A variety of automatic film processors are commercially available (Figure 9-7). Some automatic processors are limited to certain sizes of x-ray film, whereas others are capable of processing several different sizes of x-ray film. Some automatic film processors are restricted to use under safelight conditions, whereas others, with **daylight loaders**,

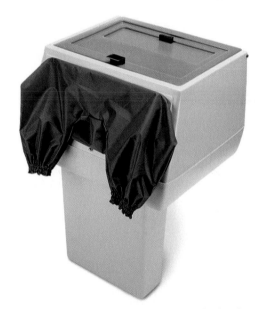

FIGURE 9-8 A daylight loader, which may be attached to the top of an automatic processor. (Courtesy Air Techniques Inc., Melville, NY.)

or light-shielded compartments, can be used in a room with white light (Figure 9-8). Automatic processors also vary in plumbing requirements and replenishment systems.

Automatic processing is often preferred over manual film processing for the following reasons:
   1. Less processing time is required.
   2. Time and temperatures are automatically controlled.
   3. Less equipment is used.
   4. Less space is required.

Automatic film processing has a number of advantages. The major advantage is the time saved; an automatic processor requires only 4 to 6 minutes to develop, fix, wash, and dry a film, whereas manual film processing techniques require approximately 1 hour. Another advantage is the automatic control of time and temperature; the automatic processor maintains the correct temperature of solutions and controls the processing time, thus contributing to the uniformity of film processing.

Although digital imaging is becoming more commonplace, many offices using digital imaging maintain automatic processing equipment in the event of a computer failure. When the automatic processor and special processing solutions are properly maintained, this equipment consistently produces high-quality radiographs, and operator error is less likely to occur.

Equipment Requirements

The automatic processor uses a roller transport system to move the unwrapped dental x-ray film through the developer, fixer, water, and drying compartments. Each component of the automatic processor contributes to the mechanism of automatic film processing and has a specific function (Figure 9-9), as follows:

- The **processor housing** encases all the component parts of the automatic processor.
- The **film feed slot** is an opening on the outside of the processor housing used to insert unwrapped films into the automatic processor.
- The **roller film transporter** is a system of rollers used to move the film rapidly through the developer, fixer, water, and drying compartments. The rollers are propelled by motor-driven gears or belts. The primary function of the rollers is to move the film through the automatic processor. In addition to moving the film, the rollers produce a wringing action that removes the excess solution from the emulsion as the film moves

from compartment to compartment. This "wringing action" eliminates the need for an additional rinse step between the developer and fixer solutions. The motion of the rollers also gently agitates the processing solutions, contributing to the uniformity of the processing.

- The **developer compartment** holds the developer solution. The developer solution used in an automatic processor is a specially formulated, highly concentrated chemical solution designed to react at temperatures between 80° F and 95° F. As a result of the high temperatures, development occurs rapidly. The developer solution used in manual film processing is not the same as the developer used in automatic film processing and should never be used in an automatic processor.
- The **fixer compartment** holds the fixer solution. The film is transported directly from the developer solution into the fixer *without* a rinsing step. The fixer solution used in an automatic processor is a specially formulated, highly concentrated chemical solution that contains additional hardening agents. In the fixer solution, the film is rapidly fixed or "cleared" and then hardened. The fixer solution used in manual film processing is not the same as the fixer used in automatic film processing and should *never* be used in an automatic processor.
- The **water compartment** holds circulating water. Water is used to wash the films after fixation. After washing, the wet film is transported from the water compartment to a drying chamber.
- The **drying chamber** holds heated air and is used to dry the wet film.
- A **replenisher pump** and **replenisher solutions** are used to maintain proper solution concentration and levels automatically in some automatic processors, whereas other processors require the operator to add the necessary replenishing solutions.

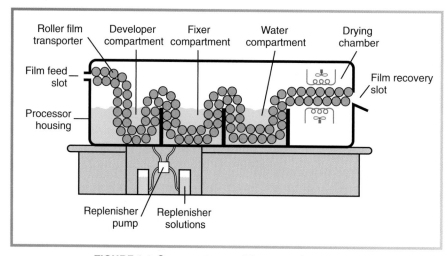

FIGURE 9-9 Component parts of the automatic processor.

- The **film recovery slot** is an opening on the outside of the processor housing where the dry, processed radiograph emerges from the automatic processor.

Step-by-Step Procedures

Before processing, the exposed dental x-ray film and automatic processor (without daylight loader) must be present in the darkroom. Specific infection control procedures that pertain to automatic film processing are detailed in Chapter 15. For procedural steps, see Procedure 9-3.

Care and Maintenance

The automatic processor and automatic processing solutions must be carefully maintained. The manufacturer's recommendations for care and maintenance must be followed meticulously.

PROCEDURE 9-3 **Automatic Film Processing**

1. Prepare the darkroom.
   - If a daylight loader is not part of the automatic processor, the films must be processed in the darkroom.
   - Close and lock the door of the darkroom, turn off the overhead white light, and turn on the safelights.
2. Prepare the films.
   - For intraoral films, carefully unwrap each exposed film over a clean work surface using proper infection control procedures (see Chapter 15).
   - Dispose of all film packet wrappings.
   - For extraoral films, carefully remove the film from the cassette.
   - Handle all films by the edges only.
3. Insert the films.
   - Insert each unwrapped film into the film feed slot of the processor, one at a time.
   - Allow at least 10 seconds between insertions of films.
   - Alternate sides or slots, whenever possible.
   - Make certain that films are straight as they are inserted. (When films are turned sideways or inserted too quickly, they overlap during processing. Overlapped films result in nondiagnostic radiographs.)
4. Process and retrieve the films.
   - After the films have been inserted into the automatic processor, allow 4 to 6 minutes for automated processing to occur.
   - Retrieve the processed radiographs from the film recovery slot on the outside of the automatic processor.

Automatic Processor

The automatic processor requires routine preventive maintenance. Without proper cleaning and replenishment, the automatic processor will malfunction. A cleaning and replenishment schedule must be established and followed strictly to ensure optimum automatic processor performance.

Depending on the volume of films processed, the automatic processor requires daily or weekly cleaning. An extraoral-size cleaning film used to clean the rollers of the automatic processor must be run through the processor at the beginning of each day. A **cleaning film** removes any residual gelatin or dirt from the rollers. Each week the rollers must be removed from the automatic processor, cleaned in warm running water, and then soaked for 10 to 20 minutes. The manufacturer's recommendations for daily and monthly cleaning of the automatic processor must be carefully followed.

Processing Solutions

Processing solution levels in the automatic processor must be checked at the beginning of each day and replenished as necessary. Failure to add **replenisher** results in exhausted solutions and nondiagnostic radiographs. Processing solutions in the automatic processor must be replaced every 2 to 6 weeks, depending on the number of films processed and the replenishment schedule. The manufacturer's recommendations for the changing of solutions must be carefully followed.

THE DARKROOM

The primary function of a **darkroom** is to provide a completely darkened environment in which x-ray film can be handled and processed to produce diagnostic radiographs. The darkroom must be properly designed and well equipped.

Room Requirements

A well-planned darkroom makes processing easier. The ideal darkroom is the result of careful planning and must have the following characteristics:

1. Convenient location
2. Adequate size
3. Correct lighting equipment
4. Ample work space with adequate storage
5. Temperature and humidity control

Location and Size

The location of the darkroom must be convenient; ideally, it should be located near the area where x-ray units are installed. The darkroom must be large enough to accommodate film processing equipment and to allow ample work space. A darkroom should measure at least 16 to 20 square feet and provide enough space for one person to work comfortably. The size of the darkroom is determined by the following factors:

1. Volume of radiographs processed
2. Number of persons using the room
3. Type of processing equipment used (processing tanks versus automatic processor)
4. Space required for duplication of films and storage

Lighting

As the term "darkroom" suggests, this room must be completely dark and must exclude all visible white light. The term **light-tight** is often used to describe the darkroom. To be considered light-tight, no light leaks can be present. Any white light that "leaks" into the darkroom (e.g., from around a door or through a vent) is termed a **light leak**. In a darkroom, when all the lights are turned off and the door is closed, no white light should be seen. Any white light coming around the door, through a vent or keyhole, or through a wall or ceiling seam is a light leak and must be corrected with weather stripping or black tape. As previously discussed, x-ray film is extremely sensitive to visible white light. Any leaks of white light in the darkroom cause film "fogging." A fogged film appears dull gray, lacks contrast, and is nondiagnostic.

Two types of lighting are essential in a darkroom, as follows:

- **Room lighting.** Incandescent room lighting is required for procedures not associated with the act of processing films. An overhead white light that provides adequate illumination for the size of the room is necessary to perform tasks such as cleaning, stocking materials, and mixing chemicals.
- **Safelighting.** The special type of lighting used to provide illumination in the darkroom is termed *safelighting*. It is a low-intensity light composed of long wavelengths in the red-orange portion of the visible light spectrum. Safelighting provides sufficient illumination in the darkroom to carry out processing activities safely without exposing or damaging the film. Safelighting does not rapidly affect unwrapped x-ray film and does not cause film fogging.

A safelight typically consists of a lamp equipped with a low-wattage bulb (7.5 or 15 watts) and a safelight filter. A **safelight filter** removes the short wavelengths in the blue-green portion of the visible light spectrum that are responsible for exposing and damaging x-ray film. At the same time, a safelight filter permits the passage of light in the red-orange range; consequently, the illumination in a darkroom is red. Most x-ray films have a reduced sensitivity to this red-orange range and are not affected by minimal exposure to the safelight.

Under safelight conditions, it is necessary to maintain an adequate safelight illumination distance and to keep film handling times to a minimum. Films that are unwrapped too close to the safelight or exposed to safelight illumination for more than 2 to 3 minutes appear fogged. A safelight must be placed a minimum of 4 feet (1.2 meters) away from the film and work area (Figure 9-10), and unwrapped

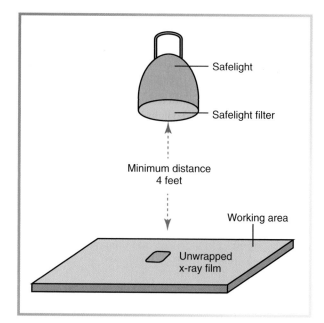

FIGURE 9-10 A minimum distance of 4 feet must exist between the safelight and the work area.

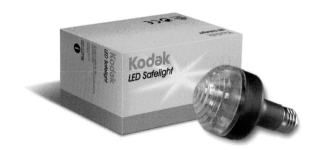

FIGURE 9-11 Safelights are available for intraoral and extraoral films. (Courtesy Carestream Health, Inc., Rochester, NY.)

films must be processed immediately under safelight conditions.

A number of safelights with different types of filters are available for use in the darkroom. Some safelights are used exclusively with intraoral films, some are used exclusively with extraoral films, and others are designed for use with both (Figure 9-11). For example, a good universal safelight filter recommended for use in a darkroom in which both extraoral screen films and intraoral films are processed is the GBX-2 safelight filter by Kodak. Recommendations for specific safelights and filters depend on the type of film (intraoral or extraoral) and are provided by the film manufacturer; such information is indicated on the outside of the film package.

Miscellaneous Requirements

The **darkroom work space** must include an adequate counter area where films can be unwrapped before processing. A clean, organized work area is essential; the work area must be kept absolutely clean, dry, and free of processing chemicals, water, dust, and debris. If an unwrapped film comes into contact with any such substance before processing, an "artifact" results, and the quality of the dental radiograph is compromised.

The **darkroom storage space** must include ample room for chemical processing solutions, film cassettes, and other miscellaneous radiographic supplies. Storage of unopened boxes of film in the darkroom is *not* recommended; a reaction between the fumes from chemical processing solutions and the film emulsion may occur that will result in film fogging. Boxes of opened extraoral film, however, must be stored in the darkroom. A light-tight storage drawer is necessary to protect opened boxes of unexposed extraoral film.

The temperature and **humidity level** of the darkroom must be controlled to prevent film damage. A room temperature of 70° F is recommended; if the room temperature exceeds 90°F, film fogging results. A relative humidity level of between 50% and 70% should be maintained. When humidity levels are too high, the film emulsion does not dry. When humidity levels are too low, static electricity becomes a problem and causes film artifacts.

The **darkroom plumbing** must include both hot and cold running water along with mixing valves to adjust the water temperature in the processing tanks. A utility sink with running water is also useful in the darkroom. Other miscellaneous darkroom requirements include boxed gloves, a wastebasket for the disposal of all film wrappings and contaminated gloves, and an x-ray viewbox that is used to examine radiographs.

Waste Management

Developer

Used developer is not typically a hazardous waste. It can be discharged to a sanitary sewer system. Unused developer may be hazardous because of a high pH. Check the material safety data sheet (MSDS) for the pH of the solution. If it is >12.5, it is considered hazardous. It is important to remember that developer is caustic and should be handled with care. If any question remains, the local sewer authority should be contacted prior to discharging. *Never* discharge used or unused developer to a septic system.

Fixer

Fixer solutions and rinse waters following fixer baths generally contain silver at concentrations of >5.0 ppm making them hazardous. Solutions should be run through a silver recovery unit to remove silver. After the silver is removed, the solutions may be discharged to the sanitary sewer system. Recovered silver must be disposed of via an approved waste carrier for recycling or disposal. If a silver recovery unit is not available, a company may be contacted to pick up the untreated fixer solutions. Store such solutions in labeled containers. *Never* discharge the fixer solution into a septic system.

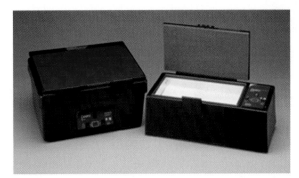

FIGURE 9-12 Examples of film duplicators. (Courtesy Dentsply RINN Corporation, Elgin, IL.)

Film

Developed films do not require special handling and may be disposed of along with normal office trash. Undeveloped film packets contain silver and lead; such packets should be collected in an approved waste container. When the container is full, an approved waste carrier or supplier should be contacted for removal. Lead foils may be collected separately in recycling containers that are located in the darkroom. When full, the container should be sent for recycling.

FILM DUPLICATION

An identical copy of an intraoral or an extraoral radiograph is made through the process of film duplication. Duplicate radiographs may be used when referring patients to specialists, for insurance claims, and as teaching aids (see Chapter 7). The dental radiographer must be familiar with the equipment requirements for film duplication and with the procedural steps for film duplication.

Equipment Requirements

The duplication of film requires the use of a **film duplicator** and **duplicating film**. A film duplicator is a light source that is commercially available from manufacturers, such as the Dentsply Rinn Corporation (Figure 9-12). A film duplicator provides a diffused light source that evenly exposes the special duplicating film.

Step-by-Step Procedures

Before film duplication, the films to be duplicated, the duplicating film, and the film duplicator must be present in the darkroom. Film duplication must take place in a light-tight darkroom. For procedural steps, see Procedure 9-4.

PROCESSING PROBLEMS AND SOLUTIONS

Processing problems may result in nondiagnostic radiographs. As described in Chapter 8, a diagnostic radiograph provides a great deal of information. Diagnostic images have proper density and contrast, have sharp outlines, and

PROCEDURE 9-4   **Film Duplication**

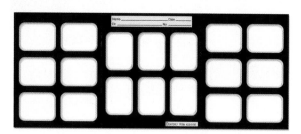

FIGURE 9-13 An x-ray "organizer," on which films are placed for duplication. (From Miles DA, Van Dis ML, Jensen CW, Ferretti A: *Radiographic imaging for dental auxiliaries*, ed 3, Philadelphia, 1999, Saunders.)

1. Arrange the radiographs.
   - Place the dental radiographs to be duplicated on the light screen of the film duplicator.
   - Use manufacturer-supplied film organizers to arrange the films and block out extraneous light (Figure 9-13).
2. Place the duplicating film.
   - Place the duplicating film on top of the arranged radiographs.
   - Place the emulsion side down. *Note:* The emulsion side will appear dull and gray or lavender in color.
3. Secure the duplicator lid.
   - Close the lid of the film duplicator, and fasten it securely to ensure adequate contact between the radiographs and the duplicating film. *Note:* To

prevent blurring of the image, good contact must be maintained between the duplicating film and the films that are being duplicated.
   - Without good contact, the duplicate film appears fuzzy and shows less detail than the original film.
4. Set the timer.
   - Select the exposure time, set the adjustable timer, and activate the light source to expose the duplicating film. *Note:* The exposure time is controlled by an adjustable timer on the film duplicator.
   - The adjustable timer controls the amount of light emitted from the film duplicator; the light passes through the radiographs and exposes the duplicating film. The longer the duplicating film is exposed to light, the lighter it appears. This is the opposite of x-ray film; x-ray film appears darker with longer exposure to light.
   - Exposure time depends on the type of duplicator used and the density of the radiographs being duplicated.
5. Process the film.
   - Process the duplicating film using manual processing techniques or the automatic processor.
6. Label the duplicate radiograph.
   - Label the processed duplicate radiographs with the patient's name and date of exposure.
   - Also, label the radiographs to indicate the patient's right (R) and left (L) sides.

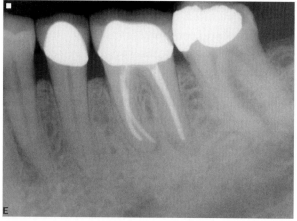

FIGURE 9-14 A diagnostic radiograph with images that exhibit proper density and contrast.

are of the same shape and size as the object radiographed (Figure 9-14).

Processing problems may occur for a number of reasons, including the following:
- Time and temperature errors (Table 9-4)
- Chemical contamination errors (Table 9-5)
- Film handling errors (Table 9-6)
- Lighting errors (Table 9-7)

Processing errors may cause a partial or total absence of images or obscure images that are present. Films that appear light, dark, yellow-brown, or fogged are the result of processing errors. Films that appear scratched or contaminated with dirt, saliva, or fingerprints are the result of faulty film handling during processing. Reticulation and fingernail and static artifacts may also result from poor processing and film handling techniques.

Many processing errors can be attributed to one or more causes. The dental radiographer must be able to recognize the appearance of common processing errors, identify potential causes of such errors, and know what steps are necessary to correct such problems.

Time and Temperature

Underdeveloped Film
- *Appearance.* The film appears light (Figure 9-15).
- *Problems.* **Underdeveloped films** may result from the following:
  - Inadequate development time
  - Inaccurate timer

TABLE **9-4**	Time and Temperature: Problems and Solutions		
Example	**Appearance**	**Problems**	**Solutions**
Underdeveloped film	Light	Inadequate development time	Check development time.
		Developer solution too cool	Check developer temperature.
		Inaccurate timer or thermometer	Replace faulty timer or thermometer.
		Depleted or contaminated developer solution	Replenish developer with fresh solutions as needed.
Overdeveloped film	Dark	Excessive developing time	Check development time.
		Developer solution too hot	Check developer temperature.
		Inaccurate timer or thermometer	Replace faulty timer or thermometer.
		Concentrated developer solution	Replenish developer with fresh solutions, as needed.
Reticulation of emulsion	Cracked	Sudden temperature change between developer and water bath	Check temperature of processing solutions and water bath; avoid drastic temperature differences.

TABLE **9-5**	Chemical Contamination: Problems and Solutions		
Example	**Appearance**	**Problems**	**Solutions**
Developer spots	Dark or black spots	Developer comes in contact with film before processing	Use a clean work area in the darkroom.
Fixer spots	White or light spots	Fixer comes in contact with film before processing	Use a clean work area in the darkroom.
Yellow-brown stains	Yellow-brown color	Exhausted developer or fixer	Replenish chemicals with fresh solutions, as needed.
		Insufficient fixation time	Use adequate fixation time.
		Insufficient rinsing	Rinse for a minimum of 20 minutes.

TABLE **9-6**	Film Handling: Problems and Solutions		
Example	**Appearance**	**Problems**	**Solutions**
Developer cutoff	Straight white border	Undeveloped portion of film due to low level of developer	Check developer level before processing; add solution if needed.
Fixer cutoff	Straight black border	Unfixed portion of film due to low level of fixer	Check fixer level before processing; add solution if needed.
Overlapped films	White or dark areas appear on film where overlapped	Two films contacting each other during processing	Separate films so that no contact takes place during processing.
Air bubbles	White spots	Air trapped on the film surface after being placed in the processing solutions	Gently agitate film racks after placing in processing solutions.
Fingernail artifact	Black crescent-shaped marks	Film emulsion damaged by operator's fingernail during rough handling	Gently handle films holding them on the edges only.
Fingerprint artifact	Black fingerprint	Film touched by fingers that are contaminated with fluoride or developer	Wash and dry hands thoroughly before processing films.
Static electricity	Thin, black, branching lines	Occurs when a film packet is opened quickly	Open film packets slowly.
		Occurs when a film pack is opened before radiographer touches a conductive object	Touch a conductive object before unwrapping films.
Scratched film	White lines	Soft emulsion removed from film by a sharp object	Use care when handling films and film racks.

TABLE 9-7 Lighting: Problems and Solutions

Example	Appearance	Problems	Solutions
Light leak	Exposed area appears black	Accidental exposure of film to white light	Examine film packets for defects before using. Never unwrap films in the presence of white light.
Fogged film	Gray; lack of detail and contrast	Improper safelighting	Check filter and bulb wattage of safelight.
		Light leaks in darkroom	Check darkroom for light leaks.
		Outdated films	Check the expiration date on film packages.
		Improper film storage	Store films in a cool, dry, protected area.
		Contaminated solutions	Avoid contaminated solutions by covering tanks after each use.
		Developer solution too hot	Check temperatures of developer.

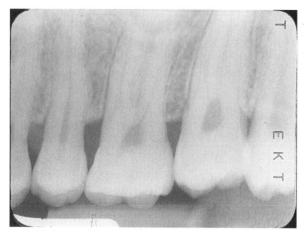

FIGURE 9-15 An underdeveloped film appears light.

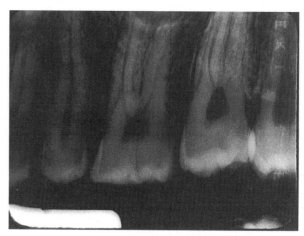

FIGURE 9-16 An overdeveloped film appears dark.

- Low developer temperature
- Inaccurate thermometer
- Depleted or contaminated developer solution
- *Solution.* To prevent underdeveloped films, do the following:
  - Check the temperature of the developer as well as the time the film must remain in the developer solution.
  - Increase the time the film remains in the developer, as needed.
  - Replace faulty and inaccurate thermometers and timers.
  - When the developer solution is depleted or contaminated, replace it.

Overdeveloped Film

- *Appearance.* The film appears dark (Figure 9-16).
- *Problems.* **Overdeveloped films** may result from the following:
  - Excess development time
  - Inaccurate timer
  - High developer temperature
  - Inaccurate thermometer
  - Concentrated (overactive) developer solution

- *Solution.* To prevent overdeveloped films, do the following:
  - Check the temperature of the developer and the time that the film should remain in the developer solution.
  - Decrease the time the film remains in the developer, as needed.
  - Replace faulty and inaccurate thermometers and timers.
  - If the developer solution is overactive, replace it.

Reticulation of Emulsion

- *Appearance.* The film appears cracked (Figure 9-17).
- *Problem.* **Reticulation of emulsion** results when a film is subjected to a sudden temperature change between the developer solution and the water bath.
- *Solution.* To prevent the reticulation of emulsion, do the following:
  - Check the temperatures of the processing solutions and of the water bath.
  - Avoid drastic temperature differences between the developer and the water bath.

Chemical Contamination

Developer Spots

- *Appearance.* Dark spots appear on the film (Figure 9-18).
- *Problem.* **Developer spots** are seen when the developer solution comes in contact with the film before processing.
- *Solution.* To avoid developer spots, do the following:
  - Use a clean work area in the darkroom.
  - To ensure a clean working surface, place a paper towel on the work area before unwrapping films.

Fixer Spots

- *Appearance.* White spots appear on the film (Figure 9-19).
- *Problem.* **Fixer spots** are the result of fixer solution coming in contact with the film before processing.
- *Solution.* To avoid fixer spots, do the following:
  - Use a clean work area in the darkroom.
  - To ensure a clean working surface, place a paper towel on the work area before unwrapping films.

Yellow-Brown Stains

- *Appearance.* The film appears yellowish brown (Figure 9-20).
- *Problems.* **Yellow-brown films** result from the following:
  - Use of exhausted developer or fixer
  - Insufficient fixation time
  - Insufficient rinsing
- *Solution.* To prevent yellow-brown films, do the following:
  - Replace the depleted developer and fixer solutions with fresh chemicals.
  - Make certain that films have adequate fixation time and adequate rinse time.
  - Rinse processed films for a minimum of 20 minutes in circulating cool water.

Film Handling

Developer Cutoff

- *Appearance.* A straight white border appears on the film (Figure 9-21).

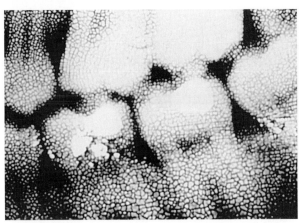

FIGURE 9-17 A film with a damaged emulsion appears cracked.

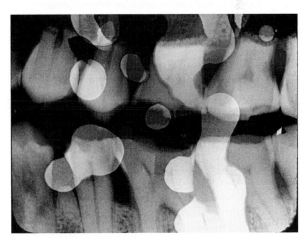

FIGURE 9-19 Fixer spots appear light or white.

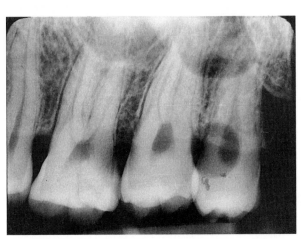

FIGURE 9-18 Developer spots appear dark or black.

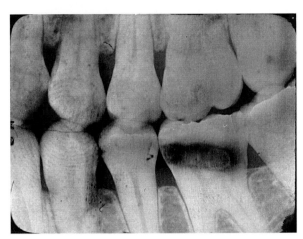

FIGURE 9-20 A number of processing errors may result in a yellow-brown film.

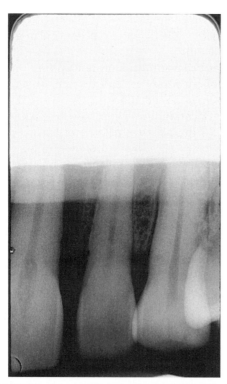

FIGURE 9-21 Developer cutoff appears as a straight white border on a film.

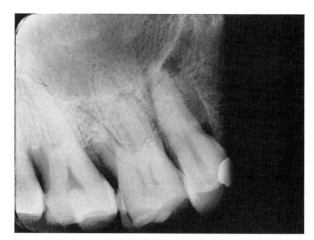

FIGURE 9-22 Fixer cutoff appears as a straight black border on a film.

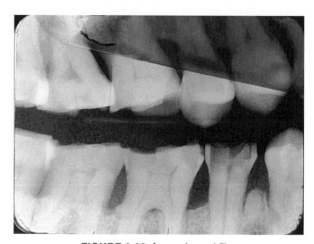

FIGURE 9-23 An overlapped film.

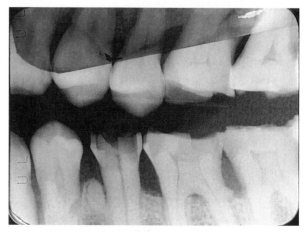

FIGURE 9-24 An overlapped film.

- *Problem.* **Developer cutoff** results from a low level of developer solution and represents an undeveloped portion of the film. If the developer solution level is low, the films clipped at the very top of the film rack may not be completely immersed in the developer solution.
- *Solution.* To avoid developer cutoff, do the following:
  - Check the developer level before processing films.
  - Add proper replenisher solution, if necessary.
  - Make certain that all films on the film rack are completely immersed in the developer solution.

Fixer Cutoff
- *Appearance.* A straight black border appears on the film (Figure 9-22).
- *Problem.* **Fixer cutoff** results from a low level of fixer solution and represents an unfixed portion of the film. If the fixer solution is low, the films clipped at the very top of the film rack may not be completely immersed in the fixer solution.
- *Solution.* To avoid fixer cutoff, do the following:
  - Check the fixer level before processing films.
  - Add proper replenisher solution if necessary.
  - Make certain that all films on the film rack are completely immersed in the fixer solution.

Overlapped Films
- *Appearance.* White or dark areas appear on films where overlap has occurred (Figures 9-23 and 9-24).

- *Problem.* **Overlapped films** occur when two films come into contact with each other during manual or automatic processing techniques. Films that overlap in the developer have white areas that represent an undeveloped portion of the film. Films that overlap in the fixer have black areas that represent an unfixed portion of the film.

- *Solution.* To avoid overlapped films, care should be taken to ensure that no film is permitted to come into contact with another film during processing.

Air Bubbles

- *Appearance.* White spots appear on the film (Figure 9-25).
- *Problem.* **Air bubbles** are seen when air is trapped on the film surface after the film is placed in the processing solution. Air bubbles prevent the chemicals from affecting the emulsion in that area.
- *Solution.* To avoid air bubbles, gently agitate and stir film racks after placing them in the processing solution.

Fingernail Artifact

- *Appearance.* Black, crescent-shaped marks appear on the film (Figure 9-26).
- *Problem.* A **fingernail artifact** is seen when the film emulsion is damaged by the operator's fingernail during rough handling of the film.
- *Solution.* To prevent a fingernail artifact, handle the film gently, holding it on the edges only.

Fingerprint Artifact

- *Appearance.* A black fingerprint appears on the film (Figure 9-27).
- *Problem.* A **fingerprint artifact** is seen when the film has been touched by fingers contaminated with fluoride or the developer.
- *Solution.* To prevent fingerprint artifacts, do the following:
  - Wash and dry hands thoroughly before processing films.
  - Work in a clean area to avoid contaminating the hands.
  - Handle the films by holding them on the edges only.

Static Electricity

- *Appearance.* Thin, black branching lines appear on the film (Figure 9-28).
- *Problem.* **Static electricity** may result from the following:
  - Opening a film packet quickly
  - Opening a film packet before touching another object such as the film processor or countertop in a carpeted office

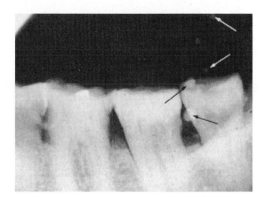

FIGURE 9-25 Air bubbles appear as tiny white spots (*arrows*). (From Langlais RP: *Exercises in oral radiology and interpretation,* ed 4, St. Louis, 2004, Saunders.)

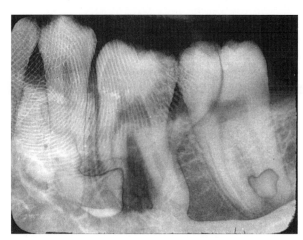

FIGURE 9-27 A black fingerprint artifact appears on the film.

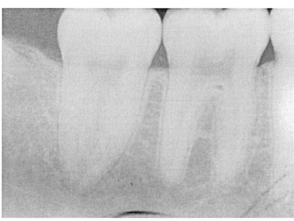

FIGURE 9-26 A fingernail artifact appears as a black, crescent-shaped mark.

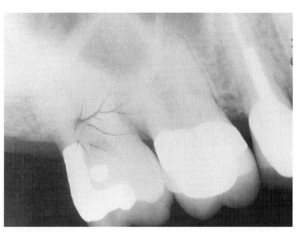

FIGURE 9-28 Static electricity appears as black branching lines.

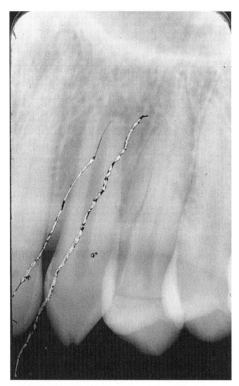

FIGURE 9-29 Scratches appear as thin white lines.

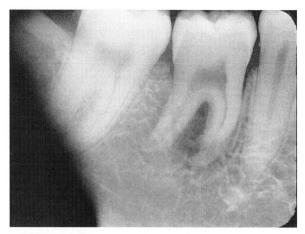

FIGURE 9-30 Portion of the film exposed to light appears black.

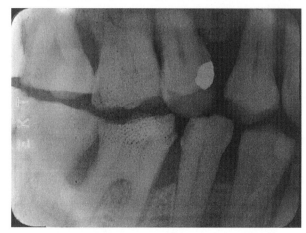

FIGURE 9-31 A fogged film appears gray and lacks detail and contrast.

Static electricity occurs most frequently during periods of low humidity.
- *Solution.* To prevent static electricity, do the following:
  - Always open film packets slowly.
  - In a carpeted office, touch a conductive object before unwrapping films.

Scratched Film
- *Appearance.* White lines appear on the film (Figure 9-29).
- *Problem.* A **scratched film** results when the soft film emulsion is removed from the film base by a sharp object, such as a film clip or film hanger.
- *Solution.* To prevent a scratched film, do the following:
  - Use care when placing a film rack in the processing solutions.
  - Avoid contact with other film hangers.

Lighting
Light Leak
- *Appearance.* The exposed area appears black (Figure 9-30).
- *Problems.* A **light leak** results from the following:
  - Accidental exposure of the film to white light
  - Torn or defective film packets that expose a portion of the film to light
- *Solution.* To prevent light leaks, do the following:
  - Examine film packets for minute tears or defects before use.
  - Do not use film packets that are torn or defective.
  - Never unwrap films in the presence of white light.

Fogged Film
- *Appearance.* The film appears gray and lacks image detail and contrast (Figure 9-31).
- *Problems.* **Fogged films** result from the following:
  - Improper safelighting and light leaks in the darkroom
  - Improper film storage
  - Outdated films
  - Contaminated processing solutions
  - High developer temperature
- *Solution.* To prevent fogged films, do the following:
  - Check the filter and bulb wattage of the safelight.
  - Minimize film exposure to the safelight, and check the darkroom for light leaks.
  - Check the expiration date on film packages, and store films in a cool, dry, protected area.
  - Avoid contamination of processing solutions by replacing tank covers after each use.
  - Always check the temperature of the developer before processing films.

SUMMARY

- Film processing refers to a series of steps that produce a visible permanent image on a dental radiograph.
- The pattern of stored energy on an exposed film is termed the *latent image*; this image remains invisible until it undergoes processing.
- The visible image that results on a dental radiograph is made up of black, white, and gray areas.
- Manual film processing includes five steps: (1) development, (2) rinsing, (3) fixation, (4) washing, and (5) drying.
- A chemical solution known as the *developer* is used in the development process to reduce the exposed, energized silver halide crystals to chemically black metallic silver.
- The developer solution contains four basic ingredients: (1) developing agent, (2) preservative, (3) accelerator, and (4) restrainer.
- After development, a water bath is used to wash or rinse the film.
- After rinsing, fixation takes place.
- The fixer solution contains four basic ingredients: (1) fixing agent, (2) preservative, (3) hardening agent, and (4) acidifier.
- After fixation, a water bath is used to wash the film and remove all excess chemicals from the emulsion.
- The final step in film processing is drying the film. Films must be completely dried before they can be handled for mounting and viewing.
- Manual processing is a simple method used to develop, rinse, fix, and wash dental x-ray films. The essential equipment is a processing tank, which is divided into compartments for the developer solution, water bath, and fixer solution.
- Automatic processing is another simple way to process dental x-ray film. The essential equipment required is the automatic processor, which automates all film-processing steps.

- A darkroom is a completely darkened room, where x-ray film can be handled and processed to produce diagnostic radiographs. The ideal darkroom should be conveniently located, of adequate size, equipped with correct lighting and ventilation, and arranged with ample work space and storage.
- The darkroom must be light-tight and must include proper safelighting. Safelighting provides illumination in the darkroom to perform processing activities safely without exposing or damaging the film.
- An identical copy of an intraoral or extraoral radiograph is made through the process of film duplication. Duplication of film requires the use of a film duplicator and a duplicating film.
- A number of processing problems may result in nondiagnostic films. Processing problems may result from time and temperature errors (see Table 9-4), chemical contamination errors (see Table 9-5), film handling errors (see Table 9-6), and lighting errors (see Table 9-7).
- The dental radiographer must be able to recognize the appearance of common processing errors, identify the potential causes of such errors, and know what steps are necessary to correct such problems.

BIBLIOGRAPHY

Frommer HH, Savage-Stabulas JJ: Film processing: the darkroom. In *Radiology for the dental professional*, ed 9, St Louis, 2011, Mosby.

Haring JI, Lind LJ: Film exposure, processing, and technique errors. In *Radiographic interpretation for the dental hygienist*, Philadelphia, 1993, Saunders.

Johnson ON, Thomson EM: Dental x-ray film processing. In *Essentials of dental radiography for dental assistants and hygienists*, ed 8, Upper Saddle River, NJ, 2007, Pearson.

Miles DA, Van Dis ML, Jensen CW, Ferretti A: Film processing and quality assurance. In *Radiographic imaging for the dental team*, ed 4, St. Louis, 2009, Saunders.

White SC, Pharoah MJ: Processing x-ray film. In *Oral radiology: principles of interpretation*, ed 6, St Louis, 2009, Mosby.

QUIZ QUESTIONS

MULTIPLE CHOICE

___ 1. The first step in manual film processing is:
   a. development
   b. rinsing
   c. fixation
   d. washing
   e. drying

___ 2. In manual film processing, the rinsing step is necessary because:
   a. rinsing removes the silver halide crystals from the emulsion
   b. rinsing slows down the fixation process
   c. rinsing removes the developer from the film and stops the development process
   d. rinsing thoroughly removes all excess chemicals from the emulsion
   e. rinsing reduces the energized silver halide crystals to black metallic silver

____ 3. The film emulsion is hardened during:
   a. development
   b. rinsing
   c. fixation
   d. washing
   e. drying

____ 4. The hydroquinone in the developer brings out the
   _____ tones, whereas the Elon in the
   developer brings out the _____ tones on a
   dental radiograph.
   a. black; white
   b. white; black
   c. gray; gray
   d. white; gray
   e. black; gray

____ 5. In manual film processing, the optimal
   temperature for the developer solution is:
   a. 55° F
   b. 68° F
   c. 78° F
   d. 80° F
   e. 90° F

____ 6. The size of a darkroom is determined by all the
   following factors except:
   a. volume of radiographs processed
   b. type of processing equipment used
   c. humidity level of the room
   d. space required for duplication of films
   e. number of persons using the room

____ 7. Any leaks of white light into the darkroom will
   cause:
   a. film fogging
   b. film reticulation
   c. overdeveloped films
   d. underexposed films
   e. any of the above

____ 8. The safelight must be placed a minimum of what
   distance from the film and the work area?
   a. 1 foot
   b. 2 feet
   c. 3 feet
   d. 4 feet
   e. 5 feet

____ 9. The GBX-2 safelight filter by Kodak is
   recommended for:
   a. intraoral films only
   b. extraoral screen films only
   c. extraoral nonscreen films only
   d. intraoral and extraoral films
   e. none of the above

____ 10. Unopened boxes of radiographic film should not
   be stored in the darkroom because:
   a. chemical fumes from processing solutions may
      fog the film
   b. continued exposure to the safelight is not
      recommended
   c. the box may have a tear that may expose the
      film
   d. processing solutions could splash onto the
      boxes of film
   e. all of the above

____ 11. The thermometer for manual processing should be
   placed in the:
   a. developer solution
   b. water bath
   c. fixer solution
   d. either a or c
   e. all of the above

____ 12. At 68° F, what is the optimal development time for
   manual film processing?
   a. 2 minutes
   b. 3 minutes
   c. 4 minutes
   d. 5 minutes
   e. 6 minutes

____ 13. All the following factors affect the life of the
   processing solutions except:
   a. number of films processed
   b. care in preparation of solutions
   c. type of safelight filter used
   d. age of solutions
   e. proper care and maintenance of the automatic
      processor

____ 14. A replenisher is added to the processing solution
   to:
   a. compensate for the loss of solution strength
   b. ensure uniform results between solution
      changes
   c. compensate for the loss of volume of solution
   d. compensate for oxidation
   e. all of the above

____ 15. How often should the processing tank be cleaned?
   a. once per week
   b. once per month
   c. once per day
   d. whenever solutions are changed
   e. none of the above

____ 16. Which of the following can be used to clean the
   processing tank?
   a. commercial tank cleaner
   b. hydrochloric acid and water solution
   c. abrasive-type cleansers
   d. both a and b
   e. all of the above

___ **17.** A breakdown of chemicals in the processing
solution that results from exposure to air is
termed:
a. reduction
b. selective reduction
c. oxidation
d. replenishment
e. none of the above

___ **18.** The superconcentrated solution that is added to
the processing solution to compensate for the
effects of oxidation is termed the:
a. acidifier
b. hardener
c. oxidizer
d. replenisher
e. emulsifier

MATCHING
*For questions 19 to 28, match each component part of the
automatic processor with its function.*
a. Opening used to insert films
b. Opening where processed films emerge
c. Holds fixer solution
d. Heated air is used to dry wet films
e. Holds developer solution
f. Solutions used to maintain proper concentration and
levels of developer and fixer
g. Moves the film through the automatic processor
h. Encases component parts of automatic processor
i. Delivers developer and fixer solution to compartments
j. Holds circulating water

___ **19.** processor housing
___ **20.** film/feed slot
___ **21.** roller film transporter
___ **22.** film recovery slot
___ **23.** drying chamber
___ **24.** water compartment
___ **25.** fixer compartment
___ **26.** developer compartment
___ **27.** replenisher solutions
___ **28.** replenisher pump

FILL IN THE BLANK
29. List the two equipment requirements for film
duplication.

_____

_____

30. Discuss how exposure time affects the density of
duplicating film.

_____

_____

MATCHING
*For questions 31 to 36, describe the appearance of the
processing error using one of the following words:*
a. light
b. white
c. black
d. dark
e. gray

___ **31.** fogged film
___ **32.** overdeveloped film
___ **33.** underdeveloped film
___ **34.** light leak
___ **35.** developer cutoff
___ **36.** fixer cutoff

IDENTIFICATION
*For questions 37 to 45, describe or identify the processing error
that causes the following:*

37. Black spots

_____

_____

38. White spots

_____

_____

39. Yellow-brown stains

_____

_____

40. Cracked appearance

_____

_____

41. Straight white border

_____

_____

42. Straight black border

_____

_____

43. Black, crescent-shaped marks

_____

_____

44. Thin, black branching lines

_____

_____

45. White lines

_____

_____

TRUE OR FALSE

For questions 46 to 50, identify each statement as true or false.

____ **46.** Film fogging results from improper safelighting.

____ **47.** Yellow-brown stains result from insufficient development time.

____ **48.** Developer cutoff appears as a straight black border across the film.

____ **49.** To avoid static electricity, touch a conductive object before unwrapping a film.

____ **50.** Torn or defective film packets may allow a portion of the film to be exposed to light.

chapter 10

Quality Assurance in the Dental Office

OUTLINE

QUALITY CONTROL TESTS
    Equipment and Supplies
    Film Processing
    Digital Imaging

QUALITY ADMINISTRATION PROCEDURES
OPERATOR COMPETENCE

LEARNING OBJECTIVES

After completion of this chapter, the student will be able to do the following:

- Define the key words associated with quality assurance in the dental office
- List quality control tests and quality administration procedures that should be included in the quality assurance plan
- Discuss the purpose and frequency of testing dental x-ray machines
- Describe the tests used to check for fresh film and adequate film-screen contact; discuss the frequency of testing and the interpretation of test results
- Describe the test used to check for darkroom light leaks and proper safelighting. Discuss the frequency of testing and the interpretation of test results
- Describe the test used to check the automatic processor; discuss the frequency of testing and the interpretation of test results

- List the three tests used to check the strength of the developer solution
- Describe the preparation of the reference radiograph and the standard stepwedge radiograph; discuss the use of these radiographs to compare densities and to monitor the strength of the developer solution
- Describe the test used to check the strength of the fixer; discuss the frequency of testing and the interpretation of test results
- Discuss the basic elements of a quality administration plan
- Detail the importance of operator competence in dental radiographic procedures

KEY TERMS

Normalizing device
Quality administration
Quality assurance

Quality control tests
Radiograph, reference

Stepwedge
Viewbox

Quality assurance refers to special procedures that are used to assure (i.e., ensure) the production of high-quality diagnostic radiographs. A quality assurance plan includes both quality control tests and quality administration procedures (Box 10-1). Although the dentist is ultimately responsible for the overall quality assurance plan, the dental radiographer can play an important role in the implementation and administration of such a plan. The dental radiographer must be knowledgeable about the quality assurance program used in the dental office.

The purpose of this chapter is to introduce the dental radiographer to quality control tests that are used to monitor dental x-ray equipment, supplies, and film processing. Quality administration procedures and operator competence for the dental office are also discussed.

QUALITY CONTROL TESTS

Quality control tests are specific tests that are used to maintain and monitor dental x-ray equipment, supplies, and film processing. To avoid excess exposure of patients and personnel to x-radiation, the dental radiographer must have a clear understanding of the quality control procedures used to test specific equipment, supplies, and film processing in the dental office.

Equipment and Supplies

Quality control tests are necessary to monitor dental x-ray machines, dental x-ray film, screens and cassettes, and viewing equipment. To produce diagnostic-quality radiographs consistently, dental x-ray equipment and supplies must always function properly and be kept in good repair.

Dental X-Ray Machines

All dental x-ray machines must be inspected and monitored periodically. Some state and local regulatory agencies provide dental x-ray equipment inspection services as part of their registration and licensing procedures. Dental x-ray machines must also be calibrated—or adjusted for accuracy—at regular intervals. A qualified technician must calibrate dental x-ray equipment to ensure consistent x-ray machine performance and the production of diagnostic radiographs.

The American Academy of Dental Radiology recommends a number of annual tests for dental x-ray machines. These tests are designed to identify minor malfunctions, including machine output variations, inadequate collimation, tubehead drift, timing errors, and inaccurate kilovoltage and milliamperage readings (Box 10-2).

Annual tests for dental x-ray machines can be performed by the dentist, dental hygienist, dental assistant, or manufacturer's service representative. Most of the tests require some basic testing materials, film, and test logs to record the results.

Dental X-Ray Film

As discussed in Chapter 7, the dental x-ray film must be properly stored, protected, and used before the expiration date. For quality control purposes, when each box of film is opened, it should be tested for freshness.

The following fresh film test is recommended to check a newly opened box of film:

1. *Prepare the film.* Unwrap one unexposed film from a newly opened box.
2. *Process the film.* Use fresh chemicals to process the unexposed film.

The results of the fresh film test can be interpreted as follows:

- *Fresh film.* If the processed film appears clear with a slight blue tint, the film is fresh and has been properly stored and protected. Proceed with the use of this film.
- *Fogged film.* Film that has expired, has been improperly stored, or has been exposed to radiation appears fogged. If the film is fogged, it should not be used.

Screens and Cassettes

Extraoral intensifying screens used within a cassette holder should be periodically examined for the presence of any dirt and scratches. Screens should be cleaned on a monthly basis with commercially available cleaners recommended by the screen manufacturer. After cleaning the screen, an antistatic solution should be applied to it. Screens that have scratches should be replaced.

Cassette holders must be examined every month for worn closures, light leaks, and warping, all of which may result in fogged and blurred radiographs; these cassettes must be repaired or replaced. Cassettes must also be checked for adequate film-to-screen contact.

The following film-to-screen contact test is recommended:

1. Insert one film between the screens in the cassette holder.
2. Place a wire mesh test object on top of the loaded cassette.
3. Position the position-indicating device (PID) using a 40-inch target-film distance while directing the central ray perpendicular to the cassette.
4. Expose the film using 10 mA, 70 kVp, and 15 impulses.
5. Process the exposed film.
6. Check the film on a viewbox in a dimly lit room at a distance of 6 ft.

FIGURE 10-1 Illustrations of film-to-screen contact. *Left*, Cassette exhibiting good film-screen contact. *Right*, Cassette exhibiting poor film-screen contact. (Courtesy Carestream Health, Inc., Rochester, NY.)

The results of the film-screen contact test can be interpreted as follows:
- *Adequate contact.* If the "wire mesh" image seen on the film exhibits a uniform density, good film-to-screen contact has taken place. Proceed with cassette and screen use.
- *Inadequate contact.* If the wire mesh image seen on the film exhibits varying densities, poor film-to-screen contact has taken place. Areas of poor film-to-screen contact appear darker than good contact areas (Figure 10-1). Cassettes that provide inadequate film-to-screen contact and exhibit areas of poor contact in the central position must be repaired or replaced.

Viewing Equipment

The **viewbox**, or illuminator, is a light source that is used to view dental radiographs (Figure 10-2). A working viewbox is a necessary piece or equipment for the interpretation of dental radiographs. The viewbox contains fluorescent light bulbs that emit light through an opaque plastic or plexiglass front. The viewbox should emit a uniform and subdued light when it is functioning properly. A photographic light meter can be used to determine proper viewing brightness.

The viewbox should be periodically examined for the presence of dirt on the plexiglass surface and any discoloration. The surface of the viewbox should be wiped clean every week. Permanently discolored plexiglass surfaces must be replaced. Any blackened fluorescent light bulbs must also be replaced.

Film Processing

Film processing is one of the most critical areas in quality control and requires daily monitoring. Processing problems have the potential to result in a large number of nondiagnostic radiographs. Quality control tests must be performed routinely to determine whether the conditions for film processing are acceptable.

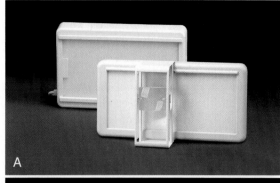
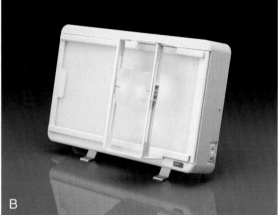
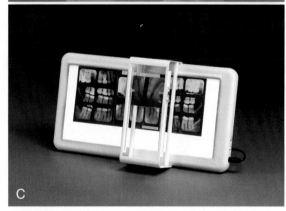

FIGURE 10-2 Examples of viewboxes in sizes to accommodate most dental viewing needs. (Courtesy Dentsply Rinn, Elgin, IL.)

Darkroom Lighting

The darkroom must be checked for light-tightness every month and proper safelighting every 6 months. The following light leak test is recommended for the darkroom:
1. Prepare the darkroom. Close the darkroom door, and turn off all lights, including the safelight.
2. Examine the darkroom. Once your eyes become accustomed to the darkness, observe the areas around the door, the seams of the walls and ceiling, the vent areas, and the keyhole for light leaks.

The results of the light leak test can be interpreted as follows:
- *No light leaks.* If the darkroom is light-tight, no visible light is seen. Proceed with film processing.

- *Light leaks.* Light leaks, if present, are seen around the door, through the seams of the walls or ceiling, or through a vent or keyhole. Light leaks must be eliminated by using weather stripping or black tape before proceeding with film processing.

Only *after* the light-tightness of the darkroom has been established can the safelighting be checked. The following safelighting test, often referred to as the *coin test*, is recommended:

1. Prepare the darkroom. Turn off all the lights in the darkroom, including the safelight.
2. Prepare the film. Unwrap one unexposed film. Place it on a flat surface at least 4 ft from the safelight. Place a coin on top of the film.
3. Turn on the safelight. Allow the film and the coin to be exposed to the safelight for 3 to 4 minutes.
4. Remove the coin, and process the film.

The results of the safelighting test can be interpreted as follows:

- *Proper safelighting.* If no visible image is seen on the processed radiograph, the safelighting is correct. Proceed with film processing.
- *Improper safelighting.* If the image of the coin and a fogged background appear on the processed radiograph, the safelight is not safe to use with that type of film (Figure 10-3). As discussed in Chapter 9, to avoid safelighting problems, the dental radiographer must use the film manufacturer's recommended safelight filters and bulb wattages. In addition, the film must be unwrapped at least 4 ft away from the safelight. Safelighting problems must be corrected before proceeding with film processing.

Processing Equipment

Processing equipment must be meticulously maintained and monitored daily. As discussed in Chapter 9, the thermometer and timer must be checked for accuracy with manual processing techniques. The temperature and level of the water bath, the developer, and the fixer solutions must also be monitored when manual processing techniques are used. The processing time and temperature recommendations of the film manufacturer must be strictly followed.

If automatic processing equipment is used, the water circulation system must be checked, and the solution level, the replenishment system, and the temperatures must be monitored. The manufacturer's procedure and maintenance directions must be followed carefully. Each day, two test films should be processed in the automatic processor. The following automatic processor test films are recommended:

1. *Prepare the films.* Unwrap two unexposed films; expose one to light.
2. *Process both films* in the automatic processor.

The results of the automatic processor test films can be interpreted as follows:

- *Functioning processor.* If the unexposed film appears clear and dry, and if the film exposed to light appears

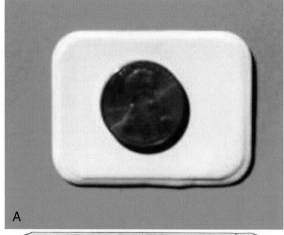

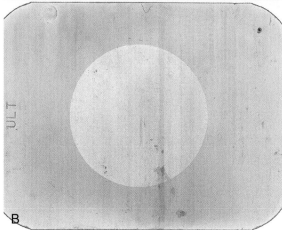

FIGURE 10-3 Coin test for safelighting. **A,** Coin placed on unexposed film under safelight. **B,** Developed film showing outline of coin indicating that safelight intensity is too great and is not safe. (From Bird DL, Robinson DS: *Modern dental assisting*, ed 10, St Louis, 2012, Saunders.)

black and dry, the automatic processor is functioning properly. Proceed with processing.

- *Nonfunctioning processor.* If the unexposed film does not appear clear and dry, and if the exposed film does not appear completely black and dry, the processing solutions and dryer temperature must be checked. Corrections must be made before proceeding with processing.

Processing Solutions

The most critical component of film processing quality control is the monitoring of the processing solutions. As discussed in Chapter 9, the processing solutions must be replenished daily and changed every 3 to 4 weeks as recommended by the manufacturer. As an alternative to using the calendar to determine the freshness of solutions, quality control tests can be used to monitor the strength of the developer and fixer solutions. Processing solutions must be evaluated each day before any patient films are processed.

Developer Strength. When the developer solution loses strength, the time–temperature recommendations of the

TABLE 10-1	Quality Control Tests for Film Processing		
Day	**Solution Strength**	**Quality Control Tests**	**Test Results**
1	Use fresh, full-strength processing solutions.	*Reference radiograph:* Using correct exposure factors, expose and process one film. This film becomes the "reference radiograph."	The reference radiograph demonstrates optimal film contrast and density.
		Stepwedge radiograph: Expose 20 stepwedge films; process one film. This film becomes the "standard radiograph."	The standard radiograph demonstrates optimal film contrast and density.
2, 3, etc.	Fresh processing solutions weaken with time and use; exhausted solutions result.	*Reference radiograph:* Each day, expose and process one film to compare with the reference radiograph.	Compare the daily film with the reference radiograph: 1. If densities match, continue processing. 2. If densities do not match, replace processing solutions.
		Stepwedge radiograph: Each day, process one of the previously exposed stepwedge films.	Compare the daily film with the standard radiograph: 1. If densities match, continue processing. 2. If the densities differ by more than two steps on the stepwedge, replace processing solutions.

manufacturer can no longer be used as the standard of measurement. An easy way to check the strength of the developer solution is to compare film densities to a standard. One of the following tests can be used (Table 10-1):

- Reference radiograph
- Stepwedge radiographs
- Normalizing device

Reference Radiograph. A **reference radiograph** is one that is processed under ideal conditions and then used to compare the film densities of radiographs that are processed daily. The following steps can be taken to create a reference radiograph:

1. *Prepare the film.* Use fresh film to make a reference radiograph.
2. *Expose the film,* using correct exposure factors.
3. *Process the film,* using fresh chemicals at the recommended time and temperature.
4. *View the reference radiograph and the daily radiographs side by side on a viewbox.* Compare the densities on the reference radiograph with the densities on the daily radiographs.

Comparison of daily radiographs with the reference radiograph can be interpreted as follows:

- *Matched densities.* If the densities seen on the reference radiograph match the densities seen on the daily radiographs, the developer solution strength is adequate. Proceed with processing.
- *Unmatched densities.* If the densities seen on the daily radiographs appear *lighter* than those seen on the reference radiograph, the developer solution is either weak

or cold. If the densities seen on the daily radiographs appear *darker* than those seen on the reference radiograph, the developer solution is either too concentrated or too warm. Weakened or concentrated developer solution must be replaced. If the developer solution is too cool or too warm, the temperature must be adjusted.

Stepwedge Radiographs. As described in Chapter 8, a **stepwedge** is a device constructed of layered aluminum steps. Aluminum stepwedges are commercially available and may be purchased from a number of sources, including Margraf Dental Manufacturing Inc. (www.margrafcorp.com). When a stepwedge is placed on top of a film and then exposed to x-rays, the different steps absorb varying amounts of x-rays. When processed, different film densities are seen on the dental radiograph as a result of the stepwedge (see Figure 8-6). The following steps can be taken to create stepwedge radiographs:

1. *Prepare the film.* Use a total of 20 fresh films to create a supply of films for daily testing. Place an aluminum stepwedge on top of one film.
2. *Expose the film.* Repeat with the remaining films using the same stepwedge and exposure factors.
3. *Using fresh chemicals, process only one of the exposed films.* This processed radiograph will exhibit different densities as a result of the stepwedge and is known as the *standard stepwedge radiograph.*
4. *Store the remaining 19 exposed films in a cool, dry area protected from x-radiation.*
5. *Each day, after the chemicals have been replenished, process one of the exposed stepwedge films.*

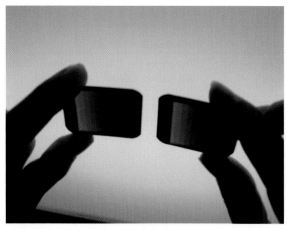

FIGURE 10-4 The daily stepwedge film should appear identical to the control (standard) film. (From Miles DA, Van Dis ML, Razmus TF: *Basic principles of oral and maxillofacial radiology*, Philadelphia, 1992, Saunders.)

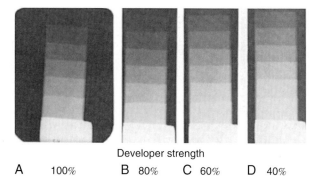

Developer strength

A   100%   B   80%   C   60%   D   40%

FIGURE 10-5 Four radiographs of stepwedges that were exposed at the same time and processed at different times. **A,** Radiograph processed when the processing chemicals were changed and complete development of image was obtained. **B,** Radiograph processed 2 weeks later, when developer solution was weaker by 20%. A 20% increase in developing time is needed to obtain full development of latent image. **C,** Radiograph processed 4 weeks later, when the developer was 60% of original strength. Full development requires a 40% increase in developing time. **D,** Radiograph processed in developer of 40% strength showing obvious underdevelopment of latent image. (From Manson-Hing LR: *Fundamentals of dental radiography*, ed 3, Philadelphia, 1990, Lea & Febiger.)

6. *View the standard radiograph and the daily radiograph side by side on a viewbox.* Compare the densities seen on the daily radiograph with the densities seen on the standard radiograph.

Comparison of the daily stepwedge radiograph with the standard stepwedge radiograph can be interpreted as follows:

- *Matched densities.* Use the middle density seen on the standard stepwedge radiograph for comparison. If the density seen on the standard radiograph matches the density seen on the daily radiograph, the developer solution strength is adequate (Figure 10-4). Proceed with processing.
- *Unmatched densities.* If the density on the daily radiograph differs from that on the standard radiograph by more than two steps on the stepwedge, the developer solution is depleted (Figure 10-5). The developer solution must be changed before proceeding with processing.

Normalizing Device. A dental radiographic normalizing and monitoring device can be used to monitor developer strength and film density. The **normalizing device** is commercially available. A current source for the dental radiographic normalizing and monitoring device is Xray Quality Control in Vail, Colorado (www.xrayqc.com).

Fixer Strength. As discussed in Chapter 9, the fixer solution removes the unexposed silver halide crystals on the film that result in "clear" areas on the processed dental radiograph. When the fixer solution loses strength, the film takes a longer time to clear or becomes transparent in the unexposed areas. When the fixer is at full strength, a film should clear within 2 minutes, without agitation. To monitor fixer strength, the following clearing test can be used:

1. *Prepare the film.* Unwrap one film and immediately place it in the fixer solution.
2. *Check the film for clearing.* Measure the amount of time the film takes to clear.

The results of the clearing test can be interpreted as follows:

- *Fast clearing.* If the film clears in 2 minutes, the fixer is of adequate strength. Proceed with processing.
- *Slow clearing.* If the film is not completely clear after 2 minutes, re-immerse it in the fixer solution. If the film does not completely clear in 3 to 4 minutes, the fixer solution is depleted. The fixer solution must be replaced before proceeding with processing.

Digital Imaging

Just as quality assurance procedures for conventional x-ray film and processing solutions are necessary, quality assurance protocols for offices that use digital imaging are also required. Along with annual tests for the calibration of the imaging equipment, the receptors (whether for direct or indirect imaging) also require periodic examination for scratching, bending, and general wear-and-tear. Since the traditional x-ray film is used one time and the digital sensors and imaging plates are re-used multiple times, greater care in handling and cleaning of the sensors is necessary. Imaging sensors that are damaged by debris or bending show the same artifacts repeatedly when the sensors are re-exposed to radiation. Dental professionals who use direct digital imaging must also inspect the wired connection for any signs of separation from the sensor or deterioration. (See Chapter 25 for more information on digital imaging.)

Performance testing and monitoring of digital radiography equipment must be done in accordance with equipment manufacturer specifications. Commercial kits that are available include a set of test objects, which can be used quickly and easily on an ongoing basis to check imaging performance, particularly those aspects that are subject to deterioration. Such kits allow for the following checks: erasure cycle efficiency, image retention, sensitivity, uniformity, scaling errors, blurring artifacts, and resolution and may be obtained from CSP Medical (www.cspmedicalstore.com).

QUALITY ADMINISTRATION PROCEDURES

Quality administration refers to the management of the quality assurance plan in the dental office. Although many of the technical aspects of the quality assurance plan (e.g., quality control tests) may be delegated to the dental radiographer, the dentist is ultimately responsible for overall quality assurance. The basic elements of a quality administration program include the following:

- Description of the plan
- Assignment of duties
- Monitoring schedule
- Maintenance schedule
- Record-keeping log
- Plan for evaluation and revision
- In-service training

A detailed, written description of the quality assurance plan used in the dental office should be on file and made available to all participating staff members. The standards of quality must be outlined by the dentist. Each staff member involved in the quality assurance plan must understand the standards of quality as well as the purpose and importance of maintaining quality control of radiographic procedures. A detailed, written assignment of quality assurance duties should also be on file and made available to all participating staff members. Each staff member assigned to perform a duty must understand the purpose and importance of that specific duty. Although the dentist may serve as the administrator of the quality assurance program, an assigned staff member may oversee the daily quality control testing and results.

A written monitoring schedule detailing all quality control tests and the frequency of testing for all dental x-ray equipment, supplies, and film processing should be posted in the office. A written maintenance schedule for the routine service and inspection of dental x-ray machines and processing equipment should also be posted in the office.

A record-keeping log of all quality control tests, including the specific test performed, the date performed, and the test results, should be carefully maintained and kept on file in the dental office. In addition, a log for processing solutions, which lists the dates of solution replacement, replenishment, and processor or tank cleaning, should be maintained. Examples of record-keeping logs can be found in a pamphlet titled *Quality Control Tests for Dental Radiography*.

A written plan for the periodic evaluation and revision of the existing quality assurance program should also be part of the quality administration plan. Finally, periodic in-service training of staff members to upgrade and improve x-ray exposure techniques and film processing procedures is recommended.

OPERATOR COMPETENCE

The dentist is ultimately responsible for the diagnostic quality of *all* dental radiographs exposed in his or her office, regardless of who actually exposes and processes the film. Therefore, the dentist relies on the competence of the dental radiographers. Each dental radiographer must be competent in both exposure and processing techniques.

If the operator (dental radiographer) produces a nondiagnostic image, the radiograph must be retaken. All retakes expose the patient to additional x-radiation, so the number of retakes must be kept to an absolute minimum. Operator errors that require retakes should all be recorded. The use of a log to record retakes aids in identifying recurring problems that require attention. Continuing education courses or individualized instruction are useful to upgrade and improve the competence of the dental radiographer.

SUMMARY

- A quality assurance plan ensures the production of high-quality radiographs and includes both quality control tests and quality administration procedures.
- Quality control tests are used to monitor dental x-ray equipment, supplies, and film processing. The following quality control tests are recommended:
  1. *X-ray machines.* Dental x-ray machines should be tested for minor malfunctions, output variations, collimation problems, tubehead drift, timing errors, and inaccurate kilovoltage and milliamperage readings (see Box 10-2). These tests should be performed once a year.
  2. *X-ray film.* The fresh film test can be used to determine whether dental x-ray film is fresh and has been properly stored and protected. This test should be performed each time a new box of film is opened.
  3. *Screens and cassettes.* Cassettes should be examined every month for adequate closure, light leaks, and warping. The film-to-screen contact test can be used to determine the adequacy of contact. This test should be performed periodically. More frequent testing is required if the screens and cassettes are used often.
  4. *Darkroom lighting.* The light leak test can be used to evaluate the darkroom for light leaks every month. The safelighting test can be used to check for proper safelighting conditions and should be performed every 6 months.
  5. *Processing equipment.* Manual and automatic processing equipment must be carefully maintained and monitored daily for potential problems. With manual processing techniques, thermometer and timer must be accurate, and temperature and level of the water bath, developer, and fixer solutions must be checked. Automatic processor test films can be used to check the functioning of the automatic processor. These tests and checks must be performed daily.
  6. *Processing solutions.* The developer strength can be monitored by a reference radiograph, stepwedge

TABLE 10-2   Monitoring Schedule

	Daily	Weekly	Monthly	Yearly	Other	Comments
DENTAL X-RAY MACHINES						
All quality-control tests (see Box 10-2)				X		Upon installation, inspection by a qualified expert
DENTAL X-RAY FILM						
Rotate stock					X	As new film arrives
Fresh film test					X	As a new box of film is opened
SCREENS AND CASSETTES						
Clean			X			
Inspect			X			
Contact test			X			
DARKROOM						
Light leak test			X			
Safelight test					X	Every 6 months
PROCESSING EQUIPMENT AND SOLUTIONS						
Temperature check–solutions	X					
Quality control tests	X					
Replenish solutions	X					
Drain and clean					X	At regular intervals, at least every 3 weeks
Change solutions					X	As indicated by quality control tests
VIEWBOX						
Clean		X				

radiographs, or a normalizing device. The fixer solution can be checked by performing a clearing test. These tests must be performed daily.

- Quality administration procedures include a description of the quality assurance plan, the assignment of duties, a monitoring schedule (Table 10-2), a maintenance schedule, record-keeping logs, a plan for evaluation and revision, and in-service training.
- The dentist is ultimately responsible for the overall quality assurance plan. In addition, the dentist is responsible for the diagnostic quality of all radiographs, regardless of who exposes and processes the films.
- To ensure the production of diagnostic radiographs, the dentist depends on the skill of competent dental radiographers who are competent in both exposure and processing techniques.

BIBLIOGRAPHY

American Dental Association Council on Scientific Affairs: The use of dental radiographs: update and recommendations. *JADA* 137(9):1304–1312, 2006.

Frommer HH, Savage-Stabulas JJ: Film processing: The darkroom. In *Radiology for the dental professional*, ed 8, St Louis, 2005, Mosby.

Frommer HH, Savage-Stabulas JJ: Patient protection. In *Radiology for the dental professional*, ed 8, St. Louis, 2005, Mosby.

Johnson ON, Thomson EM: Identifying and correcting faulty radiographs. In *Essentials of dental radiography for dental assistants and hygienists*, ed 8, Upper Saddle River, NJ, 2007, Pearson.

Johnson ON, Thomson EM: Radiation protection. In *Essentials of dental radiography for dental assistants and hygienists*, ed 8, Upper saddle River, NJ, 2007, Pearson.

Johnson ON, Thomson EM: Quality assurance in dental radiography. In *Essentials of dental radiography for dental assistants and hygienists*, ed 8, Upper Saddle River, NJ, 2007, Pearson.

Lusk LT: Peak performance, *RDH Natl Mag Dent Hygiene Professionals* 14(3):32, 37–38, 1994.

Miles DA, Van Dis ML, Jensen CW, Ferretti A: Film processing and quality assurance. In *Radiographic imaging for the dental team*, ed 4, St. Louis, 2009, Saunders.

White SC, Pharoah MJ: Health physics. In *Oral radiology: principles and interpretation*, ed 6, St. Louis, 2009, Mosby.

QUIZ QUESTIONS

MULTIPLE CHOICE

_____ 1. Calibration of dental x-ray equipment can be performed by a dentist, dental hygienist, or dental assistant.
  a. true
  b. false

_____ 2. Annual tests for dental x-ray machines can be performed by a dentist, dental hygienist, or dental assistant.
  a. true
  b. false

_____ 3. For quality control purposes, each new box of unopened film should be tested for film freshness and fogging before it is used.
  a. true
  b. false

_____ 4. After processing, fresh film that has been properly stored and protected will appear _____.
  a. fogged
  b. clear with a slight blue tint
  c. clouded with a blue tint
  d. dark blue
  e. totally black

_____ 5. After performing the film-screen contact test, a wire mesh image of uniform density appears. These results indicate _____.
  a. adequate film-screen contact
  b. inadequate film-screen contact

_____ 6. When functioning properly, a viewbox should emit a uniform and brilliant light.
  a. true
  b. false

_____ 7. One of the most critical areas of quality control that requires daily monitoring is _____.
  a. examination of the fluorescent bulbs inside the viewbox
  b. cleaning the extraoral intensifying screens
  c. examination of the darkroom for light-tightness
  d. processing of films
  e. all of the above

_____ 8. The coin test is used to check _____.
  a. proper safelighting
  b. strength of the processing solution
  c. film density
  d. film-to-screen contact
  e. beam collimation

_____ 9. The following must be closely monitored with manual processing techniques:
  a. temperature of the water bath
  b. levels of the processing solutions
  c. accuracy of the timer
  d. accuracy of the thermometer
  e. all of the above

_____ 10. On the average, processing solutions should be changed _____.
  a. once each day
  b. once each week
  c. every 3 to 4 weeks
  d. every 8 to 10 weeks
  e. every 3 to 4 months

_____ 11. On the average, processing solutions should be replenished _____.
  a. once each day
  b. once each week
  c. every 3 to 4 weeks
  d. every 8 to 10 weeks
  e. every 3 to 4 months

_____ 12. Fresh films and fresh chemicals must be used when preparing reference radiographs.
  a. true
  b. false

_____ 13. A reference radiograph is used to check _____.
  a. proper safelighting
  b. light-tightness of the darkroom
  c. strength of the fixer solution
  d. strength of the developer solution.
  e. none of the above

_____ 14. The densities seen on the daily radiograph appear lighter than the densities seen on the reference radiograph; this result indicates that _____.
  a. the developer solution is too weak
  b. the developer solution is too concentrated
  c. the developer solution is too cold
  d. either a or c
  e. either b or c

_____ 15. The clearing test is used to monitor _____.
  a. developer strength
  b. fixer strength
  c. accuracy of the timer
  d. film density
  e. none of the above

_____ 16. Regardless of who actually exposes and processes radiographs, the dentist is ultimately responsible for the diagnostic quality of all dental radiographs.
  a. true
  b. false

part III

Dental Radiographer Basics

Chapter 11   Dental Radiographs and the Dental Radiographer, 121
Chapter 12   Patient Relations and the Dental Radiographer, 125
Chapter 13   Patient Education and the Dental Radiographer, 130
Chapter 14   Legal Issues and the Dental Radiographer, 135
Chapter 15   Infection Control and the Dental Radiographer, 140

Dental Radiographs and the Dental Radiographer

OUTLINE

DENTAL RADIOGRAPHS
    Importance of Dental Radiographs
    Uses of Dental Radiographs
    Benefits of Dental Radiographs
    Information Found on Dental Radiographs

THE DENTAL RADIOGRAPHER
    Knowledge and Skill Requirements
    Duties and Responsibilities
    Professional Goals

LEARNING OBJECTIVES

After completion of this chapter, the student will be able to do the following:

- Define the key words
- Discuss the importance of dental radiographs
- List the uses of dental radiographs
- Discuss the benefits of dental radiographs
- List examples of common dental conditions that may be evident on a dental radiograph

- Discuss the knowledge and skill requirements of the dental radiographer
- List the responsibilities that may be assigned to the dental radiographer
- Discuss the professional goals of the dental radiographer

KEY TERMS

Radiograph, dental
Radiographer, dental

The dental radiographer must understand the importance of dental radiographs and the reasons why dental radiographs are a necessary component of comprehensive patient care. As discussed throughout this text, the dental radiographer must have both sufficient knowledge and technical skills to perform dental radiographic procedures. In addition to background knowledge and technical skills, an understanding of the responsibilities and professional goals of the dental radiographer is necessary.

The purpose of this chapter is to review the importance and benefits of dental radiographs and the knowledge and skill requirements of the dental radiographer. The role of the dental radiographer is defined, and his or her duties and responsibilities are described. In addition, the professional goals of the dental radiographer are outlined.

DENTAL RADIOGRAPHS

A **dental radiograph** is a two-dimensional representation of a three-dimensional object produced by the passage of x-rays through teeth and supporting structures. The dental radiographer must have a thorough understanding of the value and importance of dental radiographs. In addition, the dental radiographer must be familiar with the uses of dental radiographs, the benefits of dental radiographs, and the information that can be found on dental radiographs.

Importance of Dental Radiographs

Dental radiographs are a necessary component of comprehensive patient care. In dentistry, a radiographic examination is essential for diagnostic purposes. Radiographs enable the dental professional to identify many conditions that may otherwise go undetected; dental radiographs allow the dental practitioner to see many conditions that are not apparent clinically. An oral examination without dental radiographs limits the dental practitioner's knowledge to what is seen only clinically, that is, teeth and soft tissues. With the use of dental radiographs, the dental professional gains a great deal of information about teeth and supporting bone structures.

Uses of Dental Radiographs

Dental radiographs have many and varied uses. One of the most important uses of dental radiographs is for detection of diseases, lesions, and conditions of the teeth and bones that cannot be identified by clinical examination alone. Many diseases and conditions produce no clinical signs or symptoms and are typically discovered only through the use of dental radiographs.

Dental radiographs are also used for confirming suspected diseases and for assisting in the localization of lesions and foreign objects. Radiographs provide essential information during routine dental treatment; for example, the dentist relies on radiographs during root canal procedures. Dental radiographs can be used to examine the status of teeth and bone during growth and development. Dental radiographs are indispensable for showing changes secondary to trauma, caries, and periodontal disease.

Dental radiographs are an essential component of the patient record. A radiograph contains a vast amount of information, much more than a written record does. An initial radiographic examination provides baseline information about the patient. Each radiograph serves to document the patient's condition at a specific time. Any subsequent radiographs can be used for comparative purposes. Follow-up radiographs can be compared with initial radiographs and examined for changes resulting from treatment, trauma, or disease.

Benefits of Dental Radiographs

The primary benefit of dental radiographs to the patient is detection of disease, as mentioned earlier. When radiographs are properly prescribed (see Chapter 5), exposed, processed, and scanned, their benefit far outweighs the risk of small doses of x-radiation (see Chapter 4).

Through the proper use of dental radiographs, the dental professional can minimize and prevent problems, such as tooth-related pain or the need for surgical procedures. Thus, the dental professional can save the patient time and money while maintaining the patient's oral health.

Information Found on Dental Radiographs

A number of conditions related to teeth and jaws produce no clinical signs or symptoms and can only be detected on dental radiographs. Some of the more common diseases, lesions, and conditions found on dental radiographs include the following:

- Missing teeth
- Extra teeth
- Impacted teeth
- Dental caries
- Periodontal disease
- Tooth abnormalities
- Retained roots
- Cysts and tumors

Radiographs can be used to educate the dental patient about some of these common conditions that are only detected through the use of dental radiographs.

THE DENTAL RADIOGRAPHER

The **dental radiographer** is any person who positions, exposes, and processes dental x-ray image receptors. In the typical dental practice, the dental radiographer is a dental auxiliary, either a dental hygienist or a dental assistant. The dental radiographer must have sufficient knowledge as well as technical skills to perform dental radiographic procedures and have a thorough understanding of his or her responsibilities and professional goals.

Knowledge and Skill Requirements

To be a competent dental radiographer, background knowledge of dental radiography is essential. The purpose of the first 10 chapters of this text has been to provide the dental radiographer with adequate background information to perform dental radiographic procedures. The dental radiographer must have a basic understanding of radiation history (Chapter 1) and a working knowledge of radiation physics (Chapter 2), radiation characteristics (Chapter 3), radiation biology (Chapter 4), and radiation protection (Chapter 5). In addition, the dental radiographer must be familiar with dental x-ray equipment (Chapter 6), dental x-ray film (Chapter 7), dental x-ray image characteristics (Chapter 8), dental x-ray film processing (Chapter 9), and quality assurance in the dental office (Chapter 10).

In addition to background information, the dental radiographer must master the knowledge of patient management basics (Chapters 12 to 15). Most important, the dental radiographer must be proficient in technique concepts and the technical skills used in dental radiography (Chapters 16 to 24).

Duties and Responsibilities

The dental auxiliary is a member of the dental team and has an important role in the practice. Each auxiliary employed in the dental office is assigned specific duties and responsibilities. The assigned duties and responsibilities vary, depending on the size and nature of the dental practice and the individual qualifications of the auxiliary. Assigned responsibilities in regard to dental radiography may include the following:

- Positioning and exposure of dental x-ray imaging receptors
- Processing of dental x-ray films
- Data retrieval of digital images
- Mounting and identification of dental radiographs
- Education of patients about dental radiography
- Maintenance of darkroom facilities and processing equipment
- Implementation and monitoring of quality control procedures

- Ordering of dental x-ray equipment and related supplies

Professional Goals

The dental radiographer must have pride in his or her work, always strive for professional improvement, have defined professional goals, and be committed to achieving those goals. Priority goals for the dental radiographer include patient and operator protection, patient education, operator competence and efficiency, and production of quality radiographs.

Patient Protection

Patient protection must be a top priority and a primary concern of the dental radiographer. Whenever the dental radiographer performs radiographic procedures on patients, the lowest possible level of x-radiation must be used. Retakes resulting in unnecessary patient exposure to x-radiation must be avoided at all times. Patient protection techniques used before exposure include the proper prescription of dental radiographs and the use of proper equipment. During exposure, use of the thyroid collar, the lead apron, a fast film, and beam alignment devices can protect the patient from excessive exposure to radiation. In addition, proper selection of exposure factors and good technique protect the patient. After the films are exposed to x-rays, meticulous handling and processing techniques are critical for the production of diagnostic radiographs. Specific patient protection techniques are discussed in Chapter 5.

Operator Protection

Operator protection must also be a primary concern for the dental radiographer. To avoid occupational exposure to x-radiation, the dental radiographer must always avoid the primary beam and maintain an adequate distance, proper position, and proper shielding from x-rays during the procedure. Radiation monitoring also protects the dental radiographer. Specific operator protection recommendations are discussed in Chapter 5.

Patient Education

Patient education is another priority for the dental radiographer. The dental radiographer must play an active role in the education of patients concerning radiation exposure, patient protection, and the value and uses of dental radiographs (see Chapter 13).

Operator Competence

Operator competence must always be a concern of the dental radiographer, who must strive to maintain or improve professional competence by attending continuing education courses and lectures, studying professional books and journals, and reviewing and updating radiographic techniques.

Operator Efficiency

The dental radiographer must be committed to performing his or her assigned duties in a time-efficient manner. He or she must always work carefully but quickly when positioning and exposing dental x-ray image receptors. Patients always appreciate the auxiliary who does not waste time and who works in a competent and efficient manner.

Production of Quality Radiographs

The dental radiographer must be committed to producing high-quality diagnostic radiographs and must constantly strive to achieve perfection with each dental radiograph. To produce the perfect dental radiograph, the radiographer must carefully position and expose the image receptor, correctly process it, and properly mount and identify the finished radiograph. The dental radiographer can take great professional pride in producing perfect dental radiographs.

Quality Care

When the dental radiographer attains professional goals such as those outlined earlier, the patient receives the highest quality of care possible. Quality care benefits not only the patient but also the profession of dentistry.

SUMMARY

- The dental radiographer must understand the importance of dental radiographs and why dental radiographs are a necessary component of comprehensive patient care.
- Dental radiographs are essential for diagnostic purposes and enable the dental professional to identify many conditions that may otherwise go undetected.
- Although dental radiographs have many uses, the primary use is detection of diseases, lesions, and conditions of the teeth and bones.
- Dental radiographs are obtained to benefit the patient. The primary benefit is disease detection; the benefit of disease detection far outweighs the risk of small doses of radiation.
- Much information can be obtained from a radiographic examination. Numerous conditions related to teeth and jaws produce no clinical signs or symptoms and can only be detected on dental radiographs.
- The dental radiographer is any person who positions, exposes, and processes dental x-ray image receptors. The dental radiographer must have both sufficient knowledge and technical skills to perform dental radiographic procedures.
- Responsibilities of the dental radiographer include positioning, exposure, and processing of films; mounting and identification of radiographs; education of patients; maintenance of darkroom facilities and equipment; implementation and monitoring of quality control procedures; and ordering of equipment and supplies.
- Priority goals for the dental radiographer include patient protection, operator protection, patient education,

operator competence, operator efficiency, and production of high-quality radiographs.

BIBLIOGRAPHY

Frommer HH, Savage-Stabulas JJ: Patient management and special problems. In *Radiology for the dental professional*, ed 8, St. Louis, 2005, Mosby.

Haring JI, Lind LJ: The importance of dental radiographs and interpretation. In *Radiographic interpretation for the dental hygienist*, Philadelphia, 1993, Saunders.

Johnson ON, Thomson EM: Patient relations and education. In *Essentials of dental radiography for dental assistants and hygienists*, ed 8, Upper Saddle River, NJ, 2007, Pearson.

QUIZ QUESTIONS

TRUE OR FALSE

____ 1. Localization of foreign objects is the most important use of dental radiographs.

____ 2. The benefit of disease detection does not outweigh the risk of small doses of x-radiation.

____ 3. Through the use of dental radiographs, the dental professional can detect diseases, lesions, and conditions of the jaws that cannot be identified clinically.

____ 4. A radiograph contains less information than a written record.

____ 5. Missing, extra, and impacted teeth can be identified on a dental radiograph.

____ 6. The dental radiographer is any person who positions, exposes, and processes dental x-ray receptors.

____ 7. The dental radiographer is assigned only to position and expose dental x-ray imaging receptors.

____ 8. The dental radiographer may be assigned to monitor quality control procedures.

____ 9. Patient and operator protection must be primary concerns of the dental radiographer.

____ 10. Operator competence is maintained by performing dental radiography duties.

chapter 12

Patient Relations and the Dental Radiographer

OUTLINE

INTERPERSONAL SKILLS
    Communication Skills
    Facilitation Skills

PATIENT RELATIONS
    First Impressions and Patient Relations
    Chairside Manner and Patient Relations
    Attitude and Patient Relations

LEARNING OBJECTIVES

After completion of this chapter, the student will be able to do the following:

- Define the key words associated with patient relations
- Discuss verbal, nonverbal, and listening skills, and explain how each can be used to enhance communication
- Discuss how facilitative skills can be used to enhance patient trust
- Define a relationship of trust between the dental professional and the patient
- Discuss the importance of first impressions, chairside manner, and attitude, and explain how each can enhance patient relations

KEY TERMS

Chairside manner
Communication
Facilitation skills

Interpersonal skills
Patient relations

Patient relations are important for all dental professionals. The dental radiographer needs good interpersonal skills to communicate with patients and establish trusting relationships. Communicating with dental patients may be the most demanding professional challenge that a dental radiographer encounters. The purpose of this chapter is to discuss specific interpersonal skills that enhance communication between the dental radiographer and the patient and to review the importance of patient relations.

INTERPERSONAL SKILLS

Skills that promote good relationships between individuals are termed **interpersonal skills**. (The term *interpersonal* is defined as "between persons.") The dental radiographer must have effective interpersonal skills not only to establish trusting relationships with dental patients but also to promote patient confidence. Technical skills alone are not sufficient for providing optimal patient care. Interpersonal skills must be used in conjunction with technical skills to enhance the quality of patient care.

Communication Skills

Communication is a crucial interpersonal skill. **Communication** can be defined as the process by which information is exchanged between two or more persons. Effective communication is the basis for developing a successful radiographer–patient relationship.

Verbal Communication Skills

Verbal communication involves the use of language. The dental radiographer's choice of words is important when talking with the dental patient. Certain words detract from the professional image of the dental radiographer. For example, the term *pull* sounds less professional than *extract*, and the word *fix* sounds less professional than *repair* or *restore*. Some words used in the dental setting (e.g., *cut, drill, scrape, zap*) are associated with negative images and must be avoided. In addition, excessive use of technical words may cause confusion and result in miscommunication. The dental radiographer should always choose words that can be easily understood by the patient.

Careless use of language can contribute to miscommunication between the dental radiographer and the patient. The use of unnecessary words (e.g., "you know," "it's like," "I mean") may make it difficult for the patient to understand exactly what the radiographer is saying. Excessive use of slang can also increase the chance of misunderstanding.

The delivery of speech is important in verbal communication. The dental radiographer should always speak in a pleasant and relaxed manner. In the dental clinical setting, the use of a soft tone of voice is preferred by patients, as it is soothing and effective in conveying warmth and concern. The use of a loud tone of voice is not appropriate and is often associated with fear, anger, or excitement. The dental radiographer should avoid speaking in a rushed or tense manner as well.

Nonverbal Communication Skills

Nonverbal communication involves the use of body language. Nonverbal messages that the dental radiographer conveys through posture, body movement, and eye contact are important when working with patients in the dental clinical setting.

Nonverbal messages can be substituted for verbal messages. For example, a nod of the head indicates agreement, whereas a shake of the head signals disagreement. Nonverbal behavior can also be used to enhance communication. For example, if the statement "It's nice to see you" is accompanied by a smile, consistency exists between the verbal and nonverbal messages; the verbal message is enhanced by the nonverbal message. When nonverbal messages are consistent with verbal messages, the patient is more likely to relax and trust the dental professional. When nonverbal messages are not consistent with verbal messages, however, the patient is more likely to respond with apprehension and mistrust.

Posture and *body movement* are important nonverbal cues that convey the attitude of the dental radiographer. An attentive posture and leaning slightly toward the patient, with relaxed, still hands, are nonverbal cues associated with interest and warmth. Conversely, a slumped posture and leaning away from the patient, with arms folded across the chest and fingers tapping, are nonverbal cues that signal indifference and coldness. Patients are more likely to understand and remember information presented by an interested health professional than by a professional whose nonverbal cues signal indifference.

Eye contact is another nonverbal means of communication that is important in the dental setting. When listening to a patient, the dental radiographer should always maintain direct eye contact with the patient; the eyes should not wander. Direct eye contact is associated with interest and attention and plays a powerful role in the initiation and development of interpersonal relationships. A lack of eye contact is often interpreted as indifference or lack of concern.

Listening Skills

Listening involves more than just hearing; listening refers to the receiving and understanding of messages. When listening to a patient, the dental radiographer must receive and understand the information being presented. Careful listening results in better communication and less chance for misunderstandings. The radiographer with good listening skills understands what the patient has said and, in turn, is able to communicate that understanding to the patient.

The good listener communicates attention and interest. When listening to a patient, the dental radiographer can use nonverbal cues such as a nod of the head or facial expressions to convey appropriate emotional responses. To communicate interest, the dental radiographer can paraphrase what the patient has just stated to confirm what has been heard.

To enhance communication, sometimes the dental radiographer may want to summarize the feelings of the patient rather than paraphrase the information that has been presented. When a patient is fearful and upset, the dental radiographer conveys interest and concern for the patient when he or she can summarize and emphasize the patient's feelings.

When listening to a patient, the dental radiographer should give undivided attention to the patient. The dental radiographer should never interrupt or correct the patient, finish the patient's sentences, look at a clock or watch, or distract the patient by fidgeting or playing with objects.

Facilitation Skills

Facilitation skills are interpersonal skills used to ease communication and develop a trusting relationship between the dental professional and the patient. (The term *facilitation* is defined as "the act of making something easier.") In a trusting relationship, the patient feels cared for and understood by the dental professional. In the dental clinical setting, trust involves the belief in the patient that the dental professional will interact in a beneficial way and not in a harmful way. A trusting relationship facilitates the delivery of patient care by reducing worry and psychological stress in the patient. When a patient trusts the dental professional, the patient is more likely to provide information, cooperate during procedures, comply with prescribed treatment, and return for further treatment.

Facilitative skills that enhance patient trust include encouraging questions, answering questions, responding with action, and expressing warmth. The dental radiographer must encourage each patient to ask questions. Many patients may be hesitant to ask questions because they may be feeling intimidated by the dental professional or apprehensive about the dental visit. Inviting a patient to ask questions enhances communication. In addition, the dental radiographer must be prepared to answer the patient's questions directly. Whenever a patient asks a question, the dental radiographer should respond with accurate information in a direct manner and use language that can be easily understood by the patient.

The dental radiographer must be prepared to respond with action or carry out patient requests. For example, if a patient requests a glass of water, the dental radiographer can respond by providing a glass of water to the patient. The patient feels cared for when the dental radiographer responds to such requests with the desired action. In addition, the dental radiographer must respond to patients with *warmth*, which can be communicated through voice and facial expression. The dental radiographer who responds to patients with warmth is friendly and smiling and shows interest in the patient. Warmth communicates that the professional cares for the patient as a person.

PATIENT RELATIONS

In dentistry, the term **patient relations** refers to the relationship between the patient and the dental professional. Patient relations are important to all dental professionals: the dentist, the dental hygienist, and the dental assistant.

First Impressions and Patient Relations

The relationship between the patient and the dental professional begins with first impressions. The patient's first impression of the dental team most often involves the dental auxiliary, specifically the auxiliary's appearance and greeting.

The professional appearance of the dental auxiliary is important. The dental auxiliary should always wear a clean uniform and be well groomed. Strict attention must be paid to personal hygiene, including handwashing and maintaining fresh breath. In addition, the dental auxiliary should never eat, drink, or chew gum while working with patients (Boxes 12-1 and 12-2).

In many offices, the dental auxiliary is the first dental professional to meet and greet the patient. The dental auxiliary should always greet patients in the reception room before escorting them to the treatment area. Patients should always be greeted by name. The dental auxiliary should address the patient using the patient's proper title (Miss, Ms., Mrs., Mr., Dr., Rev., etc.) and last name. If uncertain about the correct pronunciation of the name, the dental auxiliary should find out the correct pronunciation from the patient. The dental auxiliary should always introduce himself or herself to the patient, using both name and title. A typical first greeting is given below:

EXAMPLE
Hello, Mrs. Davis. My name is Kate Miller, and I'm the dental assistant who will be working with you today. It's a pleasure to meet you. If you'll follow me to the patient treatment area, we can get started with today's appointment.

Chairside Manner and Patient Relations

The relationship between the patient and the dental professional develops as the professional works with the patient. **Chairside manner** refers to the way a dental professional conducts himself or herself at the patient's chairside. The dental auxiliary must develop a relaxing chairside manner that makes the patient feel comfortable and at ease.

The dental auxiliary must also convey a confident chairside manner. The patient must be confident about the auxiliary's ability to perform radiographic procedures. The dental radiographer must avoid comments such as "Oops!" and other statements that indicate a lack of control. The patient must feel that the operator is in control of all procedures being performed. One way to convey operator confidence is to explain to the patient exactly which procedures are about to be performed and then answer any questions the patient may have about the procedures.

In most dental offices, the dental auxiliary is responsible for performing radiographic procedures. However, some patients may be apprehensive about allowing a dental auxiliary to perform such procedures because they are accustomed to the dentist performing all procedures, including radiographic procedures. As a result, these patients may object to a dental auxiliary performing any services for them. In such cases, the dental auxiliary must try to establish a relationship with the patient by explaining the concept of the dental team. The dental auxiliary can educate and orient the patient to the dental team members and their respective roles and

BOX **12-1**	**Helpful Hints**
Personal grooming	Be well groomed. Hair should be brushed. Use of a deodorant is a must. In addition, dental professionals must pay careful attention to maintaining fresh breath.
Clothing	All clothing should be clean—without stains—and pressed.
Shoes/Socks	Pay attention to your shoes. They should be polished and clean. Always wear socks with shoes. Open-toed shoes are inappropriate for health professional environments.
Eating and drinking	Never chew gum, eat mints, eat, or drink while working with patients.
Manners	To make sure your manners are appropriate, take a business etiquette class.

BOX **12-2** **First Impressions Checklist**
• Find out the patient's preferred name, and use it.
• Upon the patient's arrival, offer a warm welcome—both verbally and through body language.
• Introduce yourself to each patient with a smile and a handshake.
• Introduce other staff members to the new patient.
• Wear a nametag; knowing your name gives the patient a sense of belonging.
• Ask your patient questions, and then *listen*.

responsibilities. The dentist may then reinforce such information and reassure the patient before the dental auxiliary performs the radiographic procedures.

Patient relations and management skills with regard to persons with specific dental needs is discussed further in Chapter 24, specifically patients with physical or developmental disabilities, as well as pediatric, endodontic, and edentulous patients.

Attitude and Patient Relations

The attitude of the dental auxiliary will affect patient relations. Attitude can be defined as "a position of the body, or manner of carrying oneself, indicative of a mood." The attitude of all dental auxiliaries must be professional and should include such attributes as courtesy, patience, and honesty. The dental auxiliary must be courteous and polite toward all patients at all times. Patience, which includes both tolerance and understanding, is important, especially when dealing with an uncooperative or difficult patient. Honesty is also a vital part of a professional attitude. Some procedures are uncomfortable in dental radiography, and the dental auxiliary must be honest and inform the patient of the potential discomfort.

SUMMARY

- Communication is an important interpersonal skill and the basis for developing a successful radiographer–patient relationship.
- Verbal communication involves the use of language. The dental radiographer's choice of words is very important; words that detract from the professional image of

dentistry and words associated with negative images must be avoided.
- Nonverbal communication involves the use of body language and includes messages conveyed by posture, body movement, and eye contact. A patient will respond positively toward the dental professional whose nonverbal cues signal interest and warmth; a patient is less likely to respond to a dental professional whose nonverbal cues signal indifference and coldness.
- Communication also involves listening skills. The dental radiographer with good listening skills understands what the patient has said and is able to communicate that understanding to the patient. The good listener communicates both attention and interest.
- Facilitation skills make communication easier and develop a trusting relationship between the patient and the dental professional. Facilitative skills include encouraging patient questions, answering patient questions, responding to patient requests, and communicating with warmth.
- Patient relations refers to the relationship between the patient and the dental professional. The dental auxiliary must develop a relaxing and confident chairside manner that makes the patient feel comfortable.

BIBLIOGRAPHY

Frommer HH, Savage-Stabulas JJ: Patient management and special problems. In *Radiology for the dental professional*, ed 9, St. Louis, 2011, Mosby.

Johnson ON, Thomson EM: Patient relations and education. In *Essentials of dental radiography for dental assistants and hygienists*, ed 8, Upper Saddle River, NJ, 2007, Pearson.

QUIZ QUESTIONS

TRUE OR FALSE

_____ 1. Skills that promote a good relationship between individuals are termed *facilitation skills.*

_____ 2. Technical skills alone are sufficient for providing optimal patient care.

_____ 3. The excessive use of technical words may confuse the patient and result in miscommunication.

_____ 4. The delivery of speech is important in verbal communication; the dental radiographer should speak in a pleasant, relaxed manner.

_____ 5. Nonverbal behavior cannot be used to enhance communication.

_____ 6. If verbal messages are consistent with nonverbal messages, the patient is likely to respond with apprehension and mistrust.

_____ 7. Patients are more likely to understand a dental professional whose nonverbal cues signal indifference.

_____ 8. Eye contact plays a powerful role in the development of interpersonal relationships.

_____ 9. Listening involves only hearing.

_____ 10. When listening to a patient, the dental radiographer can use facial expressions to convey appropriate emotional responses.

_____ 11. Interpersonal skills are skills that are used to make communication easier and develop a trusting relationship between the patient and the dental professional.

_____ 12. When a patient trusts the dental professional, the patient is more likely to comply with the prescribed treatment and return for further treatment.

_____ 13. The appearance of the dental auxiliary is important.

_____ 14. In many offices, the dental auxiliary is the first person to meet and greet the patient.

_____ 15. A patient should always be greeted by his or her first name.

_____ 16. It is appropriate for the dental auxiliary to chew gum while working with patients.

___ **17.** The dental auxiliary must develop a fast-paced, confident chairside manner.

___ **18.** In most dental offices, the dental auxiliary is responsible for performing radiographic procedures.

___ **19.** The attitude of the dental radiographer affects patient relations.

___ **20.** The dental radiographer does not need to be courteous if a patient is uncooperative or difficult.

chapter 13

Patient Education and the Dental Radiographer

OUTLINE

IMPORTANCE OF PATIENT EDUCATION
METHODS OF PATIENT EDUCATION
COMMON QUESTIONS AND ANSWERS
    Necessity Questions
    Exposure Questions

Safety Questions
Digital Imaging Questions
Miscellaneous Questions

LEARNING OBJECTIVES

After completion of this chapter, the student will be able to do the following:

- Summarize the importance of educating patients about dental radiographs
- List the three methods that can be used by the dental radiographer to educate patients about dental radiographs
- Answer common patient questions about the need for dental radiographs, x-ray exposure, the safety of dental x-rays, digital imaging, and other miscellaneous concerns

The dental radiographer must be able to educate patients about the importance of dental radiographs and also be prepared to answer common questions asked by patients about the need for dental radiographs, x-ray exposure, the safety of dental x-rays, and miscellaneous concerns. The purpose of this chapter is to discuss the importance of patient education, to describe different methods of patient education, and to review common patient questions and answers about dental radiography.

IMPORTANCE OF PATIENT EDUCATION

Educating dental patients about the importance of dental radiographs is critical, yet patient education is often overlooked by dental professionals. Many patients do not understand the value of dental radiographs. Often, the patient is simply told that "dental x-rays are required by the dentist," and little additional information is provided. As a result, many patients fear the use of x-radiation. Others believe that dental radiographs are a way for the dentist to make extra money. To address such fears and misconceptions, the dental radiographer must be prepared to educate the patient about the value of dental radiographs.

Many patients have heard or read about the damaging effects of x-radiation. Newspaper articles, magazine articles, and television magazine shows often highlight the damaging effects of radiation and cast doubt on the necessity and benefit of radiographic examinations. Such reports are often misleading and are not well researched. As a result, these reports cause the patient to fear the use of x-radiation and to avoid all radiation exposure.

Because of the presence of such misinformation, the dental radiographer must take the time to educate the patient. In some instances, the patient may have to be completely re-educated. The dental radiographer must be prepared to explain exactly why dental radiographs are important, how dental radiographs are used, and how they are beneficial. In addition, the dental professional must be able to discuss common conditions and lesions that can be detected only through the use of dental radiographs (see Chapters 4 and 11).

Comprehensive dental health education is one of the greatest services that a dental professional can provide to the patient. Education enhances understanding. A patient who is knowledgeable about the importance of dental radiographs is more likely to realize the benefit of dental radiographs, accept the prescribed treatment, and follow prevention plans.

Patient education is also likely to decrease fears of x-ray exposure, increase cooperation, and increase motivation for regular dental visits.

METHODS OF PATIENT EDUCATION

Patient education about dental radiographs can be accomplished in a number of ways. The dental radiographer can use an oral presentation, printed literature, or a combination of both to educate the dental patient.

An oral presentation, in conjunction with sample dental images, can be used to communicate the importance of dental radiographs. For example, the dental radiographer can show the patient a prepared series of radiographs illustrating typical normal and abnormal conditions. Through the use of such radiographs, the dental radiographer includes a visual component in the educational process; visual aids enhance patient comprehension. A prepared oral presentation with visual aids allows the patient to develop greater confidence in the expertise of the dental radiographer. A prepared presentation also communicates to the patient that the dental radiographer is organized and competent.

The use of digital imaging may further aid in patient education. This helps patients view their own periapical, bitewing, or extraoral images on a computer monitor or television screen instead of looking at detailed information on mounted radiographs. The use of digital imaging helps explain concepts such as caries, periodontal changes, or oral diseases (Figure 13-1).

Printed information about dental radiographs is useful to educate the dental patient as well. Brochures can be placed in the reception area of the dental office or handed to patients before the radiographic examination. The pamphlet *Dental X-rays: Your Dentist's Advice*, for example, discusses dental x-rays and how dental radiographs benefit the patient. This and other brochures about dental radiographs and x-ray exposure can be obtained from the American Dental Association and the Bureau of Radiologic Health. Printed literature about dental radiographs can also be custom designed by the dental professional and then printed for use in the dental office.

A combination of an oral presentation and printed literature is probably the most effective method of educating the dental patient about dental radiographs. The use of both approaches can stimulate a question-and-answer type of discussion about dental radiographs.

COMMON QUESTIONS AND ANSWERS

The dental radiographer must be prepared to answer common questions about the need for dental radiographs, x-ray exposure, safety of dental x-rays, digital imaging, and other concerns. Many patients ask the dental auxiliary, rather than the dentist, questions about x-radiation. The dental radiographer can answer many of the patient's questions. However, some questions must be answered only by the dentist; such questions must be established by the dentist and understood by all members of the dental team. For example, questions about diagnosis must be answered only by the dentist.

Necessity Questions

Patients often ask questions about the need for dental x-rays, the frequency of dental x-rays for adults and children, the refusal of dental x-rays, and the use of dental x-rays from a previous dentist. Examples of questions and answers follow:

Question: Are dental x-rays really necessary?

Answer: Yes. Many diseases and conditions such as tooth decay, gum disease, cysts, and tumors cannot be detected simply by looking into your mouth. Many diseases and conditions produce no signs or symptoms. Without dental x-rays, these conditions may go unnoticed for a long time. As these conditions progress, extensive damage and pain may occur; these, in turn, may result in more extensive and costly treatment. Some oral diseases can even affect your general health or become life threatening.

Dental radiographs are always taken to benefit you, the patient; the primary benefit is disease detection. Through the use of dental radiographs, conditions and diseases that cannot be detected in any other way can be identified early. Early identification and treatment minimize and prevent problems, such as pain and the need for surgical procedures.

Question: How often should I have dental x-rays?

Answer: The first step to limiting the amount of radiation that you receive is the proper prescribing, or ordering, of dental radiographs. Decisions about the number, type, and frequency of dental x-rays are determined by the dentist based on your individual needs. Guidelines published by the American Dental Association are used by the dentist to aid in prescribing the number, type, and frequency of dental radiographs.

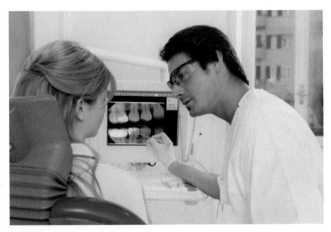

FIGURE 13-1 Dentist and patient reviewing digital images on a large computer moitor helps to facilitate patient education. (Courtesy of DEXIS, Des Plaines, Ill.)

Because every patient's dental condition is different, the frequency of radiographic examinations is also different. The frequency of your dental x-ray examinations is based on your individual needs. No set interval exists between x-ray examinations. For example, a patient with tooth decay or gum disease needs more frequent radiographic examinations than a patient without such diseases.

Question: How often should children have dental x-rays?

Answer: The interval between radiographic examinations should be based on the individual needs of the child. Because every child's dental condition is different, the frequency of radiographic examinations is different as well. There is no set interval between x-ray examinations. For example, a child with tooth decay needs more frequent radiographic examinations than a child without tooth decay.

Question: Can I refuse x-rays and be treated without them?

Answer: No. When you refuse dental x-rays, the dentist cannot treat you. The standard of care requires that the dentist refuse treatment when a patient refuses x-rays that are necessary. Treatment without necessary radiographs is considered negligent. No document can be signed to release the dentist from liability. For example, if you were to sign a paper stating that you refused dental x-rays but released the dentist from any and all liability, you would be consenting to negligent care. Legally, you cannot consent to negligent care.

Question: Instead of taking x-rays now, can you use the x-rays from my previous dentist?

Answer: Yes. Previous dental radiographs can be used, provided they are recent and of acceptable diagnostic quality. Additional dental radiographs may be necessary, however, based on your individual needs. If your previous dental radiographs, even if recent, are not of diagnostic quality, you will have to have another radiograph taken.

Exposure Questions

Patients often ask questions about x-ray measurement, amounts of x-ray exposure, the use of the lead apron during exposure, dental x-radiation during pregnancy, and the reason for the dental radiographer leaving the room during exposure. Examples of questions and answers follow:

Question: How are x-rays measured?

Answer: Special units are used to measure x-ray exposure and absorption. The radiation that reaches the surface of the skin is measured in *roentgen* units. The unit for dose, or the amount of energy absorbed by a tissue, is termed *radiation absorbed dose (rad)*. Because of the small quantities of radiation used during radiographic procedures, very small multiples of these radiation units are used. The prefix *milli-*, meaning "one one-thousandth," is used to express the small quantities of exposure in milliroentgens and the dose in millirads.

Question: How much radiation will I receive from dental x-rays?

Answer: Because no amount of radiation is considered safe, strict guidelines are followed to limit the amount of x-radiation. For example, the dentist custom-orders your x-rays on the basis of your individual needs. During exposure, a thyroid collar, a lead apron, fast film, digital imaging, and a beam alignment device will be used to protect you from excess radiation. Good exposure technique and careful processing are also used to limit your exposure to x-radiation.

The actual amount of x-radiation received will vary depending on the film speed, the technique used, and exposure factors. For example, when a single intraoral D-speed film is exposed, the x-rays expose a small area of skin, and the exposure to the skin of the face is about 250 milliroentgens. With faster F-speed film, a single intraoral film results in a surface skin exposure of 125 milliroentgens. The use of digital imaging reduces the radiation dose even further. For dental x-rays to produce permanent skin damage, such as skin cancer, exposures in the range of thousands of roentgens are needed. Such exposures are inconceivable in dental radiography and are not possible with dental x-ray equipment.

Question: Why do you use a lead apron?

Answer: A lead apron and a thyroid collar are used to protect reproductive, blood-forming, and thyroid tissues from scatter radiation. The lead acts as a shield and actually prevents the radiation from reaching these radiosensitive organs. The lead apron protects you from unnecessary radiation exposure.

Question: Is it safe to take dental x-rays during pregnancy?

Answer: When a lead apron is used during dental radiographic procedures, the amount of radiation received in the gonadal region is nearly zero. No detectable exposure to the embryo or fetus occurs with the use of the lead apron. The American Dental Association, together with the Food and Drug Administration, has stated in the Guidelines for Prescribing Dental Radiographs that the recommended guidelines "do not need to be altered because of pregnancy." Although scientific evidence indicates that dental x-ray procedures can be performed during pregnancy, many dentists elect to postpone such x-ray procedures because of patient concerns.

Question: Why do you leave the room when x-rays are used?

Answer: When you are exposed to x-rays, you receive the diagnostic benefit of the dental radiographs; I do not receive any benefit. An individual should only be exposed to x-radiation when the benefit of disease detection outweighs the risk of exposure. Since I do not benefit from your x-ray exposure, I must use proper protection measures. One of the most effective ways for me to limit my x-ray exposure is to maintain adequate distance and shielding, which is why I step out of the room during your x-ray exposure.

Safety Questions

Patients often ask questions about the safety of dental x-rays and wonder whether dental x-rays cause cancer. Examples of questions and answers follow:

Question: Are dental x-rays safe?

Answer: All x-rays are harmful to living tissue. The amount of x-radiation used in dental radiography is small, but biologic damage does occur. No amount of radiation is considered safe. As a result, dental x-rays must be prescribed only when the benefit of disease detection outweighs this risk of harm.

Question: Will dental x-rays cause cancer?

Answer: Not a single recorded case of a patient developing cancer from diagnostic x-rays exists. The radiation exposure that occurs during a dental x-ray examination is very small, and the chance that it will contribute to or cause cancer is extremely low. For example, the potential risk of dental radiography inducing a fatal cancer has been estimated to be 3 in one million. The risk of a person developing cancer spontaneously is much higher, or 3300 in one million. When these two numbers are compared, it is evident that when cancer occurs, it is much more likely to be unrelated to radiation exposure.

Digital Imaging Questions

Question: What are the advantages of digital imaging?

Answer: Digital imaging requires less exposure to radiation which benefits you, the patient. Digital information can be stored, transmitted, and manipulated electronically. Digital imaging also gives us instant images that are environmentally friendly, as no processing chemicals are used.

Question: Are there any risks associated with digital imaging?

Answer: Because radiation is involved, a certain amount of risk does exist. With digital radiography, your exposure is less than with traditional x-rays. Your radiation exposure time may be reduced by 50% to 80%.

Miscellaneous Questions

Question: Can a panoramic x-ray be taken instead of a complete series?

Answer: No. A panoramic radiograph cannot be substituted for a complete series of dental radiographs. A complete series of dental radiographs is required when information about the details of the teeth and surrounding bone are needed. A panoramic radiograph does not clearly reveal changes in teeth, as in tooth decay, or the details of the supporting bone. The panoramic radiograph is useful for showing the general condition of a patient's teeth and bone.

Question: Who owns my dental radiographs?

Answer: All your dental records, including the dental radiographs, are the property of the dentist. As a patient, however, you have the privilege of reasonable access to your dental records. For example, you can request a copy of your dental radiographs or request that a copy be sent to a dentist of your choice. Digital images may also be electronically sent to a referring doctor. The dentist usually retains the original dental radiographs as part of the patient record.

SUMMARY

- The dental radiographer must be able to educate patients about dental radiographs. A patient who is knowledgeable about the importance of dental radiographs is more likely to have reduced fears about x-ray exposure, realize the benefits of dental radiographs, accept prescribed treatment, and follow prevention plans.
- The dental radiographer can use an oral presentation, printed literature, or a combination (probably the most effective method) to educate the dental patient about radiographs.
- The dental radiographer must be prepared to answer common patient questions about the need for dental radiographs, x-ray exposure, safety of dental x-rays, digital imaging, and miscellaneous concerns.
- Some patient questions such as those about diagnosis must be answered only by the dentist, and these questions must be established by the dentist and understood by the dental team.

BIBLIOGRAPHY

Frommer HH, Savage-Stabulas JJ: Operator protection. In *Radiology for the dental professional*, ed 9, St. Louis, 2011, Mosby.

Frommer HH, Savage-Stabulas JJ: Patient protection. In *Radiology for the dental professional*, ed 9, St. Louis, 2011, Mosby.

Haring JI, Lind LJ: The importance of dental radiographs and interpretation. In *Radiographic interpretation for the dental hygienist*, Philadelphia, 1993, Saunders.

Johnson ON, Thomson EM: Patient relations and education. In *Essentials of dental radiography for dental assistants and hygienists*, ed 8, Upper Saddle River, NJ, 2007, Pearson.

Thunthy KH: X-rays: Detailed answers to frequently asked questions, *Compend Contin Educ Dentistry* 14(3):394–398, 1993.

QUIZ QUESTIONS

ESSAY

1. Summarize the importance of educating dental patients about dental radiographs.
2. List the three methods the dental radiographer can use to educate patients about dental radiographs.

SHORT ANSWER

3. Are dental x-rays really necessary?

_____

_____

4. How often should adults have dental x-rays?

_____

_____

5. How often should children have dental x-rays?

_____

_____

6. Can a patient refuse dental x-rays and be treated without them?

_____

_____

7. Can radiographs from a previous dentist be used instead of taking dental x-rays?

_____

_____

8. How are x-rays measured?

_____

_____

9. How much radiation is received from dental x-rays?

_____

_____

10. Why is a lead apron used during x-ray exposure?

_____

_____

11. Can dental x-rays be taken during pregnancy?

_____

_____

12. Why does the dental radiographer leave the room during x-ray exposure of the patient?

_____

_____

13. Are dental x-rays safe?

_____

_____

14. Will dental x-rays cause cancer?

_____

_____

15. Can a panoramic x-ray be taken instead of a complete series?

_____

_____

16. Who owns the dental radiographs—the dentist or the patient?

_____

_____

chapter 14

Legal Issues and the Dental Radiographer

OUTLINE

LEGAL ISSUES AND DENTAL RADIOGRAPHY
    Federal and State Regulations
    Licensure Requirements
LEGAL ISSUES AND THE DENTAL PATIENT
    Risk Management
    Malpractice Issues

Patient Records
Patients Who Refuse Dental Radiographs

LEARNING OBJECTIVES

After completion of this chapter, the student will be able to do the following:

- Define key words associated with legal issues
- List federal and state regulations affecting the use of dental x-ray equipment
- Describe the general application of federal and state regulations as they affect the dental auxiliary
- Describe licensure requirements for exposing dental radiographs
- Define the legal concept of informed consent

- Describe ways to obtain informed consent from a patient
- Discuss the legal significance of the dental record
- Describe the legal implications of patient refusal to have dental x-radiation
- Discuss how confidentiality laws affect the information in the dental record
- Describe the patient's rights with regard to the dental record

KEY TERMS

Confidentiality
Disclosure
Informed consent
Liability

Malpractice
Negligence
Risk management
Self-determination

Standard of care
Statute of limitations

The dental auxiliary must be aware of the legal implications of dental radiography. The dental auxiliary must be knowledgeable about, and comply with, laws that govern the use of ionizing radiation in dentistry. Furthermore, because dental radiography has implications for patient care, including the diagnosis of dental disease and treatment planning, the possibility of negligent care exists when dental radiographs are not properly exposed or used.

The purpose of this chapter is to discuss general legal concepts, including various regulations as they apply to the dental radiographer who performs dental radiographic procedures for patient care, as well as confidentiality and documentation.

LEGAL ISSUES AND DENTAL RADIOGRAPHY

Federal and State Regulations

Both federal and state regulations control the use of dental x-ray equipment. The federal government has established requirements, including safety precautions, for the use of dental x-ray machines made and sold in the United States. For example, the Consumer-Patient Radiation Health and Safety Act outlines requirements for the safe use of dental x-ray equipment. This federal law also establishes guidelines for the proper maintenance of x-ray equipment and requires persons who perform dental radiographic procedures to be properly trained and certified.

In addition to federal laws, state, county, and city laws may affect the use of dental x-ray equipment. Most states have laws that require regular inspection of dental x-ray equipment, for example, every 5 years. Some state laws also require that the dental radiographer be trained and certified or licensed to practice dental radiography.

Licensure Requirements

State laws regulate dental radiograph exposures. In most cases, the licensed dentist and the dental hygienist are not legally required to obtain additional certification to perform dental radiographic procedures. The certification required for dental assistants for dental radiography varies from state to state. Consequently, it is the responsibility of the dental auxiliary to become informed about the specific requirements relating to dental radiography in his or her particular state. These requirements may include the following:

1. Obtaining additional certification in dental radiography
2. Performing dental radiographic procedures only under the direct supervision of the dentist
3. Following restrictions concerning the types of dental radiographs that may be legally used.

LEGAL ISSUES AND THE DENTAL PATIENT

Risk Management

Risk management is extremely important in dental radiography. **Risk management** refers to the policies and procedures that should be followed by the dental radiographer to reduce the chances of a patient taking legal action against the dental radiographer or the supervising dentist.

Informed Consent

Persons seeking health care services, including dental care, have the right to **self-determination**; they have the legal right to make choices about the care they receive, including the opportunity to consent to or to refuse treatment. Therefore, before receiving treatment, the dental patient should be informed of the various aspects of the proposed treatment, including diagnostic procedures such as dental radiography.

It is the responsibility of the dentist to discuss both diagnostic and treatment procedures with the patient. All patients must be informed of the need for dental radiographs. Information provided to the patient should include the following:

1. Purpose and potential benefits of the radiographs
2. Person responsible for performing the radiographic procedure
3. Number and type of radiographs used
4. Possible harm that may result if dental radiographs are not taken

5. Risks associated with x-ray exposure
6. Alternative diagnostic aids that may serve the same purpose as radiographs

This process of informing the patient about the particulars of dental radiography is termed **disclosure**. The disclosure process must be conducted by a competent dental professional. In many states, the prescription of dental radiographs is the responsibility of the dentist, and the auxiliary is the person who performs the radiographic procedure under the dentist's supervision. In such cases, the dentist should be involved in the disclosure process and should be available to answer any patient questions.

It is important to standardize the disclosure process so that patients receive enough information to make informed choices. Patients must also be given the opportunity to ask questions and have their questions answered before the procedure. Informed consent must be obtained from all patients. In the case of a patient who is a minor (generally, those under 18 years of age) or declared to be "legally incompetent," informed consent must be obtained from a legal guardian. It is important that the person who provides the disclosure not misrepresent any of the information disclosed or threaten the patient into giving consent. The person disclosing information should use language that the patient can understand easily.

After the disclosure process has been completed, the patient may give or withhold consent for the dental radiographic procedure. **Informed consent** is defined as consent given by a patient following complete disclosure. Although the governing standards for informed consent may vary from state to state, certain recognized elements of informed consent can be summarized as follows:

1. Purpose of the procedure and who will perform it
2. Potential benefits of receiving the procedure
3. Possible risks involved in having the procedure performed, as well as the possible risks of not having it performed
4. Opportunity for the patient to ask questions and obtain complete information

A written consent form including these four elements may be used in obtaining informed consent.

If informed consent is not obtained from a patient before the dental radiographic procedure, a patient may legally claim malpractice or negligence. A patient's consent to dental procedures is generally presumed valid if it is obtained in a manner consistent with state laws, if it follows disclosure rules, and if it is obtained freely from the appropriate individual. Lack of informed consent may be shown by the following:

- Complete lack of consent from the patient
- Consent obtained from an individual who has no legal right to give it (e.g., minor, incompetent adult)
- Consent obtained from an individual who is under the influence of drugs or alcohol
- Consent obtained by misrepresentation or fraudulent means

- Consent given by an individual under duress
- Consent obtained after incomplete disclosure

Liability

When procedures are performed by a dental auxiliary, legal accountability (**liability**) is presumed to lie with both the supervising dentist and the dental auxiliary. According to state laws, dentists are legally accountable (liable) to supervise the performance of dental auxiliaries. Even though dental auxiliaries work under the supervision of a licensed dentist, they are also legally liable for their own actions. The trend in dental negligence or malpractice actions has historically been to sue the supervising dentist alone; however, the dentist and the dental auxiliary have both been sued for the actions of the dental auxiliary in some cases.

Malpractice Issues

Dental **malpractice** results when the dental practitioner is negligent in the delivery of dental care. **Negligence** in dental treatment occurs when the diagnosis made or the dental treatment delivered falls below the standard of care. The **standard of care** can be defined as the quality of care that is provided by dental practitioners in a similar locality under the same or similar conditions.

Negligent care may result from the action or lack of action of either the dentist or the dental auxiliary. Because dental radiographs are an essential part of diagnosis and treatment planning, negligence may result from the action or inaction of the dental radiographer. For example, if informed consent is not obtained from the patient before a dental radiographic procedure, negligence may be claimed, except in the case of implied consent. Negligence may also be claimed if radiographs are exposed improperly and the patient is injured in some way as a direct result. Examples of such negligence include the incorrect number of radiographs being exposed or the radiographs being nondiagnostic.

State laws govern the duration of time within which a patient may bring a malpractice action against the dentist or the auxiliary. This time is known as the **statute of limitations**. In many states, this period begins when the patient discovers (or should have discovered) that an injury has occurred as a result of dental negligence. In such cases, the statute of limitations may not begin until years after the dental negligence occurred. Frequently, it is not until a patient seeks care from another dentist that he or she becomes aware that previous dental treatment may have been negligent. For example, if dental radiographs are not exposed properly, dental disease may go undiagnosed and untreated. Years later, the patient may be informed that he or she has an irreversible condition (e.g., advanced periodontal disease), which might have been prevented or more successfully treated with early detection. Even though such a dental disease is not life threatening, the lack of diagnosis and treatment may result in significant harm to the patient. Examples of harm may include loss of self-esteem, emotional distress, loss of income, and expenses incurred in seeking additional dental treatment.

Patient Records

A dental record must be established for every patient, and dental radiographs are an integral part of such a record. The dental record must accurately reflect all aspects of patient care. Complete dental records are important to ensure continuity of patient care and to provide legal documentation of a patient's condition.

Documentation

It is essential that the dental record include the following:
1. Informed consent
2. Number and type of radiographs exposed (including re-takes)
3. Rationale for these radiographs
4. Diagnostic information obtained from the interpretation of the radiographs

The prescription and the evaluation of radiographs are typically the responsibility of the dentist; therefore, entries in the dental record should be made by the dentist or under the dentist's supervision. Entries made in the dental record should never be erased or blocked out. If an error is made, a clean line should be drawn through the error and the correct entry added to the record.

Confidentiality

All the information contained in the dental record, including dental radiographs, is *confidential*, or private, to the extent that state laws do not otherwise require disclosure. State **confidentiality** laws protect this information and generally prohibit the transfer of this information to nonprivileged persons. A *nonprivileged person* is an individual who is not directly involved in the treatment of the patient. It is not appropriate for any dental professional to discuss a patient's care with another patient or with office staff members who are not involved in the treatment of the patient. Likewise, sharing dental radiographs with others not involved in the patient's care is considered a violation or breach of confidentiality laws.

Ownership and Retention of Dental Radiographs

Legally, dental radiographs are the property of the dentist, even though the patient or an insurance company may have paid for them. The basis for this ownership of dental radiographs is that radiographs are indispensable to the dentist as part of the patient's record.

Patients do have a right to reasonable access to their records. This includes the right to have their complete dental records, including copies of the radiographs, forwarded to another dentist. When transferring to another dentist, a patient can request in writing that his or her dental records be forwarded to that dentist. Duplicates of the radiographs should be made and forwarded and the originals retained. Digital images may be sent electronically, and the patient's written request should be placed in the dental record as evidence of the patient's directive. It is generally not advisable to release a copy of the dental record, including dental radiographs, directly to the patient. Instead, this information should be forwarded directly to the dentist who is assuming responsibility for the patient's care.

Dental records and dental radiographs should be retained indefinitely. Because of varying state laws on the statute of limitation, it is not often possible to know when to destroy or discard a patient record. Therefore, patient records should be stored carefully to maintain the integrity of these materials. All dental professionals must be aware of the importance and significance of maintaining patient records in good condition.

Patients Who Refuse Dental Radiographs

Some patients may refuse dental radiographic procedures. When this occurs, the situation must be carefully considered by the dentist. The dentist must then decide whether an accurate diagnosis can be made and treatment provided without a radiograph. In most cases, patient refusal of dental radiographs compromises the patient's diagnosis and treatment, and the dentist cannot treat the patient.

As discussed in Chapter 13, every effort should be made to educate the patient about the importance and usefulness of dental radiographs. No document can be signed to release the dentist from liability. For example, if the patient signs a release or waiver that states that he or she is taking responsibility for any injury that may result, and then an injury does result from negligence (e.g., failure to take dental radiographs), the patient's consent may be invalidated. Legally, the patient cannot consent to negligent care; such consent is invalid.

Table 14-1 lists several Web sites that provide specific information on topics presented in this chapter.

SUMMARY
- Dental auxiliaries must understand their legal obligations with regard to dental radiography.
- The dentist is responsible for prescribing and interpreting dental radiographs, whereas the dental auxiliary is most often responsible for the exposure and processing of such radiographs.
- The dental auxiliary may also be responsible for disclosing the requisite information and obtaining informed consent from the patient before performing the radiographic procedure.

TABLE 14-1   Internet Resources

Organization	Web Site
American Academy of Oral and Maxillofacial Radiology	www.aaomr.org
American Dental Association	www.ada.org
American Dental Hygiene Association	www.adha.org
American Dental Assistants Association	www.dentalassistant.org
U. S. Department of Labor, Occupational Safety and Health Administration	www.osha.gov
U. S. Food and Drug Administration	www.fda.gov

- In many states, dental auxiliaries are employees who work under the supervision of a licensed dentist, who is liable for the actions of these dental personnel. Dental auxiliaries are responsible for their own actions in providing patient care.
- The dental record must include documentation of informed consent and the radiographic procedure (e.g., number and type of films, rationale for exposure, interpretation).
- Legally, dental radiographs are the property of the dentist. The patient does have reasonable access to his or her dental radiographs.
- In most cases, the dentist cannot treat a patient who refuses dental radiography; refusal compromises diagnosis and treatment. No document can be signed that releases the dentist from liability.

BIBLIOGRAPHY

American Dental Association: *Survey of legal provisions for delegating expanded functions to dental assistants and dental hygienists*, Chicago, 1995, American Dental Association.

Bundy AL: *Radiology and the law*, Rockville, MD, 1988, Aspen.

Frommer HH, Savage-Stabulas JJ: Legal considerations. In *Radiology for the dental professional*, ed 9, St. Louis, 2011, Mosby.

Miles DA, Van Dis ML, Jensen CW, Ferretti A: Radiation biology and protection. In *Radiographic imaging for the dental team*, ed 4, St. Louis, 2009, Saunders.

QUIZ QUESTIONS

MULTIPLE CHOICE

___ 1. Informed consent is based on the concept that a patient receives:
   a. some disclosure
   b. no disclosure
   c. complete disclosure
   d. enough disclosure

___ 2. The process of informing the patient about the particulars of exposing dental radiographs is termed:
   a. consent
   b. liability
   c. disclosure
   d. discussion

___ **3.** A dental assistant may have to take an additional certification or licensure examination to expose dental radiographs.
   a. true
   b. false
___ **4.** The right to self-determination means that the patient has the right to consent to or refuse treatment.
   a. true
   b. false
___ **5.** Which of the following may be liable for the actions of a dental auxiliary?
   a. the dentist
   b. the dental auxiliary
   c. both a and b
   d. neither a nor b
___ **6.** The improper exposure of dental radiographs may result in:
   a. phobia
   b. malpractice
   c. standard of care
   d. malfeasance

___ **7.** It is best to retain dental records for 6 years.
   a. true
   b. false
___ **8.** The following must be disclosed to the patient before obtaining informed consent:
   a. the purpose of the procedure and who will perform it
   b. the potential benefits of receiving the procedure
   c. the possible risks in having the procedure performed, as well as the risk of not having the procedure performed
   d. all of the above
___ **9.** Incomplete disclosure to the patient before obtaining his or her informed consent may:
   a. validate the consent
   b. serve as partial consent
   c. invalidate the consent
   d. none of the above
___ **10.** The dental record is a legal document.
   a. true
   b. false

chapter 15

Infection Control and the Dental Radiographer

OUTLINE

INFECTION CONTROL BASICS
    Rationale for Infection Control
    Infection Control Terminology
GUIDELINES FOR INFECTION CONTROL PRACTICES
    Personal Protective Equipment
    Hand Hygiene and Care of Hands
    Sterilization and Disinfection of Instruments

Cleaning and Disinfection of Dental Unit and
    Environmental Surfaces
INFECTION CONTROL IN DENTAL RADIOGRAPHY
    Infection Control Procedures Used Before Exposure
    Infection Control Procedures Used During Exposure
    Infection Control Procedures Used After Exposure
    Infection Control Procedures Used for Processing

LEARNING OBJECTIVES

After completion of this chapter, the student will be able to do the following:

- Define the key terms associated with infection control
- Describe the rationale for infection control
- Describe the three possible routes of disease transmission
- Describe the conditions that must be present for disease transmission to occur
- Discuss personal protective equipment (PPE), hand hygiene, sterilization and disinfection of instruments, and the cleaning and disinfection of the dental unit and environmental surfaces.
- Describe the infection control procedures that are necessary before x-ray exposure.
- Describe the infection control procedures that are necessary during x-ray exposure

- Describe the infection control procedures that are necessary for digital imaging
- Describe the infection control procedures that are necessary after x-ray exposure
- Describe the infection control procedures that are necessary for processing
- Discuss film handling in the darkroom—with and without barrier envelopes
- Discuss film handling without barrier envelopes using the daylight loader of an automatic processor

KEY TERMS

Antiseptic
Asepsis
Barrier envelope
Bloodborne pathogens
Disinfect
Disinfectant, high-level
Disinfectant, intermediate-level
Disinfectant, low-level

Disinfection
Exposure, occupational
Exposure, parenteral
Exposure incident
Infectious waste
Instrument, critical
Instrument, noncritical

Instrument, semicritical
Pathogen
Personal protective equipment (PPE)
Sharp
Standard precautions
Sterilization
Sterilize

Infectious diseases present a significant hazard in the dental environment, and dental professionals are at an increased risk for acquiring such diseases. Therefore, infection control is a major concern in dentistry. Infection control protocols are used in dentistry to minimize the potential for disease transmission. To protect themselves as well as their patients, dental professionals must understand and use infection control protocols.

The infection control practices used in dentistry apply to radiographic procedures as well. The purpose of this chapter is to present the rationale for infection control and the associated terminology, to review the guidelines from the Centers for Disease Control and Prevention (CDC), and to describe in detail the step-by-step infection control procedures used in dental radiography.

INFECTION CONTROL BASICS

To understand infection control practices, the dental professional must first understand the purpose of infection control and the terminology that is frequently used in infection control protocols.

Rationale for Infection Control

The primary purpose of infection control procedures is to prevent the transmission of infectious diseases. Infectious diseases may be transmitted from a patient to the dental professional, from the dental professional to a patient, and from one patient to another patient. The use of recommended infection control guidelines can greatly reduce the transmission of infectious diseases.

Before the dental professional can use infection control practices to prevent disease transmission, an understanding of how disease transmission occurs in the dental environment is necessary. Disease transmission involves pathogens; a **pathogen** is a microorganism capable of causing disease. Dental professionals and dental patients may be exposed to a variety of pathogens that are present in oral or respiratory secretions. These pathogens may include the following:

- Cold and flu viruses and bacteria
- Cytomegalovirus (CMV)
- Hepatitis B virus (HBV)
- Hepatitis C virus (HCV)
- Herpes simplex virus (HSV-1, HSV-2)
- Human immunodeficiency virus (HIV)
- *Mycobacterium tuberculosis*

In the dental environment, the general routes of disease transmission can be described as follows:

- Direct contact with pathogens present in saliva, blood, respiratory secretions, or lesions
- Indirect contact with contaminated objects or instruments
- Direct contact with airborne contaminants present in spatter or aerosols of oral and respiratory fluids

For an infection to occur by one of these routes of transmission, the following three conditions must be present:

1. A susceptible host
2. A pathogen with sufficient infectivity and numbers to cause infection
3. A portal through which the pathogen may enter the host

Effective infection control practices are intended to alter one of these three conditions, thereby preventing disease transmission.

Infection Control Terminology

An understanding of the terminology related to infection control is important for the dental professional. The following terms are frequently used in discussions of infection control, in the infection control literature, and in infection control protocols:

Antiseptic: A substance that inhibits the growth of bacteria. This term is often used to describe handwashing or wound-cleansing procedures.

Asepsis: The absence of pathogens, or disease-causing microorganisms. This term is often used to describe procedures that prevent infection (e.g., aseptic technique).

Bloodborne pathogens: Pathogens present in blood that cause diseases in humans.

Disinfect: Use a chemical or physical procedure to inhibit or destroy pathogens. Highly resistant bacterial and mycotic (fungal) spores are not killed during disinfection procedures.

Disinfection: The act of disinfecting.

Exposure incident: A specific incident that involves contact with blood or other potentially infectious materials and that results from procedures performed by the dental professional.

Infectious waste: Waste that consists of blood, blood products, contaminated sharps, or other microbiologic products.

Occupational exposure: Contact with blood or other infectious materials that involves the skin, eye, or mucous membranes and that results from procedures performed by the dental professional.

Parenteral exposure: Exposure to blood or other infectious materials that results from piercing or puncturing the skin barrier (e.g., a needle-stick injury results in parenteral exposure).

Personal protective equipment (PPE): Includes protective attire, gloves, mask, and eyewear.

Sharps: Any objects that can penetrate the skin, including, but not limited to, needles and scalpels.

Standard precautions: Measures that include a standard of care designed to protect health care personnel and patients from pathogens that can be spread by blood or any other body fluid, excretion, or secretion.

Sterilize: The use of a physical or chemical procedure to destroy all pathogens, including highly resistant bacteria and mycotic spores.

Sterilization: The act of sterilizing.

GUIDELINES FOR INFECTION CONTROL PRACTICES

In 2003, the CDC released a publication entitled *Guidelines for Infection Control in Dental Health Care Settings*, which provides updated infection control practices for dentistry.

The recommended infection control practices are applicable to *all* settings in which dental treatment is provided (Box 15-1). These guidelines must be observed in conjunction with the practices and procedures for worker protection required by the Occupational Safety and Health

- Vaccination of dental professionals
- Use of protective attire and barrier techniques
- Handwashing and care of hands
- Proper use and care of sharp instruments and needles
- Sterilization or disinfection of instruments
- Cleaning and disinfection of the dental unit and environmental surfaces
- Disinfection of the dental laboratory
- Use and care of handpieces, anti-retraction valves, and other intraoral dental devices attached to air and water lines of dental units
- Single use of disposable instruments
- Proper handling of biopsy specimens
- Proper use of extracted teeth in dental educational settings
- Proper disposal of waste materials
- Implementation of recommendations

Administration (OSHA) in its final rule on *Occupational Exposure to Bloodborne Pathogens.* The recommended infection control practices that directly relate to dental radiography procedures include the following:

- PPE
- Handwashing and care of hands
- Sterilization or disinfection of instruments
- Cleaning and disinfection of dental unit and environmental surfaces

Personal Protective Equipment

Protective Clothing

All dental professionals must wear protective clothing (e.g., gown, lab coat, uniform) to prevent skin and mucous membrane exposure when contact with blood or other body fluids is anticipated. Protective clothing must be changed daily or changed more frequently if it is visibly soiled. Dental professionals must remove all protective garments before leaving the dental office, and the garments should be laundered according to the manufacturer's instructions.

Gloves

All dental professionals must wear medical latex or vinyl gloves to prevent skin contact with blood, saliva, or mucous membranes. The dental professional must wear new gloves for each patient. Gloves must also be worn when touching contaminated items or surfaces. Nonsterile gloves are recommended for examinations and nonsurgical procedures; sterile gloves are recommended for all surgical procedures.

In preparation for treating each patient, hands must be washed before gloves are worn. After treating each patient or after exiting the patient treatment area, the dental professional must remove and discard the gloves and wash hands immediately. Dental professionals must always wash their hands and put on new gloves between patients. During treatment, gloves must be removed and changed whenever they

are torn, cut, or punctured. Gloves should never be washed before use or disinfected for reuse. Washing or disinfection causes defects and diminishes the barrier protection provided by the gloves.

Masks and Protective Eyewear

Whenever spatter and aerosolized sprays of blood and saliva are likely, all dental professionals must use surgical masks and protective eyewear, or chin-length plastic face shields, to protect the eyes and face. The mask, when used, must be changed between patients or during treatment if it becomes wet or moist. After treatment, face shields and protective eyewear must be washed with appropriate cleaning agents. When visibly soiled, such equipment should be disinfected between patients.

Hand Hygiene and Care of Hands

Hand Hygiene

In dental radiography, *hand hygiene* is a general term that applies to routine handwashing, antiseptic hand-wash, and antiseptic hand-rub techniques. Indications for hand hygiene include the following:

- Before and after treating each patient (e.g., before glove placement and after glove removal)
- After removing gloves that are torn, cut, or punctured and before putting on new gloves
- After contact of bare hands with inanimate objects likely to be contaminated by blood, saliva, or respiratory secretions
- Before leaving the dental operatory
- When hands are visibly soiled or contaminated

In dental radiography, three different types of hand hygiene may be practiced.

- *Routine hand wash:* Water and nonantimicrobial soap (i.e., plain soap) for 15 seconds
- *Antiseptic hand wash:* Water and antimicrobial soap (e.g., chlorhexidine, iodine and iodophors, chloroxylenol [PCMX], triclosan) for 15 seconds
- *Antiseptic hand rub:* Alcohol-based product until the hands are dry

For more information on hand hygiene including hand lotions and how to store hand care products, please visit the CDC at http://www.cdc.gov/OralHealth/infectioncontrol/faq/hand.htm

Care of Hands

All dental professionals must take precautions to avoid hand injuries during dental procedures. Dental professionals with exudative or "weeping" lesions on their hands must refrain from all direct patient contact and from handling patient care equipment until the condition has resolved.

Sterilization and Disinfection of Instruments

All instruments in the dental practice can be classified into one of the following categories, depending on the risk of transmitting infection and the need to sterilize the instrument between uses:

Critical instruments: Instruments that are used to penetrate soft tissue or bone are considered *critical* and must be sterilized after each use. Examples include forceps, scalpels, bone chisels, scalers, and surgical burs. In dental radiography, no critical instruments are used.

Semicritical instruments: Instruments that contact but do not penetrate soft tissue or bone are classified as *semicritical*. These devices must also be sterilized after each use. If the instrument can be damaged by heat and sterilization is not feasible, high-level disinfection is required. Beam alignment devices are an example of a semicritical instrument used in dental radiography.

Noncritical instruments: Instruments or devices that do not come in contact with mucous membranes are considered *noncritical*. Because little risk of transmitting infection from noncritical devices exists, intermediate-level or low-level infection techniques are required for their care between patients. Examples in dental radiography include the position-indicating device (PID) of the dental x-ray tubehead, the exposure button, the x-ray control panel, and the lead apron.

Acceptable methods of sterilization include steam under pressure (autoclave), dry heat, and chemical vapor. The instructions of the manufacturers of the instruments and sterilizer must be followed. Proper functioning of sterilization cycles must be verified by periodic use of a biologic indicator, such as the spore test.

The U.S. Environmental Protection Agency (EPA) has classified certain chemicals as "sterilants–disinfectants." These EPA-registered chemicals are classified as **high-level disinfectants** and can be used to disinfect heat-sensitive semicritical dental instruments.

Cleaning and Disinfection of Dental Unit and Environmental Surfaces

After each patient has been treated, dental unit surfaces and countertops that may have been contaminated with blood or saliva must be thoroughly cleaned with disposable toweling, using an appropriate cleaning agent and water as necessary. All surfaces must then be disinfected with a suitable chemical germicide.

EPA-registered chemical germicides labeled as both hospital disinfectants and tuberculocidals are classified as **intermediate-level disinfectants** and are recommended for all surfaces that have been contaminated. Intermediate-level disinfectants include phenolics, iodophors, and chlorine-containing compounds.

EPA-registered chemical germicides that are labeled only as hospital disinfectants are classified as **low-level disinfectants** and are recommended for general housekeeping purposes, such as cleaning floors and walls.

INFECTION CONTROL IN DENTAL RADIOGRAPHY

In dentistry, treatment to all patients must be provided after taking standard precautions. **Standard precautions** include a standard of care designed to protect health care personnel and patients from pathogens that can be spread by blood or any other body fluid, excretion, or secretion. The same infection control procedures must be used for each patient. No exceptions exist, and no "extra" precautions should be used on any patients. Specific infection control procedures pertain to dental radiography and must be used for each patient.

The areas designated for the exposure and processing of dental radiographs are not routinely associated with the spatter of blood or saliva; however, transmission of infectious diseases is still possible if the equipment, supplies, film packets, digital sensors, or cassettes used for the radiographic procedure are contaminated. Therefore, specific infection control procedures that pertain to dental radiography must be used before, during, and after film exposure (Box 15-2), as well as during film processing (Procedure 15-1).

Infection Control Procedures Used Before Exposure

Before dental x-ray receptors are exposed, the treatment area must be prepared using aseptic techniques. Necessary supplies and equipment must also be prepared. After such preparations, the dental radiographer can seat the patient. At that time, the dental radiographer can also complete the final infection control procedures that are necessary before exposure.

Preparation of Treatment Area

The dental professional must prepare the surfaces that are likely to be touched during the radiographic procedure. All these surfaces should be covered with impervious, disposable materials such as plastic wrap, plastic-backed paper, or aluminum foil. This provides adequate protection while eliminating the need for surface cleaning and disinfection between patients. If disposable materials are not used, after the radiographic procedures have been completed, all contaminated areas must be disinfected with disinfecting products, following the manufacturer's instructions. Examples of surfaces that must be covered or disinfected include the following:

X-Ray Machine. The tubehead, PID, control panel, and exposure button must all be covered or disinfected.

Dental Chair. The headrest as well as the headrest adjustment and chair adjustment controls must be covered or disinfected.

Work Area. The area where x-ray supplies (e.g., film, sensors) are placed during exposure must be covered or disinfected.

Lead Apron. If contaminated, the lead apron must be wiped with a disinfectant between patients.

Preparation of Supplies and Equipment

The dental professional must also have ready all anticipated supplies and equipment, such as film, sensors, sterilized beam alignment devices, and other miscellaneous items, and must make these available in the work area.

Film. Dental x-ray films should be dispensed from a central supply area in a disposable container (e.g., coin

BOX 15-2   Checklist for Infection Control in Dental Radiography

Before Exposure
Treatment Area
The following must be covered or disinfected:
- X-ray machine
- Dental chair
- Work area
- Lead apron

Supplies and Equipment
The following must be prepared before seating the patient:
- Image receptors
- Beam alignment devices
- Cotton rolls
- Paper towel
- Disposable container

Patient Preparation
The following must be performed before putting on gloves:
- Adjusting chair
- Adjusting headrest
- Placing lead apron on patient
- Removing metallic objects in the head and neck area of patient

Radiographer Preparation
The following must be completed before exposure:
- Washing hands
- Putting on gloves
- Preparing beam alignment devices

During Exposure
Film Handling
Procedures must include the following:
- Drying receptor with paper towel following exposure
- Placing dried receptor in disposable container

Beam Alignment Devices
Handling of devices includes the following:
- Transferring beam alignment device from work area to mouth and back to work area; disassembling over a protected work area
- Never placing beam alignment devices on uncovered countertop

After Exposure
Before Glove Removal
- Disposing of all contaminated items
- Placing beam alignment devices in area designated for contaminated instruments

After Glove Removal
- Washing hands
- Removing lead apron

PROCEDURE 15-1   Steps for Film Handling During Processing

With Barrier Envelopes
- Place a disposable towel on the work surface in the darkroom.
- Place the container with contaminated films next to the towel.
- Put on gloves.
- Take one contaminated film out of the container.
- Tear open the barrier envelope.
- Allow the film to drop on the paper towel.
- Do not touch the film with gloved hands.
- Dispose of the barrier envelope.
- After all barrier envelopes have been opened, dispose of the container.
- Remove gloves, and wash hands.
- Turn out the darkroom lights, and secure the door.
- Unwrap and process films.
- Label the film mount, paper cup, or envelope with the patient's name, and use it to collect processed films.

Without Barrier Envelopes
- Place a disposable towel on the work surface in the darkroom.

- Place the container with contaminated films next to the towel.
- Put on gloves.
- Turn out the darkroom lights, and secure the door.
- Take one contaminated film out of the container.
- Open the film packet tab, and slide out the lead foil backing and black paper. Discard the film packet wrapping.
- Rotate the foil away from the black paper, and discard it.
- Without touching the film, open the black paper wrapping.
- Allow the film to drop on the paper towel.
- Do not touch the film with gloved hands.
- Discard the black paper wrapping.
- After all barrier envelopes have been opened, dispose of the container.
- Remove gloves, and wash hands.
- Process the films.
- Label the film mount, paper cup, or envelope with the patient's name, and use it to collect processed films.

envelope, paper cup). Commercially available plastic barrier envelopes that fit over intraoral films can be used to protect the film packets from saliva and minimize contamination after exposure of the film. Intraoral films may be inserted and sealed in plastic **barrier envelopes** (e.g., ClinAsept Barrier Envelopes, manufactured by Carestream Health, Inc.) before dispensing films from a central supply area (Figure 15-1).

Digital Sensors. The sensors/receptors (see Chapter 25) used in digital radiography cannot be heat sterilized. In order to avoid cross-contamination, both barrier techniques and disinfection are required. The CDC recommends cleaning and disinfecting the sensor with an EPA-registered intermediate-level disinfectant after removing the barrier and before using it on another patient. Because sensors and digital radiography components vary by manufacturer and can be expensive, manufacturers should be consulted regarding specific disinfection products and procedures. As with dental x-ray film, sensors used in indirect digital imaging should also be dispensed from a central supply area. These sensors must be wrapped in plastic barrier envelopes to protect the sensor from saliva and contamination, much like the barriers used for intraoral films (Figure 15-2). Dental offices using direct digital imaging require plastic disposable sleeves to cover both the sensor and the wire connection (Figure 15-3).

Beam Alignment Devices. Beam alignment devices should be packaged in sterilized bags and dispensed from a central supply area.

Miscellaneous Items. Other items include cotton rolls that can be used to stabilize receptor placement and paper towels that can be used to remove saliva from exposed receptors. A disposable container (e.g., paper cup or bag) labeled with the patient's name is necessary to collect the exposed receptors. All miscellaneous items should be dispensed from a central supply area.

Preparation of the Patient

The dental professional can seat the patient following preparation of the treatment area, supplies, and equipment. After seating the patient, the dental radiographer must complete the procedures discussed next *before* washing hands and putting on gloves.

Chair Adjustment. The chair must be positioned so that the patient is seated upright. The height of the chair should be adjusted to a comfortable working height for the dental radiographer.

Headrest Adjustment. The headrest must be adjusted to support the patient's head. The patient's head should be positioned with the maxillary arch parallel to the floor.

Lead Apron. The lead apron with the thyroid collar must be placed on the patient and secured before any x-ray exposure.

Miscellaneous Objects. Miscellaneous objects belonging to the patient that may interfere with film exposure (e.g., eyeglasses, chewing gum, dentures) must be removed by the patient at this time.

Preparation of the Dental Radiographer

After patient preparation and before x-ray exposure of the patient, the dental radiographer must complete some final infection control procedures.

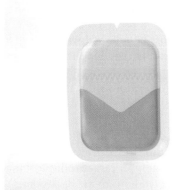

FIGURE 15-1 ClinAsept barrier films are easy to use. Exposure and processing procedures are completed in the same manner as with other intraoral films. Complete instructions are included with every carton. (Courtesy Carestream Health, Inc., Rochester, NY.)

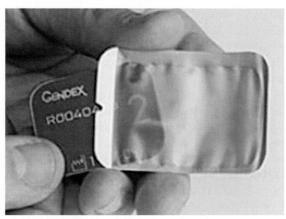

FIGURE 15-2 A plastic barrier envelope surrounds and protects this intraoral sensor. (Courtesy Gendex Dental Systems, Des Plaines, IL.)

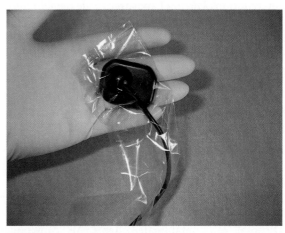

FIGURE 15-3 A plastic disposable sleeve covers both the wire and the sensor in direct digital imaging. (Courtesy Gendex Dental Systems, Des Plaines, IL.)

Handwashing. Hands must be washed with soap or an antimicrobial solution in the presence of the patient.

Gloves. Immediately after handwashing, gloves must be worn.

Mask and Eyewear. Because no aerosolized contaminants are created during radiographic exposures, the use of a surgical mask and protective eyewear is optional.

Beam Alignment Devices. If beam alignment devices are to be used during exposure, they must be removed from sterilized packages with gloved hands in the presence of the patient and then assembled over a covered work area.

Infection Control Procedures Used During Exposure

Once gloves have been put on and exposure begins, the dental radiographer should take special care to touch only covered surfaces. The best way the dental radiographer can minimize contamination is to touch as few surfaces as possible. During and immediately after exposure, the dental radiographer must handle each receptor in a manner consistent with comprehensive infection control guidelines.

Drying of Exposed Receptors. After each receptor has been placed in the patient's mouth, exposed, and removed, it must be dried with a paper towel to remove excess saliva.

Collection of Exposed Receptors. Once dried, each receptor must be placed in a disposable container (paper bag or cup) labeled with the patient's name. This container is used to collect and transport the exposed receptors to the darkroom or scanning area and must *not* be touched by gloved hands. To prevent fogging caused by scatter radiation, the container should not be placed in a room where additional receptors are being exposed. In addition, exposed receptors should never be placed in the dental radiographer's lab coat or uniform pocket.

Beam Alignment Devices. During exposure, beam alignment devices should be transferred from the covered work area to the patient's mouth and then back to the same area. Contaminated instruments should never be placed on an uncovered countertop.

Interruptions During Exposure. If the dental radiographer is interrupted (e.g., by a telephone call) and must leave the room during exposure of receptors, the radiographer must remove the gloves and wash hands before leaving the area. He or she must then rewash hands and put on new gloves before resuming the procedure.

Infection Control Procedures Used After Exposure

Immediately after the completion of receptor exposures, all contaminated items must be discarded, and any uncovered areas must be disinfected. Contaminated items must be handled in a manner consistent with recommended infection control guidelines.

Disposal of Contaminated Items. All contaminated items (cotton rolls, bite-wing tabs, cups, bags, and protective coverings) must be disposed of following local and state environmental regulations. Contaminated items must be discarded while the dental radiographer is still wearing gloves; this includes disposable materials found on protected surfaces as well. The dental radiographer must carefully unwrap all covered surfaces; the surfaces that are wrapped should not be touched by gloved hands. Ideally, the disposal of all contaminated items should take place in the presence of the patient.

Beam Alignment Devices. While still wearing gloves, the dental radiographer must remove the contaminated beam alignment devices from the treatment area and place them in an area designated for contaminated instruments.

Handwashing. After removal and disposal of all contaminated items, the radiographer must remove the gloves and discard them and wash hands.

Lead Apron Removal. After washing hands, the radiographer can remove the lead apron from the patient. Following this, the patient can be dismissed from the area.

Surface Disinfection. Any uncovered areas that were contaminated during treatment must be cleaned and disinfected using an EPA-registered hospital-grade disinfectant and utility gloves.

Infection Control Procedures Used for Processing

After the exposure of x-ray receptors, specific infection control guidelines must be followed while transporting the receptors to the darkroom, handling them, and processing them.

Film Transport. As previously described, films contaminated with saliva must be placed in a labeled disposable container after exposure. The disposable container should never be touched by gloved hands. Only after removing gloves, washing hands, dismissing the patient, and cleaning the area, should the dental radiographer carry the disposable container holding the contaminated films to the darkroom.

Darkroom Supplies. Paper towels and gloves, which are necessary for handling films before they are processed, must be available in the darkroom. Paper envelopes, paper cups, or film mounts labeled with the patient's name are used to hold films after processing, and these also should be available in the darkroom.

Film Handling with and without Barrier Envelopes. Commercially available barrier envelopes help to minimize contamination in the darkroom. Procedure 15-1 lists the recommended film-handling steps when exposed films are protected by barrier envelopes (Figure 15-4) and when films are not protected by barrier envelopes (Figure 15-5). These same steps can be applied to the handling and scanning of storage phosphor sensors used with indirect digital imaging.

Disinfection of Darkroom. Darkroom countertops and any areas touched by gloved hands must be disinfected with an EPA-registered hospital-grade disinfectant.

Daylight Loader Procedures. Infection control procedures for processing film without barrier envelopes in

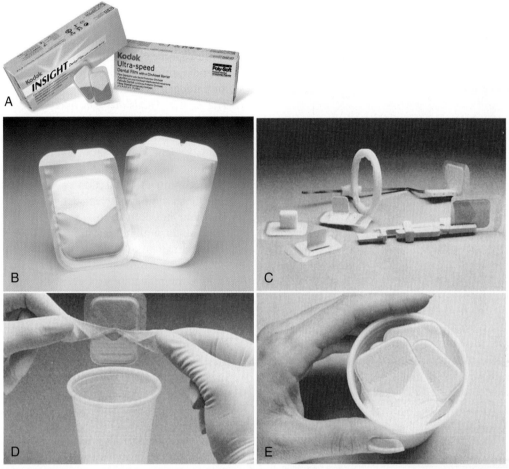

FIGURE 15-4 **A**, Packaging for barrier film. **B**, Protected and unprotected film. **C**, Bite-wing and periapical applications of protected film. **D**, Film packet removal from envelope without contamination. **E**, Uncontaminated film ready for processing. (Courtesy Carestream Health, Inc. Rochester, NY.)

automatic film processors equipped with daylight loaders include the following:

1. Place the paper cup and the vinyl or nonpowdered gloves in the daylight loader compartment.
2. Place the container with contaminated films next to the cup.
3. Close the daylight loader lid, and push hands through openings.
4. Put on gloves.
5. Take one contaminated film out of the container.
6. Open film packets as described in Film Handling without Barrier Envelopes (see Procedure 15-1).
7. Allow the film to drop onto the processor film feed slot area. (Do not touch the film with gloved hands.)
8. Dispose of film packet wrappings in the paper cup.
9. After all film packets have been opened, remove gloves and place them in the cup.
10. Feed all unwrapped films into the processor.
11. Remove hands from the daylight loader.
12. Wash hands.

13. Lift the daylight loader lid to remove and discard the cup with contaminated wrappings and the container that held contaminated films.
14. Label the film mount, paper cup, or envelope with the patient's name, and use it to collect processed films.

SUMMARY

- To protect themselves as well as their patients, dental professionals must understand and use infection control protocols. The primary purpose of infection control procedures is to prevent the transmission of infectious diseases.
- Disease transmission involves pathogens, or microorganisms that are capable of causing disease. In dentistry, disease transmission may occur as a result of one of the following:
  - Direct contact with pathogens in saliva, blood, respiratory secretions, or lesions
  - Indirect contact with contaminated objects or instruments

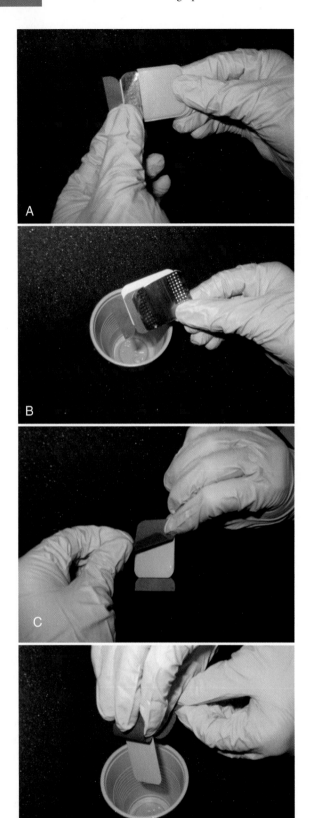

- Direct contact with airborne contaminants present in spatter or aerosols or oral and respiratory fluids
- For infection to occur, three conditions must be present: (1) susceptible host, (2) pathogen with sufficient infectivity and numbers to cause infection, and (3) portal of entry for pathogen to infect host.
- The CDC's *Guidelines for Infection Control in Dental Health Care Settings* (2003) outlines specific infection control measures that pertain to dentistry, including PPE, hand hygiene, and sterilization and disinfection of instruments.
- The recommended infection control practices are applicable to all settings in which dental treatment is provided. The same infection control procedures must be used for each patient, with no exceptions and no extra precautions for select patients.
- Infection control procedures before x-ray exposure include the preparation of (1) the treatment area (x-ray machine, dental chair, work area, lead apron), (2) the supplies and equipment (film, digital sensors, beam alignment devices, other items), (3) the patient (chair and headrest adjustment, lead apron), and (4) the radiographer (handwashing, gloves).
- Infection control practices during exposure involve drying and collecting exposed receptors, reassembly of beam alignment devices, and dealing with interruptions properly.
- Infection control procedures after exposure include disposal of contaminated items, removal of beam alignment devices, handwashing, lead apron removal, and surface disinfection.
- Infection control practices during processing involve film transport, darkroom supplies, film handling with and without barrier envelopes, disinfection of the darkroom, and daylight loaders.

BIBLIOGRAPHY

American Academy of Oral and Maxillofacial Radiology: Infection control guidelines for dental radiographic procedures. *Oral Surg Oral Med Oral Pathol* 73:248, 1992.

Centers for Disease Control and Prevention: Guidelines for infection control in dental health care settings. *MMWR* 52(RR-17):1–61, 2003.

Cottone JA, Terezhalmy GT, Molinari JA: Infection control in dental radiology. In *Practical infection control in dentistry*, Philadelphia, 1991, Lea & Febiger.

Cottone JA, Terezhalmy GT, Molinari JA: Rationale for practical infection control in dentistry. In *Practical infection control in dentistry*, Philadelphia, 1991, Lea & Febiger.

Cottone JA, Terezhalmy GT, Molinari JA: Appendix B. In *Practical infection control in dentistry*, Philadelphia, 1991, Lea & Febiger.

Frommer HH, Savage-Stabulas JJ: Infection control in dental practice. In *Radiology for the dental professional*, ed 8, St. Louis, 2005, Mosby.

White SC, Pharoah MJ: Radiographic quality assurance and infection control. In *Oral radiology: principles and interpretation*, ed 6, St. Louis, 2009, Mosby.

FIGURE 15-5 Steps used to open a size 2 film packet without contaminating film. **A,** Method for removing films from packet and not touching them with contaminated gloves. Open tab, and slide lead foil and black interleaf paper from wrapping. **B,** Rotate contaminated film packet away from black paper and foil and discard. **C,** Peel back paper wrapping away from film. **D,** Allow film to fall into a clean cup.

QUIZ QUESTIONS

MATCHING

For questions 1 to 10, match each definition with one term.

a. Disinfect
b. Sterilize
c. Asepsis
d. Infectious waste
e. Pathogen
f. Noncritical instrument
g. Critical instrument
h. Semicritical instrument
i. Parenteral exposure
j. Occupational exposure
k. Antiseptic

___ 1. Use of a chemical or physical procedure to destroy all pathogens, including spores
___ 2. Microorganism capable of causing disease
___ 3. Exposure to infectious material resulting from procedures performed by the dental professional
___ 4. Exposure to infectious materials that results from piercing or puncturing the skin
___ 5. Use of a chemical or physical procedure to destroy all pathogens, except spores
___ 6. Instrument used to penetrate soft tissue or bone
___ 7. Instrument that contacts but does not penetrate soft tissue or bone
___ 8. Instrument that does not contact mucous membranes
___ 9. Waste that consists of blood, blood products, contaminated sharps, and other microbiologic products
___ 10. Absence of pathogens

FILL IN THE BLANK

11. What is the primary purpose of infection control?

_____

_____

12. List the three possible routes of disease transmission.

_____

_____

13. List the three conditions that must be present for disease transmission to occur.

_____

_____

MULTIPLE CHOICE

___ 14. Identify the false statement concerning protective clothing:
   a. It must be worn by all dental professionals.
   b. It must be worn to prevent contact with infectious materials.
   c. It must be changed weekly.
   d. It must be removed before leaving the dental office.

___ 15. Identify the false statement concerning gloves:
   a. Gloves must be worn by all dental professionals.
   b. Gloves must be washed before use.
   c. Gloves must be worn for each patient.
   d. Gloves must be sterile for surgical procedures.

___ 16. Identify the false statement concerning masks and protective eyewear:
   a. Masks and protective eyewear are optional for dental radiographic procedures.
   b. Masks must be changed between patients.
   c. When visibly soiled, protective eyewear must be disinfected between patients.
   d. Protective shield must be worn during radiographic procedures.

___ 17. Identify the true statements concerning handwashing. Hands must be washed:
   a. before and after gloving
   b. before and after each patient
   c. after touching contaminated surfaces
   d. with plain soap for routine dental procedures
      1) 1, 2, 3, and 4
      2) 1, 2, and 3
      3) 1, 2, and 4
      4) 2, 3, and 4

___ 18. Examples of critical instruments include:
   a. beam alignment device
   b. scalpel

    c. scaler

    d. amalgam condenser

       1) 1, 2, 3, and 4

       2) 1, 2, and 3

       3) 2, 3, and 4

       4) 2 and 3

____ **19.** EPA-registered chemical germicides labeled as both hospital disinfectants and tuberculocidal agents are classified as:

    a. high-level disinfectants

    b. sterilant disinfectants

    c. low-level disinfectants

    d. intermediate-level disinfectants

____ **20.** EPA-registered chemical germicides labeled only as hospital disinfectants are classified as:

    a. high-level disinfectants

    b. sterilant disinfectants

    c. low-level disinfectants

    d. intermediate-level disinfectants

ESSAY

21. Describe the infection control procedures that are necessary before x-ray exposure.

22. Describe the infection control procedures that are necessary during x-ray exposure.

23. Describe the infection control procedures that are necessary after x-ray exposure.

24. Describe the infection control procedures that are necessary for film processing.

25. Discuss film handling in the darkroom, with and without barrier envelopes.

part IV

Technique Basics

Chapter 16 Introduction to Radiographic Examinations, 152
Chapter 17 Paralleling Technique, 155
Chapter 18 Bisecting Technique, 180
Chapter 19 Bite-Wing Technique, 210
Chapter 20 Exposure and Technique Errors, 226
Chapter 21 Occlusal and Localization Techniques, 239
Chapter 22 Panoramic Imaging, 256
Chapter 23 Extraoral Imaging, 274
Chapter 24 Imaging of Patients with Special Needs, 290

Introduction to Radiographic Examinations

OUTLINE

INTRAORAL RADIOGRAPHIC EXAMINATION
> Types of Intraoral Radiographic Examinations
> Complete Mouth Radiographic Series/Full Mouth Series
> Diagnostic Criteria for Intraoral Radiographs

EXTRAORAL RADIOGRAPHIC EXAMINATION
PRESCRIPTION OF DENTAL RADIOGRAPHS

LEARNING OBJECTIVES

After completion of this chapter, the student will be able to do the following:

- Define the key terms associated with radiographic examinations
- List the three types of intraoral radiographic examinations
- Describe the purpose and the type of receptor and technique used for each of the three types of intraoral radiographic examinations
- List the various projections that constitute a complete mouth radiographic series (CMRS)
- List the general diagnostic criteria for intraoral radiographs
- List examples of extraoral radiographic examinations
- Discuss the prescribing of dental radiographs
- Describe when prescribing a CMRS for a new patient is warranted

KEY TERMS

Complete mouth radiographic series (CMRS)
Dentulous
Edentulous
Extraoral radiographic examination
Full mouth series (FMS or FMX)

Interproximal examination
Intraoral radiographic examination
Occlusal examination
Periapical examination
Radiograph, diagnostic
Receptor, bite-wing

Receptor, extraoral
Receptor, intraoral
Receptor, occlusal
Receptor, periapical
Tooth-bearing areas

The dental radiographer must have a working knowledge of radiographic techniques. Before the discussion of the basics of the techniques, an understanding of the different types of radiographic examinations is necessary. Dental radiographic examinations may involve either intraoral projections (placed inside the mouth) or extraoral projections (placed outside the mouth).

The purpose of this chapter is to introduce the dental radiographer to the different intraoral radiographic examinations used in dentistry, to define the complete mouth radiographic series, and to describe in detail the diagnostic criteria of intraoral radiographs. In addition, the extraoral radiographic examinations used in dentistry are introduced.

INTRAORAL RADIOGRAPHIC EXAMINATION

The **intraoral radiographic examination** is a radiographic inspection of teeth and intraoral adjacent structures. Such intraoral examinations are the foundation of dental radiography. The intraoral radiographic examination requires the use of intraoral image receptors (see Chapter 7). **Intraoral receptors** are placed inside the mouth to examine the teeth and supporting structures.

Types of Intraoral Radiographic Examinations

The following three common types of examinations use intraoral radiographs:

- Periapical examination
- Interproximal examination
- Occlusal examination

Each of these examinations has a certain purpose and requires the use of a specific type of imaging receptor and technique.

Periapical Examination

Purpose. **Periapical examination** is used to examine the entire tooth (crown and root) and supporting bone.

Type of Imaging Receptor. The **periapical receptor** is used in periapical examination. The term *periapical* is derived from the Greek prefix *peri-* (meaning "around") and the Latin word *apex* (referring to the terminal end of a tooth root). Periapical images show the terminal end of the tooth root and surrounding bone as well as the crown.

Technique. Two methods are used for obtaining periapical radiographs: (1) the paralleling technique (see Chapter 17) and (2) the bisecting technique (see Chapter 18).

Interproximal Examination

Purpose. **Interproximal examination** is used to examine the crowns of both maxillary and mandibular teeth on a single image. As the term *proximal* suggests, this examination is useful in examining adjacent tooth surfaces and crestal bone.

Type of Imaging Receptor. The **bite-wing receptor** is used in interproximal examination. The bite-wing receptor has a "wing" or tab attached to it; the patient "bites" on the wing to stabilize the receptor.

Technique. The bite-wing technique (see Chapter 19) is used in interproximal examination.

Occlusal Examination

Purpose. **Occlusal examination** is used to examine large areas of the maxilla or the mandible on one image.

Type of Imaging Receptor. The **occlusal receptor** is used in occlusal examination. As the term *occlusal* suggests, the patient "occludes," or bites on, the entire receptor.

Technique. The occlusal technique (see Chapter 21) is used in occlusal examination.

Complete Mouth Radiographic Series/Full Mouth Series

The **complete mouth radiographic series (CMRS)** is also known as the **full mouth series (FMS or FMX)** or the complete series. The CMRS can be defined as a series of intraoral dental radiographs that show all the tooth-bearing areas of both jaws. **Tooth-bearing areas** are the regions of the maxilla and the mandible, where the 32 teeth of the human dentition are normally located. Tooth-bearing areas include **dentulous** areas, or areas that exhibit teeth, as well as **edentulous** areas, or areas where teeth are no longer present.

The CMRS consists of periapical radiographs alone or a combination of periapical and bite-wing radiographs. Bite-wing radiographs are used only in areas where teeth have

---

BOX 16-1	**General Diagnostic Criteria for Intraoral Images**

1. Dental images must display optimal density, contrast, definition, and detail.
2. Dental images must display the least amount of distortion possible; images must be of the same shape and size as the object being radiographed.
3. The complete mouth radiographic series (CMRS) must include images that show all tooth-bearing areas, including dentulous and edentulous regions.
4. Periapical images must show the entire crowns and roots of the teeth being examined, as well as 2 to 3 mm beyond the root apices.
5. Bite-wing images must show open contacts, or interproximal tooth surfaces that are not overlapped.

---

interproximal contact with other teeth to examine the contact areas for caries (decay). To include every tooth and all tooth-bearing areas, a range of 14 to 20 images may be included in the CMRS.

The number of images is dictated by the radiographic technique used for exposure and the number of teeth present. For example, in the patient without teeth, 14 periapical images are usually sufficient to cover the edentulous arches. In the dentulous patient, the number of periapical images varies, depending on which technique—paralleling or bisecting—is used. Receptor size is also dictated by the technique used.

Diagnostic Criteria for Intraoral Radiographs

A **diagnostic radiograph**, as described in Chapter 8, provides a great deal of information. Specific diagnostic criteria for each radiographic exposure are described in Chapters 17, 18, 19, and 21 (paralleling, bisecting, bite-wing, and occlusal, respectively). General diagnostic criteria for intraoral radiographs are listed in Box 16-1.

EXTRAORAL RADIOGRAPHIC EXAMINATION

The **extraoral radiographic examination** is a radiographic inspection of large areas of the skull or jaws. The extraoral radiographic examination requires the use of extraoral imaging receptors (see Chapter 7). **Extraoral receptors** are placed outside the mouth. Examples of common extraoral radiographs include the panoramic radiograph as well as the lateral jaw, lateral cephalometric, posteroanterior, Waters, submentovertex, reverse Towne, transcranial, and tomographic projections. Each of these extraoral examinations has a specific purpose and requires the use of certain receptors and techniques. The purposes, receptors, and techniques used in extraoral radiography are described in Chapters 22 and 23.

PRESCRIPTION OF DENTAL RADIOGRAPHS

As discussed in Chapter 5, the prescription of dental radiographs is based on the individual needs of the patient. The dentist uses professional judgment to make decisions about the number, type, and frequency of dental radiographs. Every patient's dental condition is different, and therefore every patient must be evaluated for dental radiographs on an individual basis.

For example, not all patients need a CMRS. As detailed in the Guidelines for Prescribing Dental Radiographs (see Table 5-1), a CMRS is appropriate when a new adult patient presents with clinical evidence of generalized dental disease or a history of extensive dental treatment. Otherwise, a combination of bite-wings, selected periapicals, and/or a panoramic radiograph should be prescribed on the basis of a patient's individual needs.

SUMMARY

- Dental radiographic examinations may involve either intraoral projections (placed inside the mouth) or extraoral projections (placed outside the mouth).
- The intraoral radiographic examination is a radiographic inspection of teeth and intraoral structures. The three common types of intraoral examinations are periapical, interproximal, and occlusal examinations.
- Periapical examination is used to inspect the crowns and roots of teeth as well as the supporting bone. Periapical receptors are used in periapical examination. Either the paralleling technique or the bisecting technique can be used to expose periapical receptors.
- Interproximal examination is used to examine the crowns of maxillary as well as mandibular teeth on a single image. The bite-wing receptor and the bite-wing technique are used in interproximal examination.
- Occlusal examination is used to examine large areas of the maxilla or mandible on one image. Occlusal receptors and the occlusal technique are used.
- The complete mouth radiographic series (CMRS), or full-mouth series (FMS or FMX), is an intraoral series of dental radiographs that shows all the tooth-bearing areas of the maxilla and the mandible and consists of 14 to 20 images (periapical radiographs alone or combination of periapical and bite-wing radiographs), depending on radiographic technique and number of teeth present.
- An intraoral radiograph is considered diagnostic if it shows images with optimal density, contrast, definition and detail, and minimal distortion. In addition, a diagnostic periapical radiograph shows the entire crowns and roots of the teeth being examined, and a diagnostic bite-wing radiograph should show open contacts.
- The extraoral radiographic examination is a radiographic inspection of large areas of the skull or jaws.

BIBLIOGRAPHY

Johnson ON, Thomson EM: Intraoral radiographic procedures. In *Essentials of dental radiography for dental assistants and hygienists*, ed 8, Upper Saddle River, NJ, 2007, Pearson.

Miles DA, Van Dis ML, Jensen CW, Ferretti A: Intraoral radiographic technique. In *Radiographic imaging for the dental team*, ed 4, St. Louis, 2009, Saunders.

White SC, Pharoah MJ: Intraoral radiographic examinations. In *Oral radiology: principles and interpretation*, ed 6, St. Louis, 2009, Mosby.

QUIZ QUESTIONS

MATCHING

For questions 1 to 10, match each definition with one term.

a. Dentulous
b. Edentulous
c. Periapical receptor
d. Bite-wing receptor
e. Occlusal receptor
f. Intraoral receptor
g. Extraoral receptor
h. Maxilla
i. Mandible
j. Occlude
k. Occlusion

___ 1. A receptor placed inside the mouth
___ 2. The lower jaw
___ 3. Without teeth
___ 4. To close or to bite
___ 5. A receptor used to examine a large area of the maxilla or mandible in one image
___ 6. A receptor used to examine the crowns of the maxillary and mandibular teeth on a single image
___ 7. A receptor placed outside the mouth
___ 8. With teeth
___ 9. The upper jaw
___ 10. A receptor used to examine the entire tooth and supporting bone

SHORT ANSWER

11. List the three types of intraoral radiographic examinations.
12. Describe the purpose, type of receptor, and technique used for each of the three types of intraoral radiographic examinations.
13. List the general diagnostic criteria for intraoral radiographs.
14. List examples of extraoral radiographic examinations.
15. Discuss prescription of dental radiographs.

chapter 17

Paralleling Technique

OUTLINE

BASIC CONCEPTS
    Terminology
    Principles of Paralleling Technique
    Beam Alignment Devices
    Receptors Used for Paralleling Technique
    Rules for Paralleling Technique
STEP-BY-STEP PROCEDURES
    Patient Preparation
    Equipment Preparation
Exposure Sequence for Receptor Placements
Receptor Placement for Paralleling Technique
MODIFICATIONS IN PARALLELING TECHNIQUE
    Shallow Palate
    Bony Growths
    Mandibular Premolar Region
ADVANTAGES AND DISADVANTAGES
    Advantages of Paralleling Technique
    Disadvantages of Paralleling Technique

LEARNING OBJECTIVES

After completion of this chapter, the student will be able to do the following:

- Define the key terms associated with the paralleling technique
- State the basic principle of the paralleling technique and illustrate the placement of the receptor, beam alignment device, position-indicating device (PID), and central ray
- Discuss how object–receptor distance affects the radiographic image and how target–receptor distance is used to compensate for such changes
- List the beam alignment devices that can be used with the paralleling technique
- Describe why a beam alignment device is necessary with the paralleling technique
- Identify and label the parts of the Rinn XCP instruments
- Describe the different sizes of receptors used with the paralleling technique and how each receptor is placed in the bite-block

- State the five basic rules of the paralleling technique
- Describe the patient and equipment preparations that are necessary before using the paralleling technique
- Discuss the exposure sequence for 15 periapical receptor placements using the paralleling technique
- Describe each of the 15 periapical receptor placements recommended for use with the XCP instruments
- Summarize the guidelines for periapical receptor positioning
- Explain the modifications in the paralleling technique that are used for a patient with a shallow palate, bony growths, or a sensitive premolar region
- List the advantages and disadvantages of the paralleling technique

KEY TERMS

Angle, right
Beam alignment device
Central ray
Exposure sequence
Film holder, EEZEE-Grip
Film holder, hemostat
Film holder, Precision
Film holder, Stabe

Instruments, Rinn XCP
Intersecting
Long axis (tooth)
Mandibular tori
Maxillary torus
Object–receptor distance
Palate
Parallel

Paralleling technique
Perpendicular
Receptor placement
Target–receptor distance
Teeth, anterior
Teeth, posterior
Torus, tori

In dentistry, the radiographer must master a variety of intraoral radiographic techniques. The paralleling technique is an important technique used to obtain periapical images. Before the dental radiographer can use the paralleling technique, an understanding of the basic concepts and required equipment is necessary. In addition, the dental radiographer must understand patient preparation, equipment preparation, exposure sequencing, and the receptor placement procedures used in the paralleling technique.

The purpose of this chapter is to present basic concepts and to describe patient preparation, equipment preparation, and receptor placement procedures used in the paralleling technique. This chapter also describes modifications of this technique that can be used in patients with certain anatomic conditions, outlines the advantages and disadvantages of the paralleling technique, and reviews helpful hints.

BASIC CONCEPTS

The **paralleling technique** (also known as the *extension cone paralleling [XCP] technique, right-angle technique,* and *long-cone technique*) is one method that can be used to expose periapical and bite-wing image receptors. Before the dental radiographer can competently perform the paralleling technique, a thorough understanding of the terminology, principles, and basic rules governing this technique is necessary. Knowledge of the beam alignment devices and receptors used with the paralleling technique is also required.

Terminology

An understanding of the following basic terms is necessary before describing the paralleling technique:

Parallel: Moving or lying in the same plane, always separated by the same distance and not intersecting (Figure 17-1, A)

Intersecting: To cut across or through (Figure 17-1, B)

Perpendicular: Intersecting at or forming a right angle (Figure 17-1, C)

Right angle: An angle of 90 degrees formed by two lines perpendicular to each other (Figure 17-1, D)

Long axis of the tooth: An imaginary line that divides the tooth longitudinally into two equal halves (Figure 17-2)

Central ray: The central portion of the primary beam of x-radiation

Principles of Paralleling Technique

As the term *paralleling* indicates, this technique is based on the concept of *parallelism.* The basic principles of the paralleling technique can be described as follows (Figure 17-3):

1. The receptor is placed in the mouth *parallel* to the long axis of the tooth being radiographed.

2. The central ray of the x-ray beam is directed *perpendicular* (at a right angle) to the receptor and the long axis of the tooth.

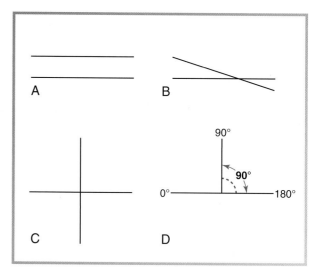

FIGURE 17-1 A, Parallel lines are always separated by the same distance and do not intersect. **B,** Intersecting lines cross one another. **C,** Perpendicular lines intersect one another to form right angles. **D,** A right angle measures 90 degrees and is formed by two perpendicular lines.

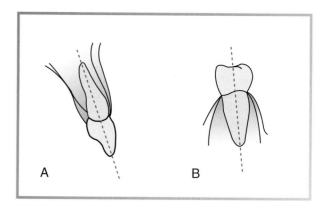

FIGURE 17-2 A, The long axis of the maxillary incisor divides the tooth into two equal halves. **B,** The long axis of a mandibular premolar divides the tooth into two equal halves.

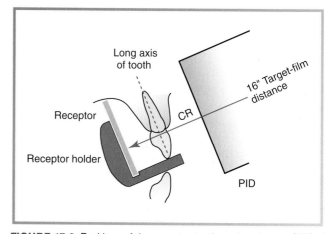

FIGURE 17-3 Positions of the receptor, teeth, and central ray (CR) of the x-ray beam in the paralleling technique. The receptor and the long axis of the tooth are parallel. The central ray is perpendicular to the tooth and the receptor. An increased target–receptor distance (16 inches) is required. *PID,* position-indicating device.

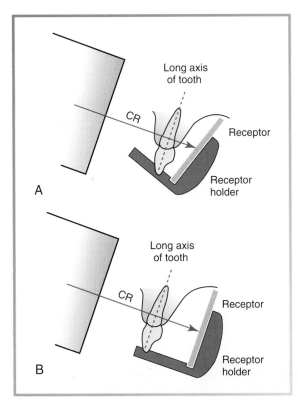

FIGURE 17-4 A, The receptor is placed close to the tooth and is not parallel to the long axis of the tooth. **B**, Increased object–receptor distance. The receptor is placed away from the tooth and is now parallel with the long axis of the tooth. *CR*, central ray.

3. A beam alignment device must be used to keep the receptor parallel with the long axis of the tooth. The patient *cannot* hold the receptor in this manner.

To achieve parallelism between the receptor and the tooth, the receptor must be placed *away* from the tooth and toward the middle of the oral cavity. Because of the anatomic configuration of the oral cavity (e.g., curvature of palate), the **object–receptor distance** (distance between receptor and tooth) must be increased to keep the receptor parallel with the long axis of the tooth (Figure 17-4). Because the receptor is placed away from the tooth, image magnification and loss of definition result. As discussed in Chapter 8, increased object–receptor distance results in increased image magnification.

To compensate for image magnification, the **target–receptor distance** (distance between source of x-rays and receptor) must also be increased to ensure that only the most parallel rays will be directed at the tooth and the receptor. As a result, a long (16-inch) target–receptor distance must be used with the paralleling technique. The paralleling technique is sometimes referred to as the "long-cone technique"; *long* refers to the length of the cone, or position-indicating device (PID), that is used. The use of a long target–receptor distance in the paralleling technique results in less image magnification and increased definition.

The American Dental Association (ADA) and the American Academy of Oral and Maxillofacial Radiology recommend the use of a rectangular collimator to reduce the amount of radiation the patient receives. Limiting the size of the x-ray beam not only reduces the amount of skin that is exposed but also results in a significant reduction of radiation to the patient, by as much as 70%. The receptor placement procedures are illustrated with a rectangular collimator attached to the end of the PID.

Beam Alignment Devices

The paralleling technique requires the use of a beam alignment instrument to position the receptor parallel to the long axis of the tooth. **Beam alignment devices** are used to position an intraoral receptor in the mouth and maintain the receptor in position during exposure (see Chapter 6). Examples of commercially available intraoral beam alignment devices include the following:

- **Rinn XCP instruments** (Dentsply Rinn Corporation, Elgin, IL). The XCP (extension cone paralleling) instruments include plastic bite-blocks, plastic aiming rings, and metal indicator arms (Figure 17-5, A). The plastic bite-blocks and aiming rings are color-coded to aid in assembly: blue instruments are used in the anterior regions, yellow instruments are used in the posterior regions, red instruments are used for bite-wing projections, and torquoise instruments are used in endodontic procedures. To reduce the amount of radiation the patient receives, a snap-on ring collimator can be added to the plastic aiming ring.
  - Rinn XCP-ORA instruments have a universal ring and arm positioning system to accommodate anterior, posterior and bitewing projections (Figure 17-5, B).
  - The Rinn Flip-Ray system uses a rotating bite-block and ring to eliminate multiple positioning parts.
  - EEZEE-Grip receptor holder, formerly known as the Snap-A-Ray. This receptor-holding device can be used in both anterior and posterior areas (Figures 17-5, D and E).
  - Stable bite blocks. The Stable bite block is a disposable receptor holder, and is designed for one time use only (Figure 17-5, F).

Some film holders are disposable (e.g., Stabe bite-block) and are designed for one-time use only. Other film holders are reusable (e.g., XCP instruments, Precision film holders, EEZEE-Grip film holder, hemostat with bite-block) and must be sterilized after each use. Additional beam alignment devices for use with imaging receptors will be discussed in Chapter 25, Digital Imaging).

Of all the film holders listed, the Rinn XCP beam alignment instruments with snap-on ring collimators and the Precision film holders are recommended for exposure of periapical receptors. These beam alignment devices are recommended because both include aiming rings that aid in the alignment of the PID with the receptor, and both significantly reduce the amount of patient exposure to radiation.

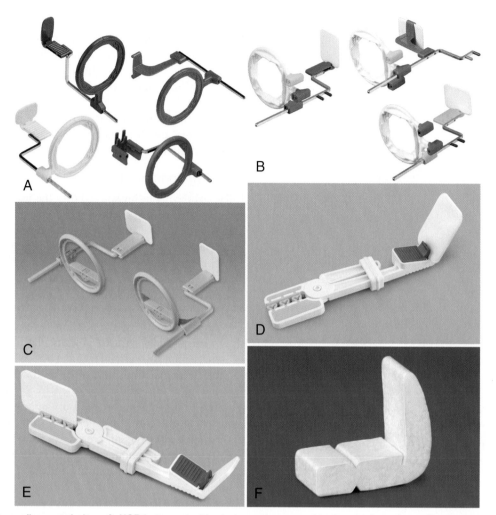

FIGURE 17-5 Beam alignment devices. **A**, XCP instruments: blue instruments are used in the anterior region, yellow instruments are used in the posterior region, red instruments are used in the bite-wing technique, and torquoise instruments are used for endodontic procedures. **B**, Rinn XCP-ORA beam alignment devices provide accurate positioning in a system with one ring and one arm for anterior, posterior, and bite-wing projections. **C**, The Rinn Flip-Ray system uses a rotating bite-block and ring to eliminate multiple beam alignment devices. **D, E**, The EEZEE Grip (formerly Snap-A-Ray) Xtra intraoral receptor holder is color coded for the anterior and posterior regions. **F**, An example of a disposable Stabe bite-block. (**A, D, E**, Courtesy Dentsply Rinn Corporation, Elgin IL.)

These instruments are simple to position and easy to sterilize. Although only the Rinn XCP beam alignment instruments are illustrated in this text, the same principles apply to all the film holders listed.

Receptors Used for Paralleling Technique

The size of the intraoral receptor used with the paralleling technique depends on the teeth being radiographed, as follows:

- In the anterior regions, size 1 receptor is used; this narrow size is needed to permit placement high in the palate without bending or curving. Size 1 is always positioned with the long portion of the receptor in a *vertical* (upright) direction.
- In the posterior regions, size 2 receptor is used. Size 2 is always placed with the long portion of the receptor in a *horizontal* (sideways) direction.

Rules for Paralleling Technique

Five basic rules should be followed when using the paralleling technique.

1. *Receptor placement.* The receptor must be positioned to cover the prescribed area of teeth to be examined. Specific placements are detailed in the Procedures sections of this chapter.
2. *Receptor position.* The receptor must be positioned parallel to the long axis of the tooth. The receptor and beam alignment device must be placed away from the teeth and toward the middle of the oral cavity (see Figure 17-3).
3. *Vertical angulation.* The central ray of the x-ray beam must be directed perpendicular (at a right angle) to the receptor and the long axis of the tooth (see Figure 17-3).

4. *Horizontal angulation.* The central ray of the x-ray beam must be directed through the contact areas between teeth (Figure 17-6).
5. *Film receptor exposure.* The x-ray beam must be centered on the receptor to ensure that all areas are exposed. Failure to center the x-ray beam results in a partial image on the receptor or a "cone-cut." Cone-cuts can be produced with either a round PID or a rectangular PID. (Figure 17-7). Cone-cuts are discussed in Chapter 20.

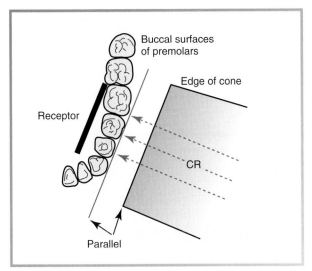

FIGURE 17-6 In this diagram, x-rays pass through the contact areas of the premolars because the central ray (CR) is directed through the contacts and perpendicular to the receptor. If the central ray is not directed through the contacts, overlap of the premolar contacts occurs.

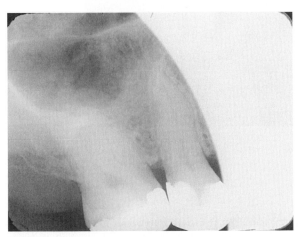

FIGURE 17-7 This image demonstrates a cone-cut, or clear, unexposed area on the image. The position-indicating device (PID) was positioned too far distally, and therefore the anterior portion of the receptor received no exposure.

STEP-BY-STEP PROCEDURES

Step-by-step procedures for the exposure of periapical receptors using the paralleling technique include patient preparation, equipment preparation, and receptor placement methods. Exposure of bite-wing receptors using the paralleling technique is discussed in Chapter 19. Before exposing any receptors using the paralleling technique, infection control procedures (as detailed in Chapter 15) must be completed.

Patient Preparation

After completion of infection control procedures and preparation of the treatment area and supplies, the patient should be seated. After seating the patient, the dental radiographer must prepare the patient before the exposure of any receptors (Procedure 17-1).

Equipment Preparation

After patient preparation, equipment must also be prepared before the exposure of any receptors (Procedure 17-2).

Exposure Sequence for Receptor Placements

When using the paralleling technique, an **exposure sequence**, or definite order for periapical receptor placement and exposure, must be followed. The dental radiographer must have an established exposure routine to prevent errors and to use time efficiently. Working without an exposure sequence may result in omitting an area or in exposing an area to x-radiation twice.

Anterior Exposure Sequence

When exposing periapical receptors with the paralleling technique, *always* begin with the **anterior teeth** (canines and incisors), for the following reasons:

PROCEDURE **17-1**	Patient Preparation for Paralleling Technique

1. Briefly explain the radiographic procedures to the patient before the procedure begins.
2. Adjust the chair so that the patient is positioned upright in the chair. The level of the chair must be adjusted to a comfortable working height.
3. Adjust the headrest to support and position the patient's head. The patient's head must be positioned such that the maxillary arch is parallel to the floor and the midsagittal (midline) plane is perpendicular to the floor.
4. Place and secure the lead apron with thyroid collar on the patient.
5. Remove all objects from the patient's mouth (e.g., dentures, retainers, chewing gum) that may interfere with the procedure. Eyeglasses must also be removed.

| PROCEDURE **17-2** | **Equipment Preparation for Paralleling Technique** |

1. Set the exposure factors (kilovoltage, milliamperage, and time) on the x-ray unit according to the recommendations of the manufacturer of the imaging receptors.
2. Open the sterilized package containing the beam alignment devices, and assemble it over a covered work area. Assembly of the anterior XCP instrument is illustrated in Figure 17-8; posterior XCP instrument assembly is illustrated in Figure 17-9. For assembly instructions on other beam alignment devices, refer to information provided by the manufacturer.

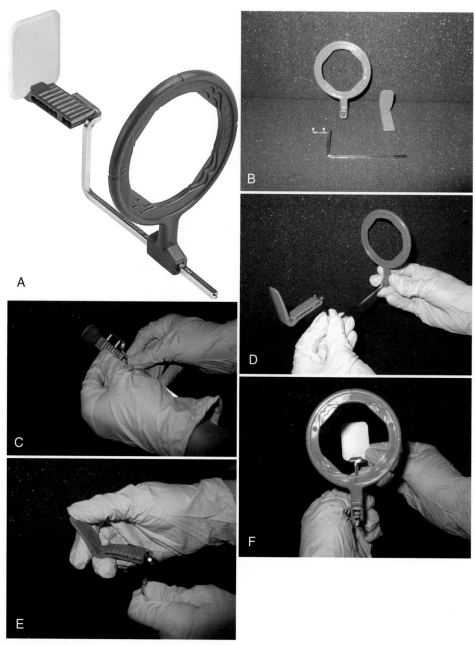

FIGURE 17-8 A, The correct assembly of the anterior XCP instrument holding an intraoral film. **B**, Parts of anterior XCP instrument. **C**, Assembly of anterior XCP instrument. The two prongs of the anterior indicator arm are inserted into the openings in the anterior bite-block, as shown. **D**, The anterior indicator arm is inserted into the opening on the anterior aiming ring, as shown. **E**, The plastic backing of bite-block is flexed to open the film slot for easy insertion of the anterior film packet. **F**, The Anterior XCP instrument is correctly assembled when the film is seen centered in the middle of the aiming ring.

PROCEDURE 17-2 **Equipment Preparation for Paralleling Technique—cont'd**

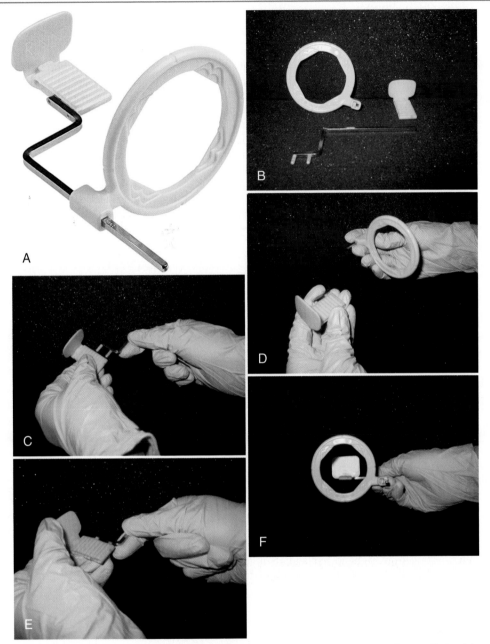

FIGURE 17-9 A, The correct assembly of the posterior XCP instrument for the maxillary left quadrant or the mandibular right quadrant. **B**, Parts of posterior XCP instrument. **C**, Assembly of posterior XCP instrument. The two prongs of the posterior indicator arm are inserted into the openings in the posterior bite-block, as shown. **D**, The posterior indicator arm is inserted into the opening on the posterior aiming ring, as shown. **E**, The plastic backing of the bite-block is flexed to open the film slot for easy insertion of the posterior film packet. **F**, The posterior XCP instrument is correctly assembled when the film is seen centered in the middle of the aiming ring.

- The receptor (size 1) used for anterior exposures is small, less uncomfortable, and easier for the patient to tolerate.
- The more tolerable anterior placements allow the patient to become accustomed to the beam alignment device used in the paralleling technique.
- Anterior placements are less likely to cause the patient to gag. Once the gag reflex is stimulated, the patient

may gag on receptor placements that might normally be tolerated. Management of the patient with a hypersensitive gag reflex is discussed in Chapter 24.

With the size 1 receptor, a total of 7 anterior placements may be used in the paralleling technique: 4 maxillary exposures and 3 mandibular exposures. If size 2 receptor is used instead, 6 anterior placements are used: 3 maxillary exposures and 3 mandibular exposures. The authors recommend the

TABLE 17-1	Exposure Sequence for Anterior Receptor Placements (with Rinn XCP Instruments): Paralleling Technique			
Exposure Number	**Arch**	**Side**	**Tooth**	**Tooth Number**
1	Maxillary	Right	Canine	6
2	Maxillary	Right	Lateral incisor	7
	Maxillary	Right	Central incisor	8
3	Maxillary	Left	Central incisor	9
	Maxillary	Left	Lateral incisor	10
4	Maxillary	Left	Canine	11
5	Mandibular	Left	Canine	22
6	Mandibular	Left	Lateral incisor	23
	Mandibular	Left	Central incisor	24
	Mandibular	Right	Central incisor	25
	Mandibular	Right	Lateral incisor	26
7	Mandibular	Right	Canine	27

use of size 1 receptors; the recommended anterior periapical exposure sequence for the Rinn XCP beam alignment instruments illustrated in this text is as follows (Table 17-1):

1. Assemble the anterior XCP instrument.
2. Begin with the maxillary right canine (tooth No. 6).
3. Radiograph all the maxillary anterior teeth from right to left.
4. End with the maxillary left canine (tooth No. 11).
5. Next, move to the mandibular arch.
6. Begin with the mandibular left canine (tooth No. 22).
7. Radiograph all the mandibular anterior teeth from left to right.
8. Finish the anterior periapical exposures with the mandibular right canine (tooth No. 27).

When the dental radiographer works from right to left in the maxillary arch and then from left to right in the mandibular arch, no wasted movement or shifting of the PID occurs (Figure 17-10).

In addition, when working from right to left and then from left to right, teeth are radiographed in ascending numerical order, as follows:

$$\text{Teeth } 6 \rightarrow 7 \rightarrow 8 \rightarrow 9 \rightarrow 10 \rightarrow 11 \text{, and then:}$$

$$\text{Teeth } 22 \rightarrow 23 \rightarrow 24 \rightarrow 25 \rightarrow 26 \rightarrow 27$$

This exposure sequence allows the dental radiographer to keep track of the last exposure easily even when interruptions occur during the procedure.

Posterior Exposure Sequence

After the anterior exposures are completed, the **posterior teeth** (premolars and molars) are radiographed. In each quadrant, *always* expose the premolar receptor first and then the molar receptor, for the following reasons:

- Premolar placement is easier for the patient to tolerate.
- Premolar placement is less likely to evoke the gag reflex.

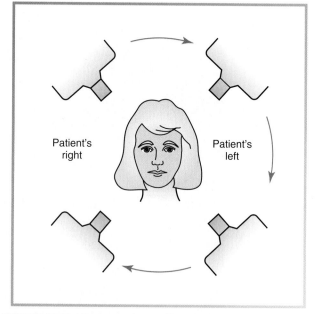

FIGURE 17-10 When exposing maxillary anterior receptors, work from the right to the left. Then, expose the mandibular anterior receptors from the left to the right. No unnecessary movements of the PID result.

Eight posterior placements may be used in the paralleling technique: 4 maxillary exposures and 4 mandibular exposures. The recommended exposure sequence for the posterior receptor placements varies, depending on the beam alignment device used. The recommended posterior periapical exposure sequence for the Rinn XCP beam alignment instruments illustrated in this text is as follows (Table 17-2):

1. Begin with the maxillary right quadrant.
2. Assemble the posterior XCP instrument for this area.
3. Expose the premolar receptor (teeth Nos. 4 and 5) first, and then expose the molar receptor (teeth Nos. 1, 2, and 3).
4. Without reassembling the XCP instrument, move to the mandibular left quadrant.

TABLE **17-2**	Exposure Sequence for Posterior Receptor Placements (with Rinn XCP Instruments): Paralleling Technique				
Exposure Number	**Arch**	**Side**	**Teeth**	**Teeth Numbers**	
1	Maxillary	Right	Premolars	4, 5	
2	Maxillary	Right	Molars	1, 2, 3	
3	Mandibular	Left	Premolars	20, 21	
4	Mandibular	Left	Molars	17, 18, 19	
5	Maxillary	Left	Premolars	12, 13	
6	Maxillary	Left	Molars	14, 15, 16	
7	Mandibular	Right	Premolars	28, 29	
8	Mandibular	Right	Molars	30, 31, 32	

5. Expose the premolar receptor (teeth Nos. 20 and 21) first, and then expose the molar receptor (teeth Nos. 17, 18, and 19).
6. Move to the maxillary left quadrant and reassemble the posterior XCP instrument over a covered work surface for this area.
7. Expose the premolar receptor (teeth Nos. 12 and 13) first, and then the molar receptor (teeth Nos. 14, 15, and 16).
8. Finish with the mandibular right quadrant.
9. Expose the premolar receptor (teeth Nos. 28 and 29) first, and then end the posterior periapical exposures with the exposure of the molar receptor (teeth Nos. 30, 31, and 32).

Receptor Placement for Paralleling Technique

In a complete mouth radiographic series (CMRS) using the paralleling technique, each periapical exposure has a pre-scribed placement. **Receptor placement**, or the specific area where the receptor must be positioned before exposure, is dictated by the specific teeth and their surrounding structures that must be included on the resultant image. Prescribed receptor placements for the anterior teeth are described in Box 17-1 and illustrated in Figure 17-11. Posterior place-ments are described in Box 17-2 and illustrated in Figure 17-12.

The specific placements described in this chapter are for a 15-receptor periapical series using size 1 receptors for ante-rior exposures and size 2 receptors for posterior exposures. Variations in placement or the number of total receptors may be recommended by other reference sources or individual practitioners. Box 17-3 lists guidelines for periapical posi-tioning used with the paralleling technique.

Anterior Receptor Placement

The anterior XCP instrument is used for all anterior receptor placements. After the anterior XCP instrument has been assembled, a size 1 receptor is inserted vertically into the bite-block and secured in the slot. Anterior placements typically include the following:
- Two maxillary canine exposures (Procedure 17-3)
- Two maxillary incisor exposures (Procedure 17-4)

BOX **17-1**	**Prescribed Placements for Anterior Periapical Exposures: Paralleling Technique**

Exposure of Maxillary Canine
The entire crown and root of the canine, including the apex and the surrounding structures, must be seen on this image. The interproximal alveolar bone and mesial contact of the canine must also be visible. The lingual cusp of the first premolar usually obscures the distal contact of the canine.

Exposure of Maxillary Incisor
The entire crowns and roots of one lateral and one central incisor, including the apices of the teeth and the surrounding structures, must be seen on this image. The interproximal alveolar bone between the central and lateral and the mesial and distal contact areas, as well as the surrounding regions of bone, must also be visible. In addition, the mesial contact of the adjacent central incisor and the mesial contact of the adjacent canine should be seen on this exposure.

Exposure of Mandibular Canine
The entire crown and root of the canine, including the apex and the surrounding structures, must be seen on this image. In addition, the interproximal alveolar bone and mesial and distal contacts must be visible.

Exposure of Mandibular Incisor
The entire crowns and roots of the four mandibular incisors, including the apices of the teeth and the surrounding structures, must be seen on this image. In addition, the contacts between the central incisors and those between the central and lateral incisors must be visible. In most cases, it is not necessary to see the distal contacts of the lateral incisors.

- Two mandibular canine exposures (Procedure 17-5)
- One mandibular incisor exposure (Procedure 17-6)

Posterior Receptor Placement

The posterior XCP instrument is used for all posterior recep-tor placements. After the posterior XCP instrument has been assembled, a size 2 receptor is inserted horizontally into the

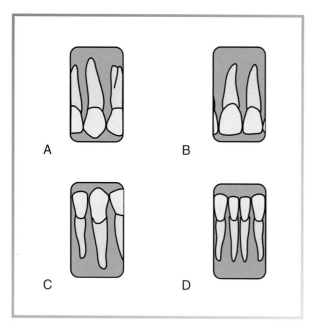

FIGURE 17-11 Prescribed placements for anterior periapical receptors. **A**, Exposure of the maxillary canine. **B**, Exposure of the maxillary lateral and central incisors. **C**, Exposure of the mandibular canine. **D**, Exposure of the mandibular lateral and central incisors.

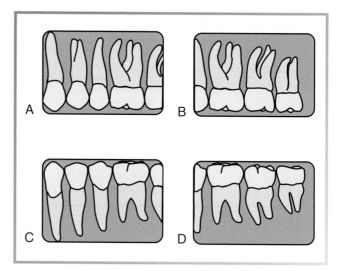

FIGURE 17-12 Prescribed placements for posterior periapical receptors. **A**, Exposure of the maxillary premolar. **B**, Exposure of the maxillary molar. **C**, Exposure of the mandibular premolar. **D**, Exposure of the mandibular molar.

BOX 17-2   **Prescribed Placements for Posterior Periapical Exposures: Paralleling Technique**

Exposure of Maxillary Premolar
All crowns and roots of the first and second premolar and of the first molar, including the apices, alveolar crests, contact areas, and surrounding bone, must be seen on this image. In addition, the distal contact of the maxillary canine must be visible in this projection.

Exposure of Maxillary Molar
All crowns and roots of the first, second, and third molars, including the apices, alveolar crests, contact areas, surrounding bone, and tuberosity region, must be seen on this image. In addition, the distal contact of the maxillary second premolar must be visible.

Exposure of Mandibular Premolar
All crowns and roots of the first and second premolars and of the first molar, including the apices, alveolar crests, contact areas, and surrounding bone, must be seen on this image. In addition, the distal contact of the mandibular canine must be visible.

Exposure of Mandibular Molar
All crowns and roots of the first, second, and third molars, including the apices, alveolar crests, contact areas, and surrounding bone, must be seen on this image. In addition, the distal contact of the mandibular second premolar must be visible.

BOX 17-3   **Guidelines for Receptor Placement with Paralleling Technique**

1. The white side of the film always faces the teeth.
2. The anterior receptors are always placed vertically.
3. The posterior receptors are always placed horizontally.
4. The identification dot on the film is always placed in the slot of the film holder, toward the occlusal end of the film. (Place the "dot in the slot.")
5. When placing the receptor in the mouth, always lead with the apical end of the receptor, and rotate the beam alignment device.
6. When positioning the beam alignment device, always place the receptor away from the teeth and toward the middle of the oral cavity.
7. When positioning the beam alignment device, always center the receptor over the area to be examined (as defined in the prescribed placements).
8. When positioning the beam alignment device, ask the patient to "slowly close" on the bite-block. Always make certain that the bite-block is stabilized by the teeth and not the lips.

bite-block and secured in the slot. Posterior placements typically include the following:

- Two maxillary premolar exposures (Procedure 17-7)
- Two maxillary molar exposures (Procedure 17-8)
- Two mandibular premolar exposures (Procedure 17-9)
- Two mandibular molar exposures (Procedure 17-10)

MODIFICATIONS IN PARALLELING TECHNIQUE

Modifications in the paralleling technique may be used to accommodate variations in anatomic conditions. Such

Text continued on p. 173

PROCEDURE 17-3 **Maxillary Canine Exposure: Paralleling Technique** (Figure 17-13)

1. Center the anterior beam alignment device and receptor on the maxillary canine.
2. Position the receptor as far away from the teeth as possible.

3. Instruct the patient to "slowly close" on the bite-block, and slide the aiming ring down the indicator arm to the skin surface. Align the PID with the aiming ring.
4. Expose the receptor.

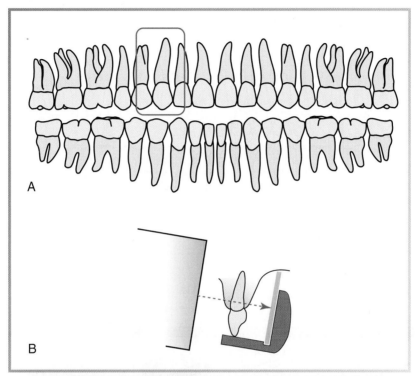

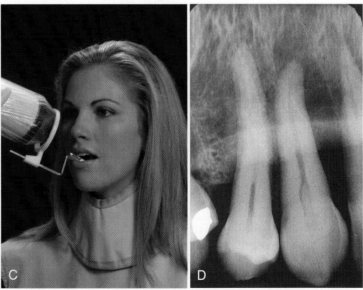

FIGURE 17-13 Exposure of the maxillary canine. **A,** Receptor placement. **B,** Relationship among the receptor, teeth, XCP instrument, and PID. **C,** Exposure of the receptor with rectangular collimation. **D,** Resultant image.

PROCEDURE 17-4   **Maxillary Incisor Exposure: Paralleling Technique** (Figure 17-14)

1. Center the anterior beam alignment device and receptor on the contact between the maxillary central incisor and the lateral incisor.
2. Position the receptor as far away from the teeth as possible.

3. Instruct the patient to "slowly close" on the bite-block, and slide the aiming ring down the indicator arm to the skin surface. Align the PID with the aiming ring.
4. Expose the receptor.

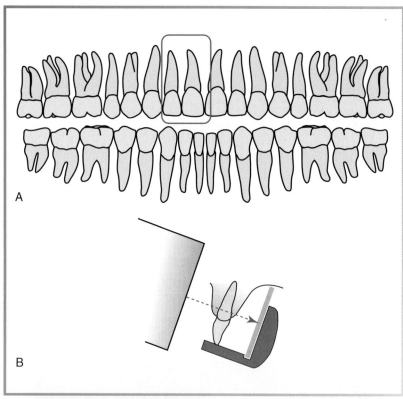

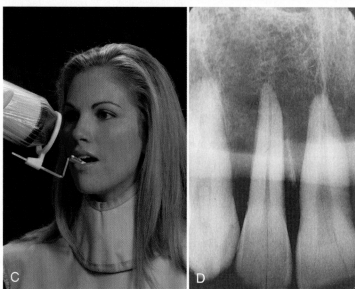

FIGURE 17-14 Exposure of the maxillary incisors. **A,** Receptor placement. **B,** Relationship among the receptor, teeth, XCP instrument, and PID. **C,** Exposure of the receptor with rectangular collimation. **D,** Resultant image.

PROCEDURE 17-5 **Mandibular Canine Exposure: Paralleling Technique** (Figure 17-15)

1. Center the anterior beam alignment device and receptor on the mandibular canine.
2. Position the receptor as far away from the teeth as possible.

3. Instruct the patient to "slowly close" on the bite-block, and slide the aiming ring down the indicator arm to the skin surface. Align the PID with the aiming ring.
4. Expose the receptor.

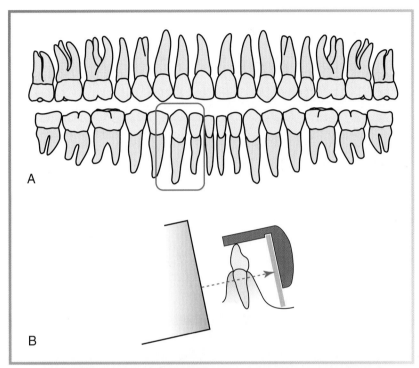

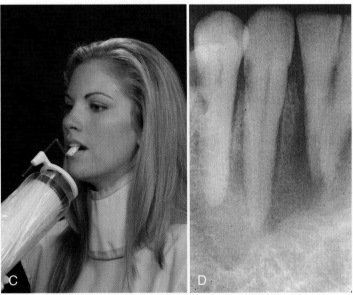

FIGURE 17-15 Exposure of the mandibular canine. **A**, Receptor placement. **B**, Relationship of receptor, teeth, XCP instrument, and PID. **C**, Exposure of receptor with rectangular collimation. **D**, Resultant image.

PROCEDURE 17-6   **Mandibular Incisor Exposure: Paralleling Technique** (Figure 17-16)

1. Center the anterior beam alignment device and receptor on the contact between the two mandibular central incisors.
2. Position the receptor as far away from the teeth as possible.

3. Instruct the patient to "slowly close" on the bite-block, and slide the aiming ring down the indicator arm to the skin surface. Align the PID with the aiming ring.
4. Expose the receptor.

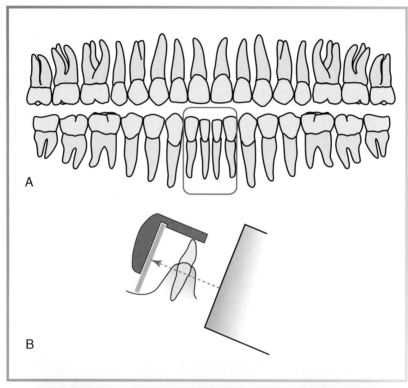

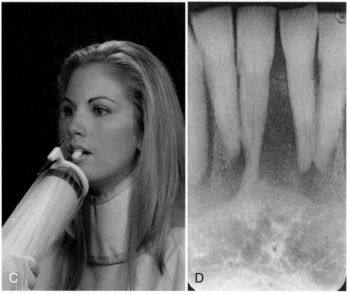

FIGURE 17-16 Exposure of the mandibular incisor. **A,** Receptor placement. **B,** Relationship among the receptor, teeth, XCP instrument, and PID. **C,** Exposure of the receptor with rectangular collimation. **D,** Resultant image.

PROCEDURE 17-7 **Maxillary Premolar Exposure: Paralleling Technique** (Figure 17-17)

1. Center the posterior beam alignment device and receptor on the maxillary second premolar; the front edge of the receptor should cover the distal half of the maxillary canine.
2. Position the receptor as far away from the teeth as possible.

3. Instruct the patient to "slowly close" on the bite-block, and slide the aiming ring down the indicator arm to the skin surface. Align the PID with the aiming ring.
4. Expose the receptor.

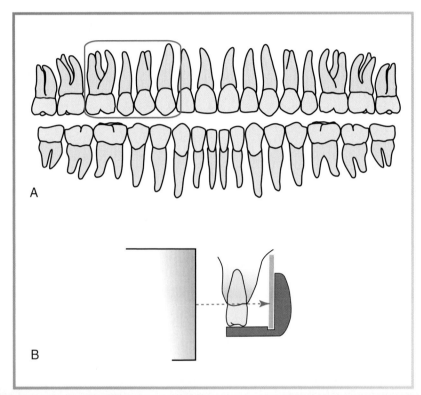

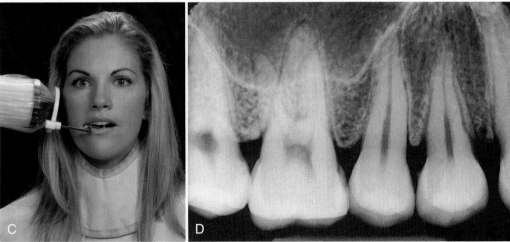

FIGURE 17-17 Exposure of the maxillary premolar. **A,** Receptor placement. **B,** Relationship among the receptor, teeth, XCP instrument, and PID. **C,** Exposure of the receptor with rectangular collimation. **D,** Resultant image.

PROCEDURE 17-8   **Maxillary Molar Exposure: Paralleling Technique** (Figure 17-18)

1. Center the posterior beam alignment device and receptor on the maxillary second molar; the front edge of the receptor should cover the distal half of the maxillary second premolar.

2. Position the receptor as far away from the teeth as possible.

3. Instruct the patient to "slowly close" on the bite-block, and slide the aiming ring down the indicator arm to the skin surface. Align the PID with the aiming ring.

4. Expose the receptor.

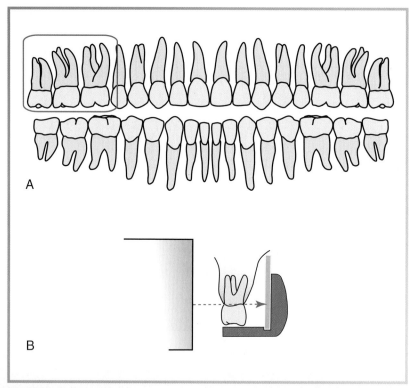

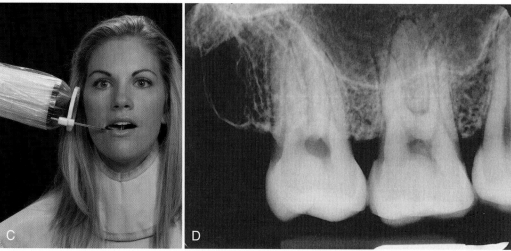

FIGURE 17-18 Exposure of the maxillary molar. **A**, Receptor placement. **B**, Relationship among the receptor, teeth, XCP instrument, and PID. **C**, Exposure of the receptor with rectangular collimation. **D**, Resultant image.

PROCEDURE 17-9 **Mandibular Premolar Exposure: Paralleling Technique** (Figure 17-19)

1. Center the on the mandibular second premolar; the front edge of the receptor should cover the distal half of the mandibular canine.
2. Position the receptor as far away from the teeth as possible.

3. Instruct the patient to "slowly close" on the bite-block, and slide the aiming ring down the indicator arm to the skin surface. Align the PID with the aiming ring.
4. Expose the receptor.

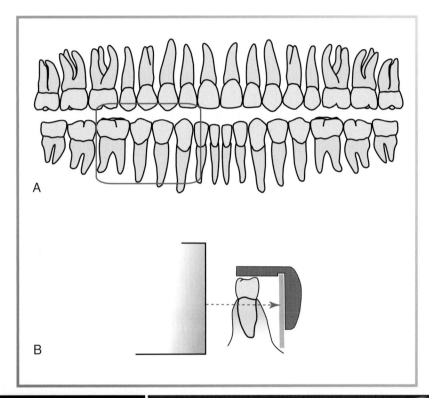

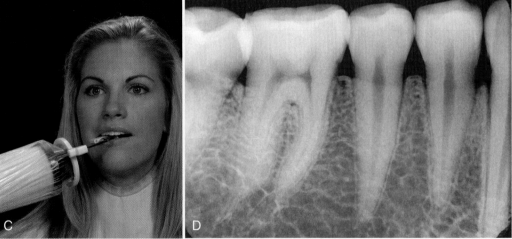

FIGURE 17-19 Exposure of the mandibular premolar. **A**, Receptor placement. **B**, Relationship among the receptor, teeth, XCP instrument, and PID. **C**, Exposure of the receptor with rectangular collimation. **D**, Resultant image.

PROCEDURE 17-10   **Mandibular Molar Exposure: Paralleling Technique** (Figure 17-20)

1. Center the posterior beam alignment device and receptor on the mandibular second molar; the front edge of the film should cover the distal half of the mandibular second premolar.
2. Position the receptor as far away from the teeth as possible.

3. Instruct the patient to "slowly close" on the bite-block, and slide the aiming ring down the indicator arm to the skin surface. Align the PID with the aiming ring.
4. Expose the receptor.
5. An example of a charting note for a full-mouth series using the paralleling technique is provided below.

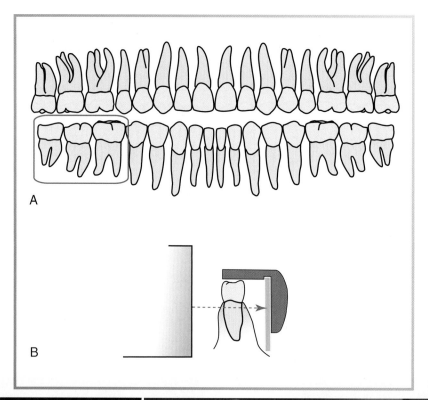

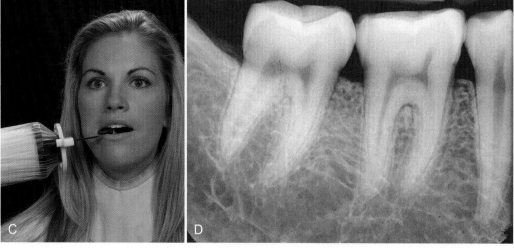

FIGURE 17-20 Exposure of the mandibular molar. **A,** Receptor placement. **B,** Relationship among the receptor, teeth, XCP instrument, and PID. **C,** Exposure of the receptor with rectangular collimation. **D,** Resultant image.

PROCEDURE **17-10**	Mandibular Molar Exposure: Paralleling Technique—cont'd

Charting a Full-Mouth Series

Date	ADA Procedure Code	Provider	Charting Notes	Comments
12/1/11	0210	LJH	Dr. Smith requested a full-mouth series of radiographs; paralleling technique used with XCP instruments; 14 periapicals and 4 bite-wings exposed; right molar bite-wing retaken because of patient movement; Insight film (19 total exposures)	Patient tolerated procedure fairly well; mandibular premolar region was difficult to place film packet because presence of bilateral tori; used the Stabe bite-block for both mandibular premolar periapical projections; patient opened her mouth before the right molar bite-wing was exposed (retake)

modifications may be necessary when a patient has a shallow palate, bony growths, or a sensitive mandibular premolar region.

Shallow Palate

Parallelism between the receptor and the long axis of the tooth is difficult to accomplish in a patient with a shallow **palate** (roof of the mouth), also known as a *low palatal vault*. In a patient with a shallow palate, tilting of the bite-block occurs, which results in a lack of parallelism between the receptor and the long axis of the tooth. If the lack of parallelism between the receptor and the long axis of the tooth does not exceed 20 degrees, the resultant image is generally acceptable (Figure 17-21). When the lack of parallelism is greater than 20 degrees, a modification in technique is necessary, as follows:

- *Cotton rolls.* To position the receptor parallel to the long axis of the tooth, two cotton rolls can be placed, one on each side of the bite-block (Figure 17-22). As a result, however, periapical coverage is reduced.
- *Vertical angulation.* To compensate for the lack of parallelism, the vertical angulation can be increased by 5 to 15 degrees more than the XCP instrument indicates. However, image distortion occurs as a result.

Bony Growths

A **torus** (plural, **tori**) is a bony growth seen in the oral cavity. A **maxillary torus** (torus palatinus) is a nodular mass of bone seen along the midline of the hard palate (Figure 17-23). **Mandibular tori** (singular, torus mandibularis) are bony growths along the lingual aspect (tongue side) of the mandible (Figure 17-24). When using the paralleling technique, maxillary and mandibular tori can cause problems with receptor placement, and modifications in technique are necessary, as follows:

- For maxillary torus, the receptor must be placed on the far side of the torus (not *on* the torus) and then exposed (Figure 17-25, A). Periapical radiographs illustrate the radiopaque borders of a maxillary torus (Figure 17-25, B).

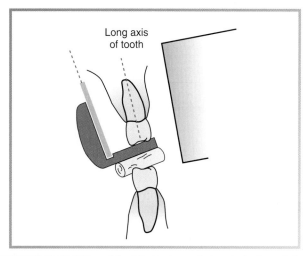

FIGURE 17-21 Tilting of the bite-block results in a lack of parallelism between the receptor and the long axis of the tooth. When the lack of parallelism is less than 20 degrees (*as shown in this diagram*), the image is generally acceptable.

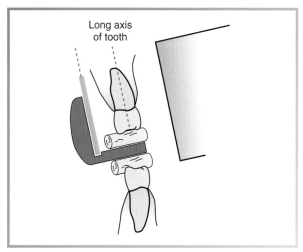

FIGURE 17-22 Two cotton rolls can be used to position the receptor parallel to the long axis of the tooth.

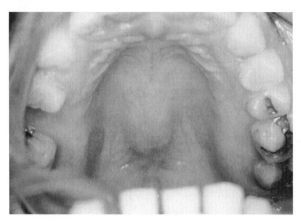

FIGURE 17-23 A maxillary torus.

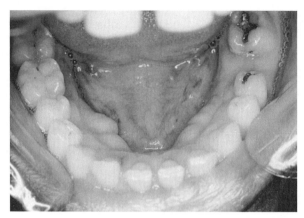

FIGURE 17-24 Mandibular tori.

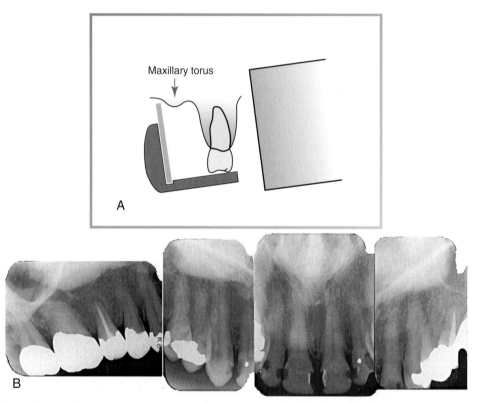

FIGURE 17-25 A, If a maxillary torus is present, the receptor must be placed on the far side of the torus and then exposed. **B,** Periapical radiographs reveal a maxillary torus as seen by the radiopaque areas superior to the apices of the teeth. (**B,** from White SC, Pharoah MJ: *Oral radiology: principles and interpretation,* ed 5, St. Louis, 2004, Mosby.)

• For mandibular tori, the receptor must be placed between the tori and the tongue (not *on* the tori) and then exposed (Figure 17-26, A). Mandibular tori are also seen radiographically as dense radiopacities (Figure 17-26, B).

Mandibular Premolar Region

The anterior floor of the mouth area can be a very sensitive region. When periapical placements cause discomfort in the mandibular premolar region, a modification in technique is necessary, as follows:

• *Receptor placement.* The receptor must be placed under the tongue to avoid impinging on muscle attachments and the sensitive lingual gingiva. When inserting the beam alignment device into the mouth, the receptor is tipped away from the tongue and toward the teeth being examined while the bite-block is placed firmly on the mandibular premolars. When the patient closes on

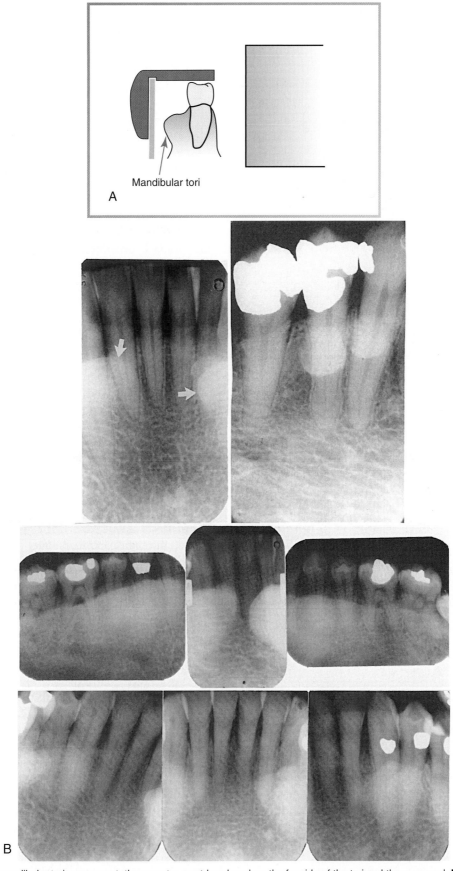

FIGURE 17-26 A, If mandibular tori are present, the receptor must be placed on the far side of the tori and then exposed. **B**, Bilateral mandibular tori are seen as dense radiopacities in the region of the canine and the first premolar. (**B**, from White SC, Pharoah MJ: *Oral radiology: principles and interpretation*, ed 5, St. Louis, 2004, Mosby.)

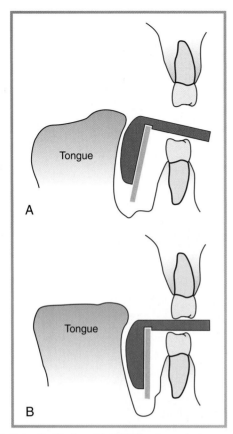

FIGURE 17-27 Positioning of the XCP instrument in the sensitive mandibular premolar area. **A,** The receptor is tipped away from the tongue while the bite-block is placed firmly on the mandibular premolars. **B,** When the patient closes on the bite-block, the receptor is moved into proper position.

the bite-block, the receptor is moved into the proper position (Figure 17-27).

- *Film.* The lower edge of the film can be gently curved, or softened, to prevent discomfort. Bending or creasing the film, however, must be avoided.

ADVANTAGES AND DISADVANTAGES

As with all intraoral techniques, the paralleling technique has both advantages and disadvantages. The advantages of the paralleling technique, however, outweigh the disadvantages.

Advantages of Paralleling Technique

The primary advantage of the paralleling technique is that it produces a radiographic image without dimensional distortion. In addition, it is uncomplicated and can be easily repeated when serial radiographs are indicated. The advantages of the paralleling technique can be summarized as follows:

- *Accuracy.* The paralleling technique produces an image that has dimensional accuracy; the image is highly

representative of the actual tooth. The radiographic image is free of distortion and exhibits maximum detail and definition.
- *Simplicity.* The paralleling technique is simple and is easy to learn and use. The use of a beam alignment device eliminates the need for the dental radiographer to determine horizontal and vertical angulations and also eliminates the chances of dimensional distortion.
- *Duplication.* The paralleling technique is easy to standardize and can be accurately duplicated, or repeated, when serial radiographs are indicated. As a result, comparisons of serial radiographs exposed using the paralleling technique have great validity.

Disadvantages of Paralleling Technique

The primary disadvantage of the paralleling technique is receptor placement. Patient discomfort may also be a problem. The disadvantages of the paralleling technique can be summarized as follows:

- *Receptor placement.* Because a beam alignment device must be used with the paralleling technique, receptor placement may be difficult for the dental radiographer. Difficulties may be encountered with the pediatric patient or with adult patients who have a small mouth or a shallow palate. Such placements become less problematic as the dental radiographer becomes more proficient at using the paralleling technique.
- *Discomfort.* The beam alignment device used to position the receptor in the paralleling technique may impinge on the oral tissues and cause discomfort for the patient.

HELPFUL HINTS

In using the paralleling technique:

- **DO** set all exposure factors (kilovoltage, milliamperage, time) before placing any receptors in the mouth.
- **DO** ask patients to remove all intraoral objects and eyeglasses before placing any receptors in the mouth.
- **DO** use a definite order (exposure sequence) when exposing receptors to avoid errors and to make efficient use of time.
- **DO** place each film in the bite-block with the "dot in the slot." The identification dot must be located at the occlusal or incisal end of the film; this facilitates film mounting and ensures that the dot will not interfere with the diagnosis in the periapical area.
- **DO** explain the radiographic procedures that will be performed; instruct patients on how to close and remain still during the exposure.
- **DO** communicate clearly with patients; patients are more likely to be tolerant of discomfort when they understand why a receptor must be placed in a specific area.
- **DO** use the word *please*; say, "Open, please."
- **DO** use praise; tell cooperative patients how much they are helping you.

▪ **DO** instruct patients to "slowly close"; when patients close slowly, the musculature relaxes and thus discomfort is reduced.

▪ **DO** align the PID such that the opening of the PID and the rectangular collimator are flush with the aiming ring of the XCP instrument.

▪ **DO NOT** bend or crimp a film packet; excessive film bending causes distortion of the image.

▪ **DO NOT** use words such as *hurt*. Instead, inform patients that the procedure will be "momentarily uncomfortable."

▪ **DO NOT** make comments such as "Oops" or other statements that indicate a lack of control in a situation. Patients will lose confidence in your abilities when they hear such comments.

▪ **DO NOT** pick up a receptor if you drop it. Leave it on the floor, as it has now become contaminated. Instead, remove it and dispose of it when you clean the treatment area.

▪ **DO NOT** allow patients to dictate how you should perform your duties. Some patients need to be handled firmly. The dental radiographer must always remain in control of the procedures.

▪ **DO NOT** begin with posterior exposures; posterior placements may cause patients to gag. Instead, always begin with anterior exposures.

▪ **DO NOT** position receptors on top of a torus (or tori); the apical regions of the teeth will not be seen on the resultant radiograph. Instead, always position receptors behind the torus (or tori).

SUMMARY

• In the paralleling technique used to obtain periapical and bite-wing images, the receptor is placed in the mouth parallel to the long axis of the tooth, and the central ray is directed perpendicular to the receptor and the long axis of the tooth. To achieve parallelism between the receptor and the tooth, the receptor must be placed away from the tooth and toward the middle of the oral cavity.

• In the paralleling technique, a beam alignment device must be used to position the receptor parallel to the long axis of the tooth. A variety of beam alignment devices are commercially available.

• The sizes of intraoral receptors used in the paralleling technique depend on the teeth being radiographed. With anterior teeth, size 1 receptors are typically used; with posterior teeth, size 2 receptors are typically used.

• The five basic rules with regard to the paralleling technique are as follows: (1) The receptor must cover the prescribed area of interest; (2) the receptor must be positioned parallel to the long axis of the tooth; (3) the central ray must be directed perpendicular to the receptor and the long axis of the tooth; (4) the central ray must be directed through the contact areas between teeth; and (5) the x-ray beam must be centered over the receptor to ensure that all areas of the receptor are exposed.

• Before the radiographic procedure using the paralleling technique begins, ensure that you take all infection control measures, prepare the treatment area and the supplies, seat the patient and explain the radiographic procedures to him or her, make the necessary chair and headrest adjustments, place the lead apron on the patient, remove any intraoral objects and eyeglasses, set the exposure factors, and assemble the beam alignment devices.

• When using the paralleling technique, always begin with anterior exposures (easier for patient to tolerate, more comfortable, less likely to cause gagging), and then move on to the posterior regions. In each quadrant, always expose the premolar receptor first and then the molar receptor.

• In a complete mouth radiographic series (CMRS) using paralleling technique, each periapical exposure has a prescribed receptor placement (see Boxes 17-1 and 17-2 and Figures 17-11 and 17-12).

• Modifications in paralleling technique may be necessary when a patient has a low or shallow palate, bony growths, or a sensitive mandibular premolar region.

• The advantages of the paralleling technique include the following: (1) it produces images with dimensional accuracy, (2) it is simple and easy to learn and use, (3) it is easy to standardize, and (4) it can be accurately repeated.

• The disadvantages of the paralleling technique are as follows: (1) placements of receptors may be difficult for the dental radiographer and (2) the beam alignment device may cause patient discomfort.

BIBLIOGRAPHY

ADA Council on Scientific Affairs: An update on radiographic practices: information and recommendations, *J Am Dent Assoc* 132:234, 2001.

Frommer HH, Savage-Stabulas JJ: Intraoral technique: the paralleling method. In *Radiology for the dental professional*, ed 9, St. Louis, 2011, Mosby.

Johnson ON, McNally MA, Essay CE: Intraoral radiographic procedures. In *Essentials of dental radiography for dental assistants and hygienists*, ed 6, Norwalk, CT, 1999, Appleton & Lange.

Johnson ON, McNally MA, Essay CE: The periapical examination. In *Essentials of dental radiography for dental assistants and hygienists*, ed 6, Norwalk, CT, 1999, Appleton & Lange.

Miles DA, Van Dis ML, Jensen CW, Williamson GF: Intraoral radiographic technique. In *Radiographic imaging for dental auxiliaries*, ed 4, Philadelphia, 2009, Saunders.

Miles DA, Van Dis ML, Razmus TF: Intraoral radiographic techniques. In *Basic principles of oral and maxillofacial radiology*, Philadelphia, 1992, Saunders.

White SC, Pharoah MJ: Intraoral radiographic examinations. In *Oral radiology: principles and interpretation*, ed 6, St. Louis, 2009, Mosby.

QUIZ QUESTIONS

MATCHING

*For questions 1 to 8, refer to Figure 17-28. Match the letters
(A to H) of the appropriate items with the descriptions below:*

___ **1.** No. 1 size receptor
___ **2.** No. 2 size receptor
___ **3.** XCP aiming ring, posterior
___ **4.** XCP aiming ring, anterior
___ **5.** XCP indicator arm, posterior
___ **6.** XCP indicator arm, anterior
___ **7.** XCP bite-block, posterior
___ **8.** XCP bite-block, anterior

FILL IN THE BLANK

9. What happens to the image when the object–receptor distance is increased?

_____

10. What piece of equipment is required to hold the receptor parallel to the long axis of the tooth in the paralleling technique?

_____

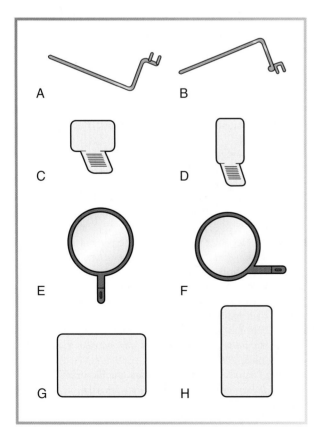

FIGURE 17-28

11. What do the letters X, C, and P refer to?

_____

12. What size receptor is typically used with the anterior XCP instrument?

_____

13. What size receptor is used with the posterior XCP instrument?

_____

14. Which beam alignment devices are recommended for use with the paralleling technique to reduce radiation exposure of the patient?

_____

15. How is the patient's head positioned before exposing receptors?

_____

MULTIPLE CHOICE

___ **16.** Why is an increased target–receptor distance required in the paralleling technique?
   a. to avoid image magnification
   b. to avoid distortion
   c. to reduce scatter radiation
   d. to improve receptor placement
___ **17.** Which of the following describes the relationship of the central ray to the receptor in the paralleling technique?
   a. 20 degrees to the long axis of the tooth
   b. 90 degrees to the receptor and long axis of the tooth
   c. 75 degrees to the long axis of the tooth
   d. 15 degrees to the receptor and the long axis of the tooth
___ **18.** Which of the following definitions is incorrect?
   a. *parallel*: always separated by the same distance
   b. *intersecting*: to cut through
   c. *right angle*: formed by two parallel lines
   d. *central ray*: central portion of the x-ray beam
___ **19.** Which of the following describes the relationship between the receptor and the long axis of the tooth in the paralleling technique?
   a. The receptor and the tooth are parallel to each other.
   b. The receptor and the tooth are at right angles to each other.

c. The receptor and the tooth are perpendicular to each other.

d. The receptor and the tooth are intersecting each other.

___ **20.** Which of the following describes the distance between the receptor and the tooth in the paralleling technique?

a. The receptor is placed as close as possible to the tooth.

b. The receptor is placed away from the tooth and toward the middle of the oral cavity.

c. Either a or b.

d. None of the above.

___ **21.** Which of the following about receptor placement is correct?

a. Anterior receptors are placed horizontally.

b. Anterior receptors are placed vertically.

c. Posterior receptors are placed horizontally

d. Posterior receptors are placed vertically

1) 1, 2, and 3
2) 2, 3, and 4
3) 2 and 3
4) 1 and 4

___ **22.** Which of the following about the exposure sequence for periapical receptors is incorrect?

a. Anterior receptors are always exposed before posterior receptors.

b. Either anterior or posterior receptors may be exposed first.

c. In posterior quadrants, the premolar receptor is always exposed before the molar receptor.

d. When exposing anterior receptors, work from the patient's right to left in the maxillary arch, and then work from left to right in the mandibular arch.

___ **23.** Which of the following about the lack of parallelism between the receptor and the long axis of the tooth is correct?

a. If the lack of parallelism is greater than 30 degrees, the image is generally acceptable.

b. If the lack of parallelism is less than 20 degrees, the image is generally acceptable.

c. If the lack of parallelism is less than 50 degrees, the image is generally acceptable.

d. If the lack of parallelism is greater than 50 degrees, the image is generally acceptable.

___ **24.** Which of the following are advantages of the paralleling technique?

a. increased accuracy

b. simplicity of use

c. ease of duplication

d. ease of receptor placement

1) 1, 2, 3, and 4
2) 1, 2, and 3
3) 2, 3, and 4
4) 1, 3, and 4

___ **25.** The advantages of the paralleling technique outweigh the disadvantages.

a. true

b. false

ESSAY

26. State the basic principle of the paralleling technique.

27. Describe why a beam alignment device must be used in the paralleling technique.

28. State the five rules of the paralleling technique.

29. Discuss the patient and equipment preparations that must be completed before using the paralleling technique.

30. Discuss the exposure sequence for 15 periapical receptor placements using the paralleling technique.

31. Describe each of the 15 periapical receptor placements that are recommended for use with the XCP instruments.

32. Summarize the guidelines for periapical receptor positioning with the paralleling technique.

33. Explain the modifications in the paralleling technique that are used for a shallow palate, bony growths, or a sensitive premolar region.

chapter 18

Bisecting Technique

OUTLINE

BASIC CONCEPTS
  Terminology
  Principles of Bisecting Technique
  Receptor Stabilization
  Receptors Used in Bisecting Technique
  Position-Indicating Device Angulation
  Rules of Bisecting Technique

STEP-BY-STEP PROCEDURES
  Patient Preparation
  Equipment Preparation
  Exposure Sequence for Receptor Placements
  Receptor Placement for Bisecting Technique
ADVANTAGES AND DISADVANTAGES
  Advantages of Bisecting Technique
  Disadvantages of Bisecting Technique

LEARNING OBJECTIVES

After completion of this chapter, the student will be able to do the following:

- Define the key terms associated with the bisecting technique
- State the rule of isometry
- State the basic principles of the bisecting technique and illustrate the location of the receptor, tooth, imaginary bisector, central ray, and position-indicating device (PID)
- List the beam alignment devices that can be used with the bisecting technique
- Describe the receptor size used with the bisecting technique
- Describe the correct and incorrect horizontal angulation
- Describe correct and incorrect vertical angulation

- State each of the recommended vertical angulation ranges used for periapical exposures in the bisecting technique
- State the basic rules of the bisecting technique
- Describe patient and equipment preparations necessary before using the bisecting technique
- Discuss the exposure sequence used for the 14 periapical receptor placements used in the bisecting technique
- Describe each of the 14 periapical receptor placements recommended for use in the bisecting technique
- List the advantages and disadvantages of the bisecting technique

KEY TERMS

Angle	Central ray	Receptor placement
Angulation	Elongation	Teeth, anterior
Angulation, horizontal	Exposure sequence	Teeth, posterior
Angulation, vertical	Foreshortening	Triangle
Beam alignment device	Hypotenuse	Triangle, equilateral
Bisect	Isometry	Triangle, right
Bisecting technique	Isometry, rule of	Triangles, congruent
Bisector, imaginary	Long axis (tooth)	

The dental radiographer must master a variety of intraoral imaging techniques. As discussed in Chapter 17, the paralleling technique is one method for exposing periapical and bite-wing images. Another intraoral method for exposing periapical images is the bisecting technique. Before the dental radiographer can use this technique, an understanding of the basic concepts, including terminology and principles, is necessary. In addition, the dental radiographer must comprehend patient preparation, equipment preparation, exposure sequencing, and receptor placement procedures used in the bisecting technique.

The purpose of this chapter is to present basic concepts and to describe patient preparation, equipment preparation, and receptor placement procedures used in the bisecting technique. This chapter also describes the advantages and disadvantages of the bisecting technique and reviews helpful hints.

BASIC CONCEPTS

The **bisecting technique** (also known as the *bisecting-angle technique* or *bisection-of-the-angle technique*) is another method that can be used to expose periapical images.

Terminology

An understanding of the following basic terms is necessary before describing the bisecting technique:

Angle: In geometry, a figure formed by two lines diverging from a common point (Figure 18-1, A).

Bisect: To divide into two equal parts (noun, bisector) (Figure 18-1, B).

Triangle: In geometry, a figure formed by connecting three points not in a straight line by three straight-line segments (Figure 18-1, C). A triangle has three angles.

Triangle, equilateral: In geometry, a triangle with three equal sides (Figure 18-1, D).

Triangle, right: In geometry, a triangle with one 90-degree angle (right angle) (Figure 18-1, E).

Triangles, congruent: Triangles that are identical and correspond exactly when superimposed (Figure 18-1, F).

Hypotenuse: In geometry, the side of a right triangle opposite the right angle (Figure 18-1, G).

Isometry: Equality of measurement.

Long axis of the tooth: An imaginary line that divides the tooth longitudinally into two equal halves (Figure 18-2).

Central ray: The central portion of the primary beam of x-radiation.

Principles of Bisecting Technique

The bisecting technique is based on a simple geometric principle known as the **rule of isometry**. The rule of isometry states that two triangles are equal if they have two equal angles and share a common side (Figure 18-3). In dental

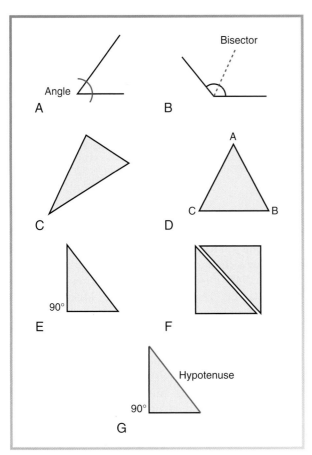

FIGURE 18-1 **A**, An angle is formed by two lines that diverge from a common point. **B**, A bisector divides an angle into equal angles. **C**, A triangle. **D**, An equilateral triangle has three equal sides (AB = BC = CA). **E**, A right triangle has one 90-degree angle. **F**, Congruent triangles are identical. **G**, The hypotenuse is the side of a right triangle opposite the right angle.

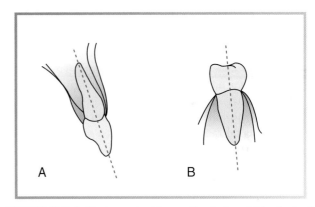

FIGURE 18-2 **A**, The long axis of the maxillary incisor divides the tooth into two equal halves. **B**, The long axis of a mandibular premolar divides the tooth into two equal halves.

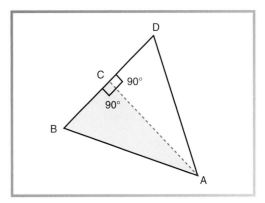

FIGURE 18-3 Angle A is bisected by line AC. Line AC is perpendicular to line BD. Angle BAC is equal to angle DAC. Angle ACB is equal to angle ACD. According to the rule of isometry, triangle BAC *(shaded)* is equal to triangle DAC.

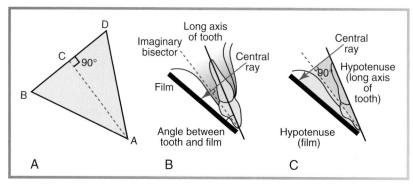

FIGURE 18-4 **A**, The receptor (line BA) is placed along the lingual surface of the tooth. At the point where the receptor contacts the tooth, the plane of the receptor and the long axis of the tooth (DA) form an angle (BAD). The imaginary bisector divides this angle into two equal angles (BAC and DAC). The central ray (BD) is directed perpendicular to the imaginary bisector and completes the third sides (BC and CD) of the two triangles. **B**, The central ray is directed at a right angle to the imaginary bisector. **C**, The two imaginary triangles that result are right triangles and congruent. The hypotenuse of each triangle is represented by the long axis of the tooth and the plane of the receptor.

imaging, this geometric principle is applied to the bisecting technique to form two imaginary equal triangles (Figure 18-4). The bisecting technique can be described as follows:

1. The receptor must be placed along the lingual surface of the tooth.
2. At the point where the receptor contacts the tooth, the plane of the receptor and the long axis of the tooth form an angle.
3. The dental radiographer must visualize a plane that divides in half, or bisects, the angle formed by the receptor and the long axis of the tooth. This plane is termed the **imaginary bisector**. The imaginary bisector creates two equal angles and provides a common side for the two imaginary equal triangles.
4. The dental radiographer must then direct the central ray of the x-ray beam perpendicular to the imaginary bisector. When the central ray is directed at an angle of 90 degrees to the imaginary bisector, two imaginary equal triangles are formed.
5. The two imaginary triangles that result are right triangles and are congruent. The hypotenuse of one imaginary triangle is represented by the long axis of the tooth; the other hypotenuse is represented by the plane of the receptor.

When the rule of isometry is followed strictly, the dental image of the tooth will be accurate. When the angle formed by the plane of the receptor and the long axis of the tooth is bisected, and the x-ray beam is directed at a right angle to the imaginary bisector, the actual tooth and the dental image of the tooth will be of the same length (Figure 18-5).

Receptor Stabilization

In the bisecting technique, beam alignment devices may be used to position and stabilize the receptor.

Beam Alignment Devices

Beam alignment devices are used to position an intraoral receptor in the mouth and maintain it in position during

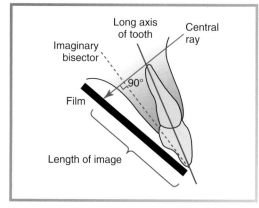

FIGURE 18-5 The image on the receptor is equal to the length of the tooth when the central ray is directed at 90 degrees to the imaginary bisector. A tooth and its image will be equal in length when two equal triangles are formed that share a common side (imaginary bisector).

exposure (see Chapter 6). Examples of commercially available intraoral beam alignment devices that can be used with the bisecting technique include the following:

- *Rinn BAI instruments* (Dentsply, Rinn Corporation, Elgin, IL). The bisecting angle instrument (BAI) includes plastic bite-blocks, plastic aiming rings, and metal indicator arms. To reduce the amount of radiation received by the patient, snap-on ring collimators can be added to the plastic aiming rings. BAIs have been designed to aid in the determination of horizontal and vertical angulations, minimize distortion from film bending, and prevent cone-cuts (Figure 18-6, A).
- *Stabe bite-block* (Rinn). This device can be used with the paralleling technique or the bisecting technique. For use with the bisecting technique, the scored front section is removed, and the receptor is placed as close to the teeth as possible (Figure 18-6, B).
- *EEZEE-Grip receptor holder* (Rinn). Formerly known as *Snap-A-Ray*, this device is used to stabilize a receptor

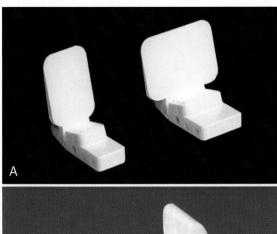

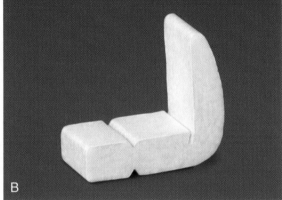

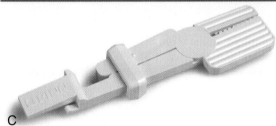

FIGURE 18-6 A, Rinn bisecting angle bite-blocks used with the bisecting technique. **B,** Stabe disposable film holders (bite-blocks). **C,** EEZEE-Grip (Snap-A-Ray) intraoral receptor holder.

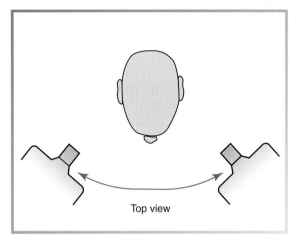

Top view

FIGURE 18-7 Horizontal angulation of the position-indicating device (PID) refers to PID placement in a side-to-side (ear-to-ear) direction. (From Haring JI, Lind LJ: *Radiographic interpretation for the dental hygienist,* Philadelphia, 1993, Saunders.)

in either the paralleling technique or the bisecting technique (Figure 18-6, C).

The Stabe bite-block is disposable and is designed for one-time use only. BAIs and the EEZEE-Grip film holder are reusable and must be sterilized after each use.

BAIs with collimators are the recommended devices for the bisecting technique because (1) aiming rings are included that aid in the alignment of the position-indicating device (PID), and (2) collimators significantly reduce the amount of patient exposure to x-radiation. BAIs are simple to assemble and position. For information about the use of BAIs or other devices available for the bisecting technique, the dental radiographer should refer to the manufacturer's instructions.

Receptors Used in Bisecting Technique

Traditionally, a size 2 intraoral receptor is used with the bisecting technique. In the anterior regions, a size 2 receptor is always placed with the long portion of the receptor in a

vertical (upright) direction. In the posterior regions, a size 2 receptor is always placed with the long portion of the receptor in a horizontal (sideways) direction.

Position-Indicating Device Angulation

In the bisecting technique, the angulation of the PID is critical. **Angulation** is a term used to describe the alignment of the central ray of the x-ray beam in horizontal and vertical planes. Angulation can be varied by moving the PID in either a horizontal direction or a vertical direction. The use of BAIs with aiming rings dictates the proper PID angulation. However, when a bite-block or other device without an aiming ring is employed, the dental radiographer must determine both horizontal and vertical angulations.

Horizontal Angulation

Horizontal angulation refers to the positioning of the PID and the direction of the central ray in a horizontal, or side-to-side, plane (Figure 18-7). The horizontal angulation does not differ according to the technique used; paralleling, bisecting, and bite-wing techniques all use the same principles of horizontal angulation.

Correct Horizontal Angulation. With correct horizontal angulation, the central ray is directed perpendicular to the curvature of the arch and through the contact areas of the teeth (Figure 18-8). As a result, the contact areas on the dental image appear "opened."

Incorrect Horizontal Angulation. Incorrect horizontal angulation results in overlapped ("unopened") contact areas (Figure 18-9). An image with overlapped interproximal contact areas cannot be used to examine the interproximal areas of the teeth and is thus nondiagnostic (Figure 18-10).

Vertical Angulation

Vertical angulation refers to the positioning of the PID in a vertical, or up-and-down, plane (Figure 18-11). Vertical

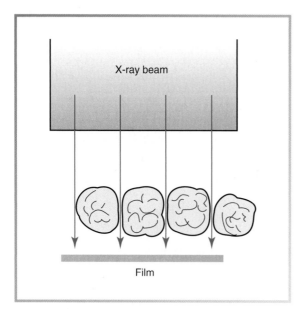

FIGURE 18-8 Correct horizontal angulation.

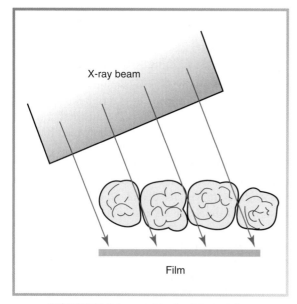

FIGURE 18-9 Incorrect horizontal angulation.

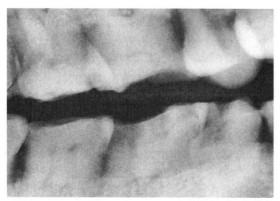

FIGURE 18-10 Overlapped contacts. (From Haring JI, Lind LJ: *Radiographic interpretation for the dental hygienist*, Philadelphia, 1993, Saunders.)

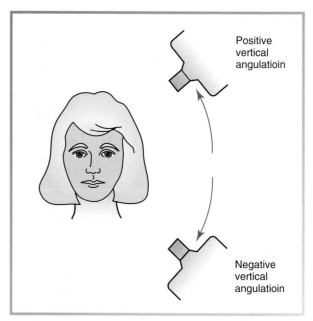

FIGURE 18-11 Vertical angulation of the position-indicating device (PID) refers to PID placement in an up-and-down (head-to-toe) direction. (From Haring JI, Lind LJ: *Radiographic interpretation for the dental hygienist*, Philadelphia, 1993, Saunders.)

angulation is measured in degrees and is registered on the outside of the tubehead. The vertical angulation differs according to the imaging technique used, as follows:

- With the paralleling technique, the vertical angulation of the central ray is directed perpendicular to the receptor and the long axis of the tooth (see Chapter 17).
- With the bisecting technique, the vertical angulation is determined by the imaginary bisector; the central ray is directed perpendicular to the imaginary bisector.
- With the bite-wing technique, the vertical angulation is predetermined; the central ray is directed at +10 degrees to the occlusal plane (see Chapter 19).

Correct Vertical Angulation. Correct vertical angulation results in a dental image that is of the same length as that of the tooth. Table 18-1 lists recommended vertical angulation ranges for the bisecting technique.

Incorrect Vertical Angulation. Incorrect vertical angulation results in a radiographic image that is not of the same length as that of the tooth; instead, the image appears longer or shorter. Elongated or foreshortened images are not diagnostic.

Foreshortened Images. Foreshortened images refer to radiographic images that appear shortened. **Foreshortening** of images results from excessive vertical angulation. When the vertical angulation is too steep, the image of the tooth appears shorter than the actual tooth (Figure 18-12). Foreshortening also occurs if the central ray is directed perpendicular to the plane of the receptor rather than to the imaginary bisector.

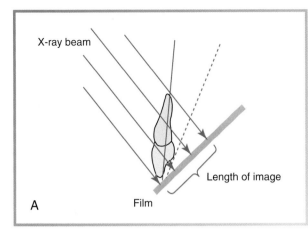

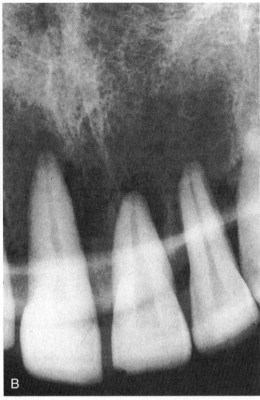

FIGURE 18-12 A, If the vertical angulation is too steep, the image is shorter than the actual tooth. **B,** Foreshortened images. (From Haring JI, Lind LJ: *Radiographic interpretation for the dental hygienist*, Philadelphia, 1993, Saunders.)

TABLE 18-1	Recommended Vertical Angulation Ranges: Bisecting Technique	
	Maxillary Teeth: Vertical Angulation (degrees)	**Mandibular Teeth: Vertical Angulation (degrees)**
Canines	+45 to +55	−20 to −30
Incisors	+40 to +50	−15 to −25
Premolars	+30 to +40	−10 to −15
Molars	+20 to +30	−5 to 0

Elongated Images. Elongated images refer to images of the teeth that appear too long. **Elongation** of images results from insufficient vertical angulation. When the vertical angulation is too flat, the image of the tooth appears longer than the actual tooth (Figure 18-13). Elongation also occurs if the central ray is directed perpendicular to the long axis of the tooth rather than to the imaginary bisector.

Rules of Bisecting Technique

Five basic rules should be followed when using the bisecting technique.

1. *Receptor placement.* The receptor must be positioned to cover the prescribed area of the tooth to be examined. Specific placements are described in the procedures.

2. *Receptor position.* The receptor must be placed against the lingual surface of the tooth. The occlusal end of the receptor must extend approximately one eighth of an inch beyond the incisal or occlusal surfaces (Figure 18-14). The apical end of the receptor must rest against the palatal or alveolar tissues.

3. *Vertical angulation.* The central ray of the x-ray beam must be directed perpendicular (at a right angle) to the imaginary bisector that divides the angle formed by the receptor and the long axis of the tooth.

4. *Horizontal angulation.* The central ray of the x-ray beam must be directed through the contact areas between teeth.

5. *Receptor exposure.* The x-ray beam must be centered on the receptor to ensure that all areas of the receptor are exposed. Failure to center the x-ray beam results in a partial image or a cone-cut.

STEP-BY-STEP PROCEDURES

Step-by-step procedures for the exposure of periapical images using the bisecting technique include patient preparation, equipment preparation, and receptor placement methods. Before exposing any receptors using the bisecting technique, infection control procedures (as detailed in Chapter 15) must be completed.

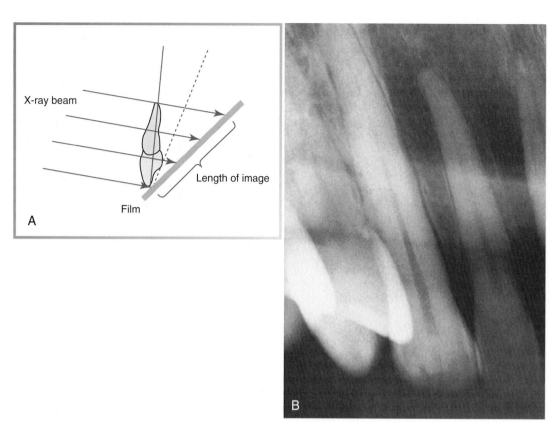

FIGURE 18-13 A, If the vertical angulation is too flat, the image is longer than the actual tooth. **B**, Elongated images. (From Haring JI, Lind LJ: *Radiographic interpretation for the dental hygienist*, Philadelphia, 1993, Saunders.)

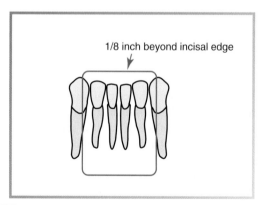

FIGURE 18-14 Approximately one eighth of an inch of the receptor must appear beyond the incisal edges of the teeth.

Patient Preparation

After completion of infection control procedures and preparation of the treatment area and supplies, the patient should be seated. After seating the patient, and before the exposure of any periapical images the dental radiographer must prepare the patient for receptor exposure (Procedure 18-1).

PROCEDURE 18-1	**Patient Preparation for Bisecting Technique**

1. Briefly explain the procedure to the patient before the procedure begins.
2. Position the patient upright in the chair. The level of the chair must be adjusted to a comfortable working height.
3. Adjust the headrest to support the patient's head. The patient's head must be positioned such that the arch that is being imaged is parallel to the floor and the midsagittal plane is perpendicular to the floor.
4. Place and secure the lead apron with thyroid collar over the patient.
5. Remove all objects from the patient's mouth (e.g., dentures, retainers, chewing gum) that may interfere with the procedure. Eyeglasses must also be removed.

Equipment Preparation

After patient preparation, the dental radiographer must complete equipment preparations before exposing any periapicals (Procedure 18-2).

PROCEDURE 18-2	Equipment Preparation for Bisecting Technique

1. Set the exposure factors (kilovoltage, milliamperage, and time) on the x-ray unit according to the recommendations of the receptor manufacturer. Either a short (8-inch) or long (16-inch) position-indicating device (PID) may be used with the bisecting technique; typically, the short PID is preferred.
2. If using a beam alignment device with the bisecting technique, open the sterilized package containing the device, and assemble it over a covered work area.

Exposure Sequence for Receptor Placements

When using the bisecting technique, an **exposure sequence,** or definite order for periapical receptor placements and exposures, must be followed. The dental radiographer must have an established exposure routine to prevent errors and use time efficiently. Working without an exposure sequence may result in omitting an area or exposing an area twice.

Anterior Exposure Sequence

When exposing periapical receptors with the bisecting technique, always begin with the **anterior teeth** (canines and incisors). The rationale for beginning in the anterior region is that anterior placements are less likely to cause the patient to gag. Once the gag reflex has been stimulated, the patient may gag on projections that could normally be tolerated. Management of the patient with a hypersensitive gag reflex is discussed in Chapter 24.

With size 2 receptors, a total of six anterior placements are used in the bisecting technique: three maxillary exposures and three mandibular exposures. The recommended anterior periapical exposure sequence for the bisecting technique is as follows (Table 18-2):

1. Begin with the maxillary right canine (tooth No. 6).
2. Expose all the maxillary anterior teeth *from right to left.*
3. End with the maxillary left canine (tooth No. 11).
4. Next, move to the mandibular arch.
5. Begin with the mandibular left canine (tooth No. 22).
6. Expose all the mandibular anterior teeth *from left to right.*
7. Finish with the mandibular right canine (tooth No. 27).

As previously discussed in Chapter 17, when the dental radiographer works from right to left in the maxillary arch and then from left to right in the mandibular arch, no wasted movement or shifting of the PID occurs (see Figure 17-10). In addition, when working from right to left and then from left to right, the teeth are exposed in ascending numerical order. This exposure sequence allows the dental radiographer easily to keep track of the last exposure if the procedure is interrupted.

TABLE 18-2	Exposure Sequence for Anterior Receptor Placement: Bisecting Technique

Exposure Number	Arch	Side	Tooth	Tooth Number
1	Maxillary	Right	Canine	6
2	Maxillary	Right	Lateral incisor	7
	Maxillary	Right	Central incisor	8
	Maxillary	Left	Central incisor	9
	Maxillary	Left	Lateral incisor	10
3	Maxillary	Left	Canine	11
4	Mandibular	Left	Canine	22
5	Mandibular	Left	Lateral incisor	23
	Mandibular	Left	Central incisor	24
	Mandibular	Right	Central incisor	25
	Mandibular	Right	Lateral incisor	26
6	Mandibular	Right	Canine	27

TABLE 18-3	Exposure Sequence for Posterior Receptor Placement: Bisecting Technique

Exposure Number	Arch	Side	Teeth	Teeth Number
1	Maxillary	Right	Premolars	4, 5
2	Maxillary	Right	Molars	1, 2, 3
3	Mandibular	Right	Premolars	28, 29
4	Mandibular	Right	Molars	30, 31, 32
5	Maxillary	Left	Premolars	12, 13
6	Maxillary	Left	Molars	14, 15, 16
7	Mandibular	Left	Premolars	20, 21
8	Mandibular	Left	Molars	17, 18, 19

Posterior Exposure Sequence

After anterior exposures, the **posterior teeth** (premolars and molars) are exposed. In each quadrant, always expose the premolar receptor first and then the molar receptor. The rationale for exposing the premolar placement first is as follows:

- Premolar placement is easier for the patient to tolerate.
- Premolar exposure is less likely to evoke the gag reflex.

Eight posterior receptor placements are used in the bisecting technique: 4 maxillary exposures and 4 mandibular exposures. The recommended posterior periapical exposure sequence for the bisecting technique is as follows (Table 18-3):

1. Begin with the maxillary right quadrant.
2. Expose the premolar receptor (teeth Nos. 4 and 5) first and then the molar receptor (teeth Nos. 1, 2, and 3).
3. Move to the mandibular right quadrant.

| BOX 18-1 | Prescribed Placements for Anterior Periapical Receptors: Bisecting Technique |

Exposure of Maxillary Canine

The entire crown and root of the canine, including the apex and the surrounding structures, must be seen on this image. The interproximal alveolar bone and mesial contact of the canine must also be visible. The lingual cusp of the first premolar usually obscures the distal contact of the canine.

Exposure of Maxillary Incisor

The entire crowns and roots of all four maxillary incisors, including the apices of the teeth and the surrounding structures, must be seen on this image. The interproximal alveolar bone between the central incisors and the central and lateral incisors must also be visible.

Exposure of Mandibular Canine

The entire crown and root of the canine, including the apex and the surrounding structures, must be seen on this image. The interproximal alveolar bone and mesial and distal contacts must also be visible.

Exposure of Mandibular Incisor

The entire crowns and roots of the four mandibular incisors, including the apices of the teeth and the surrounding structures, must be seen on this image. The contacts between the central incisors and between the central and lateral incisors must also be visible. In most cases, it is not necessary to see the distal contacts of the lateral incisors.

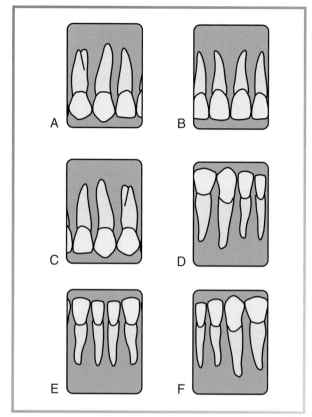

FIGURE 18-15 Prescribed placements for anterior periapicals. **A,** Exposure of the maxillary right canine. **B,** Exposure of the maxillary incisor. **C,** Exposure of the maxillary left canine. **D,** Exposure of the mandibular right canine. **E,** Exposure of the mandibular incisor. **F,** Exposure of the mandibular left canine.

4. Expose the premolar receptor (teeth Nos. 28 and 29) first and then the molar receptor (teeth Nos. 30, 31, and 32).
5. Move to the maxillary left quadrant.
6. Expose the premolar receptor (teeth Nos. 12 and 13) first and then the molar receptor (teeth Nos. 14, 15, and 16).
7. Finish with the mandibular left quadrant.
8. Expose the premolar receptor (teeth Nos. 20 and 21) first, and then finish the posterior periapical placements with exposure of the molar receptor (teeth Nos. 17, 18, and 19).

Receptor Placement for Bisecting Technique

In a complete mouth radiographic series (CMRS) using the bisecting technique, each periapical exposure has a prescribed placement. **Receptor placement,** or the specific area where the receptor must be positioned before exposure, is dictated by the teeth and surrounding structures that must be included on the resultant dental image. Prescribed placements for the anterior teeth are detailed in Box 18-1 and illustrated in Figure 18-15. Posterior placements are detailed in Box 18-2 and illustrated in Figure 18-16.

The specific placements described in this chapter are for a 14-receptor periapical series using size 2 receptors for all anterior and posterior exposures. Variations in the placement or the number of total receptors used may be recommended by other reference sources or individual practitioners (Box 18-3).

Anterior Placement

Anterior placements include the following:
- Two maxillary canine exposures (Procedure 18-3)
- One maxillary incisor exposure (Procedure 18-4)
- Two mandibular canine exposures (Procedure 18-5)
- One mandibular incisor exposure (Procedure 18-6)

Size 2 receptor is used for all anterior placements and is positioned vertically.

Posterior Placement

Posterior placements include the following:
- Two maxillary premolar exposures (Procedure 18-7)
- Two maxillary molar exposures (Procedure 18-8)
- Two mandibular premolar exposures (Procedure 18-9)
- Two mandibular molar exposures (Procedure 18-10)

| BOX 18-2 | Prescribed Placements for Posterior Periapical Receptors: Bisecting Technique |

Exposure of Maxillary Premolar
All crowns and roots of the first and second premolars and first molar, including the apices, alveolar crests, contact areas, and surrounding bone, must be seen on this image. In addition, the distal contact of the maxillary canine must be visible in this projection.

Exposure of Maxillary Molar
All crowns and roots of the first, second, and third molars, including the apices, alveolar crests, contact areas, surrounding bone, and tuberosity region, must be seen on this image. In addition, the distal contact of the maxillary second premolar must be visible in this projection.

Exposure of Mandibular Premolar
All crowns and roots of the first and second premolars and first molar, including the apices, alveolar crests, contact areas, and surrounding bone, must be seen on this image. In addition, the distal contact of the mandibular canine should be visible in this projection.

Exposure of Mandibular Molar
All crowns and roots of the first, second, and third molars, including the apices, alveolar crests, contact areas, and surrounding bone, must be seen on this image. In addition, the distal contact of the mandibular second premolar must be visible in this projection.

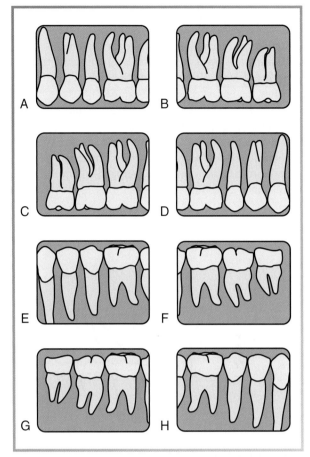

FIGURE 18-16 Prescribed placements for posterior periapicals. **A,** Exposure of the maxillary right molar. **B,** Exposure of the maxillary right premolar. **C,** Exposure of the maxillary left premolar. **D,** Exposure of the maxillary left molar. **E,** Exposure of the mandibular right molar. **F,** Exposure of the mandibular right premolar. **G,** Exposure of the mandibular left premolar. **H,** Exposure of the mandibular left molar.

| BOX 18-3 | Guidelines for Receptor Placement with Bisecting Technique |

1. When using film, the white side of the film always faces the teeth.
2. Anterior receptors are always placed vertically.
3. Posterior receptors are always placed horizontally.
4. The incisal or occlusal edge of the receptor must extend approximately one eighth of an inch beyond the teeth.
5. When positioning the receptor, always center the receptor over the area to be examined (as defined in the prescribed placements).

Size 2 receptor is used for all posterior placements and is positioned horizontally.

ADVANTAGES AND DISADVANTAGES

As with all intraoral techniques, the bisecting technique has both advantages and disadvantages. The disadvantages of the bisecting technique, however, outweigh the advantages. Therefore, the paralleling technique is preferred over the bisecting technique for the exposure of periapical images and should be used whenever possible.

Advantages of Bisecting Technique

The primary advantage of the bisecting technique is that it can be used without a beam alignment device when the anatomy of the patient (shallow palate, bony growths, sensitive mandibular premolar areas) precludes the use of such a device. Another advantage is decreased exposure time. When a short (8-inch) PID is used with the bisecting technique, a shorter exposure time is recommended.

Disadvantages of Bisecting Technique

The primary disadvantage of the bisecting technique is dimensional distortion. The disadvantages of the bisecting technique can be summarized as follows:

1. *Image distortion.* Distortion occurs when a short PID is used; a short PID causes increased divergence of x-rays, resulting in image magnification. Distortion

Text continued on p. 206

PROCEDURE 18-3 Maxillary Canine Exposure: Bisecting Technique (Figure 18-17)

1. Center the receptor on the maxillary canine.
2. Position the lower edge of the receptor parallel to the occlusal plane so that one eighth of an inch extends below the incisal edge of the canine.
3. Instruct the patient to "slowly close" on the bite-block or beam alignment device.
4. If not using a beam alignment device, establish the correct vertical angulation by bisecting the angle and directing the central ray perpendicular to the imaginary bisector.

5. If not using a beam alignment device, establish the correct horizontal angulation by directing the central ray between the contacts of the canine and the first premolar.
6. Position the position-indicating device (PID) using the correct vertical and horizontal angulations. Center the PID over the receptor to avoid cone-cutting.
7. Expose the receptor.

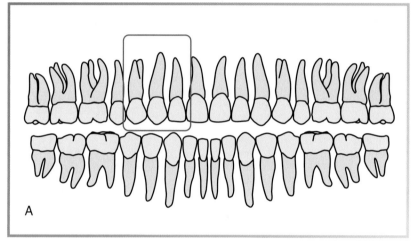

FIGURE 18-17 Exposure of the maxillary canine. **A,** Receptor placement.

PROCEDURE **18-3**   **Maxillary Canine Exposure: Bisecting Technique—cont'd**

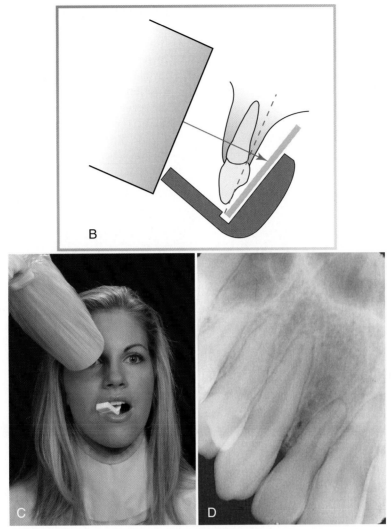

FIGURE 18-17, cont'd B, Relationship of the receptor, teeth, imaginary bisector, and central ray. **C**, Exposure of the receptor. **D**, Resultant image.

PROCEDURE 18-4   **Maxillary Incisor Exposure: Bisecting Technique** (Figure 18-18)

1. Center the receptor on the contact between the two maxillary central incisors.
2. Position the lower edge of the receptor parallel to the occlusal plane so that one eighth of an inch extends below the incisal edges of the teeth.
3. Instruct the patient to "slowly close" on the bite-block or beam alignment device.
4. If not using a beam alignment device, establish the correct vertical angulation by bisecting the angle and directing the central ray perpendicular to the imaginary bisector.
5. If not using a beam alignment device, establish the correct horizontal angulation by directing the central ray between the contacts of the central incisors.
6. Position the position-indicating device (PID) using the correct vertical and horizontal angulations. Center the PID over the receptor to avoid cone-cutting.
7. Expose the receptor.

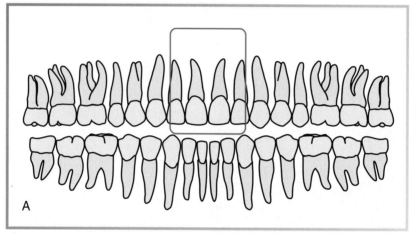

A

FIGURE 18-18 Exposure of the maxillary incisor. **A,** Receptor placement.

PROCEDURE 18-4 **Maxillary Incisor Exposure: Bisecting Technique—cont'd**

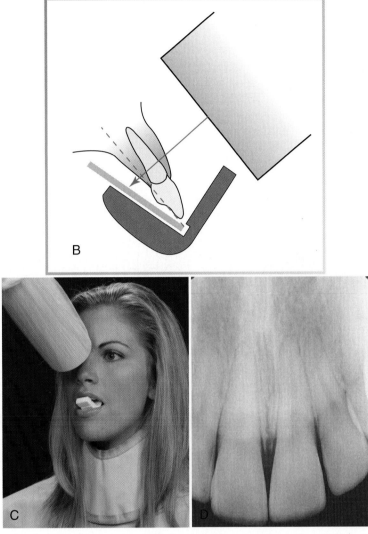

FIGURE 18-18, cont'd **B**, Relationship among the receptor, teeth, imaginary bisector, and central ray. **C**, Exposure of the receptor. **D**, Resultant image.

PROCEDURE 18-5 **Mandibular Canine Exposure: Bisecting Technique** (Figure 18-19)

1. Center the receptor on the mandibular canine.
2. Position the upper edge of the receptor parallel to the occlusal plane so that one eighth of an inch extends above the incisal edge of the canine.
3. Instruct the patient to "slowly close" on the bite-block or beam alignment device.
4. If not using a beam alignment device, establish the correct vertical angulation by bisecting the angle and directing the central ray perpendicular to the imaginary bisector.

5. If not using a beam alignment device, establish the correct horizontal angulation by directing the central ray between the contacts of the canine and first premolar.
6. Position the position-indicating device (PID) using the correct vertical and horizontal angulations. Center the PID over the receptor to avoid cone-cutting.
7. Expose the receptor.

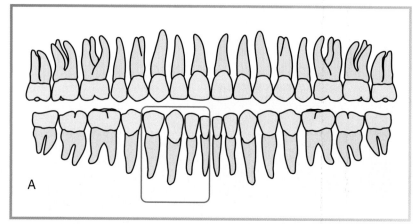

FIGURE 18-19 Exposure of the mandibular canine. **A**, Receptor placement.

PROCEDURE 18-5 | **Mandibular Canine Exposure: Bisecting Technique—cont'd**

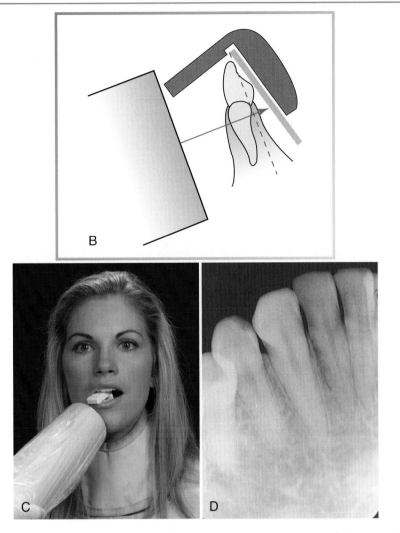

FIGURE 18-19, cont'd **B**, Relationship among the receptor, teeth, imaginary bisector, and central ray. **C**, Exposure of the receptor. **D**, Resultant image.

PROCEDURE 18-6 Mandibular Incisor Exposure: Bisecting Technique (Figure 18-20)

1. Center the receptor on the contact between the two mandibular central incisors.
2. Position the upper edge of the receptor parallel to the occlusal plane so that one eighth of an inch extends above the incisal edges of the teeth.
3. Instruct the patient to "slowly close" on the bite-block or beam alignment device.
4. If not using a beam alignment device, establish the correct vertical angulation by bisecting the angle and directing the central ray perpendicular to the imaginary bisector.
5. If not using a beam alignment device, establish the correct horizontal angulation by directing the central ray between the contacts of the central incisors.
6. Position the position-indicating device (PID) using the correct vertical and horizontal angulations. Center the PID over the receptor to avoid cone-cutting.
7. Expose the receptor.

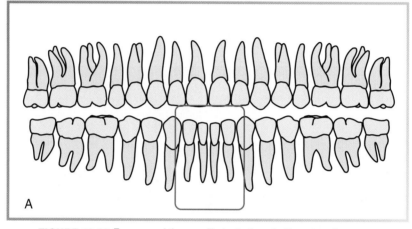

A

FIGURE 18-20 Exposure of the mandibular incisor. **A,** Receptor placement.

PROCEDURE 18-6   **Mandibular Incisor Exposure: Bisecting Technique—cont'd**

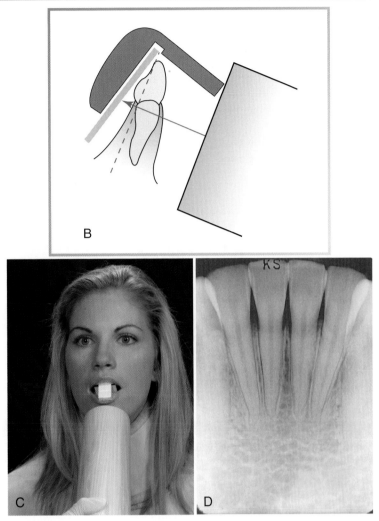

FIGURE 18-20, cont'd B, Relationship among the receptor, teeth, imaginary bisector, and central ray. **C**, Exposure of the receptor. **D**, Resultant image.

PROCEDURE 18-7 Maxillary Premolar Exposure: Bisecting Technique (Figure 18-21)

1. Center the receptor on the maxillary second premolar; the front edge of the receptor should be aligned with the midline of the maxillary canine.
2. Position the lower edge of the receptor parallel to the occlusal plane so that one eighth of an inch extends below the occlusal edges of the teeth.
3. Instruct the patient to "slowly close" on the bite-block or beam alignment device.
4. If not using a beam alignment device, establish the correct vertical angulation by bisecting the angle and directing the central ray perpendicular to the imaginary bisector.
5. If not using a beam alignment device, establish the correct horizontal angulation by directing the central ray between the contacts of the premolars.
6. Position the position-indicating device (PID) using the correct vertical and horizontal angulations. Center the PID over the receptor to avoid cone-cutting.
7. Expose the receptor.

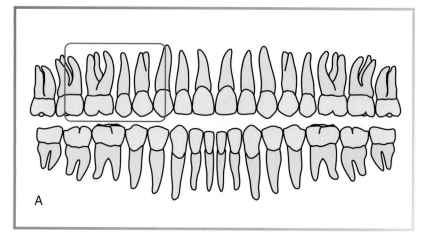

FIGURE 18-21 Exposure of the maxillary premolar. **A,** Receptor placement.

PROCEDURE 18-7   **Maxillary Premolar Exposure: Bisecting Technique—cont'd**

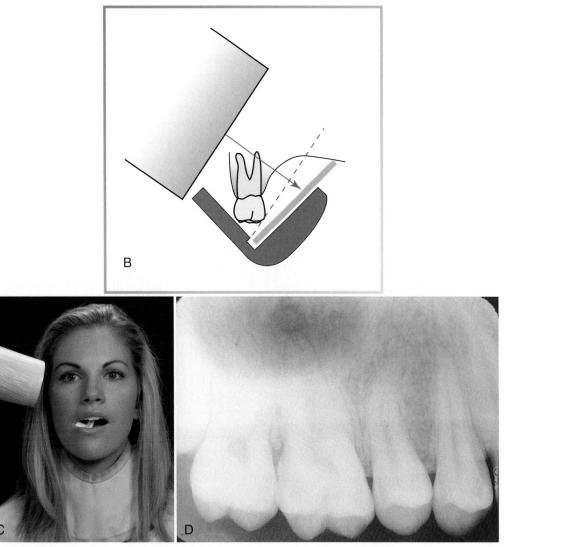

FIGURE 18-21, cont'd B, Relationship among the receptor, teeth, imaginary bisector, and central ray. **C,** Exposure of the receptor. **D,** Resultant image.

PROCEDURE 18-8   **Maxillary Molar Exposure: Bisecting Technique** (Figure 18-22)

1. Center the receptor on the maxillary second molar; the front edge of the receptor should be aligned with the midline of the maxillary second premolar.
2. Position the lower edge of the receptor parallel to the occlusal plane so that one eighth of an inch extends below the occlusal edges of the teeth.
3. Instruct the patient to "slowly close" on the bite-block or beam alignment device.
4. If not using a beam alignment device, establish the correct vertical angulation by bisecting the angle and directing the central ray perpendicular to the imaginary bisector.
5. If not using a beam alignment device, establish the correct horizontal angulation by directing the central ray between the contacts of the molars.
6. Position the position-indicating device (PID) using the correct vertical and horizontal angulations. Center the PID over the receptor to avoid cone-cutting.
7. Expose the receptor.

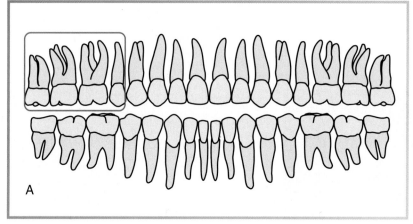

A

FIGURE 18-22 Exposure of the maxillary molar. **A,** Receptor placement.

PROCEDURE 18-8 **Maxillary Molar Exposure: Bisecting Technique—cont'd**

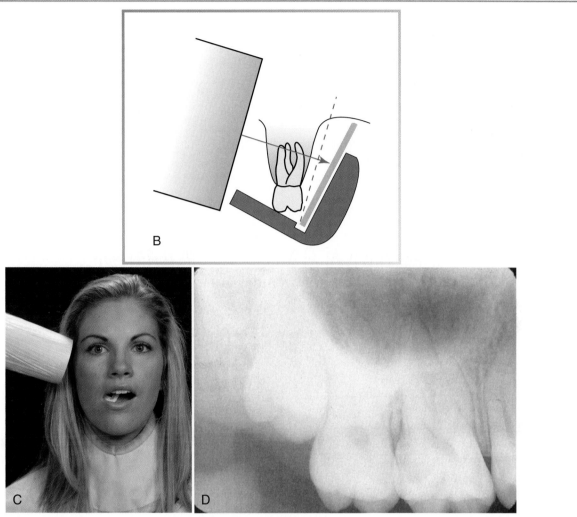

FIGURE 18-22, cont'd B, Relationship among the receptor, teeth, imaginary bisector, and central ray. **C**, Exposure of the receptor. **D**, Resultant image.

PROCEDURE 18-9   Mandibular Premolar Exposure: Bisecting Technique (Figure 18-23)

1. Center the receptor on the mandibular second premolar; the front edge of the receptor should be aligned with the midline of the mandibular canine.
2. Position the upper edge of the receptor parallel to the occlusal plane so that one eighth of an inch extends above the occlusal edges of the teeth.
3. Instruct the patient to "slowly close" on the bite-block or beam alignment device.
4. If not using a beam alignment device, establish the correct vertical angulation by bisecting the angle and directing the central ray perpendicular to the imaginary bisector.
5. If not using a beam alignment device, establish the correct horizontal angulation by directing the central ray between the contacts of the premolars.
6. Position the position-indicating device (PID) using the correct vertical and horizontal angulations. Center the PID over the receptor to avoid cone-cutting.
7. Expose the receptor.

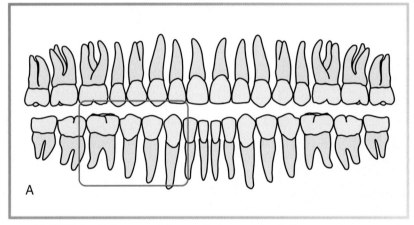

FIGURE 18-23 Exposure of the mandibular premolar. **A**, Receptor placement.

PROCEDURE 18-9   **Mandibular Premolar Exposure: Bisecting Technique—cont'd**

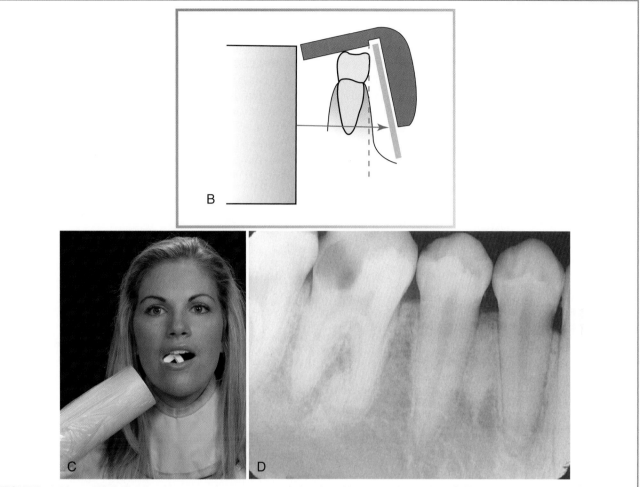

FIGURE 18-23, cont'd B, Relationship among the receptor, teeth, imaginary bisector, and central ray. **C**, Exposure of the receptor. **D**, Resultant image.

PROCEDURE 18-10   Mandibular Molar Exposure: Bisecting Technique (Figure 18-24)

1. Center the receptor on the mandibular second molar; the front edge of the receptor should be aligned with the midline of the mandibular second premolar.
2. Position the upper edge of the receptor parallel to the occlusal plane so that one eighth of an inch extends above the occlusal edges of the teeth.
3. Instruct the patient to "slowly close" on the bite-block or beam alignment device.
4. If not using a beam alignment device, establish the correct vertical angulation by bisecting the angle and directing the central ray perpendicular to the imaginary bisector.
5. If not using a beam alignment device, establish the correct horizontal angulation by directing the central ray between the contacts of the molars.
6. Position the position-indicating device (PID) using the correct vertical and horizontal angulations. Center the PID over the receptor to avoid cone-cutting.
7. Expose the receptor.
8. An example of a charting note for a full-mouth series using the bisecting technique is given below:

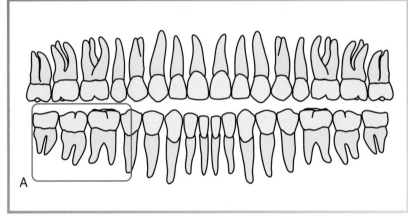

FIGURE 18-24 Exposure of the mandibular molar. **A,** Receptor placement.

PROCEDURE 18-10   Mandibular Molar Exposure: Bisecting Technique—cont'd

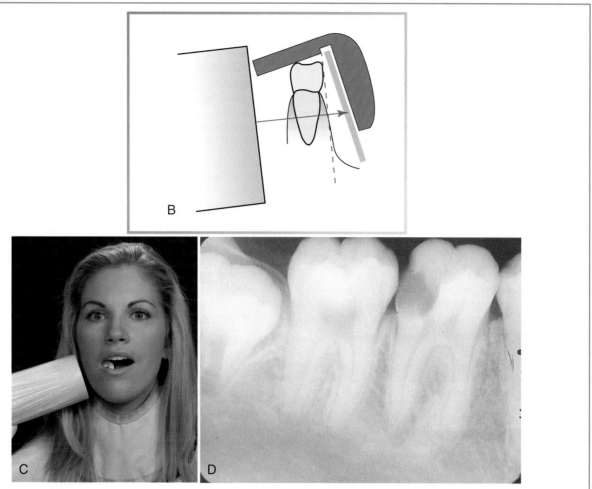

FIGURE 18-24, cont'd B, Relationship among the receptor, teeth, imaginary bisector, and central ray. **C**, Exposure of the receptor. **D**, Resultant image.

Charting a Full-Mouth Series

Date	ADA Procedure Code	Provider	Charting Notes	Comments
9/1/11	0210	LJH	Dr. Stewart requested a modified full-mouth series of radiographs; bisecting technique used with Stabe bite-block; 10 periapicals and 2 bite-wing radiographs exposed; digital PSP plates used (12 total exposures)	Patient has had all molar teeth extracted; only anterior teeth and premolars are present; patient tolerated procedure well; prefers the Styrofoam bite-block over the plastic beam alignment device; slight gag reflex noted on maxillary periapical placements; instructed patient to breathe through nose

also occurs when a tooth (three-dimensional structure) is projected onto a receptor (two-dimensional structure); structures that are farther away from the receptor appear more elongated than those closer to the receptor.

2. *Angulation problems.* Without the use of a beam alignment device and aiming ring, it is difficult for the dental radiographer to visualize the imaginary bisector and then determine the vertical angulation. Any error in vertical angulation will result in image distortion (elongation or foreshortening).

HELPFUL HINTS

In using the bisecting technique:

▪ **DO** set all exposure factors (kilovoltage, milliamperage, time) before placing any receptors in the mouth.

▪ **DO** ask patients to remove all intraoral objects and eyeglasses before placing any receptors in the mouth.

▪ **DO** use a definite order (exposure sequence) when exposing receptors to avoid errors and to make use of time in an efficient manner.

▪ **DO** explain the procedures that will be performed.

▪ **DO** instruct patients on exactly how to stabilize the bite-block and remain still during the exposure.

▪ **DO** memorize the recommended vertical angulation ranges for each periapical exposure, and use these ranges as a guide when determining PID placement.

▪ **DO** direct the central ray perpendicular to the imaginary bisector.

▪ **DO** align the opening of the PID parallel to the imaginary bisector.

▪ **DO** use the word *please*; say, "Open, please."

▪ **DO** use praise; tell cooperative patients how much they are helping you.

▪ **DO NOT** bend or crimp a film packet; bending of the film causes image distortion.

▪ **DO NOT** use words such as *hurt*. Instead, inform patients that the procedure will be "momentarily uncomfortable."

▪ **DO NOT** make comments such as "Oops." Patients will lose confidence in your abilities when they hear such comments.

▪ **DO NOT** pick up a receptor if you drop it. Leave it on the floor; it has now become contaminated. Instead,

remove it and dispose of it when you clean the treatment area.

▪ **DO NOT** allow patients to dictate how you should perform your duties. The dental radiographer must always remain in control of the procedures.

▪ **DO NOT** begin with posterior exposures; posterior placements may cause patients to gag. Instead, always begin with anterior exposures.

SUMMARY

- The bisecting technique is a technique used to expose periapical images. This technique is based on the concept of bisecting the angle formed by the receptor and the long axis of the tooth.
- In the bisecting technique, (1) the receptor is placed along the lingual surface of the tooth; (2) at the point where the receptor contacts the tooth, the plane of the receptor and the long axis of the tooth form an angle; (3) an imaginary bisector divides the angle in half, or bisects it; and (4) the central ray of the x-ray beam is directed perpendicular to the imaginary bisector.
- In the bisecting technique, beam alignment devices are used to stabilize the receptor. A variety of beam alignment devices and bite-blocks are commercially available.
- A size 2 intraoral receptor is used with the bisecting technique. For anterior exposures, the receptor is always positioned vertically; for posterior exposures, the receptor is always positioned horizontally.
- *Horizontal angulation* refers to the positioning of the PID in a side-to-side plane. With correct horizontal angulation, the central ray is directed through the contact areas of the teeth, and thus the contact areas on the image appear "opened." Incorrect horizontal angulation results in overlapped ("unopened") contacts.
- *Vertical angulation* refers to the positioning of the PID in an up-and-down plane. With the bisecting technique, the vertical angulation is determined by the imaginary bisector; the central ray is directed perpendicular to the imaginary bisector. Correct vertical angulation results in a dental image that is of the same length as that of the tooth.
- Incorrect vertical angulation results in a dental image that is not of the same length as that of the tooth. Foreshortening of images occurs with excessive vertical angulation,

whereas elongation of images results from insufficient vertical angulation.

- Five basic rules exist for the bisecting technique: (1) The receptor must cover the prescribed area of interest; (2) the receptor must be positioned with one eighth of an inch extending beyond the incisal or occlusal surfaces; (3) the central ray must be directed perpendicular to the imaginary bisector that divides the angle formed by the tooth and the receptor; (4) the central ray must be directed through the contact areas between teeth; and (5) the x-ray beam must be centered over the receptor to ensure that all areas of the receptor are exposed.

- Before receptor exposure using the bisecting technique, the dental radiographer must complete infection control procedures, prepare the treatment area and the supplies, seat the patient, explain the procedures to him or her, make chair and headrest adjustments, place the lead apron on the patient, remove intraoral objects and eyeglasses from the patient, set exposure factors, and assemble the beam alignment devices over a covered work area.

- When using the bisecting technique, the dental radiographer always begins with anterior exposures; anterior exposures are less likely to cause gagging. After anterior exposures, the posterior teeth are radiographed. In each quadrant, the premolar region is always exposed first and then the molar region.

- When exposing a complete mouth radiographic series (CMRS) using bisecting technique, each of 14 periapical exposures has a prescribed placement (see Boxes 18-2 and 18-3 and Figures 18-15 and 18-16).

- The advantages of the bisecting technique are that it can be used without a beam alignment device and that it has a shorter exposure time.

- The disadvantages of the bisecting technique are image distortion and angulation problems.

- The paralleling technique is preferred over the bisecting technique and should be used whenever possible.

BIBLIOGRAPHY

Frommer HH, Savage-Stabulas JJ: Accessory radiographic techniques: Bisecting technique and occlusal technique. In *Radiology for the dental professional*, ed 9, St. Louis, 2011, Mosby.

Johnson ON, Thomson EM: Intraoral radiographic procedures. In *Essentials of dental radiography for dental assistants and hygienists*, ed 8, Upper Saddle River, 2007, NJ, Pearson Education, Inc.

Johnson ON,Thomson EM: The periapical examination. In *Essentials of dental radiography for dental assistants and hygienists*, ed 8, Upper Saddle River, NJ, 2007, Pearson Education, Inc.

Miles DA, Van Dis ML, Razmus TF: Intraoral radiographic techniques. In *Basic principles of oral and maxillofacial radiology*, Philadelphia, 1992, Saunders.

White SC, Pharoah MJ: Intraoral radiographic examinations. In *Oral radiology: principles and interpretation*, ed 6, St. Louis, 2009, Mosby.

QUIZ QUESTIONS

MATCHING

For questions 1 to 4, refer to Figure 18-25. Match the letter (A to D) of the item shown with the description below.

___ **1.** Plane of the receptor
___ **2.** Long axis of the tooth
___ **3.** Imaginary bisector
___ **4.** Central ray

IDENTIFICATION

For questions 5 to 10, refer to Figures 18-26, 18-27, and 18-28. Write in the letter of the item defined in each question.

___ **5.** In Figure 18-26, identify the angle that is bisected correctly.
___ **6.** In Figure 18-27, identify the central ray that is correctly positioned perpendicular to the imaginary bisector.
___ **7.** In Figure 18-28, identify the position-indicating device (PID) that is aligned correctly.
___ **8.** In Figure 18-28, identify the vertical angulation that results in foreshortening.

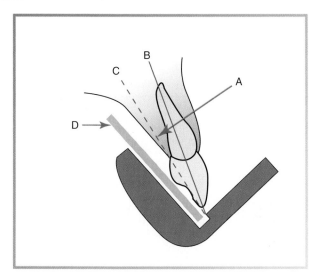

FIGURE 18-25

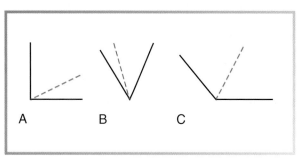

FIGURE 18-26

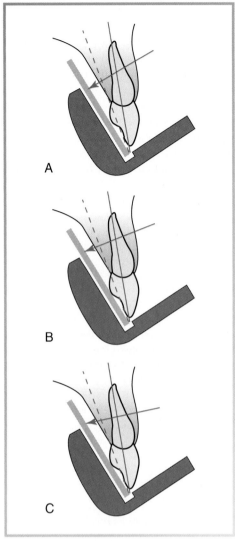

FIGURE 18-27

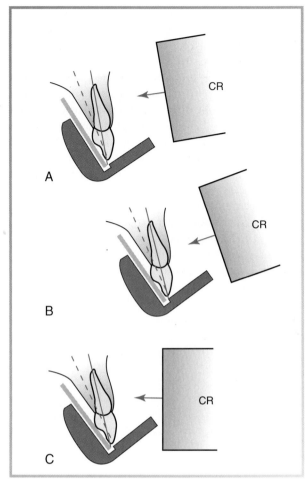

FIGURE 18-28

___ **9.** In Figure 18-28, identify the vertical angulation that results in elongation.

___ **10.** In Figure 18-28, identify the correct vertical angulation.

FILL IN THE BLANK

11. What happens to the dental image when a short (8-inch) PID is used?

_____

12. Which size receptor is used with the bisecting technique?

13. Which beam alignment device is recommended for use with the bisecting technique because it aids in the alignment of the PID and reduces patient exposure?

_____

14. How is the patient's head positioned before exposing maxillary periapicals with the bisecting technique?

_____

15. How is the patient's head positioned before exposing mandibular periapicals with the bisecting technique?

_____

MULTIPLE CHOICE

____ **16.** Which of the following describes the proper direction of the central ray in the bisecting technique?
  a. 90 degrees to the long axis of the tooth
  b. 90 degrees to the receptor and long axis of the tooth
  c. 90 degrees to the receptor
  d. 90 degrees to the imaginary bisector

____ **17.** Which of the following describes the distance between the receptor and the tooth in the bisecting technique?
  a. The receptor is placed as close as possible to the tooth.
  b. The receptor is placed away from the tooth and toward the middle of the oral cavity.
  c. The receptor is placed parallel to the tooth.
  d. None of the above.

____ **18.** Which of the following are advantages of the bisecting technique?
  a. increased accuracy
  b. simplicity of use
  c. shorter exposure time
    1) 1, 2, and 3
    2) 1 and 2
    3) 2 and 3
    4) 3 only

____ **19.** The disadvantages of the bisecting technique outweigh the advantages.
  a. true
  b. false

ESSAY

20. State the rule of isometry.
21. Discuss the significance of the shaded areas in Figure 18-29.

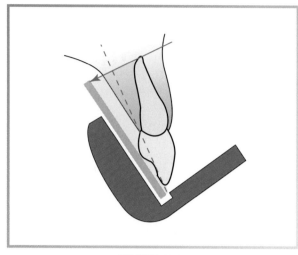

FIGURE 18-29

22. State the five rules of the bisecting technique.
23. Discuss the patient and equipment preparations that must be completed before using the bisecting technique.
24. Discuss the exposure sequence for the 14 periapical placements using the bisecting technique.
25. Describe each of the 14 periapical placements recommended for use with the bisecting technique.
26. Describe correct and incorrect horizontal angulation.
27. State the recommended vertical angulations for each maxillary periapical exposure using the bisecting technique.
28. State the recommended vertical angulations for each mandibular periapical exposure using the bisecting technique.

chapter 19

Bite-Wing Technique

OUTLINE

BASIC CONCEPTS
    Terminology
    Principles of Bite-Wing Technique
    Beam Alignment Device and Bite-Wing Tab
    Bite-Wing Receptors
    Position-Indicating Device Angulation
    Rules of Bite-Wing Technique
STEP-BY-STEP PROCEDURES
    Patient Preparation
    Equipment Preparation

Exposure Sequence for Receptor Placements
    Bitewing Receptor Placement
VERTICAL BITE-WINGS
BITE-WING TECHNIQUE MODIFICATIONS
    Edentulous Spaces
    Bony Growths

LEARNING OBJECTIVES

After completion of this chapter, the student will be able to do the following:

- Define the key terms associated with the bite-wing technique
- Describe the purpose and use of the bite-wing image
- Describe the appearance of opened and overlapped contact areas on a bite-wing image
- State the basic principles of the bite-wing technique
- List the two ways a receptor can be stabilized in the bite-wing technique and identify which one is recommended for bite-wing exposures
- List the three receptor sizes that can be used in the bite-wing technique and identify which size is recommended for exposures in the adult patient
- Describe correct and incorrect horizontal angulation
- Describe the difference between positive and negative vertical angulation

- State the recommended vertical angulation for all bite-wing exposures using a bite-wing tab
- State the basic rules for the bite-wing technique
- Describe patient and equipment preparations that are necessary before using the bite-wing technique
- Discuss the exposure sequence for a complete mouth radiographic series (CMRS) that includes both periapical and bite-wing exposures
- Describe the premolar and molar bite-wing receptor placements
- Describe the purpose and use of vertical bite-wing images
- List the number of exposures and the size of receptor used in the vertical bite-wing technique

KEY TERMS

Angulation	Bone, alveolar	Interproximal
Angulation, horizontal	Bone, crestal	Interproximal examination
Angulation, vertical	Caries	Mandibular tori
Beam alignment device	Contact areas	Negative vertical angulation
Bite-wing, horizontal	Contacts, opened	Positive vertical angulation
Bite-wing, vertical	Contacts, overlapped	Receptor, bite-wing
Bite-wing tab	Edentulous	Receptor placement
Bite-wing technique	Exposure sequence	Torus, tori

The dental radiographer must master a variety of intraoral imaging techniques. The bite-wing technique is used to examine the interproximal surfaces of teeth. A bite-wing image includes the crowns of maxillary and mandibular teeth, interproximal areas, and areas of crestal bone on the same image. Bite-wing images are used to detect interproximal **caries** (tooth decay) and are particularly useful in detecting early carious lesions that are not clinically evident. Bite-wing images are also useful in examining crestal bone levels between teeth.

Before the dental radiographer can use this important technique, an understanding of the basic concepts, including the terminology and principles relating to the bite-wing technique, is necessary. In addition, the dental radiographer must understand patient preparation, equipment preparation, exposure sequencing, and the receptor placement procedures used in the bite-wing technique.

The purpose of this chapter is to present basic concepts and to describe patient preparation, equipment preparation, and the receptor placement procedures used in the bite-wing technique. This chapter also outlines the advantages and disadvantages of the bite-wing technique and reviews helpful hints.

BASIC CONCEPTS

The **bite-wing technique** (also known as the *interproximal technique*) is a method used to examine the interproximal surfaces of teeth. Before the dental radiographer can competently use this technique, a thorough understanding of the terminology, principles, and basic rules of the bite-wing technique is necessary. In addition, a knowledge of the beam alignment devices, sizes of receptors, and angulations of the position-indicating device (PID) used with the bite-wing technique is also required.

Terminology

An understanding of the following basic terms is necessary before describing the bite-wing technique:

Interproximal: Between two adjacent surfaces.

Interproximal examination: Intraoral examination used to inspect the crowns of both maxillary and mandibular teeth on a single image.

Bite-wing receptor: Type of receptor used in interproximal examination. The bite-wing receptor has a "wing," or tab, and the patient "bites" on the wing to stabilize the receptor.

Alveolar bone: Bone that supports and encases the roots of teeth (Figure 19-1).

Crestal bone: Coronal portion of alveolar bone found between teeth; also known as the *alveolar crest* (Figure 19-2).

Contact areas: The area of a tooth that touches an adjacent tooth; the area where adjacent tooth surfaces contact each other (Figure 19-3).

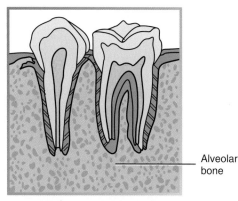

FIGURE 19-1 Alveolar bone. (Adapted from Haring JI, Lind LJ: *Radiographic interpretation for the dental hygienist*, Philadelphia, 1993, Saunders.)

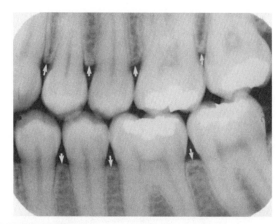

FIGURE 19-2 Crestal bone is the most coronal portion of alveolar bone found between teeth. (Adapted from Haring JI, Lind LJ: *Radiographic interpretation for the dental hygienist*, Philadelphia, 1993, Saunders.)

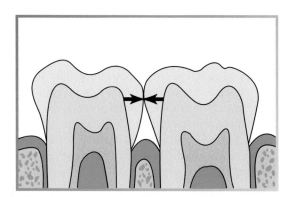

FIGURE 19-3 Contact areas are areas where adjacent tooth surfaces contact each other. (From Haring JI, Lind LJ: *Radiographic interpretation for the dental hygienist*, Philadelphia, 1993, Saunders.)

Horizontal bite-wing: The bite-wing receptor is placed in the mouth with the long portion of the receptor in a horizontal direction.

Opened contacts: On a dental image, opened contacts appear as thin radiolucent lines between adjacent tooth surfaces (Figure 19-4).

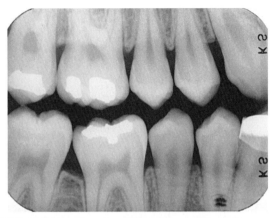

FIGURE 19-4 The opened contacts in the premolar region appear as thin radiolucent lines. Note that the occlusal plane is positioned horizontally along the midline of the long axis of the image. (From Haring JI, Lind LJ: *Radiographic interpretation for the dental hygienist*, Philadelphia, 1993, Saunders.)

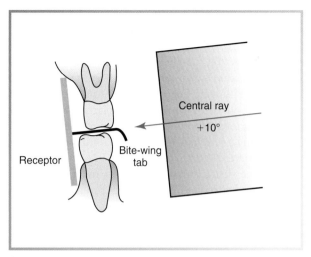

FIGURE 19-6 Positions of the receptor, bite-wing tab, and central ray in the bite-wing technique. The receptor is parallel to the crowns in the maxillary and mandibular teeth. The central ray is directed downward (+10 degrees of vertical angulation).

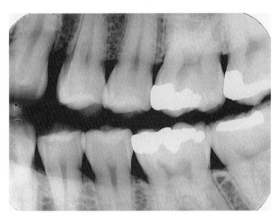

FIGURE 19-5 A nondiagnostic bite-wing image with overlapped interproximal contacts. (From Haring JI, Lind LJ: *Radiographic interpretation for the dental hygienist*, Philadelphia, 1993, Saunders.)

Overlapped contacts: On a dental image, the area where the contact area of one tooth is superimposed over the contact area of an adjacent tooth is referred to as *overlapped contacts* (Figure 19-5).

Vertical bite-wing: The bite-wing receptor is placed in the mouth with the long portion of the receptor in a vertical direction.

Principles of Bite-Wing Technique

The basic principles of the bite-wing technique can be described as follows (Figure 19-6):

1. The receptor is placed in the mouth *parallel* to the crowns of both maxillary and mandibular teeth.
2. The receptor is stabilized when the patient bites on the bite-wing tab or the bite-wing beam alignment device.
3. The central ray of the x-ray beam is directed through the contacts of teeth, using a vertical angulation of +10 degrees.

Beam Alignment Device and Bite-Wing Tab

In the bite-wing technique, either a beam alignment device or a bite-wing tab is used to stabilize the receptor.

Bite-Wing Beam Alignment Device

A **beam alignment device** is a device used to position an intraoral receptor in the mouth and maintain the receptor in position during the radiographic procedure (see Chapter 6). Beam alignment devices eliminate the need for the patient to stabilize the receptor with a bite-wing tab. An example of a commercially available intraoral bite-wing beam alignment device is the XCP bite-wing instrument; this instrument may be used to stabilize the bite-wing receptor in a horizontal or vertical direction.

- *Rinn XCP bite-wing instruments* (Rinn Corporation, Elgin, IL). The XCP bite-wing instruments include plastic horizontal and vertical bite-blocks, plastic aiming rings, and metal indicator arms (Figure 19-7, A, B). To reduce the amount of radiation the patient receives, a snap-on ring collimator can be added to the plastic aiming ring. These beam alignment devices are reusable and must be sterilized after each use.

The Rinn XCP bite-wing instruments with collimators are recommended for bite-wing exposures. These devices include aiming rings that assist in the alignment of the PID and collimators, significantly reducing the amount of radiation exposure. These instruments are simple to position and easy to sterilize. As mentioned in Chapter 17, the American Dental Association (ADA) and the American Academy of Oral and Maxillofacial Radiology recommend the use of a rectangular collimator to reduce the amount of radiation the patient receives (Figure 19-7, C). For information about the use of the Rinn XCP bite-wing instruments, the dental radiographer should refer to the instructions provided by the manufacturer.

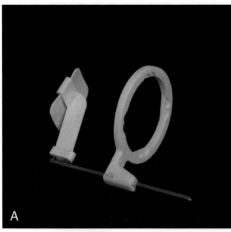

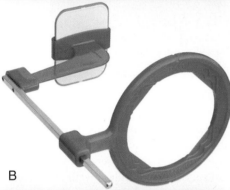

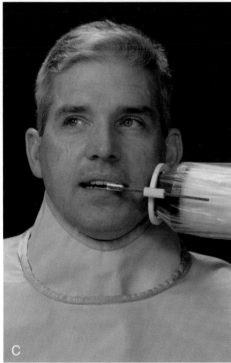

FIGURE 19-7 A, Beam alignment device for horizontal bite-wings. Note external localizing ring used for the position-aiming tube of the x-ray machine to ensure that the entire receptor is covered by the x-ray beam. **B**, Beam alignment device for vertical bite-wings. **C**, Rectangular collimation used with a bite-wing exposure.

Bite-Wing Tab

As an alternative to a beam alignment device, a receptor can be fitted with a bite-wing tab (also called a *bite loop* or *bite tab*). The **bite-wing tab** is a heavy paperboard tab or loop that is fitted around an intraoral receptor and is used to stabilize the receptor during the procedure (Figure 19-8, A). When using film, the bite-wing is oriented in the bite loop so that the tab portion extends from the white side (tube side) of the film. Bite-wing receptors may be purchased with the tabs attached, or they may be constructed by assembling a periapical receptor and a bite-wing tab. Bite-wing tabs may be used on horizontal or vertical bite-wing projections. Bite loops are available in various sizes; adhesive bite tabs are also available (Figure 19-8, B).

Bite-Wing Receptors

As described in Chapter 7, three sizes of bite-wing receptors (0, 2, and 3) are available. Table 7-2 summarizes the measurements and uses of these receptors.

- *Size 0* is used to examine the posterior teeth of children with primary dentitions. This receptor is always placed with the long portion of the receptor in a *horizontal* (sideways) direction.
- *Size 2* is used to examine the posterior teeth in adults and may be placed horizontally or vertically. For most bite-wing exposures, a size 2 receptor is placed with the long portion of the receptor in a *horizontal* direction. When a vertical posterior bite-wing exposure is indicated, a size 2 receptor is placed with the long portion of the receptor in a vertical direction.
- *Size 3* is longer and narrower than the standard size 2 receptor and is used *only* for bite-wing exposures. One receptor is exposed on each side of the arch to examine all the premolar and molar contact areas. A size 3 receptor is placed with the long portion of the receptor in a *horizontal* direction.

In the adult patient, a size 2 receptor is recommended for bite-wing exposures. The size 3 receptor is *not* recommended. With a size 3 receptor, overlapped contacts often result because of the difference in the curvature of the arch between the premolar and molar areas. In addition, the crestal bone areas may not be adequately seen on the dental images of patients with bone loss because of the narrow shape of the receptor.

Position-Indicating Device Angulation

In the bite-wing technique, the angulation of the PID is critical. As defined in Chapter 18, **angulation** is a term used to describe the alignment of the central ray of the x-ray beam in both horizontal and vertical planes. Angulation can be varied by moving the PID in a horizontal or vertical direction. Use of the XCP bite-wing instruments with aiming rings dictates the proper PID angulation. However, when a bite-wing tab is used, the dental radiographer must determine both horizontal and vertical angulations.

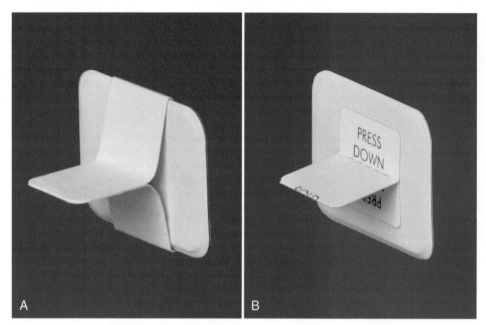

FIGURE 19-8 **A**, Bite-wing tabs. **B**, Adhesive bite-wing tabs.

Horizontal Angulation

As described in Chapter 18, **horizontal angulation** refers to the positioning of the central ray in a horizontal, or side-to-side, plane (see Figure 18-7). The bite-wing, paralleling, and bisecting techniques all use the same principles of horizontal angulation.

Correct Horizontal Angulation With correct horizontal angulation, the central ray is directed perpendicular to the curvature of the arch and through the contact areas of teeth (see Figure 18-8). As a result, the contact areas on the exposed image appear "opened" and can be examined for evidence of caries (see Figure 19-4).

Incorrect Horizontal Angulation Incorrect horizontal angulation results in overlapped ("unopened") contact areas (see Figure 18-9). An image with overlapped interproximal contact areas cannot be used to examine the interproximal areas of teeth for evidence of caries (see Figure 19-5).

Vertical Angulation

As described in Chapter 18, **vertical angulation** refers to the positioning of the PID in a vertical, or up-and-down, plane (Figure 19-9). Vertical angulation may be positive or negative and is measured in degrees as viewed on the outside of the tubehead (Figure 19-10). If the PID is positioned above the occlusal plane and the central ray is directed downward, the vertical angulation is termed **positive** (+). If the PID is positioned below the occlusal plane and the central ray is directed upward, the vertical angulation is termed **negative** (−).

Correct Vertical Angulation When a bite-wing tab is used, a vertical angulation of +10 degrees is recommended for the bite-wing image. The +10-degree vertical angulation is used to compensate for the slight bend of the upper portion of the receptor and the slight tilt of maxillary teeth (Figure 19-11).

Incorrect Vertical Angulation Incorrect vertical angulation used in the exposure of a bite-wing results in a distorted image. For example, if a negative vertical angulation is used, the occlusal surfaces of maxillary teeth are evident, and the apical regions of mandibular teeth are seen (Figure 19-12). A bite-wing image exposed with an excessive negative vertical angulation is nondiagnostic.

Rules of Bite-Wing Technique

Five basic rules must be followed when using the bite-wing technique.

1. *Receptor placement.* The bite-wing receptor must be positioned to cover the prescribed area of teeth to be examined. Specific placements are detailed in the procedures described in the next section.
2. *Receptor position.* The bite-wing receptor must be positioned parallel to the crowns of both maxillary and mandibular teeth. The receptor must be stabilized when the patient bites on the bite-wing tab or on the bite-wing beam alignment device.
3. *Vertical angulation.* When a bite-wing tab is used, the central ray of the x-ray beam must be directed at +10 degrees (see Figure 19-6).
4. *Horizontal angulation.* When a bite-wing tab is used, the central ray of the x-ray beam must be directed through the contact areas between teeth.
5. *Receptor exposure.* The x-ray beam must be centered on the receptor to ensure that all areas of the receptor are exposed. Failure to center the x-ray beam results in a partial image on the bite-wing receptor or a cone-cut.

STEP-BY-STEP PROCEDURES

Step-by-step procedures for the exposure of bite-wing receptors include patient preparation, equipment preparation, and

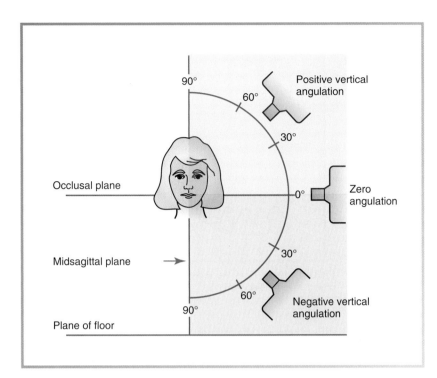

FIGURE 19-9 All vertical angulations above the occlusal plane are termed *positive*. Vertical angulations below the occlusal plane are termed *negative*. Zero angulation is achieved when the position-indicating device (PID) and the central ray are parallel to the floor.

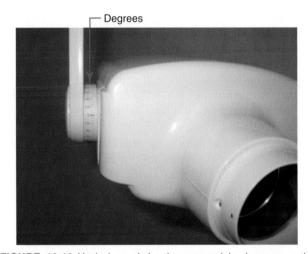

FIGURE 19-10 Vertical angulation is measured in degrees on the outside of the tubehead.

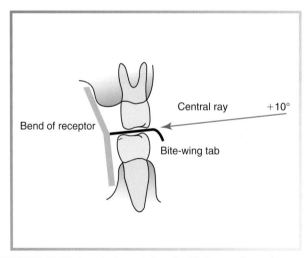

FIGURE 19-11 A vertical angulation of +10 degrees is used to compensate for the slight bend of the upper portion of the receptor and the tilt of maxillary teeth.

receptor placement methods. Before exposing any dental bite-wings, infection control procedures (as described in Chapter 15) must be completed.

Patient Preparation

After completion of infection control procedures and preparation of the treatment area and supplies, the patient should be seated. After seating the patient, the dental radiographer must prepare the patient for the radiographic procedure (Procedure 19-1).

Equipment Preparation

After patient preparation, equipment must also be prepared before exposure of any receptors (Procedure 19-2).

Exposure Sequence for Receptor Placements

When using the bite-wing technique, an **exposure sequence**, or definite order for receptor placements and exposure, must be followed. The dental radiographer must have an established exposure routine to prevent errors and make efficient use of time. Working without an exposure sequence may result in omitting an area or exposing an area twice.

As discussed in Chapter 16, a complete mouth radiographic series (CMRS) is an intraoral series of dental images that shows all the tooth-bearing areas of the maxilla and the mandible. The CMRS may consist of periapical images alone, anterior and posterior vertical bite-wings, or a combination

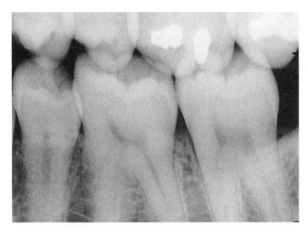

FIGURE 19-12 Negative vertical angulation.

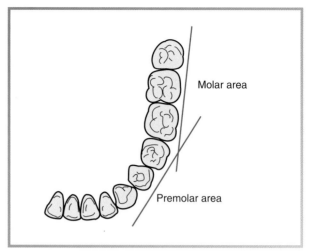

FIGURE 19-13 Note the difference in the curvature of the arch in premolar and molar areas.

| PROCEDURE 19-1 | **Patient Preparation for Bite-Wing Images** |

1. Briefly explain the imaging procedure to the patient before starting the procedure.
2. Position the patient upright in the chair. Adjust the level of the chair to a comfortable working height.
3. Adjust the headrest to support and position the patient's head. The patient's head must be positioned such that the maxillary arch is parallel to the floor and the midsagittal (midline) plane is perpendicular to the floor.
4. Place and secure the lead apron with a thyroid collar on the patient.
5. Have the patient remove all objects from the mouth (e.g., dentures, retainers, chewing gum) that may interfere with the procedure. Eyeglasses must also be removed.

| PROCEDURE 19-2 | **Equipment Preparation for Bite-Wing Images** |

1. Set the exposure factors (kilovoltage, milliamperage, and time) on the x-ray unit according to the recommendations of the receptor manufacturer.
2. If a beam alignment device is used with the bite-wing technique, open the sterilized package containing the device, and assemble the device on a covered work area.
3. If a bite-wing tab is used, attach the tab to the white side of the film, or the correct side of the receptor.

of periapical and bite-wing images. Bite-wing exposures are used only for areas where teeth have interproximal contact with other teeth.

The number of bite-wing images necessary for a patient is based on the curvature of the arch and the number of teeth present in the posterior areas. The curvature of the arch often differs between the premolar and molar areas (Figure 19-13). If the curvature of the arch differs, it is impossible to open all the posterior contact areas on one bite-wing image. Consequently, two bite-wing receptors are typically exposed on each side of the arch. Because the curvature of the arch differs in most adult patients, a total of 4 bite-wings are exposed: 1 right premolar, 1 right molar, 1 left premolar, and 1 left molar.

When posterior teeth are missing (e.g., in patients in whom the premolars have been extracted as part of orthodontic treatment), one bite-wing exposure on each side of the arch (instead of two) may be sufficient to cover the number of teeth present.

In the patient who requires both periapical and bite-wing exposures, the following exposure sequence is recommended:

1. First, expose all anterior periapical receptors (see Chapters 17 and 18).
2. Follow with posterior periapical receptors (see Chapters 17 and 18).
3. Finish with bite-wing exposures.

The sequence ends with bite-wing exposures because these receptors are relatively easy for the patient to tolerate. It is unwise to end the examination with difficult exposures (e.g., painful placements or placements that elicit the gag reflex).

In the patient who requires bite-wings only, the following exposure sequence is recommended for each side of the mouth:

1. Expose the premolar bite-wing first. (This receptor is easier for the patient to tolerate and is less likely to evoke the gag reflex.)
2. Expose the molar bite-wing last.

Bitewing Receptor Placement

When exposing bite-wings, each exposure has a prescribed placement. **Receptor placement**, or the specific area where the receptor must be positioned before exposure, is dictated by the teeth and surrounding structures that must be included on the resulting bite-wing image. The specific placements described in this chapter are for a four-receptor posterior bite-wing series using size 2 receptors and bite-wing tabs. Variations in placement, receptor size, or total number of exposures may be recommended by other reference sources or individual practitioners (Box 19-1).

Bite-Wing Receptor Placements

Receptor placements for the four posterior bite-wing exposures include the following:

- Right and left premolar exposures (Procedure 19-3)
- Right and left molar exposures (Procedure 19-4)

It is important to note that in the procedures for premolar and molar bite-wing exposures, it is recommended that the receptor be placed into the patient's mouth after both vertical and horizontal angulations have been set.

BOX 19-1 | **Guidelines for Bite-Wing Receptor Placement**

1. When using film, the white side of the film always faces the tooth. The identification dot on the film has no significance in bite-wing film placement.
2. In posterior bite-wing series, receptors are placed horizontally or vertically.
3. When positioning the receptor, always center the receptor over the area to be examined (as defined in the prescribed placements).
4. When positioning the receptor, ask the patient to "slowly bite" on the bite-wing tab or on the bite-block of the beam alignment device.

PROCEDURE 19-3 **Premolar Bite-Wing Exposure with Bite Tab** (Figure 19-14)

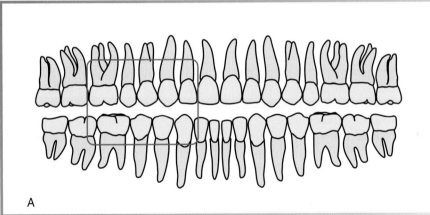

A

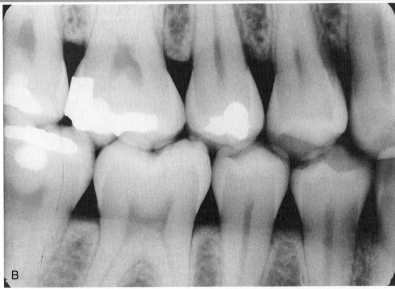

B

FIGURE 19-14 The premolar bite-wing. **A**, Receptor placement. **B**, Resultant image.

Continued

PROCEDURE 19-3   Premolar Bite-Wing Exposure with Bite Tab—cont'd

1. Set vertical angulation at +10 degrees (Figure 19-15).
2. To set the horizontal angulation, stand in front of the patient. Examine the posterior curvature of the arch. To better visualize the curvature of the arch, place your index finger along the premolar area. Align the open end of the position-indicating device (PID) parallel to your index finger and the curvature of the arch in the premolar area, and direct the central ray through the contact areas (Figure 19-16).
3. Make certain that the PID is positioned far enough forward to cover both maxillary and mandibular canines and is positioned evenly over the mandibular and maxillary arches to avoid a cone-cut. The middle of the PID should be directed at the level of the occlusal plane (Figure 19-17). After the vertical angulation, horizontal angulation, and PID position have been established, the PID should not be adjusted, and the receptor should be placed without moving the PID.
4. Fold the bite-wing tab in half, and crease it. Insert the receptor into the patient's mouth, and place the lower half of the receptor between the patient's tongue and teeth. Place the biting surface of the tab on the occlusal surfaces of mandibular teeth. Center the receptor on the mandibular second premolar; the front edge of the receptor should be aligned with the midline of the mandibular canine. Using your index finger, hold the bite-wing tab against the buccal surfaces of the premolars (Figure 19-18). Hold the tab in place during steps 5 and 6.
5. Make certain that the patient's occlusal plane is parallel to the floor. If necessary, ask the patient to lower the chin (Figure 19-19).

6. To check for cone-cut, stand directly behind the tubehead and look along the side of the PID. No portion of the receptor should be visible; the receptor should be covered by the opening of the PID (Figure 19-20). If the receptor is not visible, ask the patient to "slowly close" while you still hold the bite-wing tab. If any portion of the receptor is visible, a cone-cut will result. In such cases, the PID must be adjusted to cover the receptor. After the PID has been positioned properly, ask the patient to "slowly close" while holding the bite-wing tab.
7. Expose the receptor.

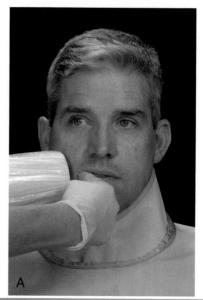

A

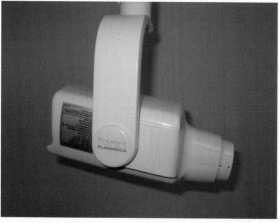

FIGURE 19-15 Vertical angulation is set at +10 degrees.

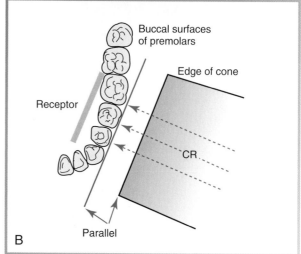

Buccal surfaces of premolars

Edge of cone

Receptor

CR

B

Parallel

FIGURE 19-16 A, To better visualize the curvature of the arch, place the index finger along the premolar area. **B,** Correct horizontal angulation of the premolar area.

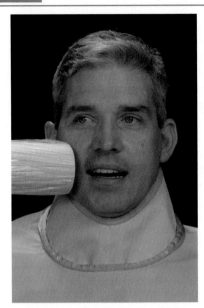

FIGURE 19-17 The middle of the position-indicating device (PID) should be directed at the level of the occlusal plane.

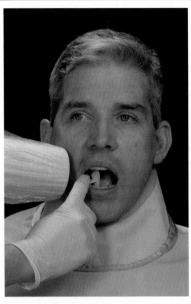

FIGURE 19-19 The patient's occlusal plane must be parallel to the floor.

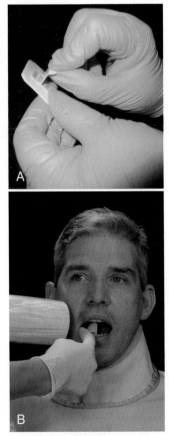

FIGURE 19-18 **A**, Crease the middle of the bite-wing tab before placing the receptor in the patient's mouth. **B**, Place the biting area of the tab on the occlusal surfaces of teeth while holding the tab against the buccal surfaces of premolars. The front edge of the receptor should be aligned with the middle of the mandibular canine.

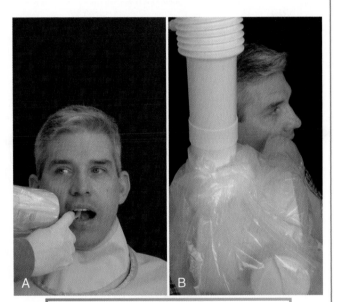

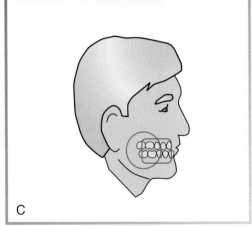

FIGURE 19-20 **A**, To check for cone-cuts, stand behind the tube-head and look along the side of the position-indicating device (PID). **B**, No portion of the receptor should be visible. **C**, A cone-cut results when any portion of the receptor is visible.

PROCEDURE 19-4   **Molar Bite-Wing Exposure with Bite Tab** (Figure 19-21)

1. Set the vertical angulation at +10 degrees (see Figure 19-15).
2. To set the horizontal angulation, stand in front of the patient. Examine the posterior curvature of the arch. To better visualize the curvature of the arch, place your index finger along the molar area. Align the open end of the position-indicating device (PID) parallel to your index finger and the curvature of the arch in the molar area, and direct the central ray through the contact areas (Figure 19-22).
3. Make certain that the PID is positioned far enough forward to cover both maxillary and mandibular second premolars and is positioned evenly over the mandibular and maxillary arches to avoid a cone-cut. The middle of the PID should be directed at the level of the occlusal plane (see Figure 19-17). After the vertical angulation, horizontal angulation, and PID position have been established, the PID should not be adjusted, and the receptor should be placed without moving the PID.
4. Fold the bite-wing tab in half, and crease it. Insert the receptor into the patient's mouth, and place the lower half of the receptor between the patient's tongue and teeth. Place the biting surface of the tab on the occlusal surfaces of mandibular teeth. Center the receptor on the mandibular second molar; the front edge of the receptor should be aligned with the midline of the mandibular second premolar. Using your index finger, hold the bite-wing tab against the buccal surfaces of the molars (Figure 19-23). Hold the tab in place during steps 5 and 6.
5. Make certain that the patient's occlusal plane is parallel to the floor. If necessary, ask the patient to lower the chin (see Figure 19-19).

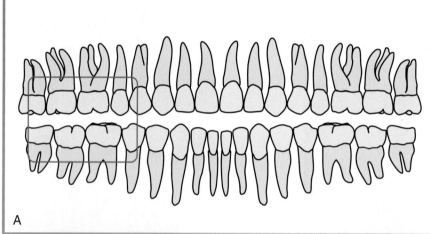

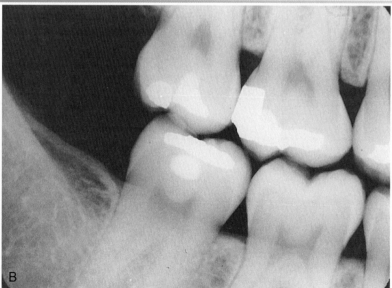

FIGURE 19-21 The molar bite-wing. **A,** Receptor placement. **B,** Resultant image.

PROCEDURE 19-4 | **Molar Bite-Wing Exposure with Bite Tab—cont'd**

6. To check for cone-cut, stand directly behind the tubehead and look along the side of the PID. No portion of the receptor should be visible; the receptor should be covered by the opening of the PID (Figure 19-24). If the receptor is not visible, instruct the patient to "slowly close" while you still hold the bite-wing tab. If any portion of the receptor is visible, a cone-cut will result. In such cases, the PID must be adjusted to cover the receptor. After the PID has been positioned properly, instruct the patient to "slowly close" while you still hold the bite-wing tab.

7. Expose the receptor.

8. An example of a charting note to document four bite-wing exposures is given below:

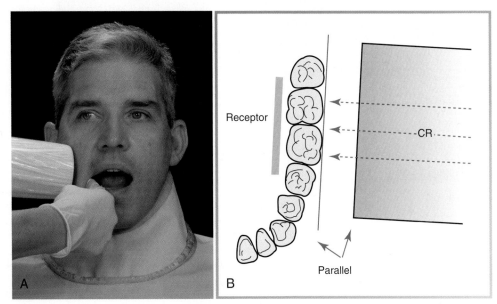

FIGURE 19-22 **A,** To better visualize the curvature of the arch, place the index finger along the molar area. **B,** Correct horizontal angulation of the molar area.

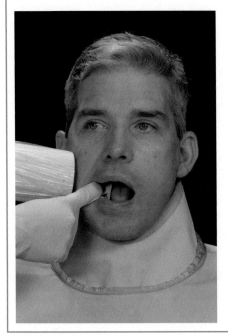

FIGURE 19-23 Place the biting area of the tab on the occlusal surfaces of teeth while holding the tab against the buccal surfaces of premolars. The front edge of the receptor should be aligned with the middle of the mandibular second premolar.

Continued

PROCEDURE 19-4   Molar Bite-Wing Exposure with Bite Tab—cont'd

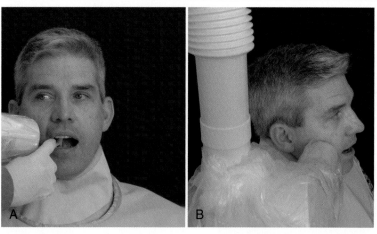

FIGURE 19-24 A, To check for cone-cuts, stand behind the tubehead and look along the side of the position-indicating device (PID). **B**, No portion of the receptor should be visible.

Charting Bite-Wing Exposures

Date	ADA Procedure Code	Provider	Charting Notes	Comments
10/23/11	0274	LJH	Dr. Campbell requested four horizontal bite-wing exposures; digital CCD sensors used (4 total exposures)	Patient recently had orthodontic appliances removed; slight cone-cut on the left premolar bite-wing but information is present on the left molar projection

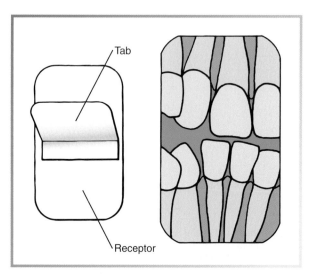

FIGURE 19-25 A vertical bite-wing image can be used to evaluate the level of supporting bone. (From Haring JI, Lind LJ: *Radiographic interpretation for the dental hygienist*, Philadelphia, 1993, Saunders.)

VERTICAL BITE-WINGS

A vertical bite-wing image can be used to examine the level of alveolar bone in the mouth. This bite-wing is placed with the long portion of the receptor in an up-and-down, or vertical, direction (Figure 19-25). Vertical bite-wings images are often used as post-treatment or follow-up images for patients with bone loss due to periodontal disease.

A modified CMRS may be performed using vertical bite-wing images. A total of 7 projections (3 anterior and 4 posterior) are used to cover the incisor, canine, premolar, and molar areas. Size 2 receptors may be used for all exposures, or a combination of size 1 (anterior teeth) and size 2 (posterior teeth) may be used. For projections in the anterior regions, a longer bite-wing tab is often necessary for the patient to be able to close completely. The patient should be instructed to bite on the tab in an end-to-end occlusal relationship (Figure 19-26).

BITE-WING TECHNIQUE MODIFICATIONS

Modifications in the bite-wing technique may be used to accommodate variations in anatomic conditions. Such modifications may be necessary in patients who have edentulous spaces or bony growths.

Edentulous Spaces

As described in Chapter 16, an **edentulous** space is an area where teeth are no longer present. An edentulous space may cause problems in bite-wing receptor placement, and a modification in technique is necessary. A cotton roll must be placed

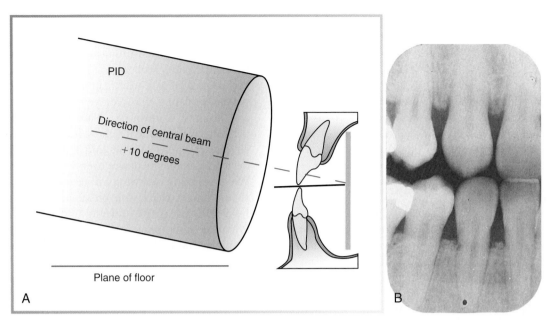

FIGURE 19-26 Anterior interproximal area. **A,** Center the receptor vertically at midline, and stabilize the patient by having him or her gently close on the tab at the incisal edges of teeth. Teeth meet the tab in the end-to-end position. Suggested vertical angulation is + 10 degrees toward the center of the receptor; horizontally, the x-ray beam is directed through the interproximal spaces. **B,** Bite-wing image of the right canine area. (Redrawn from DeLyre WR, Johnson ON: *Essentials of dental radiography for dental assistants and hygienists,* ed 4, Norwalk, CT, 1990, Appleton & Lange.)

in the area of the missing tooth (or teeth) to support the bite-wing tab or the beam alignment device. When the patient closes, opposing teeth occlude on the cotton roll and support the bite-wing tab or the beam alignment device. Failure to support the bite-wing tab or the beam alignment device results in a tipped occlusal plane on the resulting image.

Bony Growths

As described in Chapter 17, a **torus** (plural, **tori**) is a bony growth in the oral cavity. **Mandibular tori** are bony growths along the lingual aspect (tongue side) of the mandible. When using the bite-wing technique, mandibular tori may cause problems in receptor placement, and a modification in technique is therefore necessary.

The receptor must be placed *between* the tori and the tongue (not *on* the tori) and then exposed. With large tori, the receptor is pushed away from teeth. As a result, the patient bites on the very end of the bite-wing tab to stabilize the receptor, thus making it difficult for the dental radiographer to achieve correct placement. In such cases, a bite-wing beam alignment device is recommended.

HELPFUL HINTS

In using the bite-wing technique:

- **DO** set all exposure factors (kilovoltage, milliamperage, time) before placing any receptors in the mouth.
- **DO** ask patients to remove all intraoral objects and eyeglasses before placing any receptors in the patient's mouth.
- **DO** use a definite order (exposure sequence) when exposing receptors to avoid errors and to make efficient use of time.

- **DO** explain to the patient the imaging procedures to be performed.
- **DO** instruct patients on how to close on the bite-wing tab and remain still during the exposure; make certain that the patient remains closed on the bite-wing tab during the exposure.
- **DO** set the vertical angulation at +10 degrees.
- **DO** direct the central ray through the contact areas of the teeth, and align the opening of the PID parallel with the curvature of the arch.
- **DO** set vertical and horizontal angulations before placing the receptor into the patient's mouth.
- **DO** check for cone-cuts before exposing the receptor.
- **DO** use the word *please*; say, "Open, please."
- **DO** use praise; tell cooperative patients how much they are helping you.
- **DO NOT** bend or crimp a film packet; excessive film bending causes distortion of the image.
- **DO NOT** use words such as *hurt*. Instead, inform patients that the procedure will be "momentarily uncomfortable."
- **DO NOT** make comments such as "Oops." Patients will lose confidence in your abilities when they hear such comments.
- **DO NOT** pick up a receptor if you drop it. Leave it on the floor; it has now become contaminated. Instead, remove it and dispose of it when you clean the treatment area.
- **DO NOT** allow patients to dictate how you should perform your duties. The dental radiographer must always remain in control of the procedures.
- **DO NOT** begin with the molar bite-wing exposure; molar placements may cause patients to gag. Instead, always begin with the premolar bite-wing.

✳ **DO NOT** position a receptor on top of a torus (tori). Instead, always position the receptor between the torus and the tongue.

SUMMARY

- A bite-wing image includes crowns of maxillary and mandibular teeth, interproximal areas, and areas of crestal bone on the same image. Bite-wings are useful for examining the interproximal surfaces of teeth, detecting caries, and examining crestal bone levels between teeth.
- The patient bites on the wing to stabilize the bite-wing receptor.
- The bite-wing receptor is placed parallel to the crowns of both maxillary and mandibular teeth; the receptor is stabilized when the patient bites on the tab or the beam alignment device; and the central ray of the x-ray beam is directed through contacts by using a +10-degree vertical angulation.
- A beam alignment device (Rinn XCP bite-wing device with collimator is recommended) or a bite-wing tab may be used to stabilize the receptor.
- Three sizes of receptors (0, 2, and 3) can be used in the bite-wing technique; in the adult patient, a size 2 receptor is recommended.
- With correct horizontal angulation (side-to-side positioning of the PID), the central ray is directed through the contact areas of teeth; contact areas on the image appear "opened." Incorrect horizontal angulation results in overlapped ("unopened") contacts.
- A vertical angulation (up-and-down positioning of the PID) of +10 degrees is recommended for bite-wings exposed with a tab to compensate for the slight bend of the upper portion of the receptor and the slight tilt of maxillary teeth.
- Five basic rules are followed in the bite-wing technique: (1) The receptor must cover the prescribed area of interest, (2) the receptor must be positioned parallel to the crowns of maxillary and mandibular teeth and stabilized by the tab or the beam alignment device, (3) the vertical angulation must be directed at +10 degrees for receptors using bite tabs, (4) the central ray must be directed through the contact areas between teeth for receptors using bite tabs,

and (5) the x-ray beam must be centered over the receptor to ensure that all areas are exposed.
- Before receptor exposure using the bite-wing technique, the dental radiographer must complete infection control procedures, prepare treatment area and supplies, seat the patient, explain the procedures to the patient, make chair and headrest adjustments, place the lead apron on the patient, have the patient remove intraoral objects and eyeglasses, set exposure factors, and if using a beam alignment device, assemble the device over a covered work surface.
- When exposing bite-wing images only, the radiographer should always begin with premolar bite-wing exposures (easier for patients to tolerate and gagging less likely). Premolar exposures are followed by molar exposures.
- Premolar and molar bite-wing exposures have prescribed receptor placements (see Figures 19-16B, and 19-22B).
- Vertical bite-wing images can be used to examine the level of alveolar bone and are placed with the long portion of the receptor in a vertical direction. Vertical bite-wing images are often used as post-treatment exposures in the case of patients with bone loss due to periodontal disease.
- Modifications in the bite-wing technique may be necessary when a patient has edentulous spaces or bony growths.

BIBLIOGRAPHY

ADA Council on Scientific Affairs: An update on radiographic practices: information and recommendations. *J Am Dent Assoc* 132:234, 2001.

Frommer HH, Savage-Stabulas JJ: Intraoral technique: The paralleling method. In *Radiology for the dental professional*, ed 9, St. Louis, 2011, Mosby.

Johnson ON, Thomson EM: The bite-wing examination. In *Essentials of dental radiography for dental assistants and hygienists*, ed 8, Upper Saddle River, NJ, 2007, Pearson Education, Inc.

Miles DA, Van Dis ML, Jensen CW, Williamson GF: Intraoral radiographic technique. In *Radiographic imaging for dental auxiliaries*, ed 4, Philadelphia, 2009, Saunders.

Miles DA, Van Dis ML, Razmus TF: Intraoral radiographic techniques. In *Basic principles of oral and maxillofacial radiology*, Philadelphia, 1992, Saunders.

White SC, Pharoah MJ: Intraoral radiographic examinations. In *Oral radiology: principles and interpretation*, ed 6, St. Louis, 2009, Mosby.

QUIZ QUESTIONS

FILL IN THE BLANK

1. What does the term *bite-wing* refer to?

_____

2. What size receptor is recommended for use with the bite-wing technique in the adult patient?

_____

3. What size receptor is recommended for use with the bite-wing technique in the pediatric patient with primary dentition?

_____

4. How is the patient's head positioned before exposing a bite-wing receptor?

_____

5. What condition is detected by the primary use of bite-wing images?

_____

6. What size receptor is used to include all of the posterior teeth in one bite-wing exposure?

_____

7. What type of angulation is determined by the up-and-down movement of the position-indicating device (PID)?

_____

8. What type of angulation is determined by the side-to-side movement of the PID?

_____

9. When the central ray of the x-ray is not directed through the contact areas of teeth, what is seen on the resulting image?

_____

10. When does a cone-cut result?

_____

MULTIPLE CHOICE

___ 11. Which of the following describes the primary use of the bite-wing radiograph image?
   a. examination of the apical areas of teeth
   b. examination of the apical and interproximal areas of teeth
   c. examination of the interproximal areas of teeth
   d. examination of the pulp chambers of teeth

___ 12. Which of the following is the correct vertical angulation used with the bite-wing technique and the bite tab?
   a. −10 degrees
   b. −20 degrees
   c. +10 degrees
   d. +15 degrees

___ 13. Which of the following describes the relationship of the receptor to maxillary and mandibular teeth in the bite-wing technique?
   a. The receptor and teeth are parallel to each other.
   b. The receptor and teeth are at right angles to each other.
   c. The receptor and teeth are perpendicular to each other.
   d. The receptor and teeth intersect each other.

___ 14. Which of the following about receptor placement is correct?
   a. Anterior bite-wings may be placed horizontally.
   b. Anterior bite-wings may be placed vertically.
   c. Posterior bite-wings may be placed horizontally.
   d. Posterior bite-wings may be placed vertically.
      1) a, b, and c
      2) b, c, and d
      3) b and c
      4) a and d

___ 15. Which of the following about the exposure sequence for a CMRS that includes periapical and bite-wing exposures is incorrect?
   a. anterior periapicals are always exposed first.
   b. posterior periapicals are exposed after anterior periapicals.
   c. bite-wings are exposed last.
   d. none of the above.

ESSAY

16. State the basic principles of the bite-wing technique.
17. Describe the two ways to stabilize the receptor in the bite-wing technique.
18. State the basic rules of the bite-wing technique.
19. Discuss patient and equipment preparations necessary before using the bite-wing technique.
20. Discuss the exposure sequence for a CMRS that includes both periapical and bite-wing exposures.
21. Describe premolar and molar bite-wing placements.
22. Explain the modifications in the bite-wing technique that are used for patients with edentulous spaces or bony growths.
23. Describe why a +10-degree vertical angulation is used with the bite-wing technique and a bite tab.

chapter 20

Exposure and Technique Errors

OUTLINE

RECEPTOR EXPOSURE ERRORS
    Exposure Problems
    Time and Exposure Factor Problems
PERIAPICAL TECHNIQUE ERRORS
    Receptor Placement Problems
    Angulation Problems
    Position-Indicating Device Alignment Problems
BITE-WING TECHNIQUE ERRORS
    Receptor Placement Problems

    Angulation Problems
    Position-Indicating Device Alignment Problems
MISCELLANEOUS TECHNIQUE ERRORS
    Film Bending
    Film Creasing
    Phalangioma
    Double Exposure
    Movement
    Reversed Film

LEARNING OBJECTIVES

After completion of this chapter, the student will be able to do the following:

- Define the key terms associated with exposure and technique errors
- Identify and describe the appearance of the following errors: unexposed receptor, film exposed to light, underexposed receptor, and overexposed receptor
- Describe horizontal and vertical angulation
- Identify and describe the appearances of the following periapical technique errors: incorrect horizontal angulation, incorrect vertical angulation (foreshortened images and elongated images), and incorrect beam alignment (cone-cut images)

- Describe and identify proper receptor placement for bite-wing radiographs
- Identify and describe the appearances of the following bite-wing technique errors: incorrect horizontal angulation, incorrect vertical angulation, and incorrect position-indicating device (PID) alignment (cone-cut images)
- Identify and describe the appearances of the following miscellaneous technique errors: film bending, film creasing, phalangioma, double exposure, movement, and reversed film

KEY TERMS

Angulation
Angulation, horizontal
Angulation, vertical
Cone-cut

Contacts, overlapped
Elongated images
Foreshortened images
Herringbone pattern

Phalangioma
Receptor, overexposed
Receptor, underexposed

While radiographs are taken to benefit the patient, the dental radiographer must remember that only *diagnostic* images are useful. A diagnostic dental radiograph is one that has been properly placed, exposed, processed, and retrieved; errors in any one of these areas may result in nondiagnostic images. In many instances, nondiagnostic radiographs must be retaken. Retakes result in additional exposure of the patient to ionizing radiation, which is harmful to the patient.

The dental radiographer must have a working knowledge of receptor exposure, technique, and processing errors; processing errors are discussed in Chapter 9. The purpose of this chapter is to describe exposure problems and errors in periapical, bite-wing, and miscellaneous techniques.

FIGURE 20-1 An unexposed receptor appears clear.

FIGURE 20-2 A film exposed to light appears black. (From Haring JI, Lind LJ: *Radiographic interpretation for the dental hygienist*, Philadelphia, 1993, Saunders.)

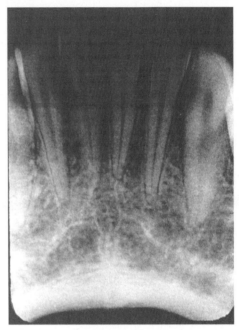

FIGURE 20-3 An overexposed receptor appears dark.

RECEPTOR EXPOSURE ERRORS

Receptor exposure errors that result in nondiagnostic images include unexposed, overexposed, and underexposed receptors, and film that is accidentally exposed to light. All these errors produce images that are too light or too dark. The dental radiographer must be able to recognize exposure errors, identify their causes, and know the necessary steps to correct such problems.

Exposure Problems

Unexposed Receptor

Appearance. The image appears clear (Figure 20-1).

Cause. The receptor was not exposed to x-radiation. Causes include failure to turn on the x-ray machine, electrical failure, and malfunction of the x-ray machine.

Correction. To ensure proper exposure of the receptor, make certain that the x-ray machine is turned on, and listen for the audible exposure signal.

Film Exposed To Light

Appearance. The image appears black (Figure 20-2).

Cause. The film was accidentally exposed to white light.

Correction. To protect the film, do not unwrap it in a room with white light. Check the darkroom for possible light leaks. Turn off all the lights in the darkroom (except for safelights) before unwrapping the film.

Time and Exposure Factor Problems

Overexposed Receptor

Appearance. The image appears dark (Figure 20-3).

Cause. The receptor was overexposed to radiation. An **overexposed image** results from excessive exposure time, kilovoltage, or milliamperage, or a combination of these factors.

Correction. To prevent overexposure, check the exposure time, kilovoltage, and milliamperage settings on the x-ray machine before exposing the receptor. Reduce exposure time, kilovoltage, or milliamperage as needed.

Underexposed Receptor

Appearance. The image appears light (Figure 20-4).

Cause. The receptor was underexposed to radiation. An **underexposed image** results from inadequate exposure time, kilovoltage, or milliamperage, or a combination of these factors.

Correction. To prevent underexposure, check the exposure time, kilovoltage, and milliamperage settings on the

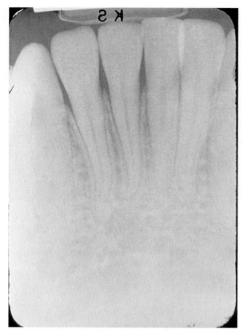

FIGURE 20-4 An underexposed receptor appears light.

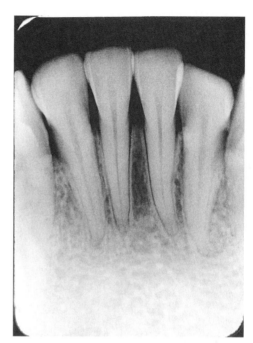

FIGURE 20-5 Correct periapical placement demonstrates the entire tooth, including the apex and surrounding structures.

x-ray machine before exposing the receptor. Increase exposure time, kilovoltage, or milliamperage as needed.

PERIAPICAL TECHNIQUE ERRORS

Just as exposure errors may result in nondiagnostic radiographs, errors in technique may also result in nondiagnostic images. Periapical technique errors include problems with receptor placement, angulation, and beam alignment. The dental radiographer must be able to recognize periapical technique errors, identify their causes, and know the necessary steps to correct such problems.

Receptor Placement Problems

Correct Receptor Placement

As described in Chapter 16, the periapical image shows the entire tooth, including the apex and surrounding structures (Figure 20-5). For a periapical image to be considered diagnostic, receptor placement must be correct. Specific periapical placements for incisors, canines, premolars, and molars are described in Chapters 17 and 18. Each periapical receptor must be positioned in a certain way to show specific teeth and related anatomic structures. In addition, the edge of the periapical receptor must be placed parallel to the incisal or occlusal surfaces of the teeth and extend one eighth of an inch beyond the incisal or occlusal surfaces.

Incorrect Receptor Placement

A nondiagnostic periapical image may result from improper placement of a receptor over the area of interest, inadequate coverage of the apical regions, or a dropped receptor corner.

Absence of Apical Structures

Appearance. No apices are seen on the image (Figure 20-6).

Cause. The receptor was not positioned in the patient's mouth to cover the apical regions of teeth. As a result, no apical structures appear on the radiograph, and an excessive margin of receptor edge exists (which appears as a black band). This error occurs with both the paralleling technique and the bisecting technique.

Correction. To make sure that apical structures appear on a periapical radiograph, make certain that no more than one eighth of an inch of the receptor edge extends beyond the incisal–occlusal surfaces of teeth. Such placement ensures adequate coverage of the apices.

Dropped Receptor Corner

Appearance. The occlusal plane appears tipped or tilted (Figure 20-7).

Cause. The edge of the receptor was not placed parallel to the incisal–occlusal surfaces of teeth. As a result, the occlusal plane appears tipped on the radiograph. If the patient is not instructed to close on the bite block to hold the receptor firmly against the tooth, a corner of the receptor may drop or slip.

Correction. To prevent a dropped receptor corner, make certain that the edge of the receptor is placed parallel to the incisal–occlusal surfaces of teeth as the patient bites his or her teeth together.

Angulation Problems

Angulation is a term used to describe the alignment of the central ray of the x-ray beam in the horizontal and vertical planes. Angulation can be varied by moving the

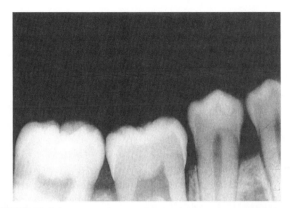

FIGURE 20-6 Improper placement; no apices are seen on this image. (From Haring JI, Lind LJ: *Radiographic interpretation for the dental hygienist*, Philadelphia, 1993, Saunders.)

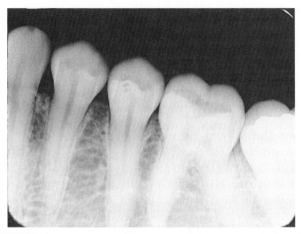

FIGURE 20-7 Improper placement; a dropped corner is seen when the edge of the receptor is not placed parallel to the incisal or occlusal surfaces of teeth.

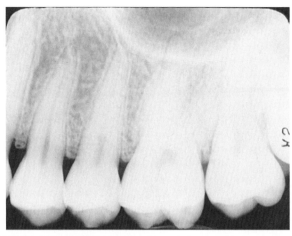

FIGURE 20-8 Incorrect horizontal angulation results in overlapped contact areas.

position-indicating device (PID) in either a horizontal or vertical direction. **Horizontal angulation** refers to the positioning of the PID in a horizontal, or side-to-side, plane. **Vertical angulation** refers to the positioning of the PID in a vertical, or up-and-down, plane. Correct horizontal and vertical angulations of periapical images are described in Chapter 18.

Incorrect Horizontal Angulation

Appearance. Overlapped contacts are seen on the image (Figure 20-8).

Cause. The central ray was not directed through the interproximal spaces. As a result, the proximal surfaces of adjacent teeth appear overlapped in the periapical image. Overlapped contacts prevent examination of the interproximal areas. This error occurs with both the paralleling technique and the bisecting technique.

Correction. To avoid overlapped contacts on a periapical image, direct the x-ray beam *through* the interproximal regions. The use of Rinn beam alignment instruments minimizes errors in horizontal angulation.

Incorrect Vertical Angulation

Incorrect vertical angulation results in a radiographic image that is not of the same length as that of the tooth; instead, the image appears either longer or shorter. Elongated or foreshortened images are nondiagnostic.

Foreshortened Images

Appearance. Teeth appear short with blunted roots on the image (Figure 20-9).

Cause. The vertical angulation was excessive (too steep). As a result, images that are shorter than the actual teeth, or **foreshortened images**, are seen on the radiograph. This error occurs more often with the bisecting technique.

Correction. To avoid foreshortened images, do not use excessive vertical angulation with the bisecting technique. The use of Rinn beam alignment instruments minimizes errors in vertical angulation.

Elongated Images

Appearance. Teeth appear long and distorted on the image (Figure 20-10).

Cause. The vertical angulation was insufficient (too flat). As a result, images that are longer than the actual teeth, or **elongated images**, are seen on the radiograph. This error occurs more often with the bisecting technique.

Correction. To avoid elongated images, use adequate vertical angulation with the bisecting technique. The use of Rinn beam alignment instruments minimizes errors in vertical angulation.

Position-Indicating Device (PID) Alignment Problems

If the PID is misaligned and the x-ray beam is not centered over the receptor, a partial image is seen on the resultant radiograph. The PID, or "cone," is said to "cut" the image. A **cone-cut** appears as a clear, unexposed area on a dental radiograph and may occur with a rectangular or round PID.

Cone-Cut with Beam Alignment Device

Appearance. A clear (unexposed) area is seen on the image (Figure 20-11).

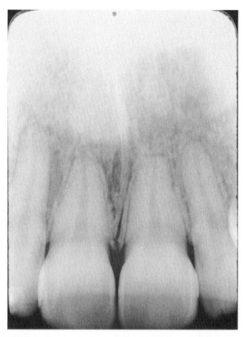

FIGURE 20-9 If the vertical angulation is too steep, the image of the tooth on the receptor is shorter than the actual tooth; the images are foreshortened.

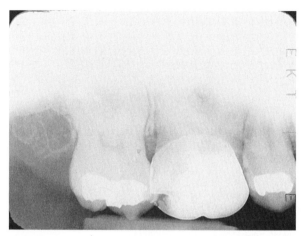

FIGURE 20-11 A cone-cut is seen when the position-indicating device (PID) is not properly aligned with the periapical beam alignment device.

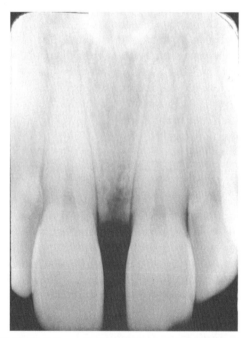

FIGURE 20-10 If the vertical angulation is too flat, the image of the tooth on the receptor is longer than the actual tooth; the images are elongated.

Cause. The PID was not properly aligned with the periapical beam alignment device, and the x-ray beam did not expose the entire receptor. As a result, a clear, unexposed area resembling the outline of the PID is seen on the radiograph.

Correction. To avoid a cone-cut on a periapical receptor when using a beam alignment device, position the PID

carefully. If a beam alignment device with an aiming ring is used, make certain that the PID and the aiming ring are aligned. If an aiming ring is not used, make certain that the x-ray beam is centered over the receptor.

Cone-Cut without Beam Alignment Device

Appearance. A clear (unexposed) area is seen on the image (Figure 20-12).

Cause. The PID was not directed at the center of the receptor, and the x-ray beam did not expose the entire receptor. As a result, a clear, unexposed area resembling the outline of the PID is seen on the radiograph.

Correction. To avoid a cone-cut on a periapical receptor when not using a beam alignment device, position the PID carefully. Make certain that the x-ray beam is centered over the receptor and that the entire receptor is covered by the diameter of the PID.

BITE-WING TECHNIQUE ERRORS

Just as errors in the periapical technique may result in non-diagnostic images, errors in the bite-wing technique may also result in images that are nondiagnostic. Bite-wing technique errors include problems with receptor placement, angulation, and beam alignment. The dental radiographer must be able to recognize bite-wing technique errors, identify their causes, and know the necessary steps to correct such problems.

Receptor Placement Problems

Correct Receptor Placement

As described in Chapter 19, the bite-wing image includes the crowns of both maxillary and mandibular teeth, the interproximal contact areas, and crestal bone. For a bite-wing image to be considered diagnostic, receptor placement must be correct. Specific bite-wing placements for premolars and molars are described in Chapter 19. In addition to placement over the prescribed areas, the radiograph must show an

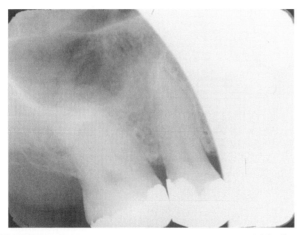

FIGURE 20-12 A cone-cut is seen as a curved unexposed (clear) area on the radiograph.

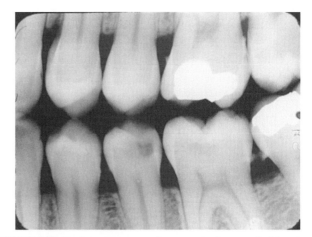

FIGURE 20-13 Correct receptor placement for the premolar bite-wing.

occlusal plane that is positioned horizontally, along the long axis of the receptor.

Premolar Bite-Wing. The premolar bite-wing must be positioned such that the resulting image shows both maxillary and mandibular premolars and the distal contact areas of both canines (Figure 20-13). To ensure that the distal surfaces of the canines are evident on the resulting radiograph, the receptor must be positioned such that the front edge of the receptor is aligned with the midline of the mandibular canine.

Molar Bite-Wing. The molar bite-wing must be positioned such that the resulting image shows both maxillary and mandibular molars. The molar bite-wing must be centered over the mandibular second molar (Figure 20-14). To ensure correct placement, the receptor must be positioned such that the front edge of the receptor is aligned with the midline of the mandibular second premolar.

Incorrect Receptor Placement

Incorrect bite-wing receptor placement may result in absence of specific teeth or tooth surfaces on an image, a tipped occlusal plane, overlapped interproximal contacts, or a distorted image. Such errors may render a bite-wing image nondiagnostic.

Premolar Bite-Wing

Appearance. The distal surfaces of canines are not visible on the image (Figure 20-15).

Cause. The bite-wing receptor was positioned too far posteriorly in the mouth; the front edge of the receptor was not placed at the midline of the mandibular canine. As a result, the distal surfaces of the canines are not seen on the radiograph.

Correction. To prevent this error, make certain that the anterior edge of the bite-wing receptor is positioned at the midline of the mandibular canine.

Molar Bite-Wing

Appearance. The third molar regions are not visible on the image (Figure 20-16).

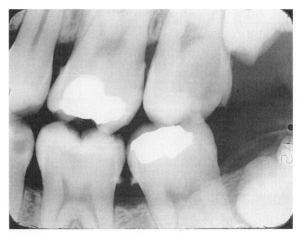

FIGURE 20-14 Correct receptor placement for the molar bite-wing.

Cause. The bite-wing receptor was positioned too far anteriorly in the mouth; the front edge of the receptor was not placed at the midline of the mandibular second premolar. As a result, the third molar areas are not seen on the radiograph.

Correction. To prevent this error, make certain that the anterior edge of the bite-wing receptor is positioned at the midline of the mandibular second premolar. *Always* center the molar bite-wing on the mandibular second molar, even when third molars are not present.

Angulation Problems

To produce diagnostic bite-wing radiographs, the dental radiographer must be prepared to choose the correct horizontal and vertical angulations. Correct horizontal and vertical angulations of bite-wing images are described in Chapter 19. Incorrect horizontal angulation results in overlapped interproximal contacts, and incorrect vertical angulation results in distorted images.

Incorrect Horizontal Angulation

Appearance. Overlapped contacts are seen on the image (Figure 20-17).

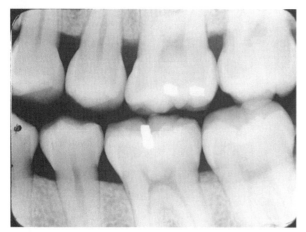

FIGURE 20-15 Incorrect receptor placement for the premolar bite-wing.

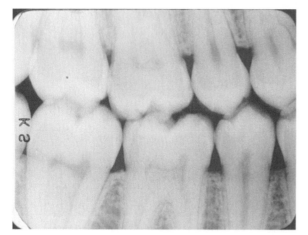

FIGURE 20-16 Incorrect receptor placement for the molar bite-wing.

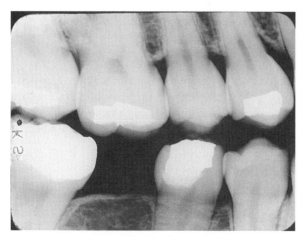

FIGURE 20-17 Overlapped interproximal contacts result from incorrect horizontal angulation.

Cause. The central ray was not directed through the interproximal spaces. As a result, the proximal surfaces of adjacent teeth appear overlapped in the bite-wing image. **Overlapped contacts** prevent examination of the interproximal areas.

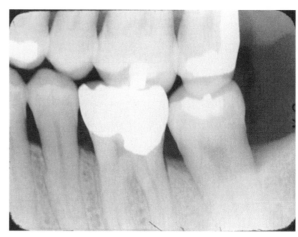

FIGURE 20-18 Incorrect vertical angulation causes the images to appear distorted.

Correction. To avoid overlapped contacts on a bite-wing image, direct the x-ray beam *through* the interproximal regions. When the contacts are opened, a thin radiolucent line is seen between the proximal surfaces of teeth. The use of Rinn bite-wing instruments minimizes errors in horizontal angulation.

Incorrect Vertical Angulation

Appearance. Images appear distorted on the radiograph (Figure 20-18).

Cause. The vertical angulation was incorrect. As a result, distorted images are seen on the radiograph. In this case, a negative vertical angulation was used. Note the occlusal surfaces of maxillary teeth and the apical regions of mandibular teeth.

Correction. To avoid incorrect vertical angulation, always use a +10-degree vertical angulation with the bite-wing technique. This vertical angulation compensates for the slight tilt of maxillary teeth and the slight lingual bend of the upper half of the receptor caused by the hard palate.

PID Alignment Problems

As previously described, if the PID is misaligned and the x-ray beam is not centered over the receptor, a partial image, known as a *cone-cut*, is seen on the bite-wing radiograph.

Cone-Cut with Beam Alignment Device

Appearance. A clear (unexposed) area is seen on the image (Figure 20-19, A). A cone-cut can also occur with a rectangular collimator and is seen as a clear area on the image (Figure 20-19, B).

Cause. The PID was not properly aligned with the bite-wing beam alignment device, and the x-ray beam did not expose the entire receptor. As a result, a clear, unexposed area resembling the outline of the PID is seen on the radiograph.

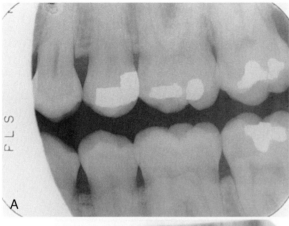

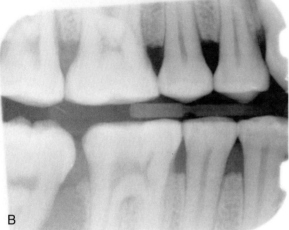

FIGURE 20-19 A, A cone-cut is seen when the position-indicating device (PID) is not properly aligned with the bite-wing beam alignment device. **B**, A cone-cut can also be produced with rectangular collimation; the PID is not properly aligned with the bite-wing beam alignment device.

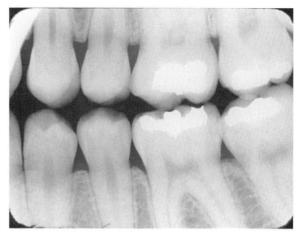

FIGURE 20-20 A cone-cut is seen as a curved unexposed (clear) area on the radiograph.

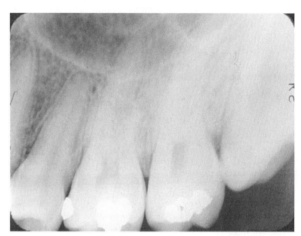

FIGURE 20-21 A bent film results in a distorted image.

Correction. To avoid a cone-cut on a bite-wing receptor when using a beam alignment device, position the PID carefully, and make certain that the PID and the aiming ring are aligned.

Cone-Cut without Beam Alignment Device

Appearance. A clear (unexposed) area is seen on the image (Figure 20-20).

Cause. The PID was not directed at the center of the receptor, and the x-ray beam did not expose the entire receptor. As a result, a clear, unexposed area resembling the outline of the PID is seen on the radiograph.

Correction. To avoid a cone-cut on a bite-wing receptor when using a beam alignment device, position the PID carefully. Make certain that the x-ray beam is centered over the receptor and that the entire receptor is covered by the diameter of the PID.

MISCELLANEOUS TECHNIQUE ERRORS

Miscellaneous technique errors, which may be seen on both periapical and bite-wing radiographs, include film bending, film creasing, phalangioma, double exposure, patient movement, and the reversed film. The dental radiographer must be able to recognize these miscellaneous errors, identify their causes, and know the necessary steps to correct such problems.

Film Bending

Appearance. Images appear stretched and distorted (Figure 20-21).

Cause. The film was bent excessively because of the curvature of the patient's hard palate. As a result, stretched and distorted images are seen on the radiograph.

Correction. To avoid film bending, always check film placement before exposure. If the film is bent because of the curvature of the hard palate, cotton rolls can be used with the paralleling technique, or the bisecting technique

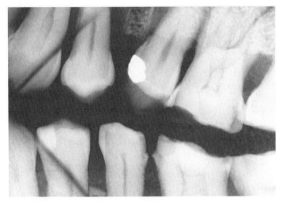

FIGURE 20-22 A film crease is seen as a thin radiolucent line on the radiograph. (From Haring JI, Lind LJ: *Radiographic interpretation for the dental hygienist*, Philadelphia, 1993, Saunders.)

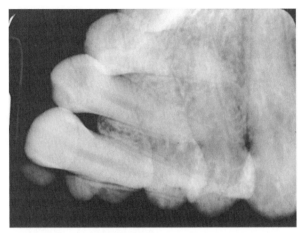

FIGURE 20-24 This image demonstrates double exposure of a receptor.

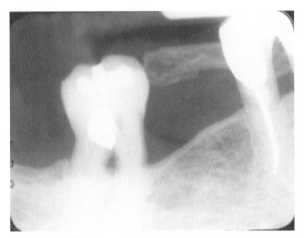

FIGURE 20-23 This example demonstrates a phalangioma; the image of the bones of a patient's finger is seen on the radiograph.

can be used. Film-holding devices are helpful in preventing film bending.

Film Creasing

Appearance. A thin radiolucent line is seen on the image (Figure 20-22).

Cause. The film was creased, and the emulsion cracked. As a result, a thin radiolucent line is seen on the radiograph.

Correction. To avoid film creasing, do not bend or crease the film excessively. Instead, gently soften the corners of the film before placing it in the patient's mouth.

Phalangioma

Appearance. An image of the patient's finger is seen on the radiograph (Figure 20-23).

Cause. The patient's finger was incorrectly positioned in front of the receptor instead of behind it. As a result, an image of the patient's finger is seen on the radiograph. The term **phalangioma** was coined by Dr. David F. Mitchell of the

Indiana University School of Dentistry; the term refers to the distal phalanx of the finger whose image is seen in the radiograph. (A *phalanx* [plural, *phalanges*] is any bone of a finger or toe.) This error occurs when the finger-holding method is used with the bisecting technique; this technique is *not* recommended by the authors of this textbook.

Correction. To avoid a phalangioma, make certain that the patient's finger used to stabilize the receptor is placed *behind* the receptor and not in front of it.

Double Exposure

Appearance. A double image is seen on the radiograph (Figure 20-24).

Cause. The same receptor was exposed twice in the patient's mouth. As a result, a double image is seen on the radiograph. A double exposure is a serious error and necessitates two retakes, one each for the two areas previously radiographed.

Correction. To avoid a double exposure, always separate exposed and unexposed receptors. Once a receptor has been exposed, place it in a designated area (e.g., a disposable cup or bag) away from unexposed receptors. If care is always taken to separate exposed receptors from unexposed receptors, this error will not occur.

Movement

Appearance. Blurred images are seen on the radiograph (Figure 20-25).

Cause. Either the tubehead or the patient moved during the exposure of the receptor. As a result, blurred images are seen on the radiograph.

Correction. To prevent movement errors, stabilize the tubehead and the patient's head before exposing the receptor, and instruct the patient to remain still. Never expose a receptor when a tubehead is drifting or a patient is moving. Reposition the tubehead, the patient, the receptor, or the PID, as necessary, and then expose the receptor.

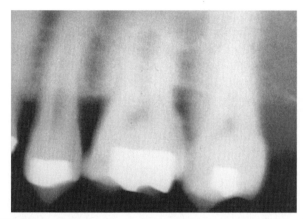

FIGURE 20-25 Movement results in a blurred image. (From Haring JI, Lind LJ: *Radiographic interpretation for the dental hygienist*, Philadelphia, 1993, Saunders.)

Reversed Film

Appearance. Light images with a herringbone pattern are seen on the radiograph (Figure 20-26).

Cause. The film was placed in the mouth backward (reversed) and then exposed. The x-ray beam was attenuated by the lead foil backing in the film packet; consequently, a decreased amount of the x-ray beam exposed the film. As a result, light images with a **herringbone pattern** (also known as the *tire-track pattern*) are seen on the radiograph. The herringbone pattern on the radiograph is representative of the actual pattern embossed on the lead foil (see Chapter 7).

Correction. To avoid a reversed film, always place the white side of the packet adjacent to the teeth. Always note the front and back sides of the film before placing it in the patient's mouth.

SUMMARY

- The dental radiographer must have a working knowledge of exposure technique errors that result in nondiagnostic images. (Processing errors are discussed in Chapter 9.)
- Exposure problems include receptors that are not exposed, accidentally exposed to white light, overexposed, or underexposed. All these errors produce nondiagnostic radiographs that are too light or too dark.
- Periapical and bite-wing technique errors include receptor placement, angulation, and PID alignment problems.

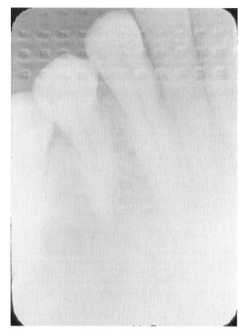

FIGURE 20-26 A reversed film causes an image that appears light with a herringbone (or tire-track) pattern. The tire-track pattern is seen on the lead-foil backing within the film packet.

- Miscellaneous technique errors include film bending, film creasing, phalangioma, double exposure, patient movement, and the reversed film.
- The dental radiographer must be able to recognize and identify the causes of exposure technique errors. In addition, the dental radiographer must know the necessary steps to correct such errors.

BIBLIOGRAPHY

Haring JI, Lind LJ: Film exposure, processing and technique errors. In *Radiographic interpretation for the dental hygienist*, Philadelphia, 1993, Saunders.

Johnson ON, Thomson EM: Identifying and correcting faulty radiographs. In *Essentials of dental radiography for dental assistants and hygienists*, ed 8, Upper Saddle River, NJ, 2007, Pearson.

Miles DA, Van Dis ML, Razmus TF: Intraoral radiographic techniques. In *Basic principles of oral and maxillofacial radiology*, Philadelphia, 1992, Saunders.

Miles DA, Van Dis ML, Williamson GF, Jensen CW: Technique/processing errors and troubleshooting. In *Radiographic imaging for the dental team*, ed 4, St. Louis, 2009, Saunders.

White SC, Pharoah MJ: Processing x-ray film. In *Oral radiology: Principles and interpretation*, ed 6, St. Louis, 2009, Mosby.

QUIZ QUESTIONS

IDENTIFICATION

For questions 1 to 10, refer to Figures 20-27 through 20-36. Identify the exposure technique error seen in each radiograph.

1. _____

2. _____

3. _____

4. _____

5. _____

6. _____

7. _____

8. _____

9. _____

10. _____

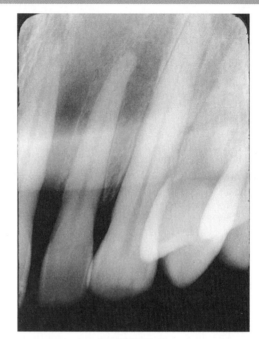

FIGURE 20-29

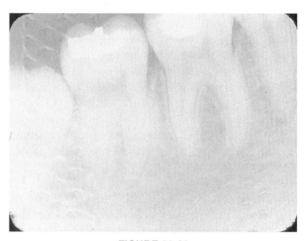

FIGURE 20-30

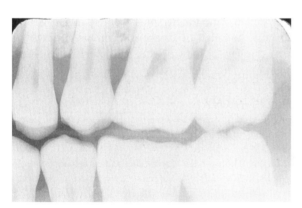

FIGURE 20-27

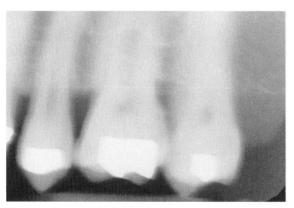

FIGURE 20-28

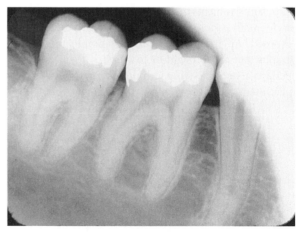

FIGURE 20-31

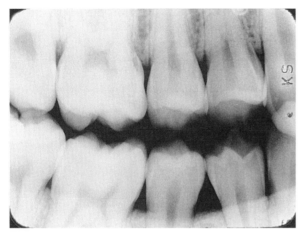

FIGURE 20-32

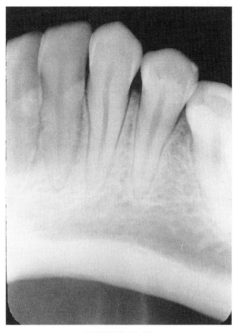

FIGURE 20-35

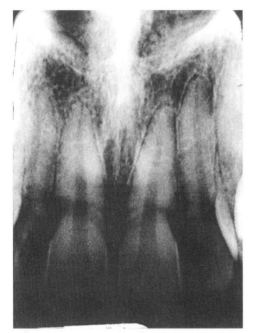

FIGURE 20-33

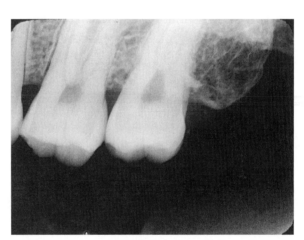

FIGURE 20-36

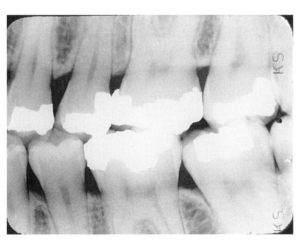

FIGURE 20-34

MATCHING

For questions 11 to 15, describe the appearance of each error using one of these words:

a. Clear
b. Black
c. Light
d. Dark

___ **11.** Overexposed image
___ **12.** Underexposed image
___ **13.** Film exposed to light
___ **14.** Unexposed receptor
___ **15.** Reversed film

MULTIPLE CHOICE

___ **16.** Too much vertical angulation results in images
that are:
   a. elongated
   b. foreshortened
   c. overlapped
   d. none of the above

___ **17.** Too little vertical angulation results in images
that are:
   a. elongated
   b. foreshortened
   c. overlapped
   d. none of the above

___ **18.** Incorrect horizontal angulation results in images
that are:
   a. elongated
   b. foreshortened
   c. overlapped
   d. none of the above

___ **19.** Which of the following errors can occur with the
bite-wing technique?
   a. elongation
   b. overlapped contacts
   c. cone-cut
   d. phalangioma
      1) 1, 2, 3, and 4
      2) 1, 2, and 3
      3) 2 and 4
      4) 2 and 3

___ **20.** Which of the following errors can occur with the
bisecting technique?
   a. elongation
   b. overlapped contacts
   c. cone-cut
   d. phalangioma
      1) 1, 2, 3, and 4
      2) 1, 2, and 3
      3) 2 and 4
      4) 2 and 3

chapter 21

Occlusal and Localization Techniques

OUTLINE

OCCLUSAL TECHNIQUE
    Basic Concepts
    Step-by-Step Procedures

LOCALIZATION TECHNIQUES
    Basic Concepts
    Step-by-Step Procedures

LEARNING OBJECTIVES

After completion of this chapter, the student will be able to do the following:

- Define the key terms associated with occlusal and localization techniques
- Describe the purpose of occlusal examination
- List the uses of occlusal examination
- Describe the patient and equipment preparations that are necessary before using the occlusal technique
- State the recommended vertical angulations for the following maxillary occlusal projections: topographic, lateral (right or left), and pediatric
- State the recommended vertical angulations for the following mandibular occlusal projections: topographic, cross-sectional, and pediatric

- State the purpose of localization techniques
- Describe the buccal object rule
- Describe the right-angle technique
- List the patient and equipment preparations that are necessary before using the buccal object rule or the right-angle technique
- Describe receptor placements for the buccal object rule and compare the resulting images
- Describe receptor placements for the right-angle technique and compare the resulting images

KEY TERMS

Buccal object rule
Localization techniques
Occlusal examination
Occlusal projection, mandibular cross-sectional
Occlusal projection, mandibular pediatric

Occlusal projection, mandibular topographic
Occlusal projection, maxillary lateral
Occlusal projection, maxillary pediatric
Occlusal projection, maxillary topographic

Occlusal surfaces
Occlusal technique
Receptor, occlusal
Right-angle technique

In addition to mastering periapical and interproximal examination techniques, the dental radiographer must also master occlusal and localization techniques. Before the dental radiographer can use these important techniques, an understanding of the basic concepts, patient preparation, equipment preparation, and receptor placement procedures is necessary.

The purpose of this chapter is to present basic concepts and to describe patient preparation, equipment preparation, and receptor placement procedures for both occlusal and localization techniques.

OCCLUSAL TECHNIQUE

The occlusal technique is used to examine large areas of the maxilla or the mandible. Before the dental radiographer can use the occlusal technique, a thorough understanding of basic concepts is necessary. In addition, a knowledge of step-by-step procedures is required.

Basic Concepts

Terminology

Before describing the principles of the occlusal technique, a number of basic terms must be defined, as follows:

Occlusal surfaces: Chewing surfaces of posterior teeth

Occlusal examination: A type of intraoral radiographic examination to inspect large areas of the maxilla or the mandible on one image.

Occlusal technique: Method used to expose a receptor in occlusal examination

Occlusal receptor: In the occlusal technique, a size 4 intraoral receptor is used. The receptor is so named because the patient "occludes," or bites, on the entire receptor. Size 4 receptors are the largest size of intraoral receptors, measuring 3 × 2.25 inches. In adults, size 4 receptors are used in occlusal examination. In children, however, size 2 receptors are typically used.

Purpose and Use

The occlusal technique is a supplementary radiographic technique that is usually used in conjunction with periapical or bite-wing images. The occlusal technique is used when large areas of the maxilla or the mandible must be visualized. The occlusal image is preferred when the area of interest is larger than a periapical receptor may cover or when the placement of intraoral receptors is too difficult for the patient. Occlusal imaging can be used for the following purposes:

- To locate retained roots of extracted teeth
- To locate supernumerary (extra), unerupted, or impacted teeth
- To locate foreign bodies in the maxilla or the mandible
- To locate salivary stones in the duct of the submandibular gland
- To locate and evaluate the extent of lesions (e.g., cysts, tumors, malignancies) in the maxilla or the mandible
- To evaluate the boundaries of the maxillary sinus
- To evaluate fractures of the maxilla or the mandible
- To aid in the examination of patients who cannot open their mouths more than a few millimeters
- To examine the area of a cleft palate
- To measure changes in the size and shape of the maxilla or the mandible

Principles

The basic principles of the occlusal technique can be described as follows:

1. When using film, it is positioned with the white side facing the arch that is being exposed.
2. The receptor is placed in the mouth between the occlusal surfaces of maxillary and mandibular teeth.
3. The receptor is stabilized when the patient gently bites on the surface of the receptor.

Step-by-Step Procedures

Step-by-step procedures for the exposure of occlusal images include patient preparation, equipment preparation, and receptor placement methods. Before exposing any occlusal receptors, infection control procedures (as described in Chapter 15) must be completed.

Patient Preparation

After completion of infection control procedures and preparation of the treatment area and supplies, the patient should be seated. After seating the patient, the dental radiographer must prepare the patient for exposure of receptors (Procedure 21-1).

Equipment Preparation

After patient preparation, equipment must also be prepared before the exposure of any receptors (Procedure 21-2).

Maxillary Occlusal Projections

Three maxillary occlusal projections are commonly used: (1) topographic, (2) lateral (right or left), and (3) pediatric.

Topographic Projection. The **maxillary topographic occlusal projection** is used to examine the palate and the anterior teeth of the maxilla (Procedure 21-3).

Lateral (Right or Left) Projection. The **maxillary lateral occlusal projection** is used to examine the palatal roots of

---

PROCEDURE 21-1   Patient Preparation for Occlusal Technique

1. Briefly explain the radiographic procedure to the patient.
2. Position the patient upright in the chair. The level of the chair must be adjusted to a comfortable working height.
3. Adjust the headrest to support and position the patient's head. For maxillary occlusal exposures, the patient's head must be positioned such that the maxillary arch is parallel to the floor and the midsagittal (midline) plane is perpendicular to the floor. For some mandibular occlusal exposures, the patient's head must be reclined and positioned such that the occlusal plane is perpendicular to the floor. For others, the patient is positioned such that the occlusal plane is parallel to the floor.
4. Place the lead apron with thyroid collar on the patient, and secure it.
5. Have the patient remove all objects from the mouth (e.g., dentures, retainers, chewing gum) that may interfere with the procedure. Eyeglasses must also be removed.

PROCEDURE 21-2   Equipment Preparation for Occlusal Technique

Set the exposure factors (kilovoltage, milliamperage, and time) on the x-ray unit according to the recommendations of the receptor manufacturer. Either a short (8-inch) or a long (16-inch) position-indicating device (PID) may be used with the occlusal technique.

PROCEDURE 21-3 **Maxillary Topographic Occlusal Projection** (Figure 21-1)

1. Position the patient such that the maxillary arch is parallel to the floor.
2. Position a size 4 film with the white side facing the maxilla and the long edge in a side-to-side direction. Insert the receptor into the patient's mouth, placing it as far posteriorly as the patient's anatomy permits.
3. Instruct the patient to bite gently on the receptor, retaining the position of the receptor in an end-to-end bite.

4. Position the position-indicating device (PID) such that the central ray is directed through the midline of the arch toward the center of the receptor.
5. Position the PID such that the central ray is directed at +65 degrees vertical angulation toward the center of the receptor. The top edge of the PID is placed between the patient's eyebrows on the bridge of the nose.

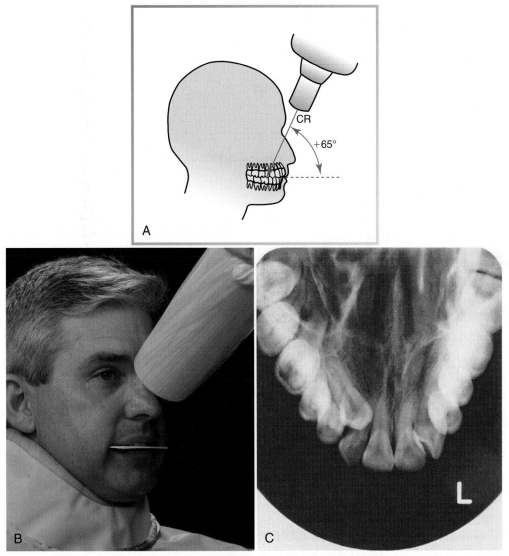

FIGURE 21-1 A, The central ray (CR) is directed at +65 degrees vertical angulation to the plane of the receptor. **B,** Relationship of the receptor and the position-indicating device (PID). **C,** Maxillary topographic occlusal projection. (**A** and **C,** Courtesy of Carestream Health Inc., Rochester, NY.)

molar teeth. It may also be used to locate foreign bodies or lesions in the posterior maxilla (Procedure 21-4).

Pediatric Projection. The **maxillary pediatric occlusal projection** is used to examine the anterior teeth of the maxilla and is recommended for use in children 5 years or younger (Procedure 21-5).

Mandibular Occlusal Projections

Three mandibular occlusal projections are commonly used: (1) topographic, (2) cross-sectional, and (3) pediatric.

Topographic Projection. The **mandibular topographic occlusal projection** is used to examine the anterior teeth of the mandible (Procedure 21-6).

Cross-Sectional Projection. The **mandibular cross-sectional occlusal projection** is used to examine the buccal and lingual aspects of the mandible. It is also used to locate foreign bodies or salivary stones in the region of the floor of the mouth (Procedure 21-7).

Pediatric Projection. The **mandibular pediatric occlusal projection** is used to examine the anterior teeth of the mandible and is recommended for use in children 5 years or younger (Procedure 21-8).

Vertical Angulations

The recommended vertical angulations for all maxillary and mandibular occlusal exposures are summarized in Table 21-1.

LOCALIZATION TECHNIQUES

A **localization technique** is a method used to locate the position of a tooth or an object in the jaws. Before the dental radiographer can use localization techniques, a thorough understanding of basic concepts is necessary. In addition, a knowledge of step-by-step procedures is required.

Basic Concepts

Purpose and Use

The dental radiograph is a two-dimensional picture of a three-dimensional object. A radiographic image depicts an object in superior–inferior and anterior–posterior relationships. The dental radiograph, however, does not depict the buccal–lingual relationship, or the depth, of an object. In dentistry, it may be necessary to establish the buccal–lingual position of a structure such as a foreign object or an impacted tooth within the jaws. Localization techniques can be used to obtain this three-dimensional information. Localization techniques may be used to locate the following:

- Foreign bodies
- Impacted teeth
- Unerupted teeth
- Retained roots
- Root positions
- Salivary stones
- Jaw fractures
- Broken needles and instruments
- Filling materials

Types of Localization Techniques

Two basic techniques are used to localize objects: (1) the buccal object rule and (2) the right-angle technique.

Buccal Object Rule. The **buccal object rule** governs the orientation of structures portrayed in two radiographs exposed at different angulations. Using proper technique and angulation, a periapical or bite-wing receptor is exposed; then, after changing the direction of the x-ray beam, a second periapical or bite-wing receptor is exposed using a different horizontal or vertical angulation. For example, a different *horizontal angulation* is used when trying to locate *vertically aligned* images (e.g., teeth treated with root canal therapy), whereas a different *vertical angulation* is used when trying to locate a *horizontally aligned* image (e.g., the mandibular canal). After the two exposures are completed, the images are compared with each other.

When the dental structure or object seen in the second image appears to have moved in the *same direction as the shift of the position-indicating device (PID)*, the structure or object in question is positioned to the lingual (Figure 21-7). For example, if the horizontal angulation is changed by shifting the PID mesially, and the object in question moves mesially on the image, then the object lies to the lingual (lingual = same).

Conversely, when the dental structure or object seen in the second image appears to have moved in the *direction opposite the shift of the PID*, the structure or object in question is positioned to the *buccal* (Figure 21-8). For example, if the horizontal angulation is changed by shifting the PID distally, and the object in question moves mesially on the image, then the object lies to the buccal (buccal = opposite).

The mnemonic "SLOB" can be used to remember the buccal object rule, as follows:

Same = Lingual; Opposite = Buccal

In other words, when the two images are compared, the object that lies to the *lingual* appears to have moved in the *same* direction as the PID, and the object that lies to the *buccal* appears to have **moved in the** opposite direction as the PID.

TABLE 21-1	Occlusal Projections and Corresponding Vertical Angulations	
Occlusal Projection	**Vertical Angulation (degrees)**
Maxillary topographic	+65
Maxillary lateral (right or left)	+60
Maxillary pediatric	+60
Mandibular topographic	−55
Mandibular cross-sectional	90
Mandibular pediatric	−55

Text continued on p. 248

PROCEDURE 21-4 | Maxillary Lateral Occlusal Projection (Figure 21-2)

1. Position the patient such that the maxillary arch is parallel to the floor.
2. Position a size 4 film with the white side facing the maxilla and the long edge in a front-to-back direction. Insert the receptor into the patient's mouth, and place it as far posteriorly as the patient's anatomy permits. Shift the receptor to the side (right or left) of the area of interest. The long edge of the receptor should extend approximately a ½ inch beyond the buccal surfaces of posterior teeth.
3. Instruct the patient to bite gently on the receptor, retaining the position of the receptor in an end-to-end bite.
4. Position the position-indicating device (PID) such that the central ray is directed through the contact areas of interest.
5. Position the PID such that the central ray is directed at +60 degrees vertical angulation toward the center of the receptor. The top edge of the PID is placed above the corner of the patient's eyebrow.

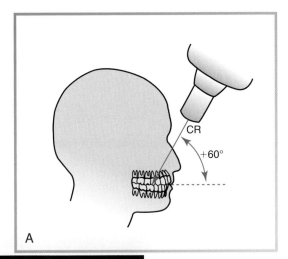

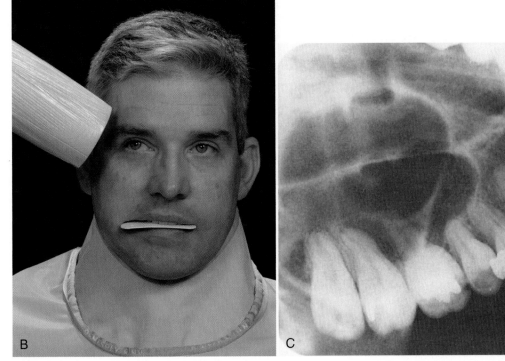

FIGURE 21-2 A, The central ray (CR) is directed at +60 degrees vertical angulation to the plane of the receptor. **B,** Relationship of the receptor and the position-indicating device (PID). **C,** Maxillary lateral occlusal projection. (**A** and **C,** Courtesy of Carestream Health Inc., Rochester, NY.)

PROCEDURE 21-5   Maxillary Pediatric Occlusal Projection (Figure 21-3)

1. Position the child such that the maxillary arch is parallel to the floor.
2. Position a size 2 film with the white side facing the maxilla and the long edge in a side-to-side direction. Insert the receptor into the child's mouth.
3. Instruct the child to bite gently on the receptor, retaining the position of the receptor in an end-to-end bite.

4. Position the position-indicating device (PID) such that the central ray is directed through the midline of the arch toward the center of the receptor.
5. Position the PID such that the central ray is directed at +60 degrees vertical angulation toward the center of the receptor. The top edge of the PID is placed between the child's eyebrows on the bridge of the nose.

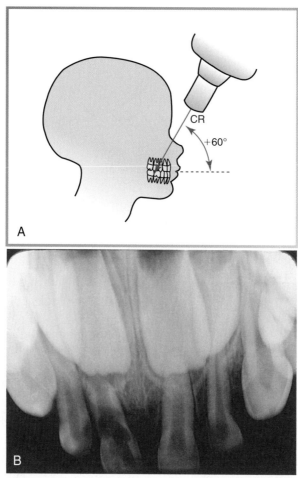

FIGURE 21-3 A, The central ray (CR) is directed at +60 degrees vertical angulation to the plane of the receptor. **B,** Maxillary pediatric occlusal projection.

PROCEDURE 21-6 Mandibular Topographic Occlusal Projection (Figure 21-4)

1. Position the patient such that the mandibular arch is parallel to the floor.
2. Position a size 4 film with the white side facing the mandible and the long edge in a side-to-side direction. Insert the receptor into the patient's mouth, placing it as far posteriorly as the patient's anatomy permits.
3. Instruct the patient to bite gently on the receptor, retaining the position of the receptor in an end-to-end bite.

4. Position the position-indicating device (PID) such that the central ray is directed through the midline of the arch toward the center of the receptor.
5. Position the PID such that the central ray is directed at −55 degrees vertical angulation toward the center of the receptor. The PID should be centered over the patient's chin.

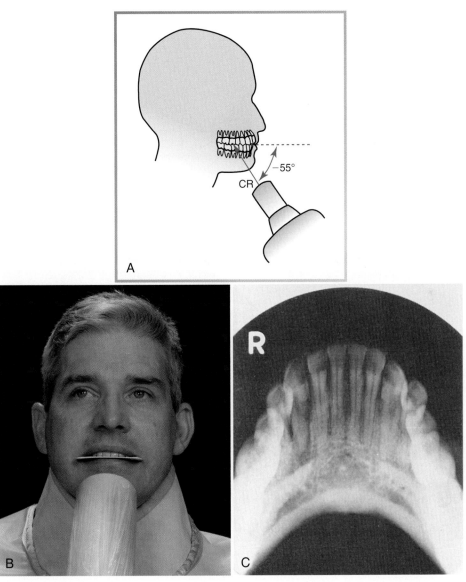

FIGURE 21-4 A, The central ray (CR) is directed at −55 degrees vertical angulation to the plane of the receptor. **B**, Relationship of the receptor and the position-indicating device (PID). **C**, Mandibular topographic occlusal projection. (**A** and **C**, Courtesy of Carestream Health Inc., Rochester, NY.)

PROCEDURE 21-7   Mandibular Cross-Sectional Occlusal Projection (Figure 21-5)

1. Recline the patient, and position him or her such that the mandibular arch is perpendicular to the floor.
2. Position a size 4 film with the white side facing the mandible and the long edge in a side-to-side direction. Insert the receptor into the patient's mouth as far posteriorly as the patient's anatomy permits.
3. Instruct the patient to bite gently on the receptor, retaining the position of the receptor in an end-to-end bite.
4. Position the position-indicating device (PID) such that the central ray is directed through the midline of the arch toward the center of the receptor.
5. Position the PID such that the central ray is directed at 90 degrees vertical angulation toward the center of the receptor. The PID should be centered approximately 1 inch below the patient's chin.

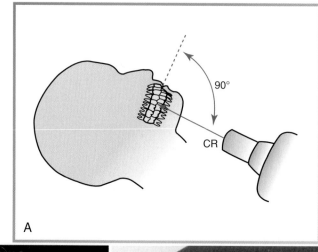

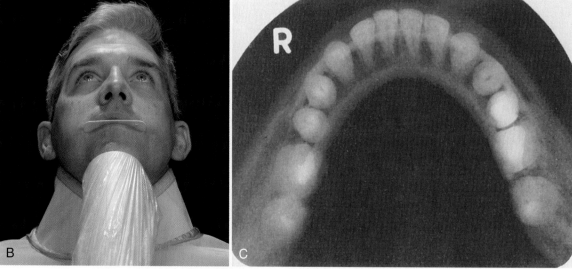

FIGURE 21-5 A, The central ray (CR) is perpendicular (90 degrees vertical angulation) to the plane of the receptor. **B**, Relationship of receptor and PID. **C**, Mandibular cross-sectional occlusal projection. (**A** and **C**, Courtesy of Carestream Health Inc., Rochester, NY.)

PROCEDURE 21-8 Mandibular Pediatric Occlusal Projection (Figure 21-6)

1. Position the child such that the mandibular arch is parallel to the floor.
2. Position a size 2 film with the white side facing the maxilla and the long edge in a side-to-side direction. Insert the receptor into the child's mouth.
3. Instruct the child to bite gently on the receptor, retaining the position of the receptor in an end-to-end bite.

4. Position the position-indicating device (PID) such that the central ray is directed through the midline of the arch toward the center of the receptor.
5. Position the PID such that the central ray is directed at −55 degrees vertical angulation. The PID should be centered over the child's chin.

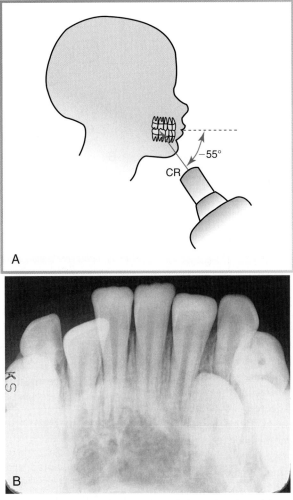

FIGURE 21-6 A, The central ray (CR) is directed at −55 degrees vertical angulation to the plane of the receptor. **B**, Mandibular pediatric occlusal projection.

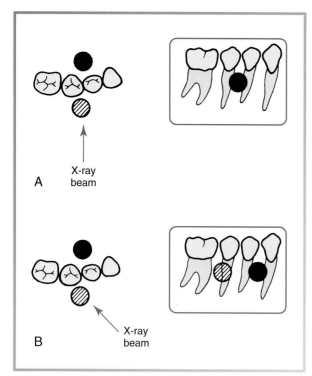

FIGURE 21-7 Buccal and lingual objects shift positions when the direction of the x-ray beam is changed. **A,** Buccal (*cross-hatched circle*) and lingual (*black circle*) objects are superimposed in the original radiograph. **B,** If the tubehead is shifted in a mesial direction, the buccal object moves distally, and the lingual object moves mesially (same direction = lingual; opposite direction = buccal). (Redrawn from Haring JI, Lind LJ: *Radiographic interpretation for the dental hygienist*, Philadelphia, 1993, Saunders.)

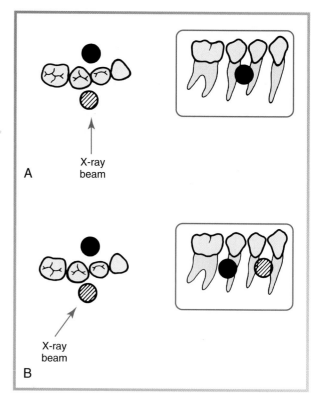

FIGURE 21-8 Buccal and lingual objects shift positions when the direction of the x-ray beam is changed. **A,** Buccal (cross-hatched circle) and lingual (black circle) objects are superimposed in the original radiograph. **B,** If the tubehead is shifted in a distal direction, the buccal object moves mesially, and the lingual object moves distally (same direction = lingual; opposite direction = buccal). (Redrawn from Haring JI, Lind LJ: *Radiographic interpretation for the dental hygienist*, Philadelphia, 1993, Saunders.)

Right-Angle Technique. The **right-angle technique** is another rule for the orientation of structures seen in two images. One periapical receptor is exposed using the proper technique and angulation to show the position of the object in superior–inferior and anterior–posterior relationships. Next, an occlusal receptor is exposed directing the central ray at a right angle, or perpendicular (90 degrees), to the receptor. The occlusal image shows the object in buccal–lingual and anterior–posterior relationships. After the two receptors have been exposed and processed, the images are compared with each other to locate the object in three dimensions (Figure 21-9). This technique is primarily used for locating objects in the mandible.

Step-by-Step Procedures

Step-by-step procedures for localization techniques include patient and equipment preparations and receptor placements and comparisons.

Patient and Equipment Preparations

Before exposing receptors using localization techniques, infection control procedures (as described in Chapter 15) and patient and equipment preparations (described earlier in this chapter) must be completed.

Receptor Placements and Image Comparisons
Buccal Object Rule

> **EXAMPLE**
>
> The buccal object rule can be used to determine the position of a tooth treated endodontically with gutta percha (an endodontic filling material) in a maxillary second premolar (Figure 21-10).
>
> 1. Position the patient in such a way that the maxillary arch is parallel to the floor.
> 2. Expose one molar periapical receptor using proper technique and angulation.
> 3. Shift the position-indicating device (PID) in a mesial direction, and expose another premolar periapical receptor.
> 4. In the second image, when the PID was moved in a mesial direction, the gutta percha moved in the opposite direction. Therefore the location of the gutta percha is in the root that lies to the buccal (buccal = opposite).

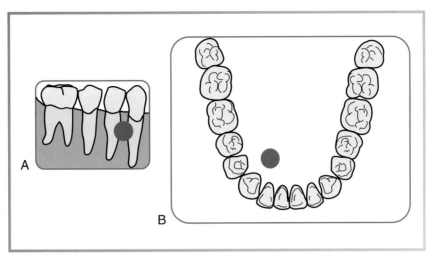

FIGURE 21-9 Right-angle technique. **A**, The object appears to be located in bone on the periapical radiograph. **B**, The occlusal image reveals that the object is actually located in soft tissue lingual to the mandible.

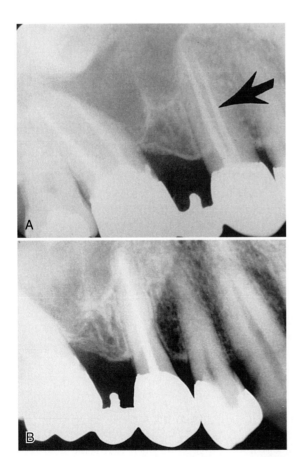

FIGURE 21-10 A, Note the two root canals filled with gutta percha in the maxillary second premolar (*arrow*). **B**, The PID was shifted in a mesial direction, so the gutta percha moved in a distal direction. The gutta percha in the original root labeled by the arrow is located on the buccal. (Radiographs courtesy of Dr. Robert Jaynes, Assistant Professor, Oral Radiology Group, The Ohio State University College of Dentistry. From Haring JI, Lind LJ: *Radiographic interpretation for the dental hygienist*, Philadelphia, 1993, Saunders.)

EXAMPLE

The buccal object rule can be used to determine the location of an impacted supernumerary (extra) tooth (Figure 21-11).
1. Position the patient in such a way that the maxillary arch is parallel to the floor.
2. Expose one central–lateral incisor periapical receptor using proper technique and angulation.
3. Shift the position-indicating device (PID) in a distal direction, and expose the canine periapical receptor.
4. In the second image, when the PID was moved in a distal direction, the impacted tooth moved in the same direction. Therefore the tooth lies to the lingual (lingual = same).

Right-Angle Technique

EXAMPLE

The right-angle technique can be used to determine the position of a radiopaque foreign object (Figure 21-12).
1. Position the patient in such a way that the maxillary arch is parallel to the floor.
2. Expose one periapical receptor using proper technique and angulation.
3. Expose an occlusal receptor, and direct the central ray perpendicular to the receptor.
4. In the occlusal image, the radiopaque foreign object is located on the buccal to side of the mandible.

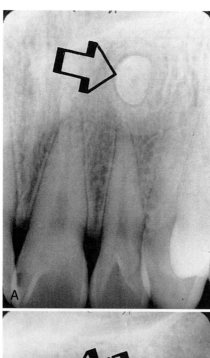

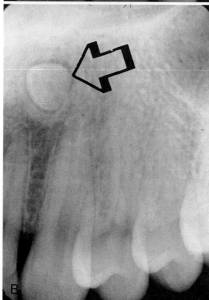

FIGURE 21-11 A, Note the impacted tooth (*arrow*). **B,** The position-indicating device (PID) was shifted in a distal direction, so the tooth moved in a distal direction. The tooth is located lingual to the adjacent teeth. (Radiographs courtesy of Dr. Robert Jaynes, Assistant Professor, Oral Radiology Group, The Ohio State University College of Dentistry.)

Buccal Object Rule and Right-Angle Technique

EXAMPLE

The patient presents to the endodontist for root canal therapy on tooth #30. A small piece of clipped orthodontic wire, which was accidentally left behind during previous treatment and was eventually covered by the buccal mucosa, is revealed by dental imaging. The buccal object rule is used to localize the orthodontic wire; the right-angle technique is also used to confirm the location, as follows:

1. Position the patient in such a way that the maxillary arch is parallel to the floor.
2. Expose one periapical image of tooth #30. A radiopaque artifact will be seen near the furcation area (Figure 21-13, A).
3. Shift the position-indicating device (PID) in a mesial direction, and expose a second periapical image. The artifact will appear to have moved in a distal direction in the second image (Figure 21-13, B).
4. To confirm the location of the radiopaque artifact, expose a mandibular cross-sectional occlusal projection (Figure 21-13, C)
5. By using both the buccal object rule and the right-angle technique, the orthodontic wire can be localized on the buccal side of the tooth and surgically removed (Figure 21-13, D).

HELPFUL HINTS

For exposing occlusal projections:

- **DO** use the exposure factors recommended by the receptor manufacturer.
- **DO** set all exposure factors (kilovoltage, milliamperage, time) before placing an occlusal receptor in the patient's mouth.
- **DO** ask the patient to remove all intraoral objects and eyeglasses before placing an occlusal receptor in the mouth.
- **DO** explain to the patient the radiographic procedure to be performed.
- **DO** instruct the patient on how to close gently on the occlusal receptor and remain still during the exposure.
- **DO** position the patient's head before placing the occlusal receptor into the mouth.
- **DO** position the occlusal film such that the white side faces the arch being exposed.
- **DO** position the receptor such that a minimal receptor edge extends beyond the teeth being exposed.
- **DO** center the occlusal receptor directly over the area of interest so that all necessary information can be recorded.
- **DO** set the vertical angulation for each occlusal projection as recommended in this chapter.

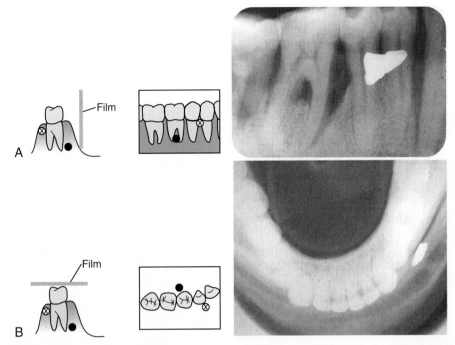

FIGURE 21-12 Right-angle localization technique. Two receptors are exposed at right angles to each other to identify the location of a foreign object. The periapical radiograph (**A**) will demonstrate the superior–inferior and anterior–posterior positions of objects. A cross-sectional mandibular occlusal radiograph (**B**) will demonstrate the anterior–posterior and buccal–lingual positions. These two radiographic views will demonstrate all three dimensions of an area, and the location of objects can thus be identified. (Redrawn from Olson SS: *Dental radiography laboratory manual*, Philadelphia, 1995, Saunders.)

SUMMARY

- The occlusal technique is a method used to examine large areas of the maxilla or the mandible. The technique is so named because the patient "occludes" or bites on the receptor.
- Size 4 intraoral receptors are used in the occlusal technique for adult patients; size 2 intraoral receptors can be used for children.
- The occlusal image is preferred when the area of interest is larger than a periapical receptor may cover or when the placement of periapical receptors is too difficult for the patient.
- Uses for occlusal images include (1) localization of roots, impacted teeth, unerupted teeth, foreign bodies, and salivary stones; (2) evaluation of the sizes of lesions, boundaries of maxillary sinus, and jaw fractures; (3) examination of patients who cannot open their mouths; and (4) measurement of changes in the size and shape of the jaws.
- (1) Film is positioned with the white side facing the arch being exposed, (2) the receptor is placed in the mouth between the occlusal surfaces of teeth, and (3) the receptor

is stabilized when the patient gently bites his or her teeth together.
- Before starting the radiographic procedure using the occlusal technique, the dental radiographer must complete infection control procedures, prepare the treatment area and supplies, seat the patient, explain the radiographic procedures to the patient, make proper chair and headrest adjustments, place the lead apron on the patient, have the patient remove any intraoral objects and eyeglasses, and set exposure factors.
- A localization technique is used to locate the position of a tooth or an object in the jaws. It can be used to determine the buccal–lingual relationship of an object or to locate foreign bodies, impacted and unerupted teeth, retained roots, root positions, salivary stones, jaw fractures, broken needles and instruments, and filling materials.
- The buccal object rule—a rule for the orientation of structures seen in two images exposed at different angles—can be used as a localization technique.
- The right-angle technique—another rule for the orientation of structures seen in two images (one periapical, one occlusal)—can also be used as a localization technique.

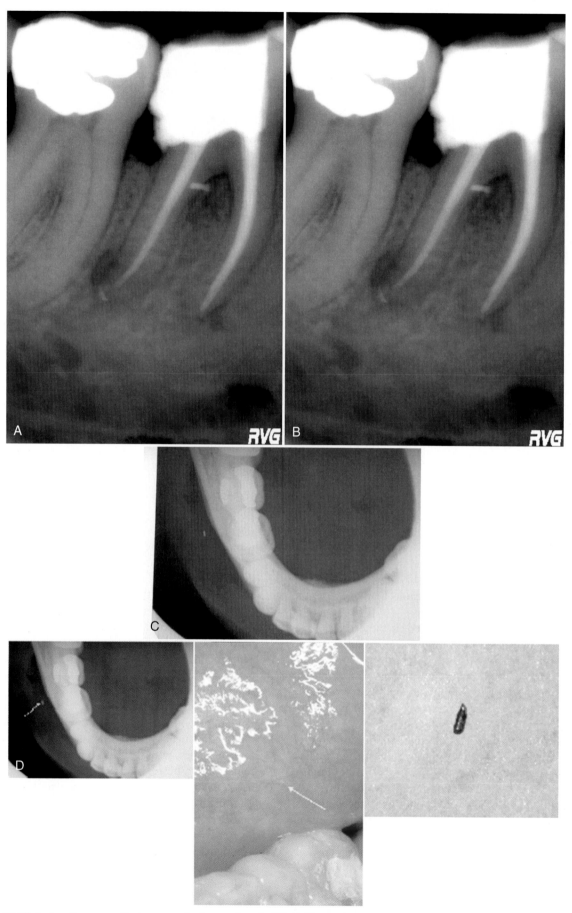

FIGURE 21-13 A, A radiopaque artifact seen on the image of tooth #30. **B**, The position-indicating device (PID) is shifted in a mesial direction, and a second image is exposed. **C**, A mandibular cross-sectional image of the same area. **D**, An arrow points to the location of the broken orthodontic wire, which is also seen in the mucosa and after surgical removal. (Courtesy of S. Craig Rhodes, DMD, Orlando, FL.)

BIBLIOGRAPHY

Frommer HH, Savage-Stabulas JJ: Accessory radiographic techniques: bisecting technique and occlusal technique. In *Radiology for the dental professional*, ed 9, St. Louis, 2011, Mosby.

Frommer HH, Savage-Stabulas JJ: Patient management and special problems. In *Radiology for the dental professional*, ed 9, St. Louis, 2011, Mosby.

Johnson ON, McNally MA, Essay CE: Mounting and introduction to interpretation. In *Essentials of dental radiography for dental assistants and hygienists*, ed 8, Upper Saddle River, NJ, 2007, Pearson Education, Inc.

Johnson ON, McNally MA, Essay CE: The occlusal examination. In *Essentials of dental radiography for dental assistants and hygienists*, ed 8, Upper Saddle River, NJ, 2007, Appleton Pearson Education, Inc.

Miles DA, Van Dis ML, Jensen CW, Ferretti A: Accessory radiographic techniques and patient management. In *Radiographic imaging for the dental team*, ed 4, Philadelphia, 2009, Saunders.

White SC, Pharoah MJ: Intraoral radiographic examinations. In *Oral radiology: principles of interpretation*, ed 6, St. Louis, 2009, Mosby.

White SC, Pharoah MJ: Projection geometry. In *Oral radiology: principles of interpretation*, ed 6, St. Louis, 2009, Mosby.

QUIZ QUESTIONS

FILL IN THE BLANK

1. What does the term *occlusal* refer to?

2. What size receptor is recommended for use with the occlusal technique in the adult patient?

3. What size receptor is recommended for use with the occlusal technique in the pediatric patient with primary dentition?

4. How is the patient's head positioned before exposing a maxillary occlusal receptor?

5. What are the uses of the occlusal image?

6. State the vertical angulation used for the maxillary topographic occlusal projection.

7. State the vertical angulation used for the maxillary lateral occlusal projection.

8. State the vertical angulation used for the mandibular topographic occlusal projection.

9. State the vertical angulation used for the mandibular cross-sectional occlusal projection.

10. State the vertical angulations used for the maxillary and mandibular pediatric occlusal projections.

SHORT ANSWER

For questions 11 to 15, use the buccal object rule, and refer to the appropriate figures.

11. In Figure 21-14, is the labeled amalgam pit buccal or lingual? Why?

12. In Figure 21-15, is the amalgam fragment between the maxillary second and third molars buccal or lingual? Why?

13. In Figure 21-16, is the impacted canine located buccal or lingual to adjacent teeth? Why?

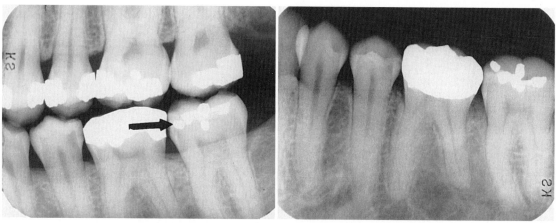

FIGURE 21-14 (Radiographs courtesy of Dr. Robert Jaynes, Assistant Professor, Oral Radiology Group, The Ohio State University College of Dentistry. From Haring JI, Lind LJ: *Radiographic interpretation for the dental hygienist*, Philadelphia, 1993, Saunders.)

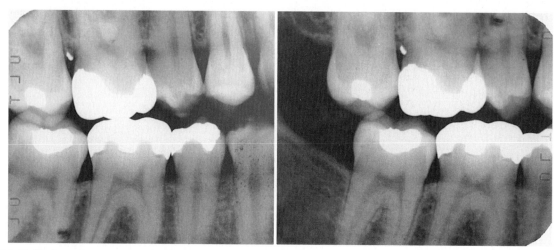

FIGURE 21-15 (Radiographs courtesy of Dr. Robert Jaynes, Assistant Professor, Oral Radiology Group, The Ohio State University College of Dentistry. From Haring JI, Lind LJ: *Radiographic interpretation for the dental hygienist*, Philadelphia, 1993, Saunders.)

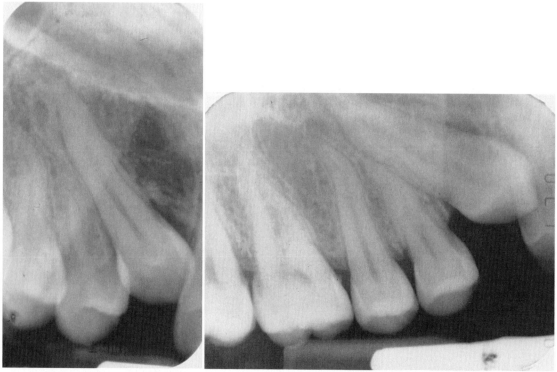

FIGURE 21-16 (Radiographs courtesy of Dr. Robert Jaynes, Assistant Professor, Oral Radiology Group, The Ohio State University College of Dentistry. From Haring JI, Lind LJ: *Radiographic interpretation for the dental hygienist*, Philadelphia, 1993, Saunders.)

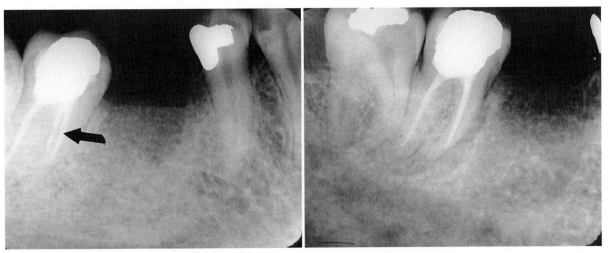

FIGURE 21-17 (Radiographs courtesy of Dr. Robert Jaynes, Assistant Professor, Oral Radiology Group, The Ohio State University College of Dentistry.)

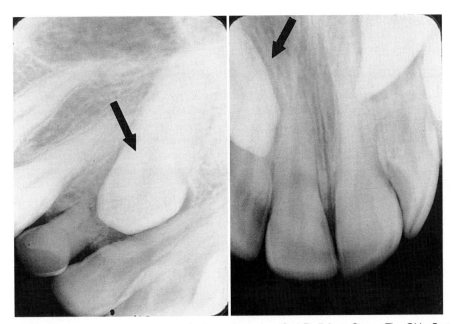

FIGURE 21-18 (Radiographs courtesy of Dr. Robert Jaynes, Assistant Professor, Oral Radiology Group, The Ohio State University College of Dentistry.)

14. In Figure 21-17, is the gutta percha in the labeled canal located on the buccal or lingual side of the tooth? Why?

_____

_____

_____

15. In Figure 21-18, is the impacted canine located buccal or lingual to adjacent teeth? Why?

_____

_____

_____

chapter 22

Panoramic Imaging

OUTLINE

BASIC CONCEPTS
    Purpose and Use
    Fundamentals
    Equipment
STEP-BY-STEP PROCEDURES
    Equipment Preparation
    Patient Preparation

    Patient Positioning
COMMON ERRORS
    Patient-Preparation Errors
    Patient-Positioning Errors
ADVANTAGES AND DISADVANTAGES
    Advantages of Panoramic Imaging
    Disadvantages of Panoramic Imaging

LEARNING OBJECTIVES

After completion of this chapter, the student will be able to do the following:

- Define the key terms associated with panoramic imaging
- Describe the purpose and uses of panoramic imaging
- Describe the fundamentals of panoramic imaging
- Describe the equipment used in panoramic imaging
- Describe patient preparation, equipment preparation, and patient-positioning procedures needed before exposing a panoramic projection

- Identify the patient-preparation and patient-positioning errors seen on panoramic images
- Discuss the causes of patient-preparation and patient-positioning errors and the necessary measures needed to correct such errors
- Discuss the advantages and disadvantages of panoramic imaging

KEY TERMS

Cassette
Collimator
Exposure factors
Film, screen
Focal trough
Frankfort plane

Ghost image
Head positioner
Midsagittal plane
Panoramic
Panoramic imaging

Receptor, panoramic
Rotation center
Screen, intensifying
Tomography
Tubehead

It is often difficult, if not impossible, to obtain adequate diagnostic information from a series of intraoral images alone. Impacted third molar teeth, jaw fractures, and large lesions in the posterior mandible cannot always be seen well enough on intraoral projections; in such cases, the panoramic image is preferred. The panoramic image allows the dental professional to view a large area of the maxilla and the mandible on a single projection.

The purpose of this chapter is to present basic concepts of panoramic imaging and to describe the patient preparation, equipment preparation, and patient positioning procedures needed to perform this procedure. In addition, this chapter describes the advantages and disadvantages of panoramic imaging and reviews helpful hints.

BASIC CONCEPTS

As the term **panoramic** suggests, a **panoramic image** shows a wide view of the maxilla and the mandible (Figure 22-1). **Panoramic imaging** is an extraoral technique that is used to examine the maxilla and the mandible on a single projection. As described in Chapter 6, an extraoral receptor is positioned *outside* the mouth during x-ray exposure. In panoramic imaging (also known as *rotational panoramic imaging*), both

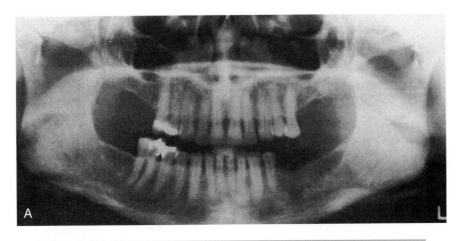

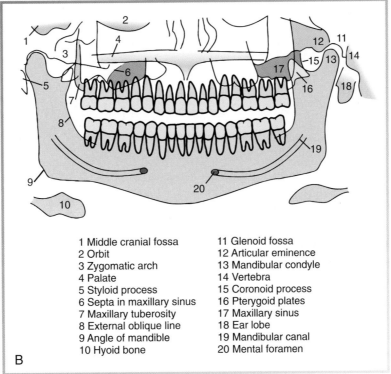

1 Middle cranial fossa	11 Glenoid fossa
2 Orbit	12 Articular eminence
3 Zygomatic arch	13 Mandibular condyle
4 Palate	14 Vertebra
5 Styloid process	15 Coronoid process
6 Septa in maxillary sinus	16 Pterygoid plates
7 Maxillary tuberosity	17 Maxillary sinus
8 External oblique line	18 Ear lobe
9 Angle of mandible	19 Mandibular canal
10 Hyoid bone	20 Mental foramen

FIGURE 22-1 A, Panoramic image. **B**, Panoramic anatomy. (**A** from Miles DA, Van Dis ML, Jensen CW, et al: *Radiographic imaging for dental auxiliaries*, ed 2, Philadelphia, 1993, Saunders; **B** from Olson SS: *Dental radiography laboratory manual*, Philadelphia, 1995, Saunders.)

the receptor and the tubehead rotate around the patient, producing a series of individual images. When such images are combined, an overall view of the maxilla and the mandible is created.

Purpose and Use

The panoramic image provides the dental radiographer with an overall view of the maxilla and the mandible and is often used to supplement bite-wing and periapical images. The panoramic image is typically used for the following purposes:

- To evaluate impacted teeth
- To evaluate eruption patterns, growth, and development

- To detect diseases, lesions, and conditions of the jaws
- To examine the extent of large lesions
- To evaluate trauma

The images on a panoramic projection are not as defined or sharp as the images seen on intraoral projections. Consequently, a panoramic image should not be used to evaluate and diagnose caries (Chapter 33), periodontal disease (Chapter 34), or periapical lesions (Chapter 35). The panoramic image should not be used as a substitute for intraoral projections.

Fundamentals

When intraoral images (e.g., periapical and bite-wing images) are exposed, the receptor and the x-ray tubehead

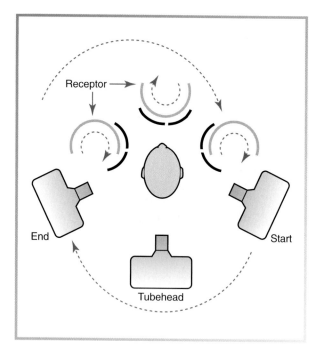

FIGURE 22-2 In panoramic imaging, the receptor and the x-ray tubehead move around the patient in opposite directions. (Courtesy of Dr. Robert M. Jaynes, Assistant Professor, Oral Radiology Group, The Ohio State University College of Dentistry.)

remain stationary. In panoramic imaging, the receptor and the x-ray tubehead move around the patient. The x-ray tube rotates around the patient's head in one direction, while the receptor rotates in the opposite direction (Figure 22-2). The patient may stand or sit in a stationary position, depending on the type of panoramic x-ray machine that is used. The movement of the receptor and the tubehead produces an image through the process known as *tomography*. *Tomo-* means section; **tomography** is an imaging technique that allows the imaging of one layer, or section, of the body while blurring the images of structures in other planes. In panoramic imaging, this image conforms to the shape of the dental arches.

Rotation Center

In panoramic imaging, the receptor and the x-ray tubehead are connected and rotate simultaneously around a patient during exposure. The pivotal point, or axis, around which the receptor and the x-ray tubehead rotate is termed the **rotation center**. Depending on the manufacturer, the number and location of the rotational centers differ. One of three basic rotation centers is used in panoramic x-ray machines (Figure 22-3), as follows:

- Double-center rotation
- Triple-center rotation
- Moving-center rotation

In all cases, the center of rotation changes as the receptor and the tubehead rotate around the patient. This rotational change allows the image layer to conform to the elliptical shape of the dental arches. The location and number of

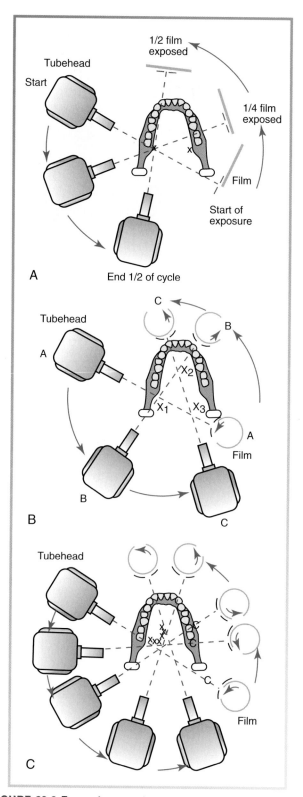

FIGURE 22-3 Types of panoramic x-ray machines. **A**, Double-center rotation machines have two rotational centers, one for the right and one for the left side of the jaws. **B**, Triple-center rotation machines have three centers of rotation and create an uninterrupted radiographic image of the jaws. **C**, Moving-center rotation machines rotate around a continuously moving center that is similar to the arches, creating an uninterrupted image of the jaws. (Redrawn from Olson SS: *Dental radiography laboratory manual*, Philadelphia, 1995, Saunders.)

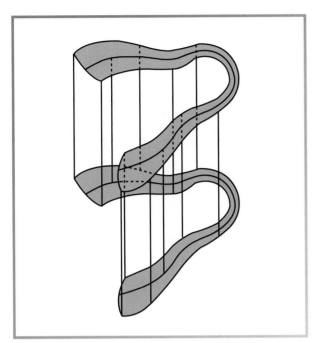

FIGURE 22-4 Example of an "image layer" or "focal trough." (Courtesy of Carestream Health, Inc. Rochester, NY.)

rotational centers influence the size and shape of the focal trough.

Focal Trough

In panoramic imaging, the focal trough is a theoretical concept used to determine where the dental arches must be positioned to obtain the clearest image (Figure 22-4). The **focal trough** (also known as the *image layer*) can be defined as a three-dimensional curved zone in which structures are clearly demonstrated on a panoramic image. The structures located within the focal trough appear reasonably well defined on the resulting panoramic image. The structures positioned inside or outside of the focal trough appear blurred or indistinct and are not readily visible on the panoramic image.

The size and shape of the focal trough vary, depending on the manufacturer of the panoramic x-ray unit. The closer the rotation center is to teeth, the narrower is the focal trough. In most panoramic x-ray machines, the focal trough is narrow in the anterior region and wide in the posterior region.

Each panoramic x-ray unit has a focal trough that is designed to accommodate the average jaw. Each manufacturer provides specific instructions about patient positioning to ensure that the teeth are positioned within the focal trough. The quality of the resulting panoramic image depends on the positioning of the patient's teeth within the focal trough and how closely the patient's maxilla and mandible conform to the focal trough designed for the average jaw.

Equipment

The use of special equipment, including the panoramic x-ray unit, the receptor, and—when using film—screen film, intensifying screens, and cassette, is necessary in panoramic imaging.

Panoramic X-Ray Units

A number of different panoramic x-ray units are available, including the Orthophos XG Plus (Sirona USA) and the Orthoralix 8500 (Gendex Dental Systems) (Figure 22-5). Panoramic units may differ with regard to the number of the rotation centers, the size and shape of the focal trough, and the type of receptor transport mechanism used. Although each manufacturer's panoramic unit is slightly different, all panoramic machines have similar components. The main components of the panoramic unit include the following (Figure 22-6):

- X-ray tubehead
- Head positioner
- Exposure controls

The panoramic x-ray **tubehead** is similar to an intraoral x-ray tubehead; each has a filament used to produce electrons and a target used to produce x-rays. The **collimator** used in the panoramic x-ray tubehead, however, differs from the collimator used in the intraoral x-ray tubehead. As described in Chapter 5, the collimator used in the intraoral x-ray machine is a lead plate with a small round or rectangular opening in the middle. The function of the collimator is to restrict the size and shape of the x-ray beam. The collimator used in the panoramic x-ray machine is a lead plate with an opening in the shape of a narrow vertical slit (Figure 22-7).

The x-ray beam emerges from the panoramic tubehead through the collimator as a narrow band. The beam passes through the patient and then exposes the receptor through another vertical slit in the cassette carrier (the metal holder that supports the cassette). The narrow x-ray beam that emerges from the collimator minimizes patient exposure to x-radiation.

The vertical angulation of the panoramic tubehead does not vary as in the case of the intraoral tubehead. The tubehead of the panoramic unit is fixed in position so that the x-ray beam is directed slightly upward. In addition, the tubehead of the panoramic unit always rotates *behind* the patient's head, while the receptor rotates in front of the patient.

Each panoramic unit has a head positioner, which is used to align the patient's teeth as accurately as possible in the focal trough. The typical **head positioner** consists of a chin rest, notched bite-block, forehead rest, and lateral head supports or guides (Figure 22-8). Each panoramic unit is different, and the operator must follow the manufacturer's instructions on how to position the patient's head in the focal trough.

Each panoramic unit has **exposure factors** that are determined by the manufacturer, who provides suggested exposure factors (milliamperage and kilovoltage) in the instruction manual for the x-ray machine. The milliamperage and kilovoltage settings are adjustable and can be varied to accommodate patients of different sizes (Figure 22-9). The exposure time, however, is fixed and cannot be changed.

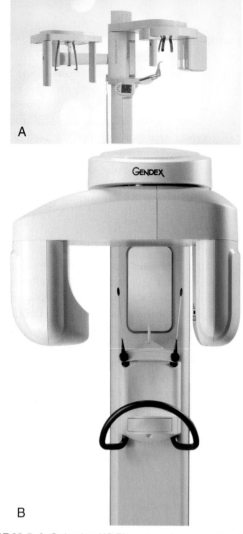

FIGURE 22-5 **A**, Orthophos XG Plus extraoral x-ray machine. **B**, Ortho-ralix 8500 extraoral x-ray machine. (**A,** Courtesy of Sirona USA, Charlotte, NC; **B,** courtesy of Gendex Dental Systems, Des Plaines, IL.)

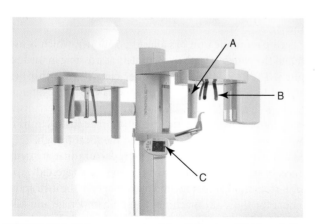

FIGURE 22-6 Main components of the Orthophos XG Plus: **A**, X-ray tubehead; **B**, head positioner; **C**, exposure controls. (Courtesy of Sirona USA, Charlotte, NC.)

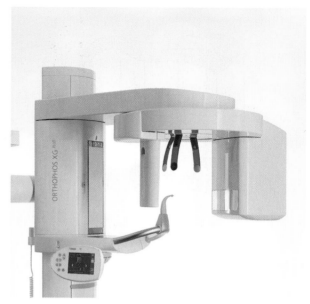

FIGURE 22-7 The collimater on the Orthophos XG Plus has a narrow slit opening. (Courtesy of Sirona USA, Charlotte, NC.)

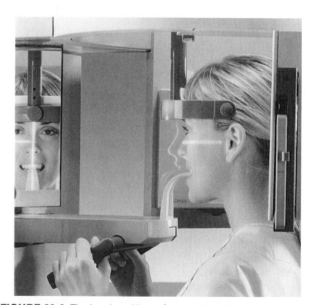

FIGURE 22-8 The head positioner (notched bite-block, forehead rest, and lateral head supports) is used to align the patient's teeth to the focal trough. (Courtesy of Sirona USA, Charlotte, NC.)

Film

Screen film is used in panoramic imaging; this film is sensitive to the light emitted from intensifying screens (see Chapter 7). A screen film is placed between two intensifying screens in a cassette holder. When the cassette holder is exposed to x-rays, the screens convert the x-ray energy into light, which, in turn, exposes the screen film. Some screen films are sensitive to green light (Kodak T-Mat G and Ortho G film), whereas others are sensitive to blue light (Kodak X-Omat RP and Ektamat G films). Blue-sensitive film must be paired with screens that produce blue light, and

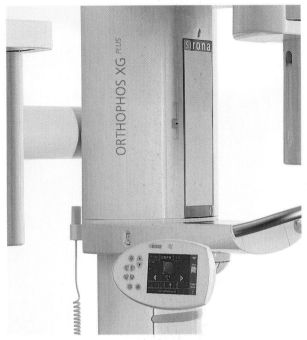

FIGURE 22-9 Exposure controls on the Orthophos XG Plus can be used to adjust exposure factors. (Courtesy of Sirona USA, Charlotte, NC.)

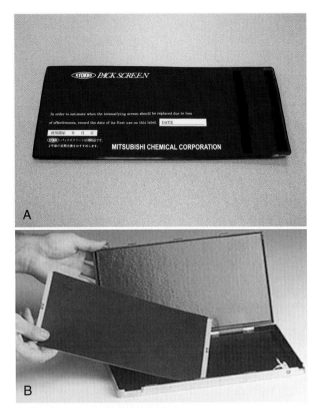

FIGURE 22-10 A, A flexible panoramic cassette has an opening at one end for the receptor. **B**, A rigid panoramic cassette. (**A**, Courtesy of Instrumentarium Dental Inc.; **B**, Courtesy of Gendex Dental Systems, Des Plaines, IL.)

green-sensitive film must be paired with screens that produce green light. The film used in panoramic imaging is available in two sizes: 5 × 12 inch and 6 × 12 inch.

Intensifying Screens

Two basic types of **intensifying screens** are used: calcium tungstate and rare earth (see Chapter 7). Calcium tungstate screens emit blue light, and the rare earth screens emit green light. Rare earth screens require less x-ray exposure than do calcium tungstate screens and are considered "faster." Consequently, rare earth screens are recommended in panoramic imaging because of less exposure of the patient to radiation.

Cassette

The **cassette** is a device that is used to hold the extraoral film and intensifying screens (see Chapter 7). The cassette may be rigid or flexible, curved or straight, depending on the panoramic x-ray unit (Figure 22-10). All cassettes must be "light-tight" to protect the film from exposure. One intensifying screen is placed on each side of the film and held in place when the cassette is closed.

The cassette must be marked to orient the finished image. Before exposure, a metal letter "R" can be attached to the front of the cassette to indicate the patient's right side; the letter "L" is used to identify the patient's left side (Figure 22-11). Special labeling may also be attached to indicate the patient's name, the dentist's name, and the date. If the cassette is not labeled before exposure, the film must be labeled

immediately after processing. A marking pen or adhesive label can be used to label the image.

STEP-BY-STEP PROCEDURES

Step-by-step procedures for the exposure of a panoramic receptor include equipment preparation, patient preparation, and patient positioning. Before exposing a panoramic receptor, infection control procedures (as described in Chapter 15) must be completed.

Equipment Preparation

The dental radiographer must complete equipment preparations *before* preparing the patient for the exposure of a panoramic receptor (Procedure 22-1).

Patient Preparation

After preparing the panoramic equipment, the dental radiographer must prepare the patient for the procedure (Procedure 22-2).

Patient Positioning

The dental radiographer must be familiar with the manufacturer's specific directions for patient positioning that

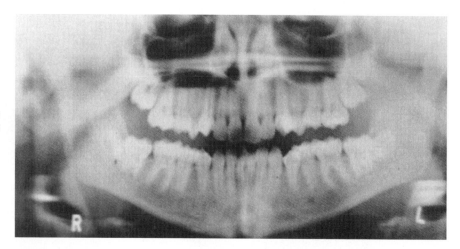

FIGURE 22-11 This panoramic image is labeled with two metal letters indicating the patient's right (R) and left (L) sides.

1. If using film, load the panoramic cassette in the darkroom under safelight conditions. One extraoral film and two intensifying screens must be placed in the cassette, and the cassette must be securely closed.
2. Cover the bite-block with a disposable plastic coverslip. If the bite-block is not covered with an impervious material (e.g., plastic coverslip), it must be sterilized between patients.
3. Set the exposure factors (kilovoltage, milliamperage) according to the manufacturer's recommendations. Adjust the machine to accommodate the height of the patient, and align all movable parts properly. The cassette must be loaded in the cassette carrier of the panoramic unit.

are included in the instruction manual. Although each manufacturer's positioning and exposure procedures are slightly different, the patient positioning steps listed here are common to all panoramic machines (Procedure 22-3).

COMMON ERRORS

To produce a diagnostic panoramic image and minimize patient exposure, mistakes must be avoided. The dental radiographer must be able to recognize common patient-preparation and patient-positioning errors and understand the necessary steps to correct these errors.

Patient-Preparation Errors

Proper patient preparation is critical in obtaining a diagnostic panoramic image. Two common patient preparation errors are (1) ghost images and (2) the lead apron artifact.

Ghost Images

Problem. If all metallic or radiodense objects (e.g., eyeglasses, earrings, necklaces, hairpins, removable partial dentures, complete dentures, orthodontic retainers, hearing aids, napkin chains) are not removed before the exposure of a panoramic receptor, it results in a ghost image that obscures diagnostic information.

A **ghost image**, which is a radiopaque artifact seen on a panoramic image, is produced when a radiodense object is penetrated twice by the x-ray beam. A ghost image resembles its real counterpart and is found on the opposite side of the image; it appears indistinct, larger, and higher than its actual counterpart. For example, a ghost image of a hoop earring appears on the opposite side of the image as a radiopacity that is larger and higher than the real hoop earring. In addition, the ghost image of the hoop earring appears blurred in both horizontal and vertical directions (Figure 22-16).

Solution. To avoid such an artifact, the dental radiographer must instruct the patient to remove all radiodense objects in the head-and-neck region before positioning the patient for panoramic radiography.

Lead Apron Artifact

Problem. If the lead apron is incorrectly placed on the patient, or if a lead apron with a thyroid collar is used during the exposure of a panoramic projection, it results in a radiopaque cone-shaped artifact that obscures diagnostic information (Figure 22-17).

Solution. To prevent such an artifact, the dental radiographer must always use a lead apron without a thyroid collar when exposing a panoramic projection. The lead apron must be placed low around the neck of the patient so that it does not block the x-ray beam.

Patient-Positioning Errors

Patient positioning is of critical importance during exposure of a panoramic projection. Because the panoramic image

PROCEDURE 22-2 Patient Preparation for Panoramic Imaging

1. Explain to the patient the imaging procedure about to be performed.
2. Place a lead apron, without a thyroid collar, on the patient, and secure it. A double-sided lead apron (one that protects the front and back of the patient) is recommended (Figure 22-12). The lead apron must be placed low around the neck so that it does not block the x-ray beam. A thyroid collar is not recommended for panoramic imaging because it blocks part of the beam and obscures important diagnostic information.
3. Have the patient remove all objects from the head-and-neck area that may interfere with the procedure. The patient must remove eyeglasses, earrings, necklaces, napkin chains, hearing aids, hairpins, and complete or partial dentures.

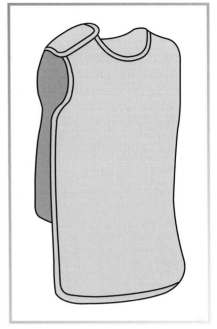

FIGURE 22-12 A double-sided lead apron is recommended for use during exposure of a panoramic receptor.

PROCEDURE 22-3 Patient Positioning for Panoramic Imaging

1. Instruct the patient to sit or stand "as tall as possible" with the back erect. The vertebral column must be perfectly straight. The spinal column is very dense; if the spine is not straight, a white shadow appears over the middle of the image and obscures diagnostic information.
2. Instruct the patient to bite on the plastic bite-block. Maxillary and mandibular anterior teeth must be in an end-to-end position in the groove (notch) on the bite-block (Figure 22-13). This groove is used to align the teeth to the focal trough. (In an edentulous patient, the radiographer must align the patient's maxillary and mandibular ridges over the notched area on the bite-block. Cotton rolls can be placed on each side of the bite-block to provide stabilization for the patient.)
3. Position the **midsagittal plane** (an imaginary line that divides the patient's face into right and left sides) perpendicular to the floor (Figure 22-14). The patient's head must not be tipped or tilted; if the midsagittal plane is not positioned perpendicular to the floor, a distorted image results.
4. Position the **Frankfort plane** (an imaginary plane that passes through the top of the ear canal and the bottom of the eye socket) parallel to the floor (Figure 22-15). When the Frankfort plane is parallel to the floor, the occlusal plane is positioned at the correct angle.

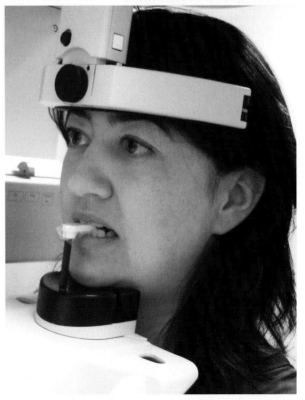

FIGURE 22-13 The patient must place his or her teeth in the grooves on the bite-block.

PROCEDURE 22-3   **Patient Positioning for Panoramic Imaging—cont'd**

5. Instruct the patient to place the tongue on the roof of the mouth. You may suggest that the patient "swallow and feel the tongue rise up to the roof of the mouth" and then instruct the patient to keep the tongue in that position during the procedure. Also, instruct the patient to close the lips around the bite-block.

6. After the patient has been positioned, instruct the patient to remain still while the machine is rotating during exposure.

7. Expose the receptor and if using film, proceed with film processing as described in Chapter 9.

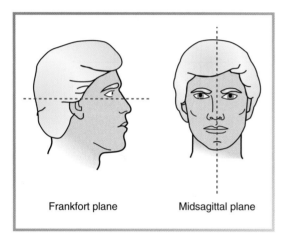

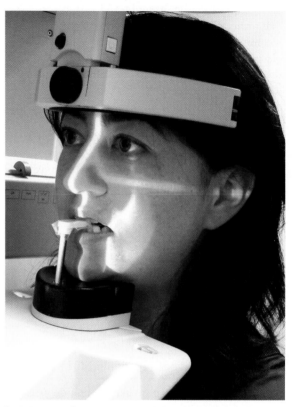

FIGURE 22-14 Frankfort and midsagittal planes. The Frankfort plane passes through the floor of the orbit and the external auditory meatus. The midsagittal plane divides the body in half into right and left sides. (From Olson SS: *Dental radiography laboratory manual*, Philadelphia, 1995, Saunders.)

FIGURE 22-15 The patient's head must be positioned such that the Frankfort plane is parallel to the floor.

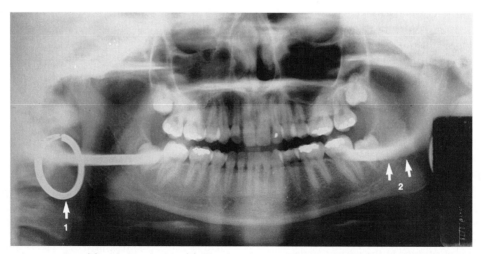

FIGURE 22-16 Large hoop earrings (1) and ghost images (2). The ghost image of the earring appears on the opposite side of the image and is enlarged and laterally distorted. (From Haring JI, Lind LJ: *Radiographic interpretation for the dental hygienist*, Philadelphia, 1993, Saunders.)

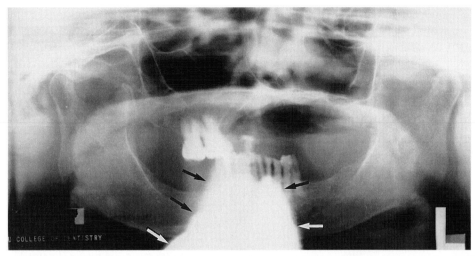

FIGURE 22-17 On a panoramic image, a lead apron artifact appears as a large cone-shaped radiopacity obscuring the mandible. (From Haring JI, Lind LJ: *Radiographic interpretation for the dental hygienist*, Philadelphia, 1993, Saunders.)

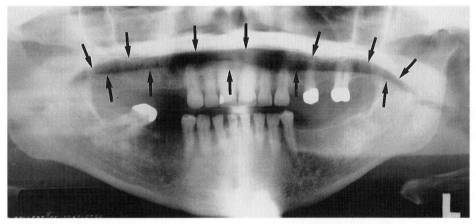

FIGURE 22-18 If the patient does not place his or her tongue on the roof of the mouth and hold it there throughout the imaging procedure, a radiolucent shadow will be superimposed over the image of the apices of maxillary teeth. (From Haring JI, Lind LJ: *Radiographic interpretation for the dental hygienist*, Philadelphia, 1993, Saunders.)

does not show the fine anatomic details seen on intraoral radiographs, even the smallest positioning error can create a distorted image.

Positioning of Lips and Tongue

Problem. If the patient's lips are not closed on the bite-block during the exposure of a panoramic projection, it results in a dark radiolucent shadow that obscures anterior teeth. If the tongue is not in contact with the palate during the exposure of a panoramic projection, it results in a dark radiolucent shadow that obscures the apices of the maxillary teeth (Figure 22-18).

Solution. To prevent such errors, the dental radiographer must instruct the patient to close the lips around the bite-block. The patient must then be instructed to swallow once; after this, the patient must be asked to raise the tongue up to the palate and hold it against the hard palate during the exposure of the projection.

Positioning of Frankfort Plane Upward

Problem. If the patient is positioned such that the chin is too high or is tipped up (Figure 22-19), the Frankfort plane is angled upward, and the following results:

1. The hard palate and floor of the nasal cavity appear superimposed over the roots of maxillary teeth.
2. A loss of detail in the maxillary incisor region occurs.
3. The maxillary incisors appear blurred and magnified.

4. A "reverse smile line" (curved downward) is seen on the image (Figure 22-20).

Solution. To prevent such an error, the dental radiographer must carefully position the patient such that the Frankfort plane is parallel to the floor.

Positioning of Frankfort Plane Downward

Problem. If the patient is positioned such that the chin is too low or is tipped down (Figure 22-21), the Frankfort plane is angled downward, and the following results:

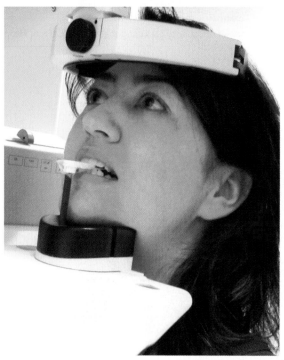

FIGURE 22-19 The patient's head is incorrectly positioned; the chin is tipped up.

1. The mandibular incisors appear blurred.
2. A loss of detail in the anterior apical region occurs.
3. The mandibular condyles may not be visible.
4. An "exaggerated smile line" (curved upward) is seen on the image (Figure 22-22).

Solution. To prevent such an error, the dental radiographer must carefully position the patient such that the Frankfort plane is parallel to the floor.

Aligning Teeth Anterior to the Focal Trough

Problem. If the patient is positioned such that the anterior teeth are not aligned to the focal trough, as indicated by the groove in the bite-block, teeth appear blurred. If the patient's teeth are too far forward on the bite-block or anterior to the focal trough (Figure 22-23), anterior teeth appear "skinny" and out of focus on the image (Figure 22-24).

Solution. To prevent such an error, the dental radiographer must position the patient such that the anterior teeth are in an end-to-end position in the groove on the bite-block. The forehead support must then be adjusted to stabilize the patient's head position and prevent the patient from sliding forward on the bite-block.

Aligning Teeth Posterior to the Focal Trough

Problem. If the patient's anterior teeth are not aligned to the focal trough, as indicated by the groove in the bite-block, the teeth appear blurred. If the patient's anterior teeth are aligned too far back on the bite-block or posterior to the focal trough (Figure 22-25), the teeth appear "fat" and out of focus on the image (Figure 22-26).

Solution. To prevent such an error, the dental radiographer must position the patient such that anterior teeth are in an end-to-end position in the groove on the bite-block.

Aligning the Midsagittal Plane

Problem. If the patient's head is not centered (Figure 22-27), the ramus and posterior teeth appear unequally magnified on the panoramic image. The side farthest from the

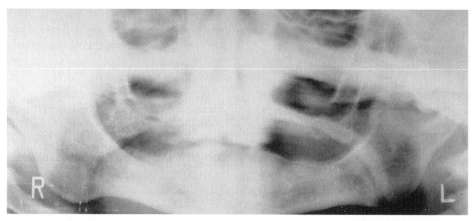

FIGURE 22-20 A "reverse smile line" is seen on a panoramic image when the patient's chin is tipped up. (From Haring JI, Lind LJ: *Radiographic interpretation for the dental hygienist*, Philadelphia, 1993, Saunders.)

receptor appears magnified, and the side closest to the receptor appears smaller (Figure 22-28).

Solution. To prevent such an error, the dental radiographer must position the patient's head such that the midsagittal plane is perpendicular to the floor while the midline is centered on the bite-stick. The lateral head supports must then be adjusted to stabilize the position of the patient's head.

Aligning the Spine

Problem. If the patient is not standing or sitting with the spine straight, the cervical spine appears as a radiopacity in the center of the image and obscures diagnostic information (Figure 22-29).

Solution. To prevent such an error, the dental radiographer must instruct the patient to stand or sit "as tall as possible" with a straight back.

ADVANTAGES AND DISADVANTAGES

As with all radiographic techniques, panoramic imaging has both advantages and disadvantages.

Advantages of Panoramic Imaging

1. *Field size.* The panoramic image covers the entire maxilla and mandible. More anatomic structures can be viewed on a panoramic image than with a complete

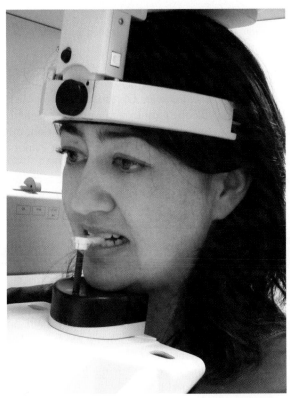

FIGURE 22-21 The patient's head is incorrectly positioned; the chin is tipped down.

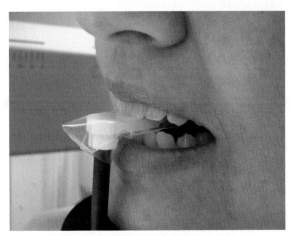

FIGURE 22-23 The patient is incorrectly positioned; the teeth have been placed too far forward on the bite-block.

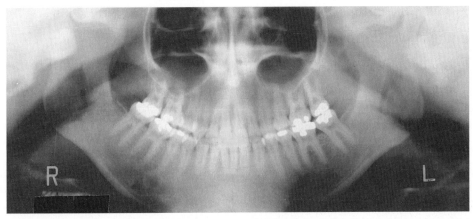

FIGURE 22-22 An "exaggerated smile line" is seen on a panoramic image when the patient's chin is tipped down. (From Haring JI, Lind LJ: *Radiographic Interpretation for the dental hygienist*, Philadelphia, 1993, Saunders.)

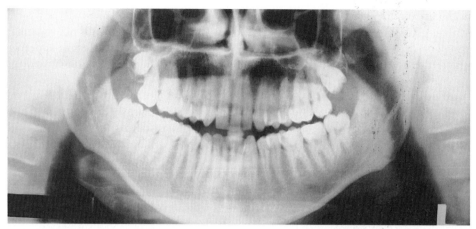

FIGURE 22-24 Anterior teeth appear narrowed and blurred on the panoramic image when the patient's teeth are positioned too far forward on the bite-block. (From Haring JI, Lind LJ: *Radiographic interpretation for the dental hygienist*, Philadelphia, 1993, Saunders.)

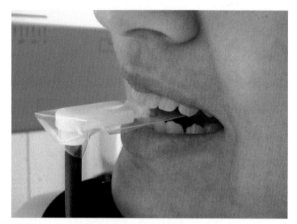

FIGURE 22-25 The patient is incorrectly positioned; the teeth have been placed too far back and not on the bite-block.

mouth radiographic series (CMRS). In addition, lesions and conditions of the jaws that may not be seen on intraoral images can be detected on a panoramic image.

2. *Simplicity.* Exposure of a panoramic receptor is relatively simple and requires minimal amounts of time and training for the dental radiographer.

3. *Patient cooperation.* The exposure of a panoramic image is more acceptable to the patient because no discomfort is involved. For example, children who may not be able to tolerate intraoral projections may find it easier to sit still during the exposure of a panoramic image (Figure 22-30).

4. *Minimal exposure.* A panoramic image involves only minimal radiation exposure of the patient.

Disadvantages of Panoramic Imaging

1. *Image quality.* The images seen on a panoramic image are not as sharp as intraoral projections because of the intensifying screens. As a result, the panoramic image cannot be used to evaluate dental caries, periodontal disease, or periapical lesions.

2. *Focal trough limitations.* Objects of interest that are located outside the focal trough cannot be seen.

3. *Distortion.* Certain amounts of magnification, distortion, and overlapping are present on a panoramic image, even when proper technique is used.

4. *Equipment cost.* The cost of a panoramic x-ray unit is relatively high compared with the cost of an intraoral x-ray unit.

HELPFUL HINTS

For exposing panoramic radiographs:

- **DO** cover the bite-block with a disposable plastic cover slip before positioning the patient.
- **DO** choose the exposure factors (kilovoltage, milliamperage) according to the manufacturer's recommendations before positioning the patient.
- **DO** briefly explain to the patient the imaging procedure that is about to be performed.
- **DO** place a lead apron without a thyroid collar on the patient, and secure it.
- **DO** ask the patient to remove all radiodense objects from the head-and-neck area before positioning the patient.
- **DO** instruct the patient to stand or sit "as straight and tall as possible."
- **DO** instruct the patient to place his or her front teeth in the deep groove on the bite-block in an end-to-end position.
- **DO** position the midsagittal plane of the patient perpendicular to the floor.
- **DO** position the Frankfort plane of the patient parallel with the floor.
- **DO** instruct the patient to close the lips on the bite-block and to swallow once; then ask the patient to place the tongue against the roof of the mouth and to maintain that position during the exposure.
- **DO** instruct the patient to remain still during the exposure.

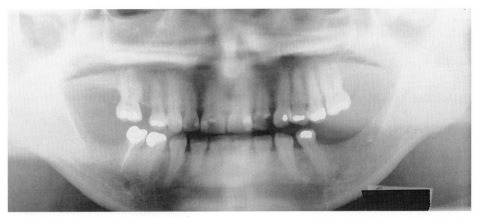

FIGURE 22-26 Anterior teeth appear widened and blurred on the panoramic image when the patient's teeth are positioned too far back on the bite-block. (From Haring JI, Lind LJ: *Radiographic interpretation for the dental hygienist*, Philadelphia, 1993, Saunders.)

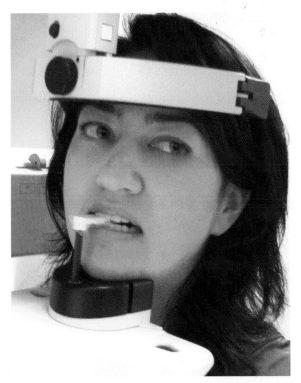

FIGURE 22-27 The patient is incorrectly positioned; the head is not centered.

SUMMARY

- The panoramic image allows the dental professional to view a large area of the maxilla and the mandible on a single projection.
- Uses of the panoramic image include (1) evaluation of impacted teeth; (2) evaluation of eruption patterns and growth and development; (3) detection of diseases, lesions, and conditions of the jaws; (4) examination of extent of large lesions; and (5) evaluation of trauma.
- The panoramic image is typically used to supplement bite-wing and periapical images and is not a substitute for intraoral projections. The panoramic image should not be used to evaluate caries, periodontal disease, or periapical lesions.
- In panoramic imaging, both the receptor and the tubehead are connected and rotate simultaneously around the patient during exposure. Rotational centers allow the image layer to conform to the elliptical shape of the dental arches. The number and locations of rotational centers influence the size and shape of the focal trough.
- The focal trough is a three-dimensional curved zone in which structures are clearly demonstrated on a panoramic image. Structures within the focal trough appear reasonably well defined, whereas structures outside the focal trough appear blurred.
- Special equipment, including the panoramic x-ray unit, the receptor, and—when using film—screen film, intensifying screens, and cassette, is necessary for the panoramic imaging procedure.
- Before preparing the patient for exposure of a panoramic projection, the following tasks must be completed: preparation of the cassette, infection control procedures, selection of the exposure factors, adjustment of the panoramic x-ray machine according to patient height and proper alignment of movable parts, and loading of the cassette into the cassette carrier.
- After preparing the equipment, the dental radiographer must prepare the patient by explaining the imaging procedure, placing the lead apron on the patient, and having the patient remove all radiodense objects from the head-and-neck region.
- The patient must then be positioned according to the manufacturer's recommendations for the alignment of the spine, teeth, the midsagittal plane, the Frankfort plane, lips, and the tongue.
- The dental radiographer must be able to identify patient-preparation and patient-positioning errors and know the necessary steps to correct such errors.
- Advantages of panoramic imaging include field size, simplicity of use, patient cooperation, and minimal patient exposure to x-radiation.

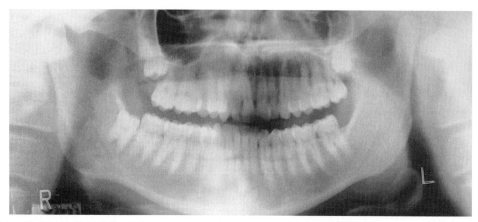

FIGURE 22-28 The patient's posterior teeth and ramus appear to be magnified on the panoramic image when the head is not centered. (From Haring JI, Lind LJ: *Radiographic interpretation for the dental hygienist*, Philadelphia, 1993, Saunders.)

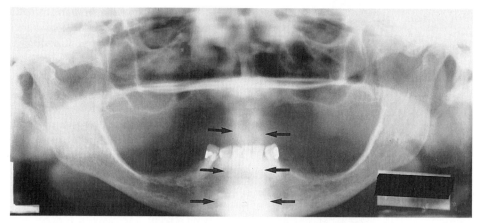

FIGURE 22-29 If the patient is not standing erect, superimposition of the cervical spine (*arrows*) may be seen at the center of the panoramic image. (From Haring JI, Lind LJ: *Radiographic interpretation for the dental hygienist*, Philadelphia, 1993, Saunders.)

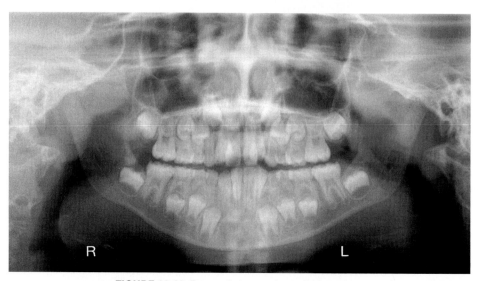

FIGURE 22-30 Panoramic image of a pediatric patient.

- Disadvantages of panoramic imaging include image quality, limitations imposed by the focal trough, image distortion, and the high cost of equipment.

BIBLIOGRAPHY

Frommer HH, Savage-Stabulas JJ: Panoramic radiography. In *Radiology for the dental professional*, ed 9, St. Louis, 2011, Mosby.

Johnson ON, McNally MA, Essay CE: Panoramic radiography. In *Essentials of dental radiography for dental assistants and hygienists*, ed 6, Norwalk, CT, 1999, Appleton & Lange.

Miles DA, Van Dis ML, Jensen CW, Williamson GF: Panoramic imaging. In *Radiographic imaging for the dental team*, ed 4, Philadelphia, 2009, Saunders.

Miles DA, Van Dis ML, Razmus TF: Plain film extraoral radiographic techniques. In *Basic principles of oral and maxillofacial radiology*, Philadelphia, 1992, Saunders.

Olson SS: Auxiliary radiographic techniques. In *Dental radiography laboratory manual*, Philadelphia, 1995, Saunders.

White SC, Pharoah MJ: Panoramic imaging. In *Oral radiology: principles of interpretation*, ed 6, St. Louis, 2009, Mosby.

QUIZ QUESTIONS

MULTIPLE CHOICE

____ 1. Which of the following describes a use of a panoramic image?
  a. diagnosis of caries
  b. evaluation of periodontal disease
  c. evaluation of impacted molars
  d. evaluation of periapical disease

____ 2. The zone in which structures are clearly demonstrated on a panoramic image is termed:
  a. the focal trough
  b. the rotation center
  c. the ghost image
  d. the midsagittal plane

____ 3. Rare earth intensifying screens are recommended in panoramic imaging because:
  a. rare earth screens emit a blue light
  b. rare earth screens provide a more diagnostic image
  c. rare earth screens require less x-ray exposure for the patient
  d. the images convert faster in automatic processors

____ 4. A thyroid collar is not recommended in panoramic imaging because:
  a. it blocks the x-ray beam and obscures information
  b. there is a relatively low dose of radiation to the thyroid gland in panoramic imaging
  c. it is impossible to sterilize the thyroid collar
  d. all of the above

____ 5. The imaginary line that passes from the bottom of the eye socket through the top of the ear canal is termed:
  a. the midsagittal plane
  b. the Frankfort plane
  c. the vertebral plane
  d. the orbital plane

MATCHING

For questions 6 to 20, match the following types of procedures with the statements given below.
  a. Panoramic imaging
  b. Intraoral imaging
  c. Both panoramic and intraoral imaging

____ 6. The receptor and the tubehead rotate around the patient.

____ 7. This type of image is used to examine the extent of large lesions.

____ 8. The dental arches must be aligned to the focal trough.

____ 9. The tubehead contains a filament used to produce electrons and a target used to produce x-rays.

____ 10. The collimator is a lead plate with an opening in the shape of a narrow vertical slit.

____ 11. The collimator is a lead plate with a small, round or rectangular opening.

____ 12. The vertical angulation of the tubehead is variable.

____ 13. A head positioner is used to position the patient's head.

____ 14. A screen film is used.

____ 15. A cassette holder with two intensifying screens is used.

____ 16. The x-ray film must be loaded into a cassette in a darkroom under safelight conditions.

____ 17. A lead apron with a thyroid collar must be placed on the patient.

____ 18. All jewelry (earrings and necklaces) must be removed before exposure.

____ 19. The midsagittal plane must be positioned perpendicular to the floor.

____ 20. The vertebral column must be perfectly straight.

ESSAY

21. Discuss the equipment preparations necessary before exposure of a panoramic projection.

22. Discuss the patient preparations necessary before exposure of a panoramic projection.
23. Discuss the patient positioning steps necessary before exposure of a panoramic projection.
24. Give examples of Frankfort plane positioning errors, and discuss what steps can be taken to correct such errors.
25. Discuss the advantages and disadvantages of panoramic imaging.

IDENTIFICATION

26. Identify the approximate age of the patient in Figure 22-31.
27. Identify the approximate age of the patient in Figure 22-32.
28. Identify the approximate age of the patient in Figure 22-33.

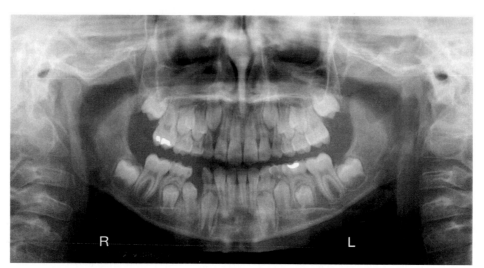

FIGURE 22-31

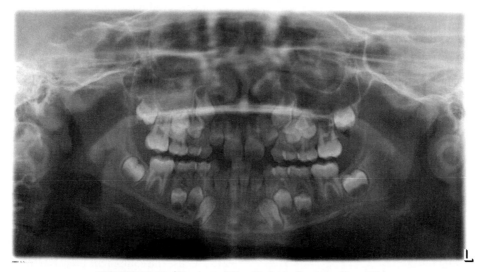

FIGURE 22-32 (Courtesy of Cary Pediatric Dentistry, Cary, NC.)

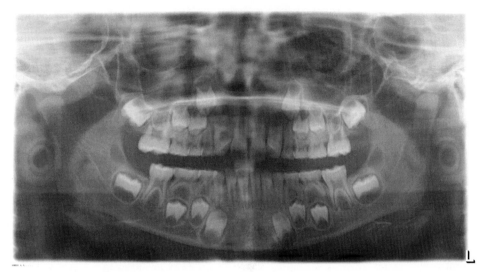

FIGURE 22-33 (Courtesy of Cary Pediatric Dentistry, Cary, NC.)

chapter 23

Extraoral Imaging

OUTLINE

BASIC CONCEPTS
    Purpose and Use
    Equipment
STEP-BY-STEP PROCEDURES
    Equipment Preparation
    Patient Preparation
    Patient Positioning

EXTRAORAL PROJECTION TECHNIQUES
    Lateral Jaw Imaging
    Skull Imaging
    Temporomandibular Joint Imaging

LEARNING OBJECTIVES

After completion of this chapter, the student will be able to do the following:

- Define the key terms associated with extraoral imaging
- Describe the purpose and uses of extraoral imaging
- Describe the equipment used in extraoral imaging
- Detail the equipment and patient preparations necessary before exposing an extraoral projection
- Identify the specific purpose of each of the extraoral projections
- Describe the head position, the receptor placement, and the beam alignment for each of the following: lateral jaw projection–body of the mandible, lateral jaw projection–ramus of the mandible, lateral cephalometric projection, posteroanterior projection, Waters projection, submentovertex projection, reverse Towne projection, and transcranial projection.

KEY TERMS

Cassette
Cephalostat
Extraoral
Extraoral imaging
Film, nonscreen
Film, screen
Grid
Image, extraoral

Lateral cephalometric projection
Lateral jaw projection–body of mandible
Lateral jaw projection–ramus of mandible
Posteroanterior projection
Radiograph, extraoral
Reverse Towne projection

Screen, intensifying
Submentovertex projection
Temporomandibular joint (TMJ)
Temporomandibular joint tomography
Tomogram
Transcranial projection
Waters projection

As discussed in Chapter 22, it is not always possible to obtain adequate diagnostic information from a series of intraoral images. Jaw fractures, impacted teeth, and large lesions cannot always be seen well enough on intraoral projections. In such cases, extraoral images can be used to view large areas of teeth and bone. The extraoral image allows the dental professional to view a large area of the jaws and the skull as a single image.

The purpose of this chapter is to present the basic concepts of extraoral imaging and describe the necessary patient and equipment preparations. In addition, this chapter introduces a number of extraoral projection techniques and describes receptor placement, patient positioning, and beam alignment for such projections.

BASIC CONCEPTS

As the term **extraoral** suggests, an **extraoral image** is one that is placed *outside the mouth* during x-ray exposure. **Extraoral imaging** is used to view large areas of the skull or

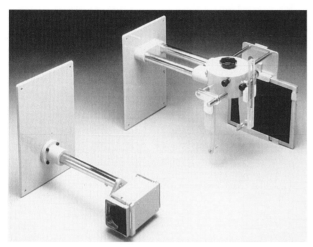

FIGURE 23-1 This unit can be used with most intraoral x-ray tube-heads. It is equipped with a collimator to allow accurate beam alignment and a head positioner to allow for proper patient positioning. (Courtesy of Wehmer Corporation, Addison, IL.)

the jaws. Many types of extraoral projections exist and are primarily used in orthodontics and oral surgery. The most common extraoral image is the panoramic projection (see Chapter 22).

Purpose and Use

The extraoral image shows an overall view of the skull and jaws. The extraoral projection is typically used for the following purposes:

- To evaluate large areas of the skull and jaws
- To evaluate growth and development
- To evaluate impacted teeth
- To detect diseases, lesions, and conditions of the jaws
- To examine the extent of large lesions
- To evaluate trauma
- To evaluate the temporomandibular joint area

In some cases, an extraoral projection is indicated because the patient has swelling or discomfort and is unable to tolerate the placement of intraoral receptors. Extraoral projections may be used alone or in conjunction with intraoral projections. As in the case of panoramic projections, extraoral images are not as defined or sharp as are intraoral projections.

Equipment
X-Ray Unit

A standard intraoral x-ray machine (see Chapter 6) may be used for a variety of extraoral images (e.g., transcranial and lateral jaw projections). To aid in patient positioning and alignment of the x-ray beam, special head-positioning and beam alignment devices can be added to the intraoral x-ray machine (Figure 23-1). Some panoramic x-ray units (see Chapter 22) may also be used for obtaining extraoral projections. In such cases, the panoramic x-ray tubehead is used in conjunction with a special extension arm and a device known as a **cephalostat**, or *craniostat* (Figure 23-2). The cephalostat

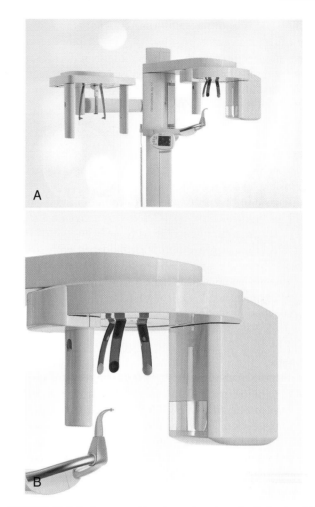

FIGURE 23-2 A, An extraoral imaging unit such as the Orthophos XG Plus contains a cephalostat for positioning the patient's head and the receptor. **B**, Example of a cephalostat. (Courtesy of Sirona USA, Charlotte, NC.)

includes a receptor holder and head positioner, which allow the dental radiographer to position both the receptor and the patient easily.

Film

When a film is used for extraoral exposures, a screen film is placed in a cassette with intensifying screens. The **screen film** is sensitive to the light emitted from intensifying screens (see Chapter 7). The use of a screen film and intensifying screens minimizes the x-ray exposure necessary to produce a diagnostic image. As discussed in Chapters 7 and 22, some screen films are sensitive to green light (Kodak T-Mat G, T-Mat L, Ortho G, and Ortho L), whereas others are sensitive to blue light (Kodak X-Omat RP and Ektamat G). Blue-sensitive film must be paired with screens that produce blue light, and green-sensitive film must be paired with screens that produce green light. Extraoral film sizes vary; the sizes most often used are 5 × 7 inch and 8 × 10 inch.

An occlusal receptor (size 4) may be used for some extraoral images (e.g., lateral jaw or transcranial projection). The occlusal film is a **nonscreen film** and does not require the use of screens for exposure. As discussed in Chapter 7, a nonscreen film requires more exposure time than does a screen film. As a result, the occlusal receptor used extraorally requires more radiation exposure than does a screen film. In addition, the occlusal film used extraorally does not cover as large an area as does a screen film.

Intensifying Screens

An **intensifying screen** is a device that converts x-ray energy into visible light; the light, in turn, exposes the screen film. As discussed in Chapters 7 and 22, calcium tungstate screens emit blue light, and rare earth screens emit green light. The screen film must be compatible with the light emitted from the screen; blue-sensitive film must be paired with screens that emit blue light, and green-sensitive film must be paired with screens that emit green light. Rare earth screens require less exposure than calcium tungstate screens. To minimize patient exposure, the fastest film and screen combination that provides a diagnostic image should be used.

Cassette

The purpose of the **cassette** is to hold the receptor in tight contact with the intensifying screen and to protect the receptor from exposure to light (see Chapter 7). Extraoral cassettes, with the exception of some panoramic cassettes, are rigid and are constructed of metal and plastic.

The cassette must be labeled before exposure to orient the finished image; a metallic "R" or "L" can be used to identify the patient's right or left side. These metallic letters must always be placed on the front of the cassette. The front side of the cassette is typically constructed of plastic and permits the passage of the x-ray beam, whereas the back side is made of metal to reduce scatter radiation. The front side is also known as the "tube side," or the side that faces the x-ray beam. The front side of the cassette must always face the patient during exposure.

Grid

A **grid** is a device used to reduce the amount of scatter radiation that reaches an extraoral film during exposure. Scatter radiation causes film fog and reduces contrast. A grid can be used to decrease film fog and increase the contrast of the image.

A grid is composed of a series of thin lead strips embedded in a material (e.g., plastic) that permits the passage of the x-ray beam. The grid is placed between the patient's head and the film. During exposure, the grid permits the passage of the x-ray beam between the lead strips. When some of the x-rays interact with the patient's tissues, scatter radiation is produced; this scatter radiation is then directed at the grid and the film at an angle. As a result, scatter radiation is absorbed by the lead strips and does not reach the surface of the film to cause film fog (Figure 23-3). To compensate for the lead strips found in the grid, exposure time must be increased. Because of this increase in exposure time, a grid should be

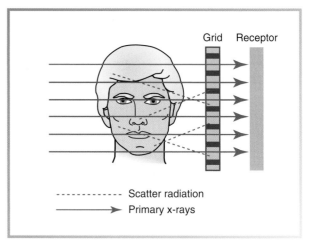

FIGURE 23-3 A grid decreases the amount of scatter radiation that reaches the extraoral receptor. (Courtesy of Dr. Robert M. Jaynes, Assistant Professor, Oral Radiology Group, The Ohio State University College of Dentistry.)

PROCEDURE 23-1	Equipment Preparation for Extraoral Imaging

1. When using a film, load the extraoral cassette in the darkroom under safelight conditions. Place one extraoral receptor between two intensifying screens, and securely close the cassette.
2. Set exposure factors (kilovoltage, milliamperage, time) according to the manufacturer's recommendations. Load the cassette into the cassette carrier.

used only when improved image quality and high contrast are necessary.

STEP-BY-STEP PROCEDURES

Step-by-step procedures for the exposure of an extraoral projection include equipment preparation, patient preparation, and patient positioning. Before exposing an extraoral projection, infection control procedures (as described in Chapter 15) must be completed. If an extraoral x-ray unit with cephalostat is used, the ear rods must be wiped with a disinfectant between patients.

Equipment Preparation

The dental radiographer must prepare the equipment before preparing a patient for the exposure of an extraoral projection (Procedure 23-1).

Patient Preparation

After preparing the equipment, the dental radiographer must prepare the patient (Procedure 23-2).

| PROCEDURE 23-2 | Patient Preparation for Extraoral Imaging |

1. Explain to the patient the procedure about to be performed.
2. Place a lead apron without a thyroid collar over the patient, and secure it. A double-sided lead apron is recommended (see Chapter 22). The lead apron must be placed low around the back of the neck so that it does not block the x-ray beam. A thyroid collar is not recommended for extraoral imaging because it blocks part of the beam and obscures important diagnostic information.
3. Have the patient remove all objects from the head-and-neck region that may interfere with exposure. The patient must remove eyeglasses, earrings, necklaces, napkin chains, hearing aids, hairpins, and complete and partial dentures.

Patient Positioning

Patient positioning varies with each extraoral projection and is discussed in the next section on specific extraoral projection techniques.

EXTRAORAL PROJECTION TECHNIQUES

A variety of projection techniques are used in extraoral imaging (Table 23-1). The purpose, receptor placement, head position, beam alignment, and exposure factors differ for each projection used in lateral jaw imaging, skull imaging, and temporomandibular joint imaging.

Lateral Jaw Imaging

Lateral jaw imaging is used to examine the posterior region of the mandible and is valuable for use in children, in patients with limited jaw opening due to a fracture or swelling, and in patients who have difficulty stabilizing or tolerating intraoral receptor placement. Although lateral jaw imaging is useful, it is important to note that because more diagnostic information is obtained from a panoramic image, it is preferred to the lateral jaw image.

As the term *lateral jaw imaging* indicates, the receptor in this extraoral projection is positioned lateral to the jaw during exposure. Lateral jaw imaging does not require the use of a special x-ray unit; a standard intraoral x-ray machine can be used. The following two techniques are used with lateral jaw projection:

- Body of mandible
- Ramus of mandible

Body of Mandible

Purpose. The purpose of the **lateral jaw projection–body of mandible** is to evaluate impacted teeth, fractures, and lesions located in the body of the mandible. This projection demonstrates the mandibular premolar and molar regions as well as the inferior border of the mandible (Figure 23-4).

Receptor Placement. The cassette is placed flat against the patient's cheek and is centered over the body of the mandible. The cassette must also be positioned parallel with the body of the mandible. The patient must hold the cassette in position, with the thumb placed under the edge of the cassette and the palm against the outer surface of the cassette.

Head Position. The head is tipped approximately 15 degrees toward the side being imaged. The chin is extended and elevated slightly.

Beam Alignment. The central ray is directed to a point just below the inferior border of the mandible on the side *opposite* the cassette. The beam is directed upward (−15 to −20 degrees) and centered on the body of the mandible. The beam must be directed perpendicular to the horizontal plane of the receptor.

Exposure Factors. Exposure factors for this lateral jaw projection vary with the receptor, intensifying screens, and equipment used.

Ramus of Mandible

Purpose. The purpose of the **lateral jaw projection–ramus of mandible** is to evaluate impacted third molars, large lesions, and fractures that extend into the ramus of the mandible. This projection demonstrates a view of the ramus from the angle of the mandible to the condyle (Figure 23-5).

Receptor Placement. The cassette is placed flat against the patient's cheek and is centered over the ramus of the mandible. The cassette is also positioned parallel with the ramus of the mandible. The patient must hold the cassette in position, with the thumb placed under the edge of the cassette and the palm placed against the outer surface of the cassette.

Head Position. The head is tipped approximately 15 degrees toward the side being imaged. The chin is extended and elevated slightly.

Beam Alignment. The central ray is directed to a point posterior to the third molar region on the side *opposite* the cassette. The beam is directed upward (−15 to −20 degrees) and centered on the ramus of the mandible. The beam must be directed perpendicular to the horizontal plane of the receptor.

Exposure Factors. Exposure factors for this lateral jaw projection vary with the receptor, intensifying screens, and equipment used.

Skull Imaging

Skull imaging is used to examine the bones of the face and skull and is most often used in oral surgery and orthodontics. Although some skull projections can be exposed using a standard intraoral x-ray machine, most require the use of an extraoral unit and a cephalostat.

Images of the skull may be difficult to interpret because of the numerous anatomic structures that exist in a very small

TABLE 23-1   Extraoral Projection Techniques

Projection	Receptor Placement	Head Position	X-Ray Beam Point of Entry
Lateral jaw, body (mandible)	Flat against cheek	Tipped 15 degrees toward side being imaged	Below inferior border of mandible
	Centered over body of mandible	Chin extended and elevated	Vertical angulation −15 to −20 degrees ⊥ to horizontal plane of cassette
Lateral jaw, ramus (mandible)	Flat against cheek	Tipped 15 degrees toward side being imaged	Posterior to third molar area
	Centered over ramus of mandible	Chin extended and elevated	Vertical angulation −15 to −20 degrees ⊥ to horizontal plane of cassette
Lateral cephalometric	Cassette ⊥ to floor	Left side near cassette	Center of cassette
	Long axis horizontal	MSP ⊥ to floor	⊥ to cassette
		FP ‖ to floor	
Posteroanterior	Cassette ⊥ to floor	Forehead and nose touch cassette	Center of cassette
	Long axis vertical	MSP ⊥ to floor	⊥ to cassette
		FP ‖ to floor	
Waters	Cassette ⊥ to floor	Chin touches cassette	Center of cassette
	Long axis vertical	Tip of nose 1−2 inches from cassette	⊥ to cassette
		MSP ⊥ to floor	
Submentovertex	Cassette ⊥ to floor	Head tipped back	Center of cassette
	Long axis vertical	Top of head touches cassette	⊥ to cassette
		MSP and FP ⊥ to floor	
Reverse Towne	Cassette ⊥ to floor	Head tipped down	Center of cassette
	Long axis vertical	Mouth open	⊥ to cassette
		Top of forehead touches cassette	
		MSP ⊥ to floor	
Transcranial	Flat against ear	MSP ⊥ to floor	2 inches above and 0.5 inch below the ear canal opening
	Centered over TMJ		Vertical angulation +25 degrees
			Horizontal angulation 20 degrees

FP, Frankfort plane; *MSP*, midsagittal plane; *TMJ*, temporomandibular joint; ⊥, perpendicular; ‖, parallel.

area; these structures often appear superimposed over each other. In many cases, multiple exposures may be necessary to obtain a clear view of the area in question. The most common skull images used in dentistry include the following:

- Lateral cephalometric projection
- Posteroanterior projection
- Waters projection
- Submentovertex projection
- Reverse Towne projection

Lateral Cephalometric Projection

Purpose. The purpose of the **lateral cephalometric projection** is to evaluate facial growth and development, trauma, and disease and developmental abnormalities. This projection demonstrates the bones of the face and skull as well as the soft tissue profile of the face (Figure 23-6).

The soft tissue outline of the face is more readily seen on the resulting image when a filter is used. A filter is placed at the x-ray source or between the patient and the receptor and serves to remove some of the x-rays that pass through the soft tissue of the face, thus enhancing the image of the soft tissue profile of the face.

Receptor Placement. The cassette is placed perpendicular to the floor in a cassette-holding device. The long axis of the cassette is positioned *horizontally*.

Head Position. The left side of the patient's head is positioned adjacent to the cassette. The midsagittal plane (an imaginary line that divides the face in half) must be aligned perpendicular to the floor and parallel to the cassette. The Frankfort plane (a line extending from the top of the ear canal to the bottom of the eye socket) is aligned parallel to the floor. The head is centered over the cassette.

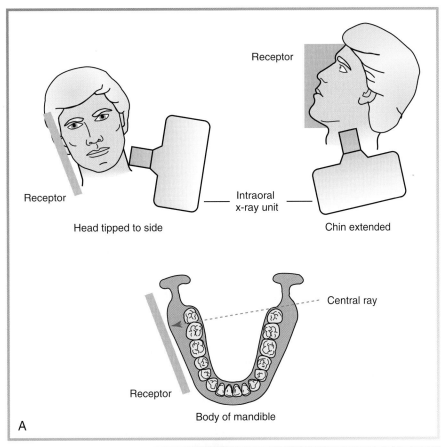

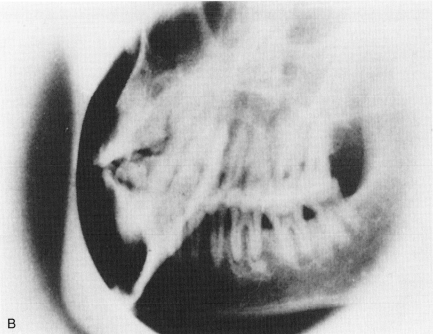

FIGURE 23-4 A, For the lateral jaw projection of the body of the mandible, proper patient positioning and receptor positioning are shown as viewed from the front and side of the patient. **B,** Example of lateral jaw image–body of mandible. (**A** and **B,** Courtesy of Dr. Robert M. Jaynes, Assistant Professor, Oral Radiology Group, The Ohio State University College of Dentistry.)

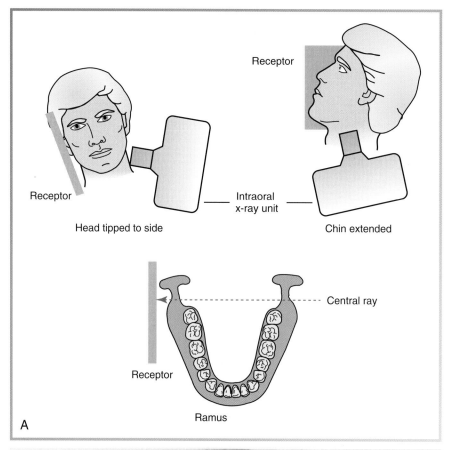

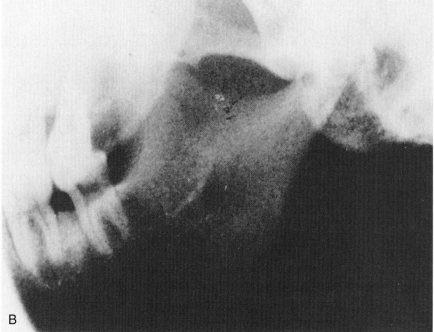

FIGURE 23-5 **A**, For the lateral jaw projection of the ramus of the mandible, proper patient positioning and receptor positioning are shown as viewed from the front and side of the patient. **B**, Example of lateral jaw image–ramus of mandible. (**A** and **B**, Courtesy of Dr. Robert M. Jaynes, Assistant Professor, Oral Radiology Group, The Ohio State University College of Dentistry.)

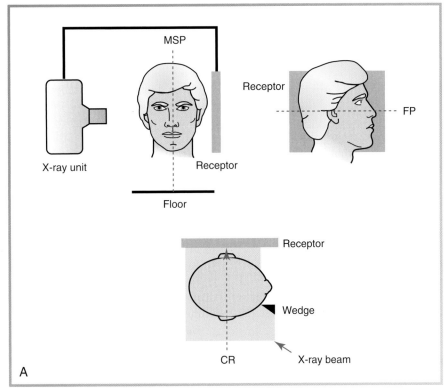

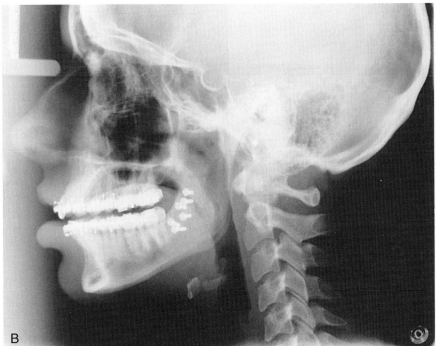

FIGURE 23-6 A, For the lateral cephalometric projection, proper patient positioning and receptor positioning are shown as viewed from the front, side, and top of the patient. *MSP*, Midsagittal plane; *FP*, Frankfort plane; *CR*, central ray. **B**, Example of lateral cephalometric image. (**A** and **B**, Courtesy of Dr. Robert M. Jaynes, Assistant Professor, Oral Radiology Group, The Ohio State University College of Dentistry.)

Beam Alignment. The central ray is directed through the center of the cassette and perpendicular to the cassette.

Exposure Factors. Exposure factors for the lateral cephalometric projection vary with the receptor, intensifying screens, and equipment used.

Posteroanterior Projection

Purpose. The purpose of the **posteroanterior projection** is to evaluate facial growth and development, trauma, and disease and developmental abnormalities. This projection also demonstrates the frontal and ethmoid sinuses, the orbits, and the nasal cavity (Figure 23-7).

Receptor Placement. The cassette is positioned perpendicular to the floor in a cassette-holding device. The long axis of the cassette is positioned *vertically*.

Head Position. The patient faces the cassette; the forehead and nose both touch the cassette. The midsagittal plane is aligned perpendicular to the floor, and the Frankfort plane is aligned parallel to the floor. The head is centered over the cassette.

Beam Alignment. The central ray is directed through the center of the head and perpendicular to the cassette.

Exposure Factors. Exposure factors for the posteroanterior projection vary with the receptor, intensifying screens, and equipment used.

Waters Projection

Purpose. The purpose of the **Waters projection** is to evaluate the maxillary sinus area. This projection also demonstrates the frontal and ethmoid sinuses, the orbits, and the nasal cavity (Figure 23-8).

Receptor Placement. The cassette is positioned perpendicular to the floor in a cassette-holding device. The long axis of the cassette is positioned *vertically*.

Head Position. The patient faces the cassette and elevates the chin; the chin touches the cassette, and the tip of the nose is positioned $\frac{1}{2}$ to 1 inch away from the cassette. The midsagittal plane must be aligned perpendicular to the floor, and the head is centered over the cassette.

Beam Alignment. The central ray is directed through the center of the head and perpendicular to the cassette.

Exposure Factors. Exposure factors for the Waters projection vary with the receptor, intensifying screens, and equipment used.

Submentovertex Projection

Purpose. The purpose of the **submentovertex projection** is to identify the position of the condyles, demonstrate the base of the skull, and evaluate fractures of the zygomatic arch. This projection also demonstrates the sphenoid and ethmoid sinuses and the lateral wall of the maxillary sinus (Figure 23-9).

Receptor Placement. The cassette is positioned perpendicular to the floor in a cassette-holding device. The long axis of the cassette is positioned *vertically*.

Head Position. The patient's head and neck are tipped back as far as possible; the vertex (top) of the skull touches the cassette. Both the midsagittal plane and the Frankfort plane are aligned perpendicular to the floor. The head is centered on the cassette.

Beam Alignment. The central ray is directed through the center of the head and perpendicular to the cassette.

Exposure Factors. Exposure factors for this projection vary with the receptor, intensifying screens, and equipment used. If the zygomatic arch is the area of interest, the exposure time is reduced to approximately one third the normal exposure time for a submentovertex projection.

Reverse Towne Projection

Purpose. The purpose of the **reverse Towne projection** is to identify fractures of the condylar neck and ramus area (Figure 23-10).

Receptor Placement. The cassette is positioned perpendicular to the floor in a cassette-holding device. The long axis of the cassette is positioned *vertically*.

Head Position. The patient faces the cassette, with the head tipped down and the mouth open as wide as possible; the chin rests on the chest, and the top of the forehead touches the cassette. The midsagittal plane must be aligned perpendicular to the floor, and the head is centered on the cassette.

Beam Alignment. The central ray is directed through the center of the head and perpendicular to the cassette.

Exposure Factors. Exposure factors for the reverse Towne projection vary with the receptor, intensifying screens, and equipment used.

Temporomandibular Joint Imaging

The **temporomandibular joint (TMJ)** is the jaw joint. As the term *temporomandibular* indicates, this joint includes the temporal bone and the mandible. The glenoid fossa and the articular eminence of the temporal bone, the condyle of the mandible, and the articular disc between the bones make up the TMJ area. This area can be very difficult to examine on an image because of multiple adjacent bony structures.

Imaging cannot be used to examine the articular disc and other soft tissue areas of the TMJ; instead, specialized imaging techniques (e.g., arthrography and magnetic resonance imaging [MRI]) must be used. Imaging, however, can be used to show bone and the relationship of the joint components. For example, changes in bone (e.g., erosions, bony deposits) can be seen on TMJ images. The following two techniques are used in TMJ imaging:

- Transcranial projection
- Temporomandibular joint tomography

Transcranial Projection (Lindblom Technique)

Purpose. The purpose of the **transcranial projection** is to evaluate the superior surface of the condyle and the articular eminence (Figure 23-11). This projection can also be used to

Text continued on page 287

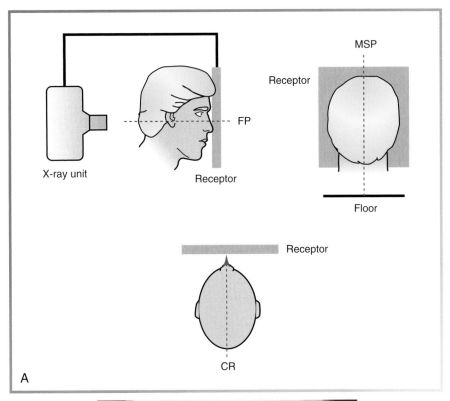

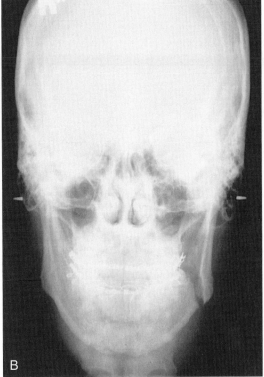

FIGURE 23-7 A, For the posteroanterior skull projection, proper patient positioning and receptor positioning are shown as viewed from the side, back, and top of the patient. *MSP*, Midsagittal plane; *FP*, Frankfort plane; *CR*, central ray. **B**, Example of a posteroanterior skull image. (**A** and **B**, Courtesy of Dr. Robert M. Jaynes, Assistant Professor, Oral Radiology Group, The Ohio State University College of Dentistry.)

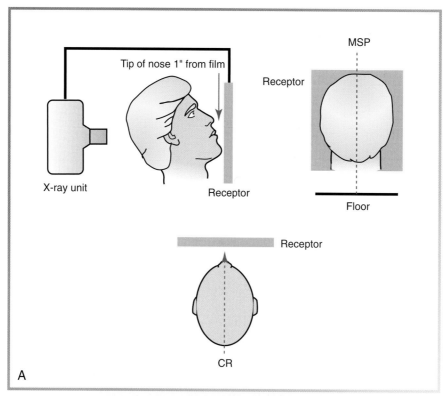

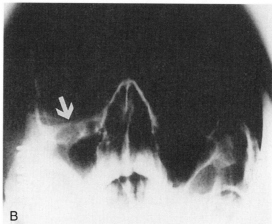

FIGURE 23-8 A, For the Waters projection, proper patient positioning and receptor positioning are shown as viewed from the side, back, and top of the patient. *MSP,* Midsagittal plane; *CR,* central ray. **B,** This case of chronic maxillary sinusitis secondary to an oroantral fistula shows thickening of the lining membrane (*arrow*) (Waters view). (**A,** Courtesy of Dr. Robert M. Jaynes, Assistant Professor, Oral Radiology Group, The Ohio State University College of Dentistry; **B,** from Pedersen GW: *Oral surgery,* Philadelphia, 1988, Saunders.)

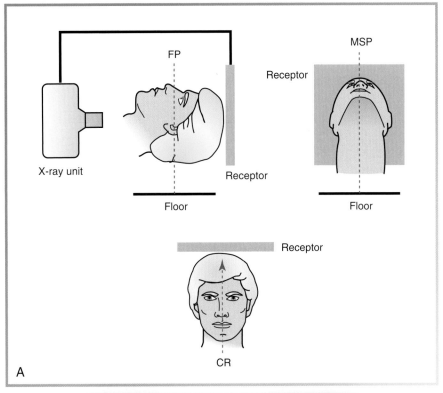

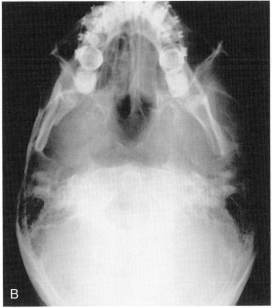

FIGURE 23-9 A, For the submentovertex projection, proper patient positioning and receptor positioning are shown as viewed from the side, front, and top of the patient. *MSP*, Midsagittal plane; *FP*, Frankfort plane; *CR*, central ray. **B**, Example of a submentovertex image. (**A** and **B**, Courtesy of Dr. Robert M. Jaynes, Assistant Professor, Oral Radiology Group, The Ohio State University College of Dentistry.)

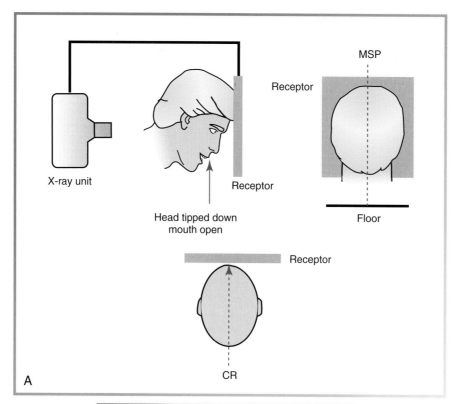

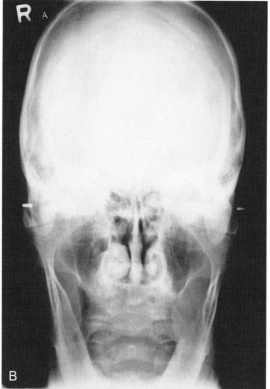

FIGURE 23-10 A, For the reverse Towne projection, proper patient positioning and receptor positioning are shown as viewed from the side, back, and top of the patient. *MSP,* midsagittal plane; *CR,* central ray. **B,** Example of a reverse Towne image. (**A** and **B,** Courtesy of Dr. Robert M. Jaynes, Assistant Professor, Oral Radiology Group, The Ohio State University College of Dentistry.)

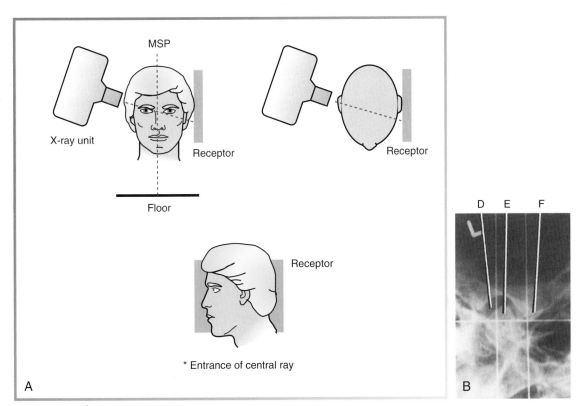

FIGURE 23-11 A, For the transcranial projection, proper patient positioning and receptor positioning are shown as viewed from the front, top, and side of the patient. *MSP,* midsagittal plane. **B,** Transcranial view of temporomandibular joint in the rest position. **D,** Glenoid fossa; **E,** head of mandibular condyle; **F,** articular eminence. (**A,** Courtesy of Dr. Robert M. Jaynes, Assistant Professor, Oral Radiology Group, The Ohio State University College of Dentistry; **B,** from Kasle MJ: *An atlas of dental radiographic anatomy,* ed 4, Philadelphia, 1994, Saunders.)

evaluate movement of the condyle when the mouth is opened and to compare the joint spaces (right versus left).

Receptor Placement. The cassette is placed flat against the patient's ear and is centered over the TMJ.

Head Position. The midsagittal plane must be aligned perpendicular to the floor and parallel to the cassette.

Beam Alignment. The central ray is directed toward a point 2 inches above and 0.5 inch behind the opening of the ear canal. The beam is directed downward (+25 degrees) and forward (20 degrees) and is centered on the TMJ that is being imaged.

Exposure Factors. Exposure factors for the transcranial projection vary with the receptor, intensifying screens, and equipment used.

The intraoral x-ray unit can be used in the exposure of a transcranial projection. Special positioning devices can be used to coordinate the alignment of the receptor, the patient's head, and the beam to obtain an accurate transcranial image. Such devices are also used to reproduce the same patient positioning in subsequent exposures, thereby permitting comparison of images.

Temporomandibular Joint Tomography

The technique of **temporomandibular joint tomography** is used to examine the TMJ. *Tomography,* as defined in Chapter 22, is a technique used to show structures located within a selected plane of tissue while blurring structures outside the selected plane. In TMJ tomography, this is accomplished by moving the receptor and x-ray tubehead in opposite directions around a fixed rotation point. The location of this rotation point determines what plane of the head will be imaged (Figure 23-12).

TMJ tomography provides the most definitive imaging of the bony components of the TMJ. As a result, the condyle, the articular eminence, and the glenoid fossa can all be examined on an image known as the **tomogram.** In addition, the tomogram can be used to estimate joint space and evaluate the extent of movement of the condyle when the mouth is open.

A special tomographic x-ray unit is required for TMJ tomography. Most dental practitioners do not purchase such specialized equipment because of the prohibitive cost. Therefore, dental patients who require TMJ tomography are usually referred to a specialized imaging facility. Further discussion about the specifics of TMJ tomography is beyond the scope of this text.

SUMMARY

- The extraoral receptor is placed outside the mouth during x-ray exposure.
- Uses of extraoral projections include (1) evaluation of large areas of skull and jaws; (2) evaluation of growth

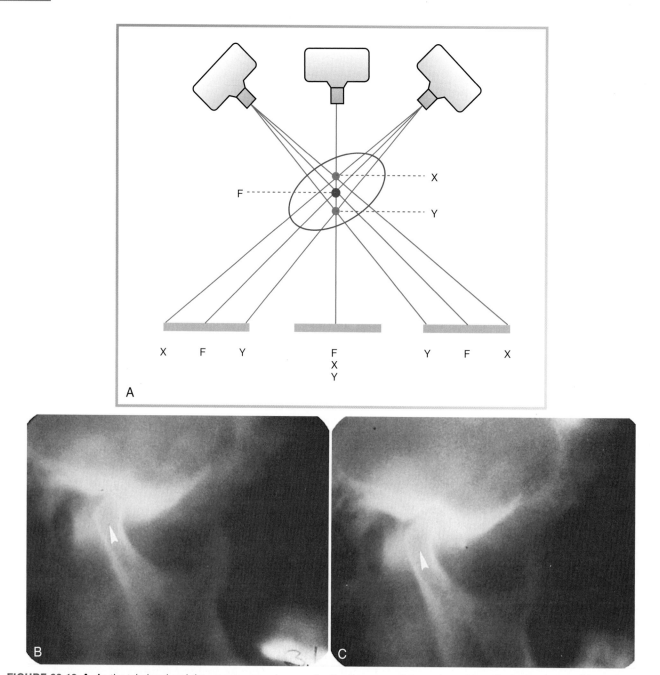

FIGURE 23-12 A, As the tubehead and the receptor move in opposite directions around the patient, objects in the image layer (*F*) appear sharp on the image. Objects on either side of the image layer (*X, Y*) are blurred. **B** and **C**, Corrected axis tomograms showing decreased joint space and posterior positioning of the left condyle (*arrowheads*) caused by the anteriorly placed meniscus. (**A**, Courtesy of Dr. Robert M. Jaynes, Assistant Professor, Oral Radiology Group, The Ohio State University College of Dentistry; **B** and **C**, From Kasle MJ: *An atlas of dental radiographic anatomy*, ed 4, Philadelphia, 1994, Saunders.)

and development; (3) evaluation of impacted teeth; (4) detection of diseases, lesions, and conditions of the jaws; (5) examination of the extent of large lesions; (6) evaluation of trauma; and (7) evaluation of the TMJ area.

- Special equipment, including the x-ray unit, receptors, screen film, intensifying screens, grid, and cassette, is necessary for extraoral imaging.

- Before preparing the patient for exposure of an extraoral projection, the cassette must be prepared, infection control procedures completed, and exposure factors selected.

- After preparing the equipment, the dental radiographer must explain the imaging procedures to the patient, place the lead apron, and have the patient remove all radiodense objects from the head-and-neck region.

- A variety of projection techniques are used in extraoral imaging; the choice depends on what information is needed.

BIBLIOGRAPHY

Danforth RA, Dus I, Mah J: 3-D volume imaging for dentistry: a new dimension. *J Calif Dent Assoc* 31(11):817–823, 2003.

Frommer HH, Savage-Stabulas JJ: Extraoral techniques. In *Radiology for the dental professional*, ed 9, St. Louis, 2011, Mosby.

Johnson ON, McNally MA, Essay CE: Extraoral radiography. In *Essentials of dental radiography for dental assistants and hygienists*, ed 8, Upper Saddle River, NJ, 2007, Pearson Education, Inc.

Miles DA, Van Dis ML, Jensen CW, Williamson GF: Extraoral radiography. In *Radiographic imaging for dental auxiliaries*, ed 4, St. Louis, 2009, Saunders.

Miles DA, Van Dis ML, Razmus TF: Plain film extraoral radiographic techniques. In *Basic principles of oral and maxillofacial radiology*, Philadelphia, 1992, Saunders.

Olson SS: Auxiliary radiographic techniques. In *Dental radiography laboratory manual*, Philadelphia, 1995, Saunders.

White SC, Pharoah MJ: Advanced imaging. In *Oral radiology: principles of interpretation*, ed 6, St. Louis, 2009, Mosby.

White SC, Pharoah MJ: Extraoral radiographic examinations. In *Oral radiology: principles of interpretation*, ed 6, St. Louis, 2009, Mosby.

QUIZ QUESTIONS

ESSAY

Describe the head position, receptor placement, and beam alignment for each of the following extraoral images:

1. Lateral jaw projection–body of mandible
2. Lateral jaw projection–ramus of mandible
3. Lateral cephalometric projection
4. Posteroanterior projection
5. Waters projection
6. Submentovertex projection
7. Reverse Towne projection
8. Transcranial projection

MULTIPLE CHOICE

____ 9. Which of the following projections is best for the examination of the maxillary sinus?
   a. lateral jaw projection
   b. reverse Towne projection
   c. Waters projection
   d. submentovertex projection

____ 10. Which of the following projections is best for the examination of fractures of the zygomatic arch?
   a. submentovertex projection
   b. reverse Towne projection
   c. Waters projection
   d. lateral cephalometric projection

____ 11. Which of the following projections is best for examination of fractures of the condylar neck?
   a. submentovertex projection
   b. Waters projection
   c. lateral cephalometric projection
   d. reverse Towne projection

____ 12. Which of the following projections is best for the examination of the soft tissue profile of the face?
   a. transcranial projection
   b. lateral cephalometric projection
   c. reverse Towne projection
   d. posteroanterior projection

____ 13. Which of the following projections is best for the examination of the condyle and articular eminence?
   a. transcranial projection
   b. posteroanterior projection
   c. Waters projection
   d. submentovertex projection

____ 14. Which of the following projections is best for the examination of fractures of the mandibular body?
   a. lateral cephalometric projection
   b. submentovertex projection
   c. lateral jaw projection
   d. transcranial projection

____ 15. Which of the following projections is best for the examination of a large lesion in the ramus?
   a. posteroanterior projection
   b. Waters projection
   c. lateral cephalometric projection
   d. lateral jaw projection

chapter 24

Imaging of Patients with Special Needs

OUTLINE

PATIENTS WITH GAG REFLEX
    Patient Management
    Extreme Cases of Gag Reflex
PATIENTS WITH DISABILITIES
    Physical Disabilities
    Developmental Disabilities

PATIENTS WITH SPECIFIC DENTAL NEEDS
    Pediatric Patients
    Endodontic Patients
    Edentulous Patients

LEARNING OBJECTIVES

After completion of this chapter, the student will be able to do the following:

- Define the key terms associated with patients who have special needs
- List the areas of the oral cavity that are most likely to elicit the gag reflex when stimulated
- List two precipitating factors responsible for initiating the gag reflex
- Describe how to control the gag reflex using operator attitude, patient and equipment preparations, exposure sequencing, and receptor placement and technique
- Describe common physical disabilities and what modifications in technique may be necessary during the imaging examination
- Describe common developmental disabilities and what modifications in technique may be necessary during the imaging examination

- List helpful hints that can be used when treating a person with a disability
- Describe the prescribing of dental images, patient and equipment preparations, recommended techniques, and patient management as they pertain to the pediatric dental patient
- Describe the use of receptor placement modifications, and recommended periapical technique during root canal procedures
- Describe the purposes of the imaging examination in the edentulous patient
- List and describe the three types of imaging examination that may be used for the edentulous patient

KEY TERMS

Disability	Endodontic	Pediatric
Disability, developmental	Endodontic patient	Pediatric patient
Disability, physical	Endodontics	Pediatrics
Edentulous	Gag reflex	Stimuli, psychogenic
Edentulous patient	Gagging	Stimuli, tactile

Not all dental imaging techniques can be successfully performed on all patients. Imaging examination techniques must often be modified to accommodate patients with special needs. The dental radiographer must be competent in altering the techniques to meet the specific diagnostic needs of individual patients.

The purpose of this chapter is to introduce the dental radiographer to the issues in dealing with patients with special needs. In addition, this chapter provides specific information on how to manage patients with a hypersensitive gag reflex, patients with physical or developmental disabilities, pediatric patients, endodontic patients, and edentulous patients.

PATIENTS WITH GAG REFLEX

The term **gagging** (also called *retching*) refers to the strong, involuntary effort to vomit. The **gag reflex** (also called the *pharyngeal reflex*) can be defined as retching that is elicited by stimulation of the sensitive tissues of the soft palate region. The gag reflex is a protective mechanism of the body that serves to clear the airway of obstruction. All patients have gag reflexes, although some are more sensitive than others. In dental imaging, a hypersensitive gag reflex is a problem that is commonly encountered.

The areas that are most likely to elicit the gag reflex when stimulated include the soft palate and the lateral posterior third of the tongue. Before the gag reflex is initiated, the following two reactions occur:

- Cessation of respiration
- Contraction of the muscles in the throat and abdomen

Precipitating factors for the initiation of the gag reflex include **psychogenic stimuli** (stimuli originating in the mind) and **tactile stimuli** (stimuli originating from touch). To suppress the gag reflex, the dental radiographer must eliminate or lessen these precipitating factors.

Patient Management

To effectively manage the patient with a hypersensitive gag reflex, the dental radiographer must be aware of the following:

- Operator attitude
- Patient and equipment preparations
- Exposure sequencing
- Receptor placement and technique

Operator Attitude

To prevent the gag reflex, the dental radiographer must convey a confident attitude. The patient must be confident of the radiographer's ability to perform imaging procedures and must be sure that the receptor will not slip and lodge in the throat. If the dental radiographer does not appear to be in complete control of the procedures, the patient interprets this as a lack of confidence. This lack of confidence may act as a psychogenic stimulus and elicit the gag reflex.

In addition, the dental radiographer must also convey patience, tolerance, and understanding. Every effort should be made to relax and reassure the patient with a hypersensitive gag reflex. The dental radiographer should explain the imaging procedures about to be performed and then compliment the patient as each exposure is completed. As the patient becomes comfortable with the imaging procedures, he or she becomes more confident and, as a result, is less likely to gag.

Patient and Equipment Preparations

Patient and equipment preparations can help prevent the gag reflex (see Chapters 17, 18, and 19). In the patient with a hypersensitive gag reflex, every effort should be made to limit the amount of time that a receptor remains in the mouth.

The longer a receptor stays in the mouth, the more likely the patient is to gag. When patient and equipment preparations are completed *before* receptor placement, valuable time is saved, and the likelihood of stimulating the gag reflex is reduced.

Exposure Sequencing

Exposure sequencing plays an important role in preventing the gag reflex. As discussed in Chapters 17 to 19, the dental radiographer should always begin with anterior exposures. Anterior receptors are easier for the patient to tolerate and are less likely to elicit the gag reflex. With posterior receptor placements, the dental radiographer should always expose the premolar receptor before the molar receptor. Of all receptor placements, *the maxillary molar receptor is the most likely to elicit the gag reflex.* In the patient with a hypersensitive gag reflex, the exposure sequence should be altered so that the maxillary molar receptors are exposed last.

Receptor Placement and Technique

Receptor placement and technique also play an important role in preventing the gag reflex. To avoid stimulating the gag reflex, *each receptor must be placed and exposed as quickly as possible.* Placement and technique modifications include the following:

- *Avoid the palate.* When placing receptors in the maxillary posterior areas, do not slide the receptor along the palate. Sliding the receptor along the palate stimulates this sensitive area and causes the gag reflex. Instead, position the receptor lingual to the teeth, and then firmly bring the receptor into contact with the palatal tissues using one decisive motion.
- *Demonstrate receptor placement.* In the areas that are most likely to elicit the gag reflex, rub a finger along the tissues near the intended area of receptor placement while telling the patient, "This is where the receptor will be positioned." Then place the receptor quickly. This technique demonstrates where the receptor will be placed and desensitizes the tissues in the area.

Extreme Cases of Gag Reflex

Occasionally the dental radiographer encounters a patient with a gag reflex that is uncontrollable. In such a patient, intraoral images are impossible to obtain. Instead, the dental radiographer must resort to extraoral images such as panoramic or lateral jaw images to obtain diagnostic information.

HELPFUL HINTS

To reduce the gag reflex:

- **NEVER** suggest gagging. The dental radiographer must never bring up the subject of gagging or ask the patient such questions as "Are you a gagger?" or "Do you gag?" The power of suggestion can act as a strong psychogenic stimulus and can, in turn, elicit the gag reflex. When the patient brings up the subject of gagging, the dental radiographer must refrain from using the terms *gag*, *gagging*, and *gagger*; instead, the radiographer should refer to the gag reflex as "a tickle in the back of the throat" when discussing the topic with the patient.

- **DO** reassure the patient. If the patient gags, the dental radiographer must remove the receptor as quickly as possible and then reassure the patient. The patient with a hypersensitive gag reflex must be reassured that such a response is not unusual. Some patients are very embarrassed, and others may even cry. The dental radiographer must always maintain control of the situation while remaining calm and understanding.
- **DO** suggest deep breathing. The dental radiographer should instruct the patient to "breathe deeply" through the nose during receptor placement and exposure. The breathing should be audible, and the dental radiographer should demonstrate it to the patient. As previously stated, respiration must cease for the gag reflex to occur; therefore, if the patient maintains breathing, the gag reflex cannot occur.
- **DO** try to distract the patient. Distraction often helps suppress the gag reflex. The dental radiographer can instruct the patient to do one of the following during receptor placement and exposure: (1) bite as hard as possible on the bite-block or the tab or (2) position a leg or arm in the air. These acts help divert the patient's attention and lessen the likelihood of the gag reflex being elicited.
- **DO** try to reduce tactile stimuli. Reducing tactile stimuli helps prevent the gag reflex. The dental radiographer can try one of the following techniques before placing and exposing the receptor: (1) giving the patient a cup of ice water to drink or (2) placing a small amount of ordinary table salt on the tip of the tongue. These techniques help confuse the sensory nerve endings and lessen the likelihood of the gag reflex being stimulated.
- **DO** use a topical anesthetic. In the patient with a severe hypersensitive gag reflex, a topical anesthetic spray may be used. The spray is used to numb the areas that elicit the gag reflex. The dental radiographer should instruct the patient to exhale while the anesthetic is sprayed on the soft palate and posterior tongue. Caution must be used to ensure that the patient does not inhale the spray, which may cause inflammation of the lungs. The topical anesthetic spray takes effect after 1 minute and lasts for approximately 20 minutes. Topical anesthetic sprays should not be used in patients who are allergic to benzocaine.

PATIENTS WITH DISABILITIES

A **disability** can be defined as a "physical or mental impairment that substantially limits one or more of an individual's major life activities." In the dental office, persons with both physical and developmental disabilities are encountered. The dental radiographer must be prepared to modify imaging techniques to accommodate persons with disabilities.

Physical Disabilities

A person with a **physical disability** may have problems with vision, hearing, or mobility. The dental radiographer must make every effort to meet the individual needs of such patients. The person with a physical disability often is accompanied to the dental office by a family member or other caregiver. Caregivers can be asked to assist the dental radiographer with communication or with the patient's physical needs. The dental radiographer must be aware of the common physical disabilities involving vision, hearing, and mobility and the necessary modifications to the procedure for patients who have such problems.

Vision Impairment

If a person is blind or visually impaired, the dental radiographer must communicate using clear verbal explanations. The dental radiographer must keep the patient informed of what is being done and explain each step of the procedure before performing it. The dental radiographer must never gesture to another person in the presence of a person who is blind. Blind persons are sensitive to this type of communication and perceive this as the dental radiographer "talking behind their backs."

Hearing Impairment

With regard to a person is deaf or hearing impaired, the dental radiographer has several options. The radiographer may ask the caregiver to act as an interpreter, use gestures or sign language, or use written instructions. When the patient can read lips, the dental radiographer must face the patient and speak clearly and slowly.

Mobility Impairment

If a person is in a wheelchair and does not have use of the lower limbs, the dental radiographer should initially ask the patient how he or she would prefer to transfer to the dental chair. The dental radiographer may offer to assist the patient in transferring to the dental chair or ask the caregiver to assist in the transfer. If a transfer is not possible, the dental radiographer may attempt to perform the necessary imaging procedures with the patient seated in the wheelchair.

If a person does not have use of the upper limbs and a beam alignment device cannot be used to stabilize receptor placement, the dental radiographer may ask the caregiver to assist with the holding of the receptor. In such cases, the caregiver must wear a lead apron and thyroid collar during exposure of the receptors. In addition, the caregiver must be given specific instructions on how to hold the receptor for the patient. As stated in previous chapters, the dental radiographer must *never* hold a receptor for a patient during an x-ray exposure.

Developmental Disabilities

A **developmental disability** is "a substantial impairment of mental or physical functioning that occurs before the age of

22 and is of indefinite duration." Examples include autism, cerebral palsy, epilepsy and other neuropathies, and mental retardation. The dental radiographer must make every effort to meet the individual needs of the patient with a developmental disability.

A person with a developmental disability may have problems with coordination or with comprehension of instructions. As a result, the dental radiographer may experience difficulties in obtaining intraoral images. If coordination is a problem, mild sedation may be useful. If comprehension is a problem, the caregiver may be asked to assist with the holding of the receptor.

It is important that the dental radiographer recognize situations in which the patient cannot tolerate intraoral exposures. In such cases, *no intraoral exposures must be done*; such exposures result only in nondiagnostic images and needless radiation exposure of the patient. In these patients, extraoral exposures (e.g., lateral jaw and panoramic) may be used.

HELPFUL HINTS

For treating a patient with a disability:

- **DO NOT** ask personal questions about a disability; such questions are inappropriate in the dental setting.
- **DO** offer assistance to a person with a disability. For example, offer to push a wheelchair or to guide a person who is blind. The person with a disability will indicate whether help is needed or not and is often specific about how the assistance should be provided. For example, a person who is blind may prefer to hold the arm of a person offering guidance rather than having an arm held.
- **DO** talk directly to the person with a disability. It is inappropriate to talk to the caregiver instead of talking to the patient; for example, instead of asking the caretaker, "Can he [or she] transfer out of the wheelchair?" the radiographer should speak directly to the patient in the wheelchair. In addition, it is inappropriate to talk to the caregiver about a person with a disability as if that person were not present; the same is also true when an interpreter accompanies a deaf person.

PATIENTS WITH SPECIFIC DENTAL NEEDS

Different patients have different diagnostic dental requirements based on specific needs. Dental imaging examination techniques must often be modified to accommodate patients with specific dental needs, including pediatric, endodontic, and edentulous patients.

Pediatric Patients

A **pediatric patient** is a child; the term **pediatric** is derived from the Greek word *pedia* meaning child. **Pediatrics** is the branch of dentistry dealing with the diagnosis and treatment of dental diseases in children. In children, dental images are useful for detecting lesions as well as conditions of teeth and bones, for showing changes secondary to caries and trauma, and for evaluating growth and development. When treating pediatric patients, the dental radiographer must be aware of the following:

- Prescribing of dental images
- Patient and equipment preparations
- Recommended techniques
- Patient management

Prescribing of Dental Images

As described in Chapter 5, the prescribing of dental images is based on individual needs of patients. The *Guidelines for Prescribing Dental Radiographs* include recommendations for both children and adults (see Table 5-1). For the pediatric patient, the prescribed number and type of dental images depend not only on the individual needs of the child but also on the age of the child and his or her ability to cooperate during the procedures.

Patient and Equipment Preparations

Patient and equipment preparations for the pediatric patient are identical to those described for the adult patient (see Chapters 17 to 19). With the pediatric patient, however, special attention must be devoted to the following preparations:

- *Explanation of procedure.* The imaging procedures that are to be performed must be explained to the child in terms that are easily understood by the child. For example, the dental radiographer can refer to the tubehead as a "camera," the lead apron as a "coat," and the image as a "picture."
- *Lead apron.* The growing tissues of a child are particularly vulnerable to the effects of ionizing radiation and must be protected. As a result, a lead apron and thyroid collar must be placed on a child before radiographic exposure.
- *Exposure factors.* Exposure factors (milliamperage, kilovoltage, time) must be reduced because of the size of the pediatric patient. A reduced exposure time is preferred; the shorter exposure time will reduce the chance of a blurred image should the child move. All exposure factors should be set according to the recommendations of the receptor manufacturer.
- *Receptor size.* As described in Chapter 7, size 0 receptor is recommended for use in the pediatric patient with a primary dentition because of the small mouth size. In the child with a transitional dentition, size 1 or 2 receptor is recommended. As described in Chapter 21, a size 2 receptor is preferred for maxillary and mandibular occlusal exposures in children.

Recommended Techniques

The techniques used to expose intraoral projections in pediatric patients are basically the same as those used in adults. With periapical projections, either the bisecting technique or the paralleling technique can be used (see Chapters 17 and

TABLE 24-1   Dental Imaging Examination of the Pediatric Patient

Dentition	Number of Projections	Type of Projection	Receptor Size
Primary (3–6 years)	1	Occlusal: maxillary	2
	1	Occlusal: mandibular	2
	2	Bite-wing	0
	2	Periapical: maxillary molar	0
	2	Periapical: mandibular molar	0
Transitional (7–12 years)	3	Periapical: maxillary anterior	1
	3	Periapical: mandibular anterior	1
	2	Bite-wing	1 or 2
	2	Periapical: maxillary molar	1 or 2
	2	Periapical: mandibular molar	1 or 2

18). In children with primary or transitional dentition, the bisecting technique is preferred because the small size of the mouth precludes the placement of a receptor beyond the apical regions of teeth. The bite-wing and occlusal techniques are also used in pediatric patients (see Chapters 19 and 21). Typical examinations of primary and transitional dentitions using these techniques are described in Table 24-1. Figures 24-1 through 24-5 provide examples of occlusal, bite-wing, and panoramic pediatric dental images.

Patient Management

Management of children requires that the dental radiographer be confident, patient, and understanding. The dental radiographer can use the helpful hints listed below in managing the pediatric patient.

HELPFUL HINTS

For managing a pediatric patient:

- **BE CONFIDENT.** Most children react favorably to the authority of a confident and capable operator. The dental radiographer must secure the child's confidence, trust, and cooperation. In addition, the dental radiographer must be patient and must not rush the imaging procedures.
- **SHOW AND TELL.** The typical child is curious. The dental radiographer can use a "show and tell" approach to prepare the patient for imaging procedures. Before beginning any exposures, the dental radiographer can show the child the equipment and materials that will be used and then describe to the child what will happen. The child should be encouraged to touch the tubehead, receptor, beam alignment device, and lead apron.
- **REASSURE THE PATIENT.** The typical child has a fear of the unknown. Because a frightened child is not cooperative, the dental radiographer must reassure the child and allay any fears about the procedures.
- **DEMONSTRATE BEHAVIOR.** With the pediatric patient, the dental radiographer can demonstrate the desired behavior to show the child exactly what to do. For example, the radiographer can demonstrate "how to hold still" and then ask the child to do the same thing.

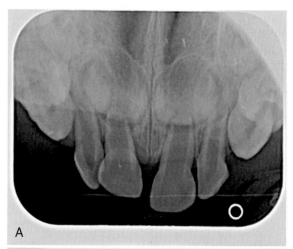

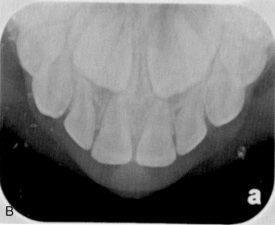

FIGURE 24-1 A & B, Examples of maxillary pediatric occlusal projections, each patient exposed with size 2 intraoral receptors. (Courtesy of Cary Pediatric Dentistry, Cary, NC.)

- **REQUEST ASSISTANCE.** If a child cannot hold still or stabilize the receptor, the dental radiographer can ask the parent or accompanying adult to provide assistance. The adult should wear a lead apron and thyroid collar and hold the receptor or the child during the x-ray exposure.
- **POSTPONE THE EXAMINATION.** Only in emergencies should a child be forced to undergo dental imaging. It is

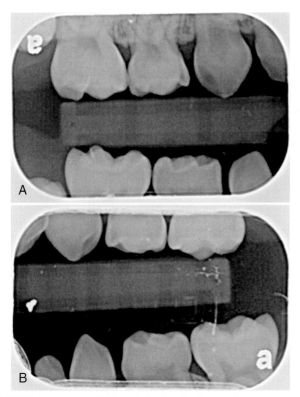

FIGURE 24-2 A & B, Right and left bite-wing images from a 5-year-old patient. (Courtesy of Cary Pediatric Dentistry, Cary, NC.)

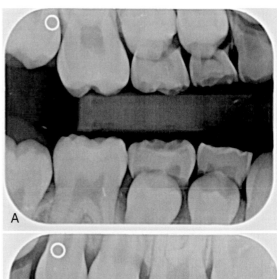

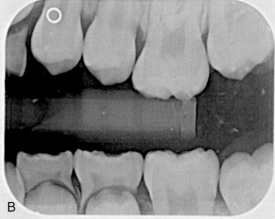

FIGURE 24-4 A & B, Right and left bite-wing images from a young teenage patient demonstrating mixed dentition. (Courtesy of Cary Pediatric Dentistry, Cary NC.)

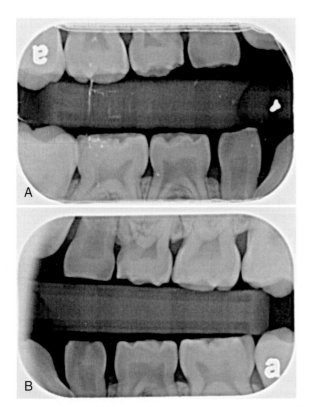

FIGURE 24-3 A & B, Right and left bite-wing images from a 6½-year-old patient. (Courtesy of Cary Pediatric Dentistry, Cary, NC.)

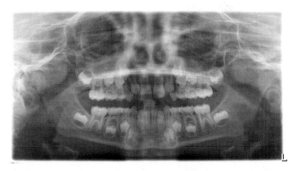

FIGURE 24-5 A panoramic dental image from a 7-year-old patient. (Courtesy of Cary Pediatric Dentistry, Cary, NC.)

much better to postpone the examination until the second or third visit rather than instill in the child a fear of visiting the dental office.

Endodontic Patients

The term **endodontic** is derived from two Greek words, *endon*, meaning "within," and *odontos*, meaning "tooth." **Endodontics** is the branch of dentistry concerned with the

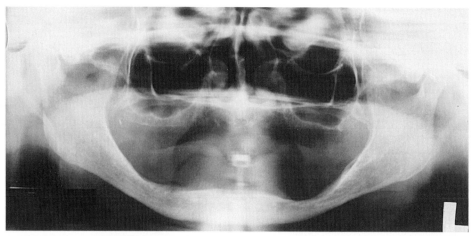

FIGURE 24-6 A panoramic image from an edentulous patient.

diagnosis and treatment of diseases of the dental pulp within the tooth. Endodontic treatment usually involves removal of the dental pulp (nerve tissue) from the pulp chamber and canals within the tooth, then filling the empty pulp chamber and canals with a material such as gutta percha or silver points. This treatment is often referred to as a *root canal procedure* or *root canal therapy*. The **endodontic patient** is one who has undergone root canal therapy.

The dental image is indispensable during root canal procedures and essential for diagnosing and managing pulpal problems. During a root canal procedure, a series of exposures is typically obtained of the same tooth; these exposures are used to evaluate the tooth before, during, and after treatment.

Receptor Placement

The dental radiographer must modify the receptor placement method for the endodontic patient. During a root canal procedure, receptor placement is difficult because of poor visualization of the tooth. The equipment used during a root canal procedure makes it difficult for the dental radiographer to visualize the area well in order to position and stabilize the receptor. Equipment used during a root canal procedure includes a rubber dam, rubber dam clamp, root canal instruments (files, reamers, broaches), and filling materials (gutta percha and silver points).

The EndoRay film holder (see Chapter 6) can be used as an aid in positioning the receptor during a root canal procedure; this holder fits around a rubber dam clamp and allows space for root canal instruments and filling materials to protrude from the tooth. A hemostat or a wooden tongue depressor may also be used to hold the receptor.

Recommended Technique

During a root canal procedure, the length of the pulp canals must be accurately measured without distortion (elongation or foreshortening). To avoid distortion, the paralleling technique (see Chapter 17) should be used whenever possible; the

use of the bisecting technique (see Chapter 18) may result in elongated or foreshortened images. With the paralleling technique, the use of a beam alignment device (e.g., EndoRay) is strongly recommended.

Edentulous Patients

Edentulous means "without teeth." The **edentulous patient**, or patient without teeth, requires a dental imaging examination for the following reasons:

- To detect the presence of root tips, impacted teeth, and lesions (cysts, tumors)
- To identify objects embedded in bone
- To establish the position of normal anatomic landmarks (e.g., mental foramen) relative to the crest of the alveolar ridge
- To observe the quantity and quality of bone that is present

The dental imaging examination of the edentulous patient may include the following projections: panoramic, periapical, or a combination of occlusal and periapical.

Panoramic Examination

A panoramic image (see Chapter 22) is the most common way of examining the edentulous jaw (Figure 24-6). The panoramic examination is quick and easy for the patient and requires only one exposure. If a panoramic image reveals any root tips, impacted teeth, foreign bodies, or lesions in the jaws, a periapical projection of that specific area must be exposed. The periapical image has more definition and permits the area in question to be examined in greater detail.

Periapical Examination

If a panoramic x-ray machine is not available, 14 periapical projections (6 anterior and 8 posterior) can be used to examine the edentulous arches (Figure 24-7). A size 2 receptor is typically used for the edentulous examination. Either the paralleling technique (see Chapter 17) or the bisecting technique (see Chapter 18) can be used for this periapical

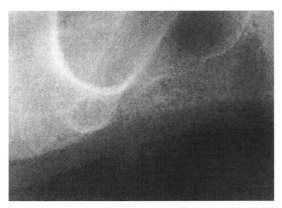

FIGURE 24-7 Projections must be exposed in all teeth-bearing areas of the mouth whether or not teeth are present. (From Olson SS: *Dental radiography laboratory manual*, Philadelphia, 1995, Saunders.)

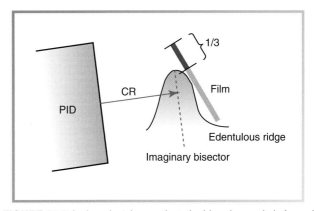

FIGURE 24-8 In the edentulous patient, the bisecting angle is formed by the ridge of bone and the receptor. The central ray (CR) is directed perpendicular to the imaginary bisector. Approximately one third of the receptor should extend beyond the edentulous ridge. *PID,* Position-indicating device.

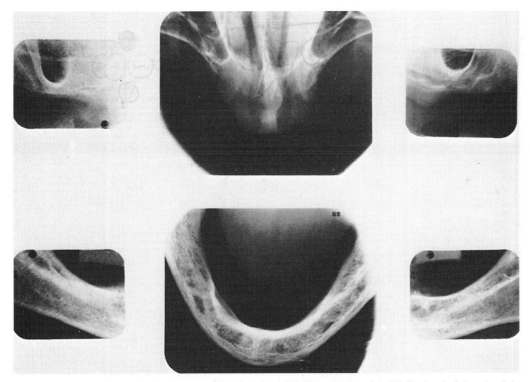

FIGURE 24-9 Mixed occlusal–periapical edentulous survey. (From Langland OE, Sippy FH, Langlais RP: *Textbook of dental radiology*, ed 2, Springfield, IL, 1984, Charles C Thomas. Courtesy of Dr. Robert Langlais.)

examination. If the paralleling technique is used, cotton rolls must be placed on both sides of the bite-block in place of the missing teeth. If the bisecting technique is used, the edentulous ridge and the receptor form the angle to be bisected (Figure 24-8). The receptor should be positioned such that approximately one third of it extends beyond the edentulous ridge. If the alveolar ridges of the patient are severely resorbed, the bisecting technique is recommended.

Occlusal–Periapical Examination

Some practitioners prefer to use both occlusal and periapical projections to examine the edentulous patient. The combined occlusal and periapical examination consists of a total of 6 exposures (Figure 24-9): 1 maxillary topographic occlusal projection (size 4 receptor), 1 mandibular cross-sectional occlusal projection (size 4 receptor), and 4 standard molar periapical exposures (size 2 receptor). As with the panoramic image, if an object is identified on an occlusal projection, a periapical projection of that specific area should be exposed.

SUMMARY

- Imaging techniques must often be modified to accommodate patients with special needs, including patients with a hypersensitive gag reflex, patients with physical or developmental disabilities, pediatric patients, endodontic patients, and edentulous patients.
- In dental imaging, the hypersensitive gag reflex is a commonly encountered problem. The areas most likely to elicit the gag reflex when stimulated include the soft palate and the posterior third of the tongue.
- The dental radiographer can effectively manage the patient with a hypersensitive gag reflex by conveying a confident attitude, completing all patient and equipment preparations before receptor placement, using proper exposure sequencing, placing and exposing receptors as quickly as possible, and using modifications in technique as necessary.
- Helpful strategies to prevent gagging include never suggesting gagging, reassuring the patient, suggesting breathing, distracting the patient, reducing tactile stimuli, and using a topical anesthetic.
- If the patient has an uncontrollable gag reflex, extraoral projections (e.g., panoramic or lateral jaw) can be used to obtain diagnostic information.
- The dental radiographer must be aware of the common physical disabilities (e.g., problems with vision, hearing, or mobility) and know the necessary modifications in technique to accommodate a person with a disability.
- The dental radiographer must also be aware of patients with specific dental needs, including pediatric patients, endodontic patients, and edentulous patients, and know the necessary modifications in technique to accommodate such patients.

- With the pediatric patient, special attention must be paid to the prescription of dental images, patient and equipment preparations, recommended techniques, and patient management.
- With the endodontic patient, the dental radiographer must be able to modify receptor placement and, at the same time, provide accurate images that measure the length of the pulp canals without distortion.
- With the edentulous patient also, the dental radiographer must be able to modify intraoral placements. Imaging is used in the edentulous patient to detect lesions, root tips, impacted teeth, and objects embedded in bone and to observe the quantity of bone present.

BIBLIOGRAPHY

Frommer HH, Savage-Stabulas JJ: Patient management and special problems. In *Radiology for the dental professional*, ed 9, St. Louis, 2011, Mosby.

Johnson ON, McNally MA, Essay CE: Managing patients with special needs. In *Essentials of dental radiography for dental assistants and hygienists*, ed 8, Upper Saddle River, NY, 2009, Pearson Education, Inc.

Johnson ON, McNally MA, Essay CE: Radiography for children. In *Essentials of dental radiography for dental assistants and hygienists*, ed 8, Upper Saddle River, NY, 2009, Pearson Education, Inc.

Miles DA, Van Dis ML, Jensen CW, Williamson GF: Accessory radiographic techniques and patient management. In *Radiographic imaging for dental auxiliaries*, ed 4, St. Louis, 2009, Saunders.

Miles DA, Van Dis ML, Razmus TF: Intraoral radiographic techniques. In *Basic principles of oral and maxillofacial radiology*, Philadelphia, 1992, Saunders.

Ohio Governor's Council on People with Disabilities: *Ten do's and don't's when you meet a person with a disability*, Catalog No G-16, Columbus, Ohio, 1990: http://gcpd.ohio.gov/index.asp: accessed October 2010

White SC, Pharoah MJ: Intraoral radiographic examinations. In *Oral radiology: Principles of interpretation*, ed 6, St. Louis, 2009, Mosby.

QUIZ QUESTIONS

TRUE OR FALSE

___ 1. The area of the oral cavity that is most likely to elicit the gag reflex when stimulated is the anterior third of the tongue.

___ 2. Breathing takes place simultaneously with the gag reflex.

___ 3. Psychogenic and tactile stimuli are precipitating factors for the gag reflex.

___ 4. Lack of operator confidence may act as a psychogenic stimulus and contribute to the gag reflex.

___ 5. The longer a receptor stays in the mouth, the more likely the patient is to gag.

___ 6. Exposure sequence does not play a role in preventing the gag reflex.

___ 7. Posterior periapical projections are always exposed before anterior periapical projections.

___ 8. The mandibular molar periapical projection is most likely to elicit the gag reflex.

___ 9. A receptor that is dragged along the palatal tissues may stimulate the gag reflex.

___ 10. The dental radiographer should ask the patient, "Are you a gagger?"

___ 11. If a patient gags, the dental radiographer should remove the receptor as quickly as possible and reassure the patient.

___ 12. If a patient is breathing during receptor placement and exposure, the gag reflex will not occur.

___ 13. Distracting the patient often helps suppress the gag reflex.

____ **14.** Increasing tactile stimuli helps prevent the gag reflex.

____ **15.** The patient with a hypersensitive gag reflex should be instructed to inhale during the application of topical anesthetic spray.

____ **16.** It is appropriate for the dental radiographer to gesture to another person in the presence of a person who is blind.

____ **17.** In the case of a person with a disability, it is appropriate for the dental radiographer to hold a receptor during x-ray exposure.

____ **18.** If the dental radiographer determines that a person cannot tolerate intraoral projections, no intraoral receptors should be exposed.

____ **19.** It is appropriate for the dental radiographer to question a patient about a disability.

____ **20.** The dental radiographer should talk to the caregiver of a patient with a disability instead of talking directly to the patient.

____ **21.** With the pediatric patient, the dental radiographer does not need to alter patient management techniques.

____ **22.** The radiographic examination should be performed on the pediatric patient regardless of the cooperation of the patient.

____ **23.** During an endodontic procedure, receptor placement is difficult because of poor visualization of the tooth.

____ **24.** The bisecting technique is recommended for the endodontic patient.

____ **24.** The panoramic examination is the imaging examination most often used in edentulous patients.

part **V**

Digital Imaging Basics

Chapter 25   Digital Imaging, 301
Chapter 26   Three-Dimensional Digital Imaging, 312

Digital Imaging

OUTLINE

BASIC CONCEPTS
    Terminology
    Purpose and Use
    Fundamentals
    Radiation Exposure
    Equipment
TYPES OF DIGITAL IMAGING
    Direct Digital Imaging
    Indirect Digital Imaging

STEP-BY-STEP PROCEDURES
    Sensor Preparation
    Sensor Placement
ADVANTAGES AND DISADVANTAGES
    Advantages of Digital Imaging
    Disadvantages of Digital Imaging

LEARNING OBJECTIVES

After completion of this chapter, the student will be able to do the following:
- Define the key terms associated with digital imaging
- Describe the purpose and use of digital imaging
- Discuss the fundamentals of digital imaging
- List and describe the equipment used in digital imaging
- List and describe the two types of digital imaging
- Describe the patient and equipment preparations required for digital imaging
- List and discuss the advantages and disadvantages of digital imaging

KEY TERMS

Analog image	Digital image	Indirect digital imaging
Bit-depth image	Digital imaging	Line pairs/millimeter (lp/mm)
Charge-coupled device	Digital subtraction	Pixel
Complementary metal oxide	Digitize	Sensor
semiconductor/active pixel sensor	Direct digital imaging	Storage phosphor imaging

For more than a century, film has been the only medium and recording device for dental radiography. Today, digital technology can be found in many aspects of a dental office, including intraoral digital cameras, digital blood pressure cuffs, and electronic patient files. Advances in technology have also produced a significant impact in the field of dental digital imaging.

Such advances in computer technology have resulted in a unique "filmless" radiography system known as **digital imaging**. Since its introduction to dentistry in 1987, digital imaging has influenced not only how dental disease is *recognized* but also how it is *diagnosed*. Digital imaging is a dependable and versatile technique that improves the diagnostic capabilities in the field of dentistry. Before the dental radiographer can use this very specialized technology, an understanding of the basic concepts, which include terminology, purpose, use, and fundamentals, is necessary. In addition, the dental radiographer must have a working knowledge of the equipment used in digital imaging.

The purpose of this chapter is to present the basic concepts of digital imaging, to introduce the types of digital imaging, and to discuss the advantages and disadvantages of digital imaging.

BASIC CONCEPTS

Digital imaging is a technique used to record radiographic images. Unlike conventional dental radiography techniques discussed in the previous chapters, no film or processing chemistry is used. Instead, digital imaging uses an electronic sensor as well as a computerized imaging system that produces radiographic images almost instantly on a computer monitor. Before the dental radiographer can use this technique competently, a thorough understanding of the terminology and fundamentals of digital imaging is necessary. Knowledge of radiation exposure, equipment, and types of digital imaging is also required.

Terminology

Analog image: Radiographic image produced by conventional film.

Bit-depth image: Number of possible gray-scale combinations for each pixel (e.g., 8 bit-depth image has gray-scale combination of 2^8, which equals 256 shades of gray).

Charge-coupled device (CCD): Solid-state detector used in many devices (e.g., fax machine, home video camera); in digital imaging, CCD is an image receptor found in the intraoral sensor.

Digital imaging: Filmless imaging system; a method of capturing a radiographic image using a sensor, breaking it into electronic pieces, and presenting and storing the image using a computer.

Digital image: An image composed of pixels.

Digital subtraction: One feature of digital imaging; a method of reversing the gray scale as an image is viewed; radiolucent images (normally black) appear white, and radiopaque images (normally white) appear black.

Digitize: In digital imaging, to convert an image into a digital form that, in turn, can be processed by a computer.

Direct digital imaging: Method of obtaining a digital image, in which an intraoral sensor is exposed to x-radiation to capture a radiographic image that can be viewed on a computer monitor.

Indirect digital imaging: Method of obtaining a digital image, in which an existing radiograph is scanned and converted into a digital form by using a CCD camera.

Line pairs/millimeter (lp/mm): Measurement used to evaluate the ability of the computer to capture the resolution (or detail) of a radiographic image.

Pixel: A discrete unit of information. In digital electronic images, digital information is contained in, and presented as, discrete units of information; also termed *picture element.*

Sensor: In digital imaging, a small detector that is placed intraorally to capture a radiographic image.

Storage phosphor imaging: Method of obtaining a digital image in which the image is recorded on phosphor-coated plates and then placed into an electronic processor, where a laser scans the plate and produces an image on a computer screen.

Purpose and Use

The purpose of digital imaging is to generate images that can be used in the diagnosis and assessment of dental disease. The images produced are diagnostically equivalent to film-based imaging and enable the dental radiographer to identify many conditions that may otherwise go undetected, as well as to see conditions that cannot be identified clinically. Similar to film-based radiographic procedures, digital imaging allows the radiographer to obtain a wealth of information about teeth and supporting structures. Uses of digital imaging include the following:

- To detect lesions, diseases, and conditions of teeth and surrounding structures
- To confirm or classify suspected disease
- To provide information during dental procedures (e.g., root canal therapy instrumentation and surgical placement of implants)
- To evaluate growth and development
- To illustrate changes secondary to caries, periodontal disease, or trauma
- To document the condition of a patient at a specific point in time

Fundamentals

The term *digital imaging* refers to a method of capturing a radiographic image using a sensor, breaking the image into electronic pieces, and presenting and storing the image using a computer. Remember that film-based images are produced when x-ray photons strike an intraoral film; the information recorded on the film is known as an *analog image.* Analog images are depicted by a continuous spectrum of gray shades between the extremes of white and black. It might be helpful to visualize a painting done entirely in black, grays, and white; these shades flow together on a canvas, and it is difficult to see where one shade ends and another begins. In digital imaging, the sensor receives the analog information and converts it to a digital image in the computer processing unit. The *digital image* is an array of picture elements, called *pixels,* with discrete gray values for each pixel. Imagine the same black, gray, and white painting just described, but in a mosaic pattern instead of the shades flowing together. Each tiny square of the mosaic is similar to an individual pixel.

Traditional film-based radiography consists of x-radiation interacting with the silver halide crystals of the emulsion, production of a latent image, and chemical processing to convert the latent image into a visible image. In digital imaging, a *sensor,* or small detector, is placed inside the mouth of the patient to capture the radiographic image. The sensor is used in place of intraoral dental film. As in conventional radiography, the x-ray beam is aimed to strike the sensor. An electronic charge is produced on the surface of the sensor; this electronic signal is *digitized,* or converted into "digital" form. The sensor, in turn, transmits this information to a computer, and the computer stores the incoming electronic signal. Data acquired by the sensor are communicated to the

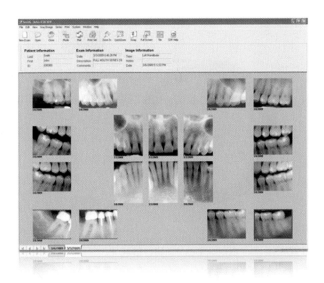

FIGURE 25-1 A full mouth series of digital images displayed on a computer monitor. (From Bird DL, Robinson DS: *Modern dental assisting,* ed 10, St. Louis, 2011, Elsevier.)

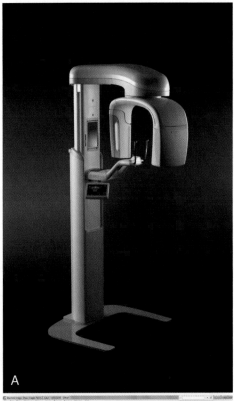

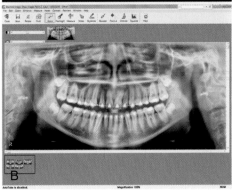

FIGURE 25-2 A, A panoramic machine used with digital imaging. (Courtesy of Progeny Dental, Lincolnshire. IL.) **B,** An example of a panoramic digital image. (Courtesy of Schick Technologies, Long Island City, NY.)

computer in analog form and are then converted into digital form by the use of an *analog-to-digital converter* (ADC). Software is used to store the image electronically. The image is displayed within seconds to minutes and may be readily manipulated to enhance the appearance for interpretation and diagnosis.

With digital imaging, the term *image* (not *radiograph* or *x-ray film*) is used to describe the pictures that are produced (Figure 25-1). Digital imaging systems are not limited to intraoral images; panoramic, cephalometric, and other extraoral images may also be obtained (Figure 25-2). For example, the extraoral film traditionally used in panoramic radiography is replaced with an electronic sensor that delivers the image information to a computer for storage in digital format. As with intraoral radiography, the extraoral images are displayed on a computer monitor and may be stored for future use.

Radiation Exposure

Digital imaging requires less x-radiation than does conventional radiography. Less x-radiation is necessary to form a digital image on the sensor because the typical sensor is more sensitive to x-radiation than is conventional film. Exposure times for digital imaging are 50% to 90% less than those required for conventional radiography. For example, the typical exposure time required to produce an image for digital imaging is 3 impulses (3/60 or 0.05 second). This exposure time is much less than the 12 impulses (12/60 or 0.2 second) required for intraoral film used in conventional radiography. With less radiation exposure, the absorbed dose to the patient is significantly reduced.

Equipment

Digital imaging requires the use of specialized equipment. The essential components of a digital imaging system include an x-radiation source, an intraoral sensor, and a computer.

X-Radiation Source

Most digital imaging systems use a conventional dental x-ray unit as the x-radiation source. The conventional x-radiation source is compatible with the digital imaging system; however, the x-ray unit timer must be adapted to allow exposures in a time frame of 1/100 of a second. A standard x-ray unit that is adapted for digital imaging can still be functional for conventional radiography (Figure 25-3).

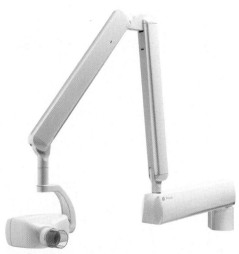

FIGURE 25-3 A conventional source of x-radiation, which is compatible with digital imaging. (Courtesy of Instrumentarium Dental Inc., Milwaukee, WI.)

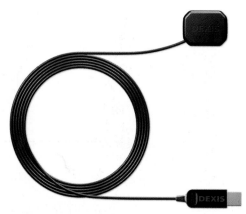

FIGURE 25-5 A wired sensor used with digital imaging showing the intraoral sensor at one end and the link to the computer at the other end. (Courtesy of DEXIS, Des Plaines IL.)

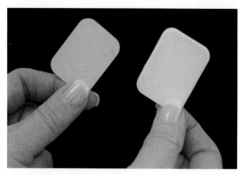

FIGURE 25-4 A #2 intraoral film, which is similar in size and shape to a sensor used in digital imaging.

Intraoral Sensor

As previously defined, the sensor is a small detector that is placed intraorally to capture the radiographic image. Some sensors are thick, bulky, and rigid, whereas others mimic conventional film in size and flexibility (Figure 25-4). Most manufacturers produce sensors similar in dimension to sizes 0, 1, 2, and 4 of intraoral films. Intraoral sensors used in digital imaging systems may be wired or wireless. The term *wired* refers to the fact that the imaging sensor is physically linked by a fiberoptic cable to a computer that records the generated signal (Figure 25-5). In wired systems, the cable varies in length from 8 to 35 feet; the shorter the cable, the more limited is the range of motion. The term *wireless* refers to an imaging sensor that is not linked by a cable; the wireless sensor sends data to the computer electronically.

The most popular types of sensor technology include the charge-coupled device and the complementary metal oxide semiconductor.

Charge-Coupled Device.
The *charge-coupled device* (CCD) is one of the most common image receptors used in dental digital imaging. The CCD technology used in digital imaging relies on a specialized fabrication process that is costly to manufacture.

The CCD is not a new technology; it was initially developed in the 1960s. Currently, CCD technology is used in many devices, including fax machines, home video cameras, microscopes, and telescopes. The CCD is a solid-state detector that contains a silicon chip with an electronic circuit embedded in it. This silicon chip is sensitive to x-radiation or light.

The electrons that compose the silicon CCD can be visualized as being divided into an arrangement of blocks or picture elements known as *pixels*. A pixel is a small box, or "well," into which the electrons produced by the x-ray exposure are deposited. A pixel is the digital equivalent of a silver crystal used in conventional radiography. As opposed to a film emulsion that contains a *random* arrangement of silver crystals, a pixel is structured in an *ordered* arrangement. The CCD is 640 × 480 individual pixels in size. Consequently, the CCD contains 307,200 pixels and functions to sense transmitted light and translate it into an electronic message.

The x-ray photons that come into contact with the CCD cause electrons to be released from the silicon and produce a corresponding electronic charge. Consequently, each pixel arrangement, or *electron potential well*, contains an electronic charge proportional to the number of electrons that reacted within the well. Furthermore, each electronic well corresponds to a specific area on the linked computer screen. When x-radiation activates electrons and produces such electronic charges, an electronic latent image is produced. The latent image is then transmitted and stored in a computer and can be converted to a visible image on screen or printed on paper.

Complementary Metal Oxide Semiconductor/Active Pixel Sensor.
Another sensor technology that is used in digital imaging is the **complementary metal oxide semiconductor/active pixel sensor** (CMOS/APS). Although the CMOS process is the standard in the making of semiconductor chips, it was not until APS was developed that CMOS became useful

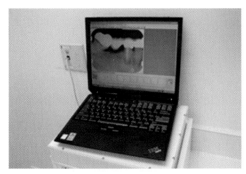

FIGURE 25-6 A digital image of the mandibular right periapical region as seen on a computer monitor.

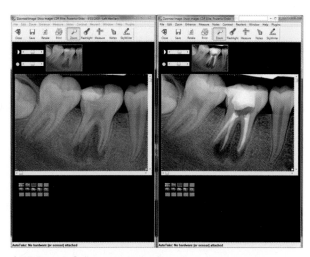

FIGURE 25-7 Split-screen technology that assists the dental professional to view several images of tooth #30 simultaneously. (Courtesy of Schick Technologies, Long Island City, NY.)

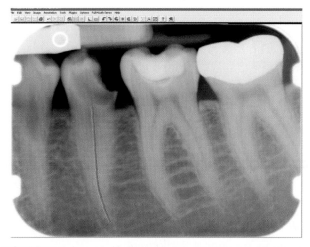

FIGURE 25-8 An example of a measurement tool as part of the imaging software. (Courtesy of Dr. Donald Tyndall, The University of North Carolina School of Dentistry, Chapel Hill, NC.)

as a sensor in dental digital imaging. The CMOS detector is silicon based and differs from the CCD detector in the way that the pixels are read. At this time, one digital imaging manufacturer uses a CMOS/APS sensor instead of a CCD and claims that it has a 25% greater resolution. Additional advantages of the CMOS/APS technology are the lower production cost of the chip and greater durability than the CCD.

Computer

A computer is used to store the incoming electronic signal. The computer is responsible for converting the electronic signal from the sensor into a shade of gray that is viewed on the computer monitor. Each pixel is represented numerically in the computer by location and the color level of the gray. The range of numbers for a pixel varies from 0 to 255, which creates 256 shades of gray, referred to as a pixel's *gray-scale resolution*. In comparison, the human eye can only perceive 32 shades of gray.

The number of possible gray-scale combinations per pixel is known as the *bit-depth image*. The bit-depth image is determined by the computer software for the digital system. For each pixel, the number of possible gray-scale combinations is 2^N; for example, an 8 bit-depth image has a gray-scale combination of 2^8, which equals 256 shades of gray. The software also allows for manipulation of the pixels, enhancing contrast and density without additional x-ray exposure of the patient.

The computer digitizes, processes, and stores information received from the sensor. The exposure can be viewed immediately on the computer monitor. An image is recorded on a computer monitor in 0.5 to 120 seconds, much less time than required for conventional film processing (Figure 25-6). This speed of image recording is extremely useful during certain dental procedures, such as the placement of surgical implants or during endodontic instrumentation. The image may be stored permanently in the computer, printed out as a hard copy for the patient record, or transmitted electronically to insurance companies or referring dental specialists.

Various computer viewing features are available with digital imaging systems. Digital systems feature split-screen technology, which allows the operator to view and compare multiple images on the same screen (Figure 25-7). This feature is helpful for comparison and for the evaluation of

progression of caries or periodontal disease. For example, caries progression can be evaluated by comparing successive bite-wing images. Digital systems also provide a feature that allows specific images to be magnified up to four times the original size. This feature is helpful when evaluating the apical area of a tooth. Many digital systems include a measurement tool as part of the imaging software. Measurement tools are valuable in therapies such as endodontic procedures or in implant treatment planning. Linear and angular measurements must be made with the proper projection geometry, avoiding such errors as elongation or foreshortening, which may distort the measurements (Figure 25-8).

TYPES OF DIGITAL IMAGING

Two methods of obtaining a digital image currently exist: (1) direct digital imaging and (2) indirect digital imaging.

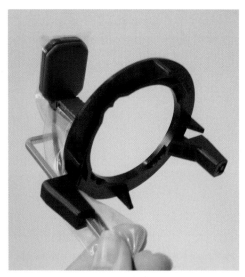

FIGURE 25-9 An anterior beam alignment device, which holds the digital sensor as well as the wire attachment. (Courtesy of DEXIS, Des Plaines, IL.)

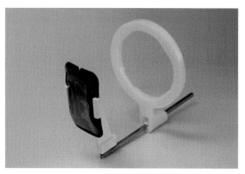

FIGURE 25-10 A beam alignment device, which holds a PSP digital sensor for a bite-wing image exposure. (Courtesy of Schick Technologies, Long Island City, NY.)

Direct Digital Imaging

The essential components of a *direct digital imaging* system include an x-ray machine, an intraoral sensor, and a computer monitor. A sensor with a fiberoptic cable linked to the computer is placed into the mouth of the patient and exposed to x-radiation (Figure 25-9). The sensor captures the radiographic image and then transmits the image to a computer monitor. Within seconds of exposing the sensor to radiation, an image appears on the computer screen. Software is then used to enhance and store the image.

Indirect Digital Imaging

Scanning Traditional Radiographs

The essential components of an *indirect digital imaging* system include a CCD camera and a computer. In the scanning method, an existing radiograph is digitized using a CCD camera. The CCD camera scans the image on the film, digitizes or converts the image, and then displays it on the computer monitor. This concept is similar in theory to scanning an image, for example, a photograph, to a computer screen. Indirect digital imaging is inferior to direct digital imaging because the resultant image is similar to a "copy" of an image versus the "original" image.

Storage Phosphor Imaging

A second type of indirect digital imaging is *storage phosphor imaging*, which is a wireless digital imaging system. Storage phosphor imaging is also referred to as *photo-stimulable phosphor imaging* (PSP). In this system, a reusable imaging plate coated with phosphors is used instead of a sensor with a fiberoptic cable. The phosphor-coated plate is flexible and is placed into the mouth in the same way as intraoral film (Figure 25-10). A phosphor-coated plate resembles an intensifying screen used to expose an extraoral film in that it

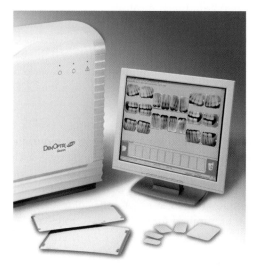

FIGURE 25-11 A storage phosphor imaging system, illustrating the laser scanning device and the intraoral and extraoral PSP digital sensors. A full mouth series of intraoral images is seen on the computer monitor. (Courtesy of Gendex Imaging, Des Plaines, IL.)

converts x-ray energy into light. The images are cleared from the plates by exposure to viewbox light for several minutes, or the images may be erased from the plates immediately after the scanning process. Once the image is erased, the plates may be wrapped in plastic and sterilized for reuse.

Storage phosphor imaging records diagnostic data on a plate after x-ray exposure and then uses a high-speed scanner to convert the information into electronic files. After exposure, the plate is removed from the mouth and placed into an electronic processor, where a laser scans the plate and produces an image that is transferred to a computer screen. Because of this step involving laser scanning, which can take 30 seconds to 5 minutes, this type of digital imaging is less rapid than direct digital imaging (Figure 25-11). The dental radiographer must take care in placing the phosphor plates in the mouth and exposing them correctly. Currently, some PSP systems are unable to distinguish images that have been exposed backward (similar to placing a film in the mouth with the colored tab facing the beam of radiation). It is

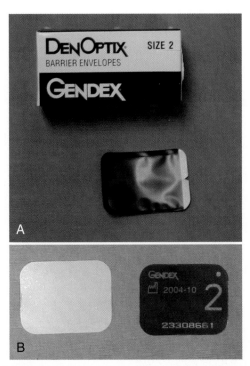

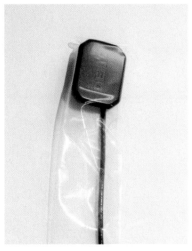

FIGURE 25-13 A wired digital sensor wrapped in a protective plastic sleeve. (Courtesy of Gendex Imaging, Des Plaines, IL.)

FIGURE 25-12 A, Barrier envelopes used to seal and protect the PSP sensors from contamination. **B,** An example of a PSP sensor, the blue side facing the teeth and the radiation source and the black side facing the tongue. (From Bird DL, Robinson DS: *Modern dental assisting,* ed 10, St. Louis, 2011, Elsevier.)

recommended that the dental radiographer view the mounted images and confirm all the findings while the patient remains seated in the dental chair.

STEP-BY-STEP PROCEDURES

Step-by-step procedures for the use of digital imaging systems vary from manufacturer to manufacturer. It is critical to refer to the manufacturer's instruction booklet for information on the operation of the system, equipment preparation, patient preparation, and exposure. Only general guidelines concerning sensor preparation and placement are provided here.

Sensor Preparation

Digital imaging involves the placement of the intraoral sensor in the mouth of the patient, using the same technique as in conventional film placement. Whether using indirect or direct digital imaging, it is important that the individual sensors are kept sterile. Storage phosphor sensors are sealed and waterproofed (Figure 25-12). For infection control purposes, sensors used in direct digital imaging *must* be covered with a disposable barrier or sleeve because they cannot withstand heat sterilization (Figure 25-13).

Sensor Placement

The sensor is held in the mouth by bite-block attachments or devices that aim the beam and sensor accurately. The *paralleling technique* is the preferred exposure method because of the dimensional accuracy of images produced and the ease of standardizing such images. Paralleling technique beam alignment devices must be used to stabilize the sensor in the mouth. As with conventional intraoral film, the sensor is centered over the area of interest. Various manufacturers have produced beam alignment devices that can be used not only with film but with wired sensors and PSP plates as well (Figure 25-14).

ADVANTAGES AND DISADVANTAGES

As with any intraoral radiographic technique, digital imaging has both advantages and disadvantages.

Advantages of Digital Imaging

1. *Superior gray-scale resolution.* A primary advantage of digital imaging is the superior gray-scale resolution that results. Digital imaging uses up to 256 (over 16,000, depending on the manufacturer) shades of gray compared with the 16 to 25 shades of gray differentiated on conventional film. This advantage is critical because diagnosis is often based on contrast discrimination. The ability to manipulate the density and contrast of the digital image without additional exposure of the patient to x-radiation is also an important advantage (Figure 25-15). In addition, studies have investigated the diagnostic capability of the intraoral sensor used in digital imaging. Digital imaging enables the dental professional to identify dental disease just as with traditional film methods. One of the ways to measure the diagnostic value of digital imaging is through its ability to capture detail, or resolution. *Line pairs/ millimeter (lp/mm)* is a measurement of the ability of the digital system to capture the detail in an image. Most digital imaging manufacturers maintain a range of 6 to 22 lp/mm. The human eye can only recognize approximately

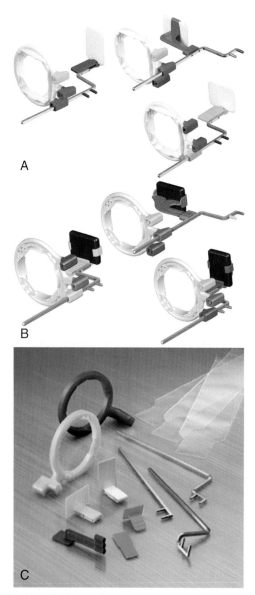

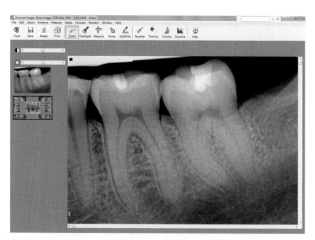

FIGURE 25-15 Magnification of a periapical image from a full mouth series, which allows the dental professional to take a closer look at teeth #18 and #19. (Courtesy of Schick Technologies, Long Island City, NY.)

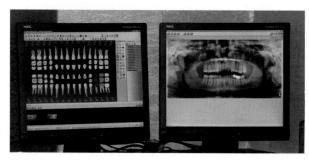

FIGURE 25-16 Two computer monitors side by side allowing the dental professional to view the patient's electronic chart and the panoramic image at the same time. (From Bird DL, Robinson DS: *Modern dental assisting,* ed 10, St. Louis, 2011, Elsevier.)

FIGURE 25-14 A, Beam alignment devices holding film for anterior, posterior, and bite-wing exposures. **B,** The same beam alignment devices now holding digital sensors for anterior, posterior, and bite-wing exposures. (Courtesy of Dentsply RINN, Elgin, IL.) **C,** Beam alignment bite-blocks manufactured with adhesive backing to hold PSP digital sensors firmly in place. (Courtesy of Schick Technologies, Long Island City, NY.)

8 lp/mm. All the current digital systems produce a diagnostically acceptable image.

2. *Reduced exposure to x-radiation.* Another primary advantage of the digital imaging system is the reduction in patient exposure to x-radiation. Decreased exposure results from the sensitivity of the CCD. The radiation exposure for digital imaging systems is 50% to 90% less than that required for E-speed film used in conventional radiography.

3. *Increased speed of image viewing.* Dental professionals as well as patients are able to view the digital images instantaneously, which allows for immediate interpretation and evaluation. Chairside viewing of the digitized image on a computer monitor within moments after exposure continues to be a compelling reason for the growing popularity of this technology.

4. *Lower equipment and film cost.* Long-term digital imaging eliminates the need for purchasing conventional film, costly processing equipment, and processing solutions. With digital imaging, darkroom and processing solutions and maintenance are unnecessary. Also, environmental costs are reduced because the disposal hazards of processing chemicals, silver salts in film emulsion, and lead foil sheets are avoided. The elimination of darkroom processing errors is also an advantage.

5. *Increased efficiency.* Dental professionals can be more productive because digital imaging does not interrupt routine patient treatment or care. Dental practices that also use electronic charting have the advantage of the operator's ability to access both patient data and digital images simultaneously (Figure 25-16). Both image storage and communication are easier with digital networking. The digital image can be incorporated into the electronic record of the patient, and the radiographic image can be

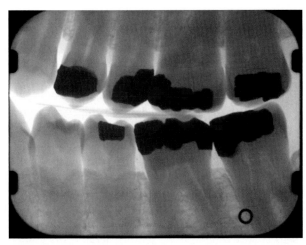

FIGURE 25-17 An example of digital subtraction of a bite-wing image. (Courtesy of Dr. Donald Tyndall, The University of North Carolina School of Dentistry, Chapel Hill, NC.)

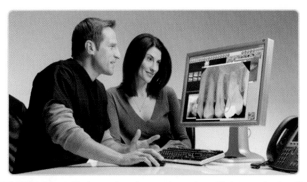

FIGURE 25-18 Patient education made easier with larger-sized radiographic image. (Courtesy of DEXIS, Des Plaines, IL.)

printed out whenever needed. Digital images can also be electronically transmitted to referring dentists and specialists, insurance companies, or consultants.

6. *Enhancement of diagnostic image.* Features such as colorization and zooming allow users to highlight conditions such as bone resorption caused by periodontal disease or to help detect small areas of decay. Another feature that can be used to enhance a diagnostic image is *digital subtraction*. With digital subtraction, the gray-scale is reversed so that radiolucent images (normally black) appear white and radiopaque images (normally white) appear black (Figure 25-17). Digital subtraction also eliminates distracting background information. For example, this feature permits the operator to remove all anatomic structures that have not changed between radiographic examinations to facilitate identification of changes in diagnostic information. Additional features commonly available in image software include brightness, contrast, sharpness, image orientation, and pseudo-color alteration.

7. *Effective patient education tool.* Digital images can be an effective tool in patient education and interaction. Patients can view radiographic images along with the operator, which facilitates dialogue and rapport and increases a patient's understanding of the disease process and acceptance of treatment modalities. In addition, the size of the digitized image on the 15-inch or 17-inch computer screen (compared with a 2-inch piece of film) makes the digital image an attractive patient education tool (Figure 25-18).

Disadvantages of Digital Imaging

1. *Initial setup costs.* The initial cost of purchasing a digital imaging system is a significant disadvantage. The cost depends on the manufacturer, the level of computer equipment currently in the office, and auxiliary features such as the intraoral camera. Maintenance and repairs must also be considered.

2. *Image quality.* At one time, image quality was a source of debate. The spatial resolution of an image is defined as the number of line pairs per millimeter (lp/mm). Conventional dental x-ray film has a resolution of 12 to 20 lp/mm. A digital imaging system using a CCD has a resolution closer to 10 lp/mm. Considering that the human eye can only perceive 8 to 10 lp/mm, a CCD system is significantly more effective in the recognition of dental disease. Many studies have reported on the ability of the digital image to capture early caries, bone loss, periapical radiolucencies, and so on. The majority of the research has shown that the digital imaging performs at least as well as, and at times even better than, traditional radiography.

3. *Sensor size and thickness.* Some digital sensors are thicker and less flexible than intraoral film. Patients may complain about the bulkiness of the sensor, which may cause discomfort or elicit the gag reflex. However, with increasing experience and familiarity with the use of these rigid sensors, sensor placement becomes less of an issue. In addition, manufacturers have produced many varieties of beam alignment devices to aid sensor placement (Figure 25-19).

4. *Infection control.* Some digital sensors cannot withstand heat sterilization. Therefore, these sensors require complete coverage with disposable plastic sleeves that must be changed between patients every time to prevent cross-contamination.

5. *Wear and tear.* The receptors used in the PSP system are vulnerable to wear and tear and may have a limited lifespan. The phosphor plates are not designed to have their edges bent or softened to accommodate individual patient anatomy. If bending or scratching of the plates occurs, permanent defects will appear on all images exposed, which may obscure diagnostic information.

6. *Legal issues.* Because the original digital image can be enhanced, it is questionable whether digital images can be used as evidence in lawsuits. To address this concern, manufacturers (for example, Kodak, with its Digital Science Dental Scanning System) have included in the software a warning feature that appears if the image displayed on the

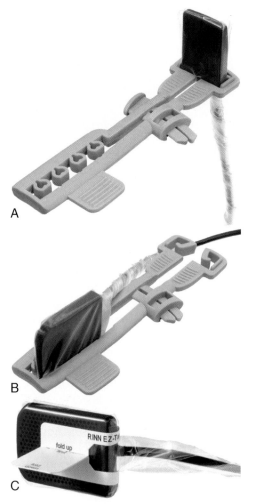

FIGURE 25-19 A, **B**, Examples of anterior and posterior beam alignment devices holding a direct digital sensor. **C**, A direct digital sensor fitted with an adhesive bite-wing tab. (Courtesy of Dentsply RINN, Elgin, IL.)

monitor is not comparable with the original image. A file copy of the original image should always be kept on the computer, even when characteristics such as density and contrast have been changed.

SUMMARY

- Digital imaging is a method of capturing a radiographic image and displaying it on a computer screen; no film is used, and no film processing chemicals are required.

- A conventional dental x-ray unit is used as the radiation source in digital imaging. A sensor or small detector is placed inside the patient's mouth, and the x-ray beam is aimed to strike the sensor. The electronic charge produced on the sensor is digitized (or converted into digital form) and can be viewed on a computer monitor.
- Advantages of digital imaging include superior gray-scale resolution, reduced patient exposure to x-radiation, increased speed of image viewing, lower equipment and receptor costs, increased time efficiency, enhanced patient education, and many viewing options to enhance the diagnostic information of the image.
- Disadvantages of digital imaging include initial setup costs of the digital system, image quality, size of the intraoral sensor, wear and tear of sensors, legal issues, and the inability to heat-sterilize the sensor.

BIBLIOGRAPHY

Brennan J: An introduction to digital radiography in dentistry. *J Orthod* 29:66–69, 2002.

Frommer HH, Savage-Stabulas JJ: Digital imaging. In *Radiology for the dental professional*, ed 9, St. Louis, 2011, Mosby.

Levato C: Are you ready for digital radiography? *Dent Pract Finance* 7:17–24, 1999.

Lusk LT: Comparison of film-based and digital radiography. *J Pract Hygiene* 7:45–50, 1998.

Miles DA, Van Dis ML, Jensen CW, Williamson GF: Digital imaging. In *Radiographic imaging for the dental team*, ed 4, St. Louis, 2009, Saunders.

Parks ET, Williamson GF: Digital radiography: An overview. *J Contemp Dent Pract* 3(4):23–39, 2002.

Razmus TF, Williamson GF: An overview of oral and maxillofacial imaging. In *Current oral and maxillofacial imaging*, Philadelphia, 1996, Saunders.

Schleyer T, et al: The technologically well-equipped dental office. *J Am Dent Assoc* 134:30–40, 2003.

Tyndall DA, Ludlow JB, Platin E, et al: A comparison of Kodak Ektaspeed Plus film and the Siemens Sidexis digital imaging system for caries detection using receiver operating characteristic analysis. *Oral Surg Oral Med Oral Pathol Oral Radiol Endod* 85:113–118, 1998.

Van der Stelt PF: Better imaging: The advantages of digital radiography. *J Am Dent Assoc* 139(3):7S–13S, 2008.

Van der Stelt PF: Filmless imaging: The uses of digital radiography in dental practice. *J Am Dent Assoc* 136(10):1379–1387, 2005.

White SC, Pharoah MJ: Digital imaging. In *Oral radiology: principles and interpretation*, ed 6, St. Louis, 2009, Mosby.

QUIZ QUESTIONS

MATCHING

For questions 1 to 9, match each term with its corresponding definition.

a. charge-coupled device
b. digital radiography
c. digital subtraction
d. digitize
e. direct digital imaging
f. indirect digital imaging
g. pixel
h. sensor
i. storage phosphor imaging

_____ 1. A small detector that is placed intraorally to capture the radiographic image.

_____ 2. An image receptor found in the intraoral sensor.

_____ 3. A form of indirect digital imaging in which the image is recorded on phosphor-coated plates and then placed into an electronic processor, where a laser scans the plate and produces an image on a computer screen.

_____ 4. To convert an image into digital form that, in turn, can be processed by a computer.

_____ 5. A method of obtaining a digital image in which an intraoral sensor is exposed to x-rays to capture a radiographic image that can be viewed on a computer monitor.

_____ 6. A discrete unit of information; a picture element.

_____ 7. A method of obtaining a digital image, in which an existing radiograph is scanned and converted into a digital form using a CCD camera.

_____ 8. A method of reversing the gray scale as a digital image is viewed.

_____ 9. A filmless imaging system; a method of capturing a radiographic image using a sensor, breaking the image into electronic pieces, and presenting and storing the image using a computer.

TRUE OR FALSE

_____ 10. In digital imaging, the term used to describe the picture that is produced is *radiograph*.

_____ 11. Digital imaging requires more x-radiation than does conventional radiography.

_____ 12. The x-radiation source used in most digital imaging systems is a conventional dental x-ray unit.

_____ 13. Compared with film emulsion, the pixels used in digital imaging are structured in an orderly arrangement.

_____ 14. All intraoral sensors can be heat-sterilized after use.

_____ 15. The preferred exposure method for intraoral digital imaging is the paralleling technique.

_____ 16. One advantage of a digital imaging system is the superior gray-scale resolution that results.

_____ 17. Digital subtraction is an advantage in digital imaging because distracting background information is eliminated from the image.

_____ 18. The manipulation of the original digital images can be considered a legal issue.

MULTIPLE CHOICE

_____ 19. Digital imaging was introduced to dentistry in:
a. 1967
b. 1977
c. 1987
d. 1997

_____ 20. Digital imaging can be used for:
a. detecting conditions of teeth and surrounding structures
b. evaluating the growth and development of jaws
c. confirmation of suspected disease
d. all of the above

_____ 21. Digital imaging requires less radiation than does conventional radiography because:
a. the sensor is larger
b. the sensor is more sensitive to x-rays
c. the exposure time is increased
d. the pixels sense transmitted light quickly

_____ 22. The method of obtaining a digital image similar to scanning a photograph to a computer screen is termed:
a. direct digital imaging
b. indirect digital imaging
c. storage phosphor imaging
d. CMOS/APS

_____ 23. The image receptor found in the intraoral sensor is termed:
a. CCD
b. pixel
c. semiconductor chip
d. software

_____ 24. Digital imaging systems can be used for:
a. bite-wing images
b. panoramic images
c. cephalometric images
d. all of the above

_____ 25. All of the following are advantages of digital imaging except:
a. digital subtraction
b. the ability to enhance the image
c. size of the intraoral sensor
d. patient education

chapter 26

Three-Dimensional Digital Imaging

OUTLINE

BASIC CONCEPTS
    Terminology
    Fundamentals
    Equipment
    Common Uses

STEP-BY-STEP PROCEDURES
    Patient Preparation
    Patient Positioning
ADVANTAGES AND DISADVANTAGES
    Advantages of Three-Dimensional Digital Imaging
    Disadvantages of Three-Dimensional Digital Imaging

LEARNING OBJECTIVES

After completion of this chapter, the student will be able to do the following:

- Define the key terms associated with three-dimensional digital imaging
- Describe the purpose and uses of three-dimensional digital imaging
- Describe the equipment used in three-dimensional digital imaging
- Detail the equipment and patient preparation necessary before exposure to x-radiation using three-dimensional digital imaging
- Identify advantages and disadvantages of three-dimensional digital imaging

KEY TERMS

Cone-beam computed tomography (CBCT)
Cone-beam volume tomography (CBVT)
DICOM data
Field of view

Multiplanar reconstruction (MPR)
Plane, axial
Plane, coronal
Plane, sagittal
Resolution, contrast

Resolution, spatial
Three-dimensional digital imaging
Three-dimensional volume rendering
Voxel

All of the radiographic images discussed until this point in this textbook have been two-dimensional images. Within the past decade, a new technology termed *cone beam computed tomography (CBCT)* that allows the viewing of structures in the oral–maxillofacial complex in three dimensions has been developed. Three-dimensional digital imaging in dentistry has become popular and is quickly becoming the desired technology because of the accurate information it provides.

BASIC CONCEPTS

As discussed in Chapter 8, geometric characteristics such as magnification, distortion, and overlap of anatomy minimize the diagnostic quality of dental images. These characteristics limit the accurate interpretation of traditional two-dimensional images (Figure 26-1). The dental professional, therefore, may not have the ability to evaluate pathology (e.g., bony and soft tissue relationships), distances to critical anatomic landmarks (e.g., maxillary sinus, mandibular canal), locations of impacted teeth, eruption patterns, or other concerns of the oral–maxillofacial complex. Three-dimensional imaging eliminates these deficiencies by providing more detailed information for the dental professional.

The purpose of this chapter is to discuss the basic concepts and indications of three-dimensional digital imaging, the equipment used, and the advantages and disadvantages of this technology. The dental radiographer has to have knowledge of the terminology and fundamentals of three-dimensional digital imaging to be able to understand this technology.

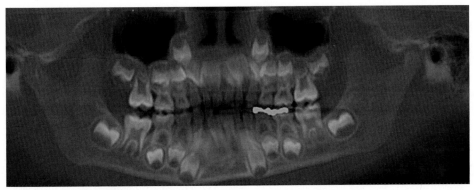

FIGURE 26-1 Panoramic image revealing mixed dentition of a 6-year-old. It is difficult to determine the eruption pattern of permanent teeth, especially in the anterior maxilla. (Courtesy of Carolina OMF Imaging, W. Bruce Howerton Jr., DDS, MS, Raleigh, NC.)

Terminology

Cone beam computed tomography (CBCT): Term used to describe computer-assisted digital imaging in dentistry; this imaging technique uses a cone-shaped x-ray beam to acquire information and present it in three dimensions.

Cone beam volume tomography (CBVT): Term used to describe computer-assisted digital imaging in dentistry; used interchangeably with *cone beam volume imaging (CBVI)*; these terms are used to differentiate this procedure from medical computed tomography (CT).

DICOM data: The universal format for handling, storing, and transmitting three-dimensional images; the acronym refers to digital imaging and communications in medicine.

Field of view: The area that can be captured when performing imaging procedures.

Multiplanar reconstruction (MPR): The reconstruction of raw data into images when imported into viewing software to create three anatomic planes of the body.

Plane, axial: A horizontal plane that divides the body into superior and inferior parts; runs parallel to the ground.

Plane, coronal: A vertical plane that divides the body into anterior and posterior sides; runs perpendicular to the ground.

Plane, sagittal: A vertical plane that divides the body into right and left sides; runs perpendicular to the ground. A midsagittal plane describes a plane that runs through the midline of the body.

Resolution, contrast: The number of gray scale colors available for each pixel in the image.

Resolution, spatial: A measurement of pixel size in multiplanar reconstruction.

Three-dimensional digital imaging: An image that demonstrates the anatomy in three dimensions.

Three-dimensional volume rendering: A three-dimensional shape that is created from two-dimensional images.

Voxel: The smallest element of a three-dimensional image; also referred to as *volume element* or *three-dimensional pixel*.

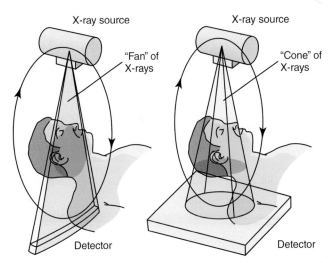

FIGURE 26-2 Cone-shaped beam used in cone-beam computed tomography (CBCT).

Fundamentals

In the past, three-dimensional imaging was performed primarily for medical procedures. Today, manufacturers of CBCT have developed three-dimensional imaging specifically to evaluate the oral–maxillofacial complex. CBCT is so named because it uses a cone-shaped x-ray beam to acquire three-dimensional information (Figure 26-2). The source of radiation in CBCT machines rotates around the head of the patient, as in panoramic radiography.

Three-dimensional imaging serves a number of diagnostic purposes for dental practitioners. Periapical and bite-wing images focus on specific teeth in the arches while using conventional imaging techniques (see Chapters 16 through 19). With CBCT, however, the area of interest in the patient's anatomy is termed the *field of view*. In a single scan, the source of radiation and the digital sensor rotate around the patient and acquire multiple images of the field of view. Manufacturers of three-dimensional imaging use a variety of sizes to accommodate the appropriate field of view for diagnostic purposes (Figure 26-3).

As the divergent rays exit the machine, some of the radiation is attenuated by the patient, and some of the radiation passes through the patient and is received by a digital receptor. The information that the receptor receives is termed *raw data*. In contrast to producing a single intraoral image, as in two-dimensional imaging, raw data are three-dimensional in volume and undergo reconstruction forming a "stack" of

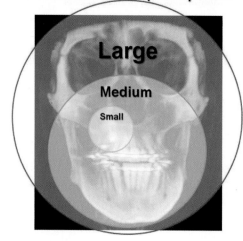

FIGURE 26-3 Examples of various sizes of the field of view.

axial images termed *DICOM images*. DICOM images are imported into the viewing software that allows the dental practitioner to see the field of view in three dimensions. Once the DICOM images are imported into the viewing software, the data are viewed in three planes: (1) axial (X) plane, (2) coronal (Y) plane, and (3) sagittal (Z) plane (Figure 26-4).

- The *axial plane* is a horizontal plane that divides the body into superior and inferior sides (Figure 26-5).
- The *coronal plane* is a vertical plane that runs perpendicular to the ground and divides the body into anterior and posterior sides (Figure 26-6).
- The *sagittal plane* is also a vertical plane that runs perpendicular to the ground and divides the body into right and left sides (Figure 26-7).

When viewed together, axial, coronal, and sagittal images are referred to as *multiplanar reconstructed images* (MPR images). Anatomic structures of the reconstructed volume provide accurate dimensional measurements of the patient with a 1:1 ratio relationship. One of the advantages of using DICOM data is that images can be shared among dental professionals, imaging centers, and referring physicians. The volume of data produced is similar to medical CT, but CBCT uses much less radiation to acquire the images.

Equipment

The use of specialized equipment is necessary for three-dimensional digital imaging. The essential components for

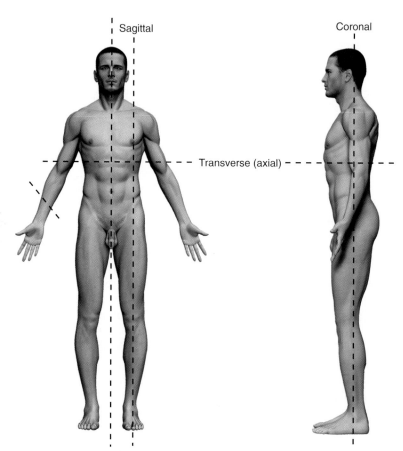

FIGURE 26-4 An illustration of the three planes: axial (or transverse) (X), coronal (Y), and sagittal (Z). (From Liebgott B: *The anatomical basis of dentistry*, ed 3, St. Louis, 2011, Mosby.)

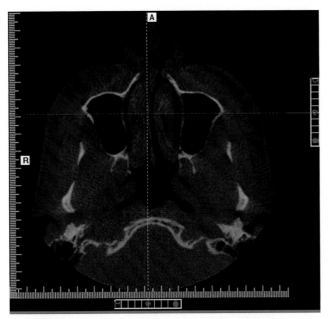

FIGURE 26-5 An axial image. (Courtesy of Carolina OMF Imaging, W. Bruce Howerton Jr., DDS, MS, Raleigh, NC.)

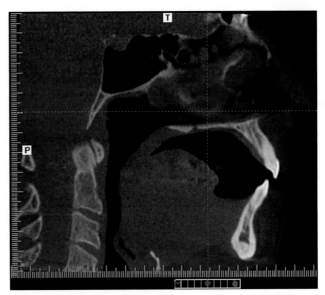

FIGURE 26-7 A sagittal image. (Courtesy of Carolina OMF Imaging, W. Bruce Howerton Jr., DDS, MS, Raleigh, NC.)

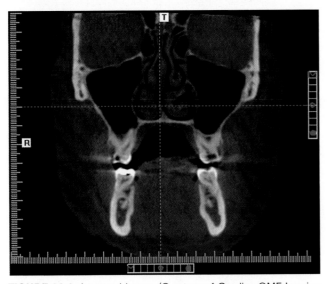

FIGURE 26-6 A coronal image. (Courtesy of Carolina OMF Imaging, W. Bruce Howerton Jr., DDS, MS, Raleigh, NC.)

this type of imaging system include a CBCT machine, a computer, and various types of viewing software.

CBCT Machine

The CBCT machine is comparable in size and appearance with a panoramic machine; with the CBCT machine also, the patient sits, stands, or is placed in a supine position during the scanning process. In a single rotation, the source of radiation and the receptor capture the field of view. The radiation that exits the patient is received by a solid-state flat panel detector and becomes the raw data that are sent to the computer. Scan times vary between 7 and 30 seconds (shorter scan times are desirable to eliminate artifacts created by patient movement). Factors that can be altered when scanning the patient are the size of field of view and resolution. *Contrast resolution* refers to the number of gray scales available, and *spatial resolution* is the measurement, in millimeters, of the size of pixels in the multiplanar reconstructed images. Spatial resolution also refers to the measurement of three-dimensional pixels in the volume of data, termed *voxels*. Choosing the appropriate field of view and the resolution is dependent on the task at hand, for example, dental implant placement, temporomandibular joint examination, orthodontic evaluation, and so on.

The number of manufacturers producing CBCT technology in dentistry is growing rapidly. The following Web site has a comprehensive list of current CBCT manufacturers, organized by sizes of the field of view: http://www.3dorthodontist.com/CBCT_Machines.html. Figure 26-8 displays several CBCT machines currently on the market.

Computer

A computer attached to the CBCT machine accepts raw data and converts them into a stack of axial images (DICOM images). The computer has a separate proprietary viewing software to import DICOM images. The technique chosen for the task at hand, which includes field of view and spatial resolution, is completed during the data reconstruction process.

Viewing Software

The viewing software allows the dental practitioner to view axial, coronal, and sagittal images, select the region of interest such as a presurgical dental implant site or the location of an impacted canine, and scroll through these images on a computer monitor to create three-dimensional information

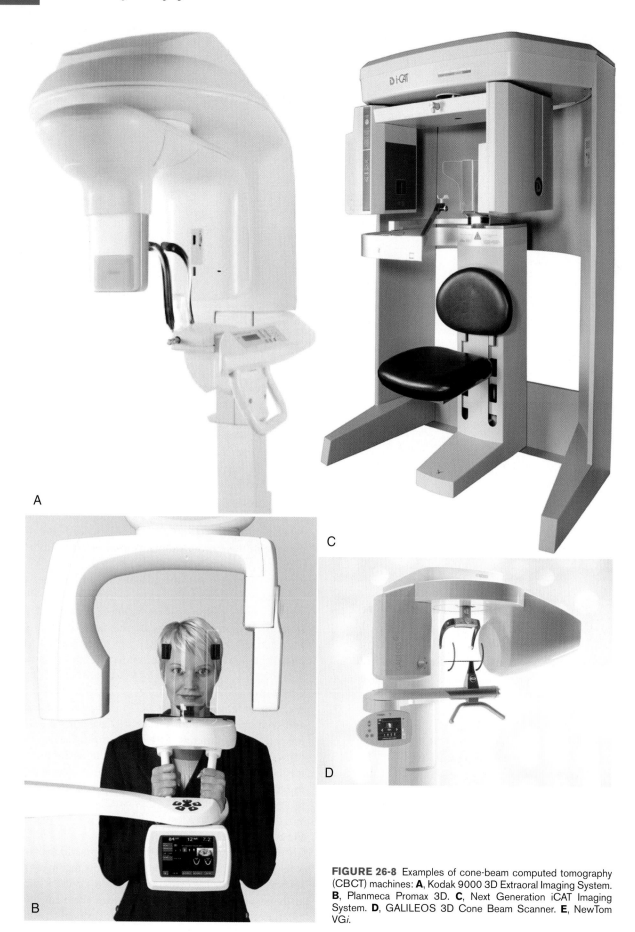

FIGURE 26-8 Examples of cone-beam computed tomography (CBCT) machines: **A**, Kodak 9000 3D Extraoral Imaging System. **B**, Planmeca Promax 3D. **C**, Next Generation iCAT Imaging System. **D**, GALILEOS 3D Cone Beam Scanner. **E**, NewTom VG*i*.

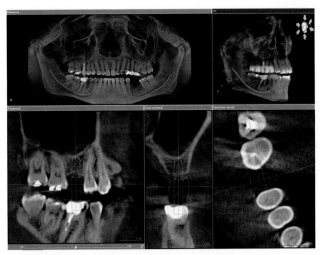

FIGURE 26-9 The diagnostic capabilities of three-dimensional cone beam imaging viewed in this example of implant placement for tooth #3. (Courtesy of Sirona Dental System, Charlotte, NC.)

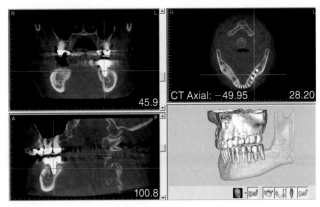

FIGURE 26-10 An implant placed in the mandible to replace tooth #19 viewed from coronal, axial, and sagittal planes to ensure secure placement in bone. (Courtesy of Carolina OMF Imaging, W. Bruce Howerton Jr., DDS, MS, Raleigh, NC.)

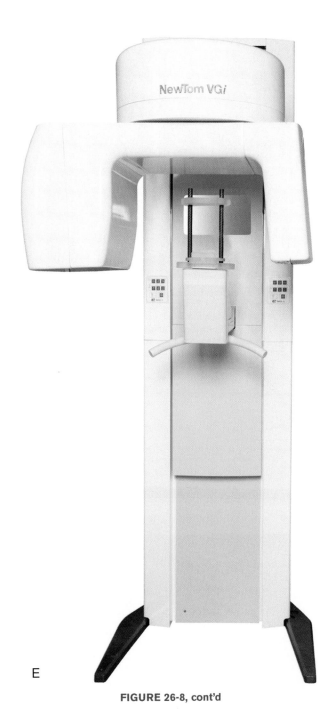

E

FIGURE 26-8, cont'd

that will assist the referring dentist or physician in diagnosis and treatment planning (Figure 26-9). Each CBCT machine has its proprietary viewing software, but many third-party DICOM viewing software packages are available with additional features.

Common Uses

Computer-generated, three-dimensional multiplanar images are new applications that greatly improve interpretation, diagnosis, and treatment planning in many aspects of dental care. Some of the common uses of three-dimensional imaging include the following: implant placement (Figure 26-10), extraction or exposure of impacted teeth (Figure 26-11), definition of anatomic structures (Figure 26-12), endodontic assessment (Figure 26-13), airway and sinus analysis (Figure 26-14), evaluation of temporomandibular joint (TMJ) disorders (Figure 26-15), orthodontic evaluation (Figure 26-16) and pathology evaluation (Figure 26-17).

It is easy to see from Figures 26-10 through Figure 26-17 that CBCT is revolutionizing the practice of dentistry. However, reviewing scans and images with CBCT also requires responsibility on the part of the dental practitioner to recognize findings and pathology outside of the region of interest, specifically outside of the maxilla and the mandible. Some such regions include the cerebral hemispheres or areas lateral to the oropharynx (for hard tissue calcifications) and the paranasal sinuses. These regions are not typically evaluated on a routine basis, although they are visible on three-dimensional imaging. Comprehensive examination and interpretation should be completed and documented with

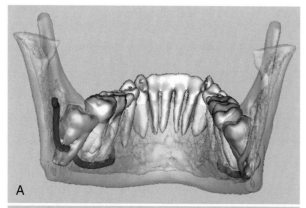

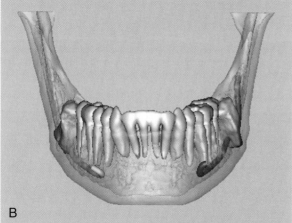

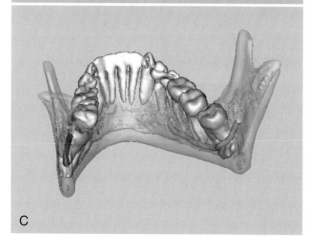

FIGURE 26-11 **A,** Impacted mandibular third molars (tooth #17 in green; tooth #32 in pink). Note the roots of #17 surrounding the mandibular canal. **B,** Teeth #17 and 32 positioned facial to the mandibular canal. **C,** Transparent mandible allowing full view of the location of the mandibular canals. (Courtesy of Carolina OMF Imaging, W. Bruce Howerton Jr., Raleigh, NC.)

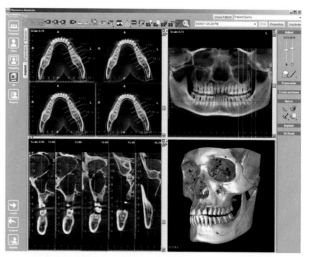

FIGURE 26-12 Planmeca Romexis 3D Explorer, the 3D image acquisition software for Planmeca ProMax 3D, which enables flexible viewing in all three relevant projections: axial, coronal, and sagittal. A rendered three-dimensional view provides a realistic overview of the anatomy, highlighting the mandibular canal in red. (Courtesy of Planmeca Oy, Helsinki, Finland.)

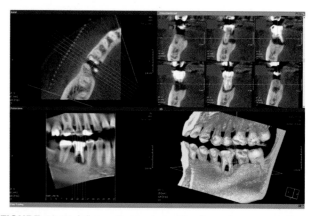

FIGURE 26-13 Inflammation and resulting bone loss surrounding a tooth with prior endodontic therapy. Multiple views, including a three-dimensional image, reveal the extent of bone loss.

the overall health of the patient in mind. Failure to do so could result in poor treatment outcomes for the dental provider and, more importantly, negative consequences for patients.

STEP-BY-STEP PROCEDURES

Patient Preparation

Depending on the guidelines from the manufacturer of the equipment, patients may be asked to sit or stand or be placed

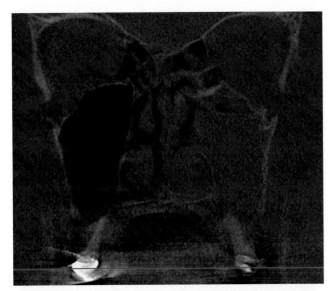

FIGURE 26-14 A portion of the maxillary sinus obliterated by mucosal thickening and inflammation as seen in this coronal image. (Courtesy of Carolina OMF Imaging, W. Bruce Howerton Jr., DDS, MS, Raleigh, NC.)

in the supine position during radiation exposure. Instructions given to the patient before the imaging procedure include the removal of all metallic items in the head-and-neck region, including jewelry, eyeglasses, and removable dental appliances. In certain instances, an intraoral radiographic guide may be placed in the patient's mouth during the scanning process. Referring specialists may also request that the scan be performed with the patient keeping the upper and lower teeth slightly apart, which would require the use of a cotton roll, gauze square, or bite registration material placed between maxillary and mandibular anterior teeth.

Patient Positioning

As with all radiographic procedures, the patient is instructed to remain very still during the exposure of three-dimensional images as well. As mentioned earlier, scan times vary from 7 to 30 seconds. Ergonomic head and chin supports have been designed for improved patient comfort. Manufacturers may install laser beams to help with proper alignment of clinical structures and to ensure correct anatomic positioning. As with most extraoral imaging procedures, patients have an open and comfortable view of the surrounding area (Figure 26-18).

ADVANTAGES AND DISADVANTAGES

Advantages of Three-Dimensional Imaging

1. *Lower radiation dose.* Compared with traditional CT procedures, cone beam imaging involves a lower radiation dose to the patient. Studies have compared the dose given

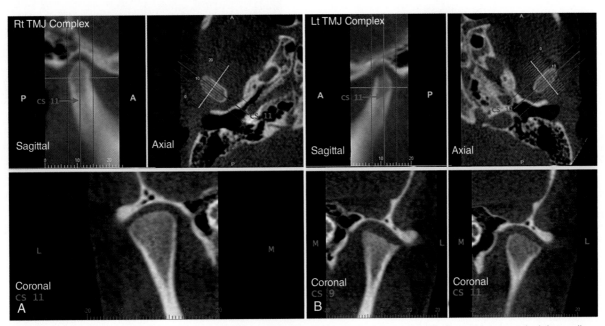

FIGURE 26-15 A, Coronal image demonstrating normal radiographic appearance of the right condyle. **B,** Coronal image on the left revealing erosion of the superior border of the mandibular condyle. (Courtesy of Carolina OMF Imaging, W. Bruce Howerton Jr., DDS, MS, Raleigh, NC.)

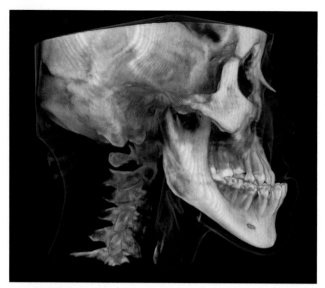

FIGURE 26-16 The Kodak 9500 3D System providing a large field of view and thus enabling the orthodontist to make a comprehensive dental and skeletal assessment of the patient before the beginning of treatment. (Courtesy of Carestream Health Inc., Rochester, NY.)

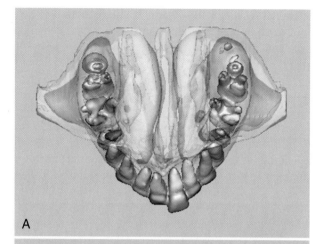

A

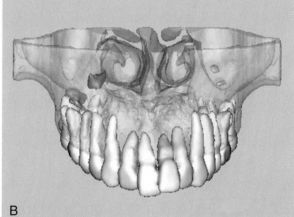

B

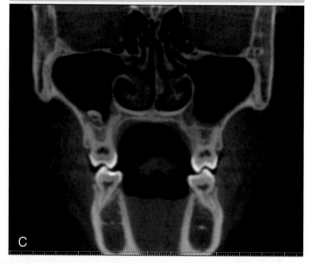

C

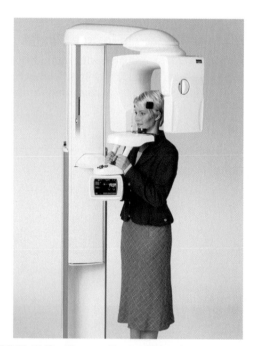

FIGURE 26-18 The Planmeca Promax 3D imaging system, which offers a comfortable and open view of the surroundings to the patient. (Courtesy of Planmeca Oy, Helsinki, Finland.)

FIGURE 26-17 A, Imaging software that allows visualization of maxillary teeth through the maxilla. **B,** Unknown objects (in green, red, yellow, turquoise, and violet) noted in the sinus near maxillary posterior teeth. A differential diagnosis included multiple osteomas. **C,** Coronal image revealing the location of the larger osteoma. (Courtesy of Carolina OMF Imaging, W. Bruce Howerton Jr., DDS, MS, Raleigh, NC.)

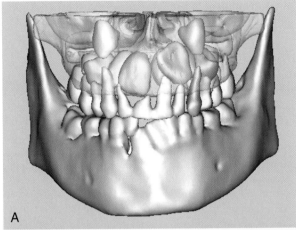

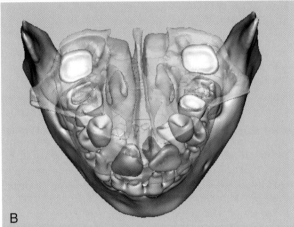

FIGURE 26-19 (Refer to the panoramic image in Figure 26-1.) **A**, Through the use of three-dimensional imaging and viewing software, the transparent maxilla revealing an inverted tooth #9 (shaded green) as well as a supernumerary tooth (shaded purple). **B**, The exact location of teeth in the anterior maxilla visualized from a superior view (looking down on the roots of the teeth). (Courtesy of Carolina OMF Imaging, W. Bruce Howerton Jr., DDS, MS, Raleigh, NC.)

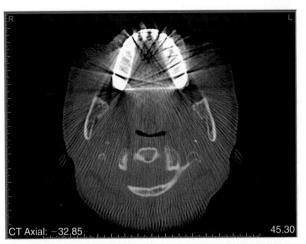

FIGURE 26-20 Streak artifacts demonstrated in this axial image of a patient with many full-coverage restorations. (Courtesy of Carolina OMF Imaging, W. Bruce Howerton Jr., DDS, MS, Raleigh, NC.)

Disadvantages of Three-Dimensional Digital Imaging

1. *Patient movement and artifacts.* Motion artifact occurs when a patient moves during the radiographic procedure. This type of artifact may occur with both two-dimensional and three-dimensional imaging. CBCT machines are equipped with devices to stabilize the head and the neck of the patient, and the patient should also be given oral instructions prior to the procedure to remain still during exposure.

   Radiation is stopped and may not reach the receptor when it interacts with an area of high attenuation, such as a metal crown, bridge, or large amalgam restoration. Streak artifacts from these types of metallic restorations may eliminate or obscure the surrounding anatomy (Figure 26-20).

2. *Size of the field of view.* If the field of view is small, findings or pathology in other regions of the oral–maxillofacial complex may be missed. The size of the field of view should capture the appropriate anatomy.

3. *Cost of equipment; need to learn a new computer language.* The cost of the setup of CBCT equipment may be prohibitive for many dental offices. CBCT machines currently range in cost from $150,000 to $300,000. In addition, becoming fully acquainted with the imaging software and correctly using DICOM data require time and dedication to learn the skills needed to create accurate three-dimensional volume images.

4. *Lack of training in interpretation of image data on areas outside the maxilla and the mandible.* Many dental professionals who incorporate this technology into their practices have not had the training required to interpret data on anatomic areas beyond the maxilla and the mandible. To ensure the correct and safe use of this technology, educational institutions are incorporating CBCT into their curricula, and continuing education courses are being offered to help dental professionals use and interpret

for a typical CBCT scan to be comparable with the dose given for three or four full-mouth series of intraoral radiographs.

2. *Brief scanning time.* With some machines, cone-beam data can be acquired with a quick 8- to 10-second scan. This short exposure time decreases the chances for motion artifacts to occur and encourages a high level of patient cooperation.

3. *Anatomically accurate images.* CBCT eliminates the superimposition of structures; magnification of measurements does not occur. Therefore, cone-beam data have a 1:1 relationship with the anatomy (Figure 26-19).

4. *Ability to save and easily transport images.* Three-dimensional images can be saved digitally in a .jpg (Joint Photographic (Experts) Group) or .bmp (bitmap) format and viewed online, placed on a compact disc (CD), or printed to paper or film. The images can also be easily e-mailed to referring dentists.

DICOM data accurately and effectively. As mentioned in Chapter 1, in 1999, the American Dental Association recognized oral and maxillofacial radiology as a specialty. Oral and maxillofacial radiologists are trained to interpret hard-tissue changes within the oral–maxillofacial complex. The American Academy of Oral and Maxillofacial Radiology has stated that CBCT and implant imaging should be performed only by a board-certified oral and maxillofacial radiologist or a dentist with adequate training and/or experience.

SUMMARY

- Three-dimensional imaging provides dental professionals with a more complete interpretive image than does traditional radiography, which can only provide two-dimensional images.
- Three-dimensional imaging serves a number of diagnostic purposes for dental practitioners.
- Anatomic structures of the reconstructed volume of data provide accurate dimensional measurements of the patient with a 1:1 ratio relationship.
- The essential components for three-dimensional imaging include a CBCT machine, a computer, and various types of viewing software.
- The advantages of three-dimensional imaging include a lower dose of radiation to the patient, a brief scanning time, anatomically accurate images, and ability to easily save and transport the images.
- The disadvantages of three-dimensional imaging include patient movement artifacts, limited size of the field of view, cost of equipment, and lack of training in interpretation of image data on areas outside of the maxilla and the mandible.

BIBLIOGRAPHY

American Academy of Oral and Maxillofacial Radiology: Directory of advanced educational programs: www.aaomr.org/adv_edu_prog.php: Accessed April 2, 2008.

American Dental Association: Dental professionals. Specialty National Organizations: www.ada.org/prof/ed/specialties/specorgs.asp: Accessed April 2, 2008.

Danforth RA, Miles DA: Cone beam volume imaging: 3D applications for dentistry. *Ir Dent* 10(9):14–18, 2007.

Howerton WB, Mora MA: Advancements in digital imaging: what is new and on the horizon? *J Am Dent Assoc* 139:20S–24S, 2008.

Ludlow JB, Davies-Ludlow LE, Brooks SL, Howerton WB: Dosimetry of 3 CBCT devices for oral and maxillofacial radiology: CB Mercuray, NewTom 3G and i-CAT, *Dentomaxillofac Radiol* 35:219–226, 2006.

Ludlow JB, Davies-Ludlow LE, White SC: Patient risk related to common dental radiographic examinations, *J Am Dent Assoc* 139:1237–1243, 2008.

Roberts JA, Drage NA, Davies J, Thomas DW: Effective dose from cone beam CT examinations in dentistry, *Br J Radiol* 82:35–40, 2009.

White SC, Heslop EW, Hollender LG, Mosier KM, Ruprecht A, Shrout MK: American Academy of Oral and Maxillofacial Radiology, ad hoc Committee on Parameters of Care: Parameters of radiologic care: an official report of the American Academy of Oral and Maxillofacial Radiology, *Oral Surg Oral Med Oral Pathol Oral Radiol Endod* 91(5):498–511, 2001.

White SC, Pharoah MJ: Cone-beam computed tomography. In *Oral radiology: principles and interpretation*, ed 6, St. Louis, 2009, Mosby.

QUIZ QUESTIONS

MATCHING

For questions 1 to 10, match each term with its corresponding definition.

a. cone-beam computer tomography
b. DICOM data
c. field of view
d. multiplanar reconstruction (MPR)
e. coronal plane
f. sagittal plane
g. contrast resolution
h. spatial resolution
i. voxel
j. three-dimensional volume rendering

___ 1. The universal format for handling, storing, and transmitting three-dimensional images.

___ 2. The smallest element of a three-dimensional image.

___ 3. A measurement of pixel size in multiplanar reconstruction.

___ 4. A vertical plane that divides the body into right and left sides; runs perpendicular to the ground.

___ 5. The reconstruction of raw data into images when imported into viewing software to create three anatomical planes of the body.

___ 6. The area that can be captured when performing imaging procedures.

___ 7. Term used to describe computer-assisted digital imaging in dentistry; this imaging technique uses a cone-shaped x-ray beam to acquire information and present it in three dimensions

___ 8. A vertical plane that divides the body into anterior and posterior sides; runs perpendicular to the ground.

___ 9. The number of gray scale colors available to be chosen for each pixel in the image.

___ 10. A three-dimensional shape that is created from two-dimensional images.

TRUE OR FALSE

___ 11. Compared with traditional computer tomography (CT) procedures, cone beam imaging provides a higher radiation dose for the patient.

____ **12.** A short exposure time decreases the chances for motion artifacts to occur, as well as encouraging a high level of patient cooperation.

____ **13.** If the field of view is small, findings or pathology in other regions of the oral and maxillofacial complex may be missed.

____ **14.** Cone-beam data are said to have a 2:1 relationship with the anatomy.

____ **15.** A disadvantage of use of cone-beam data is that many dental professionals who incorporate CBCT into their practices have not had the training required to interpret anatomy beyond the maxilla and mandible.

____ **16.** Three-dimensional imaging provides an in-depth image that gives dental professionals a more complete interpretive image than with two-dimensional scans of traditional radiography.

____ **17.** Three-dimensional imaging serves a number of diagnostic purposes for dental practitioners.

____ **18.** The American Dental Association recognized the specialty of oral and maxillofacial radiology in 2009.

MULTIPLE CHOICE

19. An area of high attenuation that could stop radiation from reaching the receptor could include which of the following?
   a. metal crown
   b. bridge
   c. large amalgam restoration
   d. all of the above

20. Advantages of the CBCT include which of the following?
   a. images can be saved digitally in a .jpg or .bmp format
   b. images can be placed on a compact disc media
   c. images can be e-mailed to referring dentists
   d. all of the above

21. The fact that the cone-beam data has a 1:1 relationship with the anatomy means that:
   a. anatomically accurate images are produced
   b. magnification of measurements does not occur
   c. CBCT eliminates the superimposition of structures
   d. all of the above

SHORT ANSWERS

22. Name some of the common uses of three-dimensional imaging.

23. Why is it important for the dental professional who uses CBCT to be a board-certified oral and maxillofacial radiologist or a dentist with adequate training or experience?

24. Prior to performing CBCT, what instructions should be given to the patient?

25. Name the essential specialized equipment necessary for three-dimensional digital imaging.

part VI

Normal Anatomy and Film Mounting Basics

Chapter 27   Normal Anatomy: Intraoral Images, 325
Chapter 28   Film Mounting and Viewing, 345
Chapter 29   Normal Anatomy: Panoramic Images, 357

Normal Anatomy: Intraoral Images

OUTLINE

DEFINITIONS OF GENERAL TERMS
    Types of Bone
    Prominences of Bone
    Spaces and Depressions in Bone
    Miscellaneous Terms

NORMAL ANATOMIC LANDMARKS
    Bony Landmarks of the Maxilla
    Bony Landmarks of the Mandible
NORMAL TOOTH ANATOMY
    Tooth Structure
    Supporting Structures

LEARNING OBJECTIVES

After completion of this chapter, the student will be able to do the following:

- Define the key terms associated with normal anatomy on intraoral images
- State the difference between cortical and cancellous bone
- Define the general terms that describe prominences, spaces, and depressions in bone
- Identify and describe the normal anatomic landmarks of the maxilla on a human skull
- Identify and describe the normal anatomic landmarks of the maxilla as viewed on dental images
- Identify and describe the normal anatomic landmarks of the mandible on a human skull

- Identify and describe the normal anatomic landmarks of the mandible as viewed on dental images
- Identify and describe the appearance of tooth anatomy as viewed on dental images
- Identify each normal landmark of the maxilla and the mandible as either radiolucent or radiopaque as viewed on a dental image
- Identify each normal anatomic landmark of a tooth as radiolucent or radiopaque as viewed on a dental image

KEY TERMS

Alveolar bone	Hamulus	Nasal septum
Alveolar crest	Incisive foramen	Nutrient canal(s)
Alveolar process	Inferior nasal conchae	Periodontal ligament space
Anterior nasal spine	Internal oblique ridge	Process
Body of mandible	Inverted Y	Pulp cavity
Canal	Lamina dura	Ramus
Cancellous	Lateral fossa	Ridge
Coronoid process	Lingual foramen	Septum, septa
Cortical	Mandibular canal	Sinus
Dentin	Maxillary sinus	Spine
Dentino-enamel junction	Maxillary tuberosity	Submandibular fossa
Enamel	Median palatal suture	Superior foramina of incisive canal
External oblique ridge	Mental foramen	Suture
Floor of nasal cavity	Mental fossa	Tubercle
Foramen	Mental ridge	Tuberosity
Fossa	Mylohyoid ridge	Zygoma
Genial tubercles	Nasal cavity	Zygomatic process of maxilla

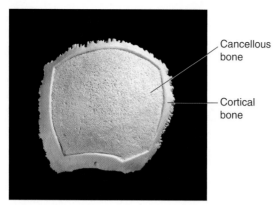

Figure 27-1 Cortical bone and cancellous bone. (From Logan BM, Reynolds PA, Hutchings RT: *McMinn's color atlas of head and neck anatomy*, Philadelphia, 2010, Mosby.).

The dental radiographer must be able to recognize the normal anatomic landmarks viewed on intraoral images. Recognition of such normal anatomic landmarks enables the radiographer to mount and interpret intraoral images accurately. Without a working knowledge of normal anatomy, the dental radiographer may incorrectly mount dental images or mistake normal anatomic structures for pathologic conditions.

Before dental images can be interpreted and normal anatomic landmarks identified, the dental radiographer must first have a thorough knowledge of the anatomy of the maxilla and the mandible. Each normal anatomic landmark seen on a periapical image corresponds to that seen on the human skull. If the dental radiographer knows the anatomy of the maxilla and the mandible as viewed on the human skull, he or she can identify the normal anatomy on a dental image.

The purpose of this chapter is to review the normal anatomy of the maxilla and the mandible as viewed on the skull and to describe the normal anatomic landmarks as viewed on intraoral images.

DEFINITIONS OF GENERAL TERMS

A number of general terms are used to describe the anatomy of the bones of the skull. Terms describing types of bone, bony prominences, and bony spaces and depressions can be used to characterize areas of the maxilla and the mandible normally seen on periapical images. The dental radiographer can use these general terms to describe areas of normal anatomy viewed on intraoral images.

Types of Bone

The composition of bone in the human body can be described as either cortical or cancellous.

Cortical Bone

The term **cortical** is derived from the Latin word *cortex* and means "outer layer." Cortical bone, also referred to as *compact bone*, is the dense outer layer of bone (Figure 27-1). Cortical

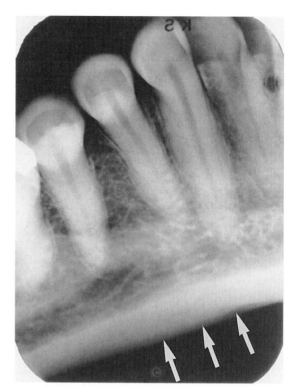

FIGURE 27-2 Cortical bone appears highly radiopaque on a dental image. (From Haring JI, Lind LJ: *Radiographic interpretation for the dental hygienist*, Philadelphia, 1993, Saunders.)

bone resists the passage of the x-ray beam and appears radiopaque on a dental image. The inferior border of the mandible is composed of cortical bone and appears radiopaque (Figure 27-2).

Cancellous Bone

The term **cancellous** is also derived from Latin and means "arranged like a lattice." Cancellous bone is the soft, spongy bone located between two layers of dense cortical bone (see Figure 27-1). Cancellous bone is composed of numerous bony trabeculae that form a latticelike network of intercommunicating spaces filled with bone marrow. The trabeculae, actual pieces of bone, resist the passage of the x-ray beam and appear radiopaque; in contrast, the marrow spaces permit the passage of the x-ray beam and appear radiolucent. The larger the trabeculations, the more radiolucent the area of cancellous bone appears. Cancellous bone appears predominantly radiolucent (Figure 27-3).

Prominences of Bone

Prominences of bone are composed of dense cortical bone and appear radiopaque on dental images. Five terms can be used to describe the bony prominences seen in maxillary and mandibular periapical images, as follows:

    Process: A marked prominence or projection of bone; an example is the coronoid process of the mandible (Figure 27-4).

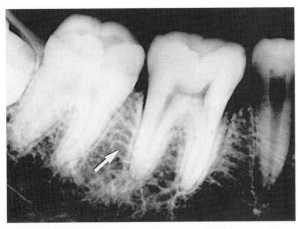

FIGURE 27-3 Cancellous bone appears predominantly radiolucent. (From Haring JI, Lind LJ: *Radiographic interpretation for the dental hygienist*, Philadelphia, 1993, Saunders.)

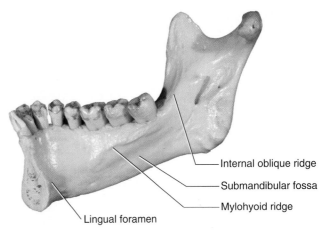

FIGURE 27-5 Internal oblique ridge, submandibular fossa, mylohyoid ridge, and lingual foramen. (From Liebgott B: *The anatomical basis of dentistry*, ed 3, St. Louis, 2011, Mosby).

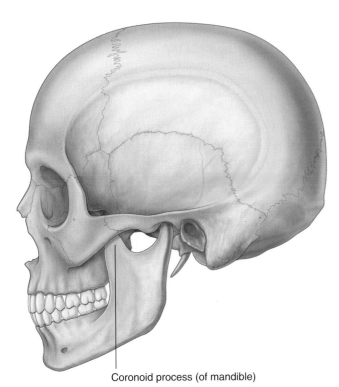

FIGURE 27-4 Coronoid process. (From Drake RL, et al: *Gray's atlas of anatomy*, Philadelphia, 2008, Churchill Livingstone).

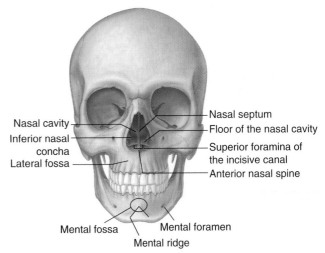

FIGURE 27-6 Anterior nasal spine, mental foramen, nasal septum, superior foramina of the incisive canal, lateral fossa, nasal cavity, the floor of the nasal cavity, inferior nasal concha, mental fossa, and mental ridge. (From Drake RL, et al: *Gray's atlas of anatomy*, Philadelphia, 2008, Churchill Livingstone).

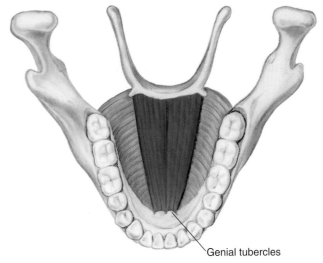

FIGURE 27-7 Genial tubercles. (From Fehrenbach MF, Herring SW: *Illustrated anatomy of the head and neck*, ed 3, St. Louis, 2007, Saunders).

Ridge: A linear prominence or projection of bone; an example is the internal oblique ridge of the mandible (Figure 27-5).

Spine: A sharp, thornlike projection of bone; an example is the anterior nasal spine of the maxilla (Figure 27-6).

Tubercle: A small bump or nodule of bone; an example is the genial tubercles of the mandible (Figure 27-7).

Tuberosity: A rounded prominence of bone; an example is the maxillary tuberosity (Figure 27-8).

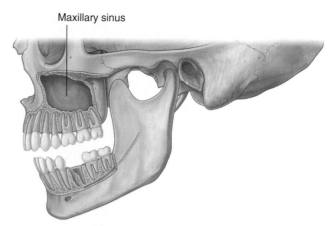

Maxillary sinus

FIGURE 27-10 Maxillary sinus. (From Drake RL, et al: *Gray's atlas of anatomy*, Philadelphia, 2008, Churchill Livingstone).

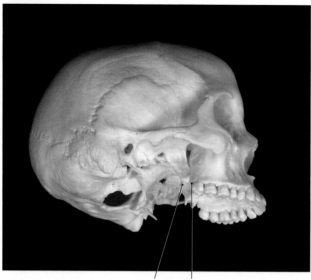

Hamulus   Maxillary tuberosity

FIGURE 27-8 The maxillary tuberosity and the hamulus. (From Logan BM, Reynolds PA, Hutchings RT: *McMinn's color atlas of head and neck anatomy*, Philadelphia, 2010, Mosby).

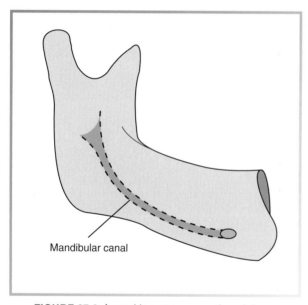

Mandibular canal

FIGURE 27-9 A canal is a passageway through bone.

Spaces and Depressions in Bone

Spaces and depressions in bone do not resist the passage of the x-ray beam and appear radiolucent on dental images. Four terms can be used to describe the spaces and depressions in bone viewed in maxillary and mandibular periapical images, as follows:

Canal: A tubelike passageway through bone that contains nerves and blood vessels; an example is the mandibular canal (Figure 27-9).

Foramen: An opening or hole in bone that permits the passage of nerves and blood vessels; an example is the mental foramen of the mandible (see Figure 27-6).

Fossa: A broad, shallow, scooped-out or depressed area of bone; an example is the submandibular fossa of the mandible (see Figure 27-5).

Sinus: A hollow space, cavity, or recess in bone; an example is the maxillary sinus (Figure 27-10).

Miscellaneous Terms

Two other general terms can be used to describe normal landmarks viewed on a dental image, as follows:

Septum: A bony wall or partition that divides two spaces or cavities. A septum may be present within the space of a fossa or sinus. A bony septum appears radiopaque, in contrast to a space or cavity, which appears radiolucent. An example is the nasal septum (see Figure 27-6).

Suture: An immovable joint that represents a line of union between adjoining bones of the skull. Sutures are found only in the skull. On dental images, a suture appears as a thin radiolucent line. An example is the median palatine suture of the maxilla (Figure 27-11).

NORMAL ANATOMIC LANDMARKS

Bony Landmarks of the Maxilla

The upper jaw is composed of two paired bones, the *maxillae* (Figure 27-12). The paired maxillae meet at the midline of the face and are often referred to as a single bone, the *maxilla*. The maxilla has been described as the architectural cornerstone of the face. All the bones of the face, with the exception of the mandible, articulate with the maxilla. The maxilla forms the floor of the orbit of the eyes, the sides and floor of the nasal cavities, and the hard palate. The lower border of the maxilla supports maxillary teeth. This section reviews bony landmarks that frequently appear in maxillary periapical images.

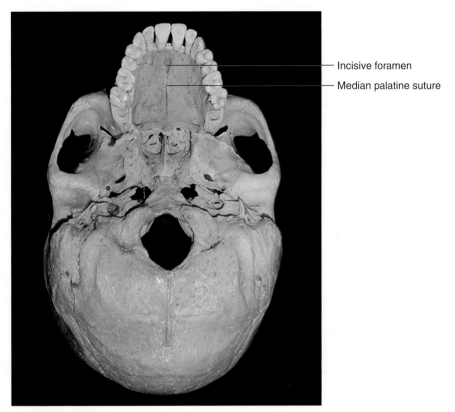

FIGURE 27-11 Median palatine suture and incisive foramen. (From Fehrenbach MF, Herring SW: *Illustrated anatomy of the head and neck*, ed 3, St. Louis, 2007, Saunders).

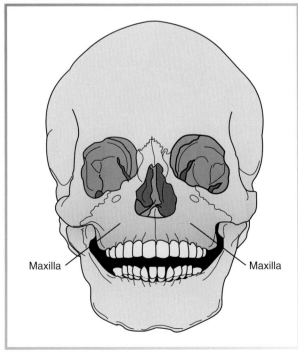

FIGURE 27-12 Paired bones of the maxilla.

Incisive Foramen

Description. The **incisive foramen** (also known as the *nasopalatine foramen*) is an opening or hole in bone located at the midline of the anterior portion of the hard palate directly posterior to maxillary central incisors (see Figure 27-11). The nasopalatine nerve exits the maxilla through the incisive foramen.

Appearance. On a maxillary periapical image, the incisive foramen appears as a small, ovoid or round radiolucent area located between the roots of the maxillary central incisors (Figure 27-13).

Superior Foramina of Incisive Canal

Description. The **superior foramina of the incisive canal** are two tiny openings or holes in bone that are located on the floor of the nasal cavity (*foramina* is the plural of *foramen*) (see Figure 27-6). The superior foramina are the openings of two small canals that extend downward and medially from the floor of the nasal cavity. These two small canals join together to form the incisive canal and share a common exit, the *incisive foramen*. The nasopalatine nerve enters the maxilla through the superior foramina, travels through the incisive canal, and exits at the incisive foramen.

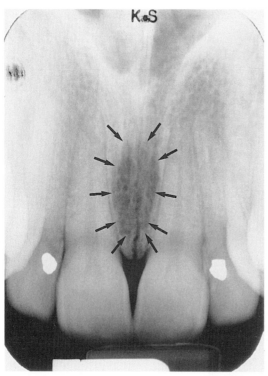

FIGURE 27-13 The incisive foramen appears radiolucent. (From Haring JI, Lind LJ: *Radiographic interpretation for the dental hygienist*, Philadelphia, 1993, Saunders.)

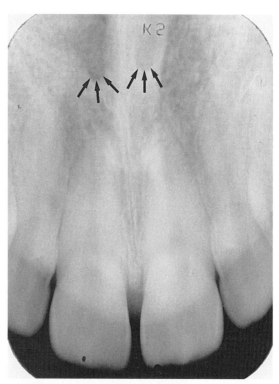

FIGURE 27-14 The superior foramina of the incisive canal appear as two small, round radiolucencies. (From Haring JI, Lind LJ: *Radiographic interpretation for the dental hygienist*, Philadelphia, 1993, Saunders.)

Appearance. On a maxillary periapical image, the superior foramina appear as two small, round radiolucencies located superior to the apices of the maxillary central incisors (Figure 27-14).

Median Palatal Suture

Description. The **median palatal suture** is the immovable joint between the two palatine processes of the maxilla. (The palatine processes of the maxilla form the major portion of the hard palate.) The median palatal suture extends from the alveolar bone between the maxillary central incisors to the posterior hard palate (see Figure 27-11).

Appearance. On a maxillary periapical image, the median palatal suture appears as a thin radiolucent line between maxillary central incisors (Figure 27-15). The median palatal suture is bounded on both sides by dense cortical bone that appears radiopaque. As the median palatal suture fuses with age, it may become less distinct on a dental image.

Lateral Fossa

Description. The **lateral fossa** (also known as the *canine fossa*) is a smooth, depressed area of the maxilla located just inferior and medial to the infraorbital foramen between maxillary canine and lateral incisors (see Figure 27-6).

Appearance. On a maxillary periapical image, the lateral fossa appears as a radiolucent area between maxillary canine and lateral incisors (Figure 27-16). In some periapical images,

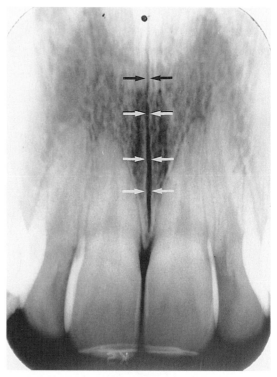

FIGURE 27-15 The median palatal suture appears as a thin radiolucent line. (From Haring JI, Lind LJ: *Radiographic interpretation for the dental hygienist*, Philadelphia, 1993, Saunders.)

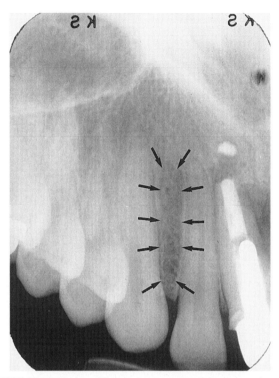

FIGURE 27-16 The lateral fossa appears as a radiolucent area between the lateral incisor and the canine. (Photo courtesy of Allyson Bowcutt.)

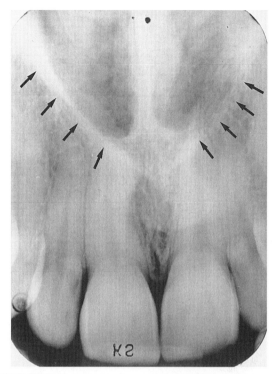

FIGURE 27-17 The nasal cavity appears as a large radiolucent area above the maxilla. (From Haring JI, Lind LJ: *Radiographic interpretation for the dental hygienist*, Philadelphia, 1993, Saunders.)

the lateral fossa may appear as a distinct radiolucency; in others, it may appear to be absent. The appearance of the lateral fossa varies depending on the anatomy of the individual.

Nasal Cavity

Description. The **nasal cavity** (also known as the *nasal fossa*) is a pear-shaped compartment of bone located superior to the maxilla (see Figure 27-6). The inferior portion, or floor, of the nasal cavity is formed by the palatal processes of the maxilla and the horizontal portions of palatine bones. The lateral walls of the nasal cavity are formed by the ethmoid bone and the maxillae. The nasal cavity is divided by a bony partition, or wall, called the *nasal septum*.

Appearance. On a maxillary periapical image, the nasal cavity appears as a large, radiolucent area superior to maxillary incisors (Figure 27-17).

Nasal Septum

Description. The **nasal septum** is a vertical bony wall or partition that divides the nasal cavity into the right and left nasal fossae (*fossae* is the plural of *fossa*) (see Figure 27-6). The nasal septum is formed by two bones—the vomer and a portion of the ethmoid bone—and cartilage.

Appearance. On a maxillary periapical image, the nasal septum appears as a vertical radiopaque partition that divides the nasal cavity (Figure 27-18). The nasal septum may be superimposed over the median palatal suture.

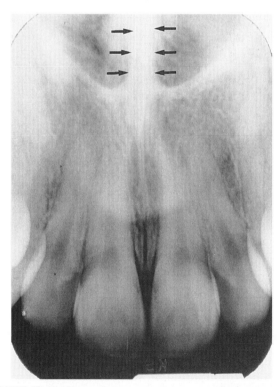

FIGURE 27-18 The nasal septum appears as a radiopaque partition that divides the nasal cavity. (From Haring JI, Lind LJ: *Radiographic interpretation for the dental hygienist*, Philadelphia, 1993, Saunders.)

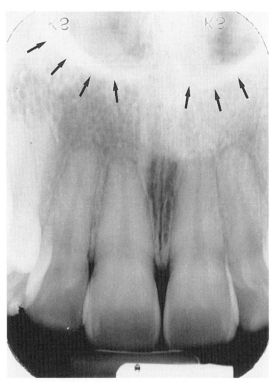

FIGURE 27-19 The floor of the nasal cavity appears as a radiopaque band. (From Haring JI, Lind LJ: *Radiographic interpretation for the dental hygienist*, Philadelphia, 1993, Saunders.)

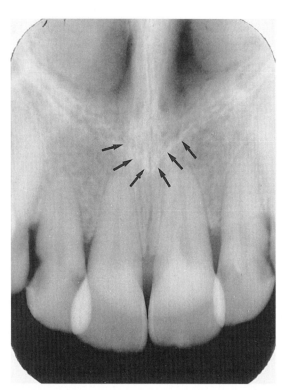

FIGURE 27-20 The anterior nasal spine appears as a V-shaped radiopacity at the midline of the floor of the nasal cavity. (From Haring JI, Lind LJ: *Radiographic interpretation for the dental hygienist*, Philadelphia, 1993, Saunders.)

Floor of Nasal Cavity

Description. The **floor of the nasal cavity** is a bony wall formed by the palatal processes of the maxilla and the horizontal portions of palatine bones (see Figure 27-6). The floor is composed of dense cortical bone and defines the inferior border of the nasal cavity.

Appearance. On a maxillary periapical image, the floor of the nasal cavity appears as a dense radiopaque band of bone superior to maxillary incisors (Figure 27-19).

Anterior Nasal Spine

Description. The **anterior nasal spine** is a sharp projection of the maxilla located at the anterior and inferior portion of the nasal cavity (see Figure 27-6).

Appearance. On a maxillary periapical image, the anterior nasal spine appears as a V-shaped radiopaque area located at the intersection of the floor of the nasal cavity and the nasal septum (Figure 27-20).

Inferior Nasal Conchae

Description. **Inferior nasal conchae** are wafer-thin, curved plates of bone that extend from the lateral walls of the nasal cavity (see Figure 27-6). Inferior nasal conchae are seen in the lower lateral portions of the nasal cavity. The term *concha* is derived from Latin and means "shell shaped" or "scroll shaped."

Appearance. On a maxillary periapical image, inferior nasal conchae appear as a diffuse radiopaque mass or projection within the nasal cavity (Figure 27-21).

Maxillary Sinus

Description. **Maxillary sinuses** are paired cavities or compartments of bone located within the maxilla (see Figure 27-10). Maxillary sinuses are located superior to maxillary premolar and molar teeth. Rarely does the maxillary sinus extend anteriorly beyond the canines. At birth, the maxillary sinus is the size of a small pea. With growth, the maxillary sinus expands and eventually occupies a large portion of the maxilla. The maxillary sinus may extend to include interdental bone, molar furcation areas, or the maxillary tuberosity region.

Appearance. On a maxillary periapical image, the maxillary sinus appears as a radiolucent area located superior to the apices of maxillary premolars and molars (Figures 27-22, and 27-23). The floor of the maxillary sinus is composed of dense cortical bone and appears as a radiopaque line.

Septa within Maxillary Sinus

Description. Bony **septa** (*septa* is the plural of *septum*) may be seen within the maxillary sinus. Septa are bony walls or partitions that appear to divide the maxillary sinus into compartments (Figure 27-24).

Appearance. On a maxillary periapical image, the septa appear as radiopaque lines within the maxillary sinus (Figure 27-25). In some periapical images, the septa appear as distinct radiopaque lines; in others, no septa are seen. The presence and number of bony septa within a maxillary sinus vary depending on the anatomy of the individual.

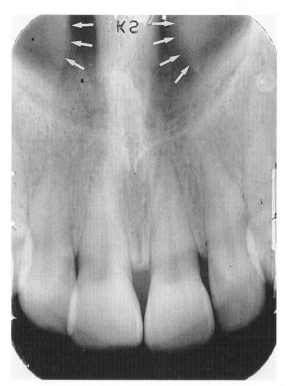

FIGURE 27-21 The inferior nasal conchae appear as diffuse radiopacities within the nasal cavity. (From Haring JI, Lind LJ: *Radiographic interpretation for the dental hygienist*, Philadelphia, 1993, Saunders.)

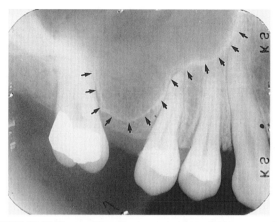

FIGURE 27-23 The maxillary sinus appears as a radiolucent area above maxillary posterior teeth. (From Haring JI, Lind LJ: *Radiographic interpretation for the dental hygienist*, Philadelphia, 1993, Saunders.)

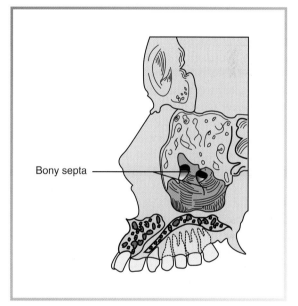

FIGURE 27-24 Septa are bony walls within the maxillary sinus.

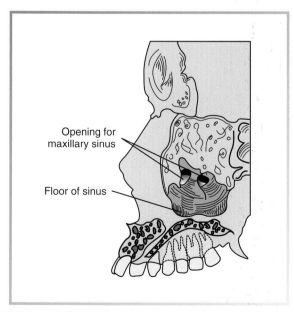

FIGURE 27-22 The maxillary sinuses are paired compartments of bone located above the maxillary posterior teeth. (From Haring JI, Lind LJ: *Radiographic interpretation for the dental hygienist*, Philadelphia, 1993, Saunders.)

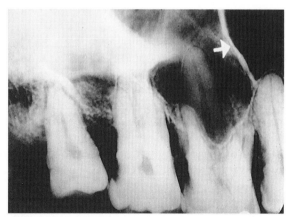

FIGURE 27-25 Septa within the maxillary sinus appear as radiopaque lines. (From Haring JI, Lind LJ: *Radiographic interpretation for the dental hygienist*, Philadelphia, 1993, Saunders.)

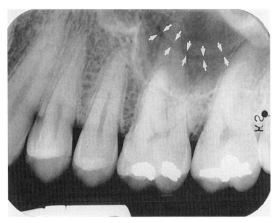

FIGURE 27-26 Nutrient canals appear as narrow radiolucent lines. (From Haring JI, Lind LJ: *Radiographic interpretation for the dental hygienist*, Philadelphia, 1993, Saunders.)

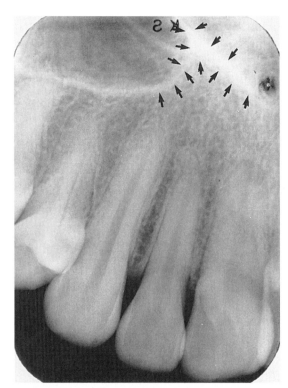

FIGURE 27-27 The inverted Y appears as a radiopaque upside-down Y. (From Haring JI, Lind LJ: *Radiographic interpretation for the dental hygienist*, Philadelphia, 1993, Saunders.)

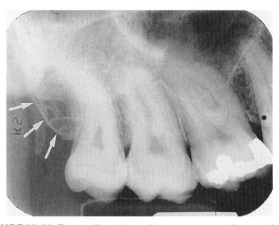

FIGURE 27-28 The maxillary tuberosity appears as a radiopaque bulge distal to the third molar region. (From Haring JI, Lind LJ: *Radiographic interpretation for the dental hygienist*, Philadelphia, 1993, Saunders.)

Nutrient Canals within Maxillary Sinus

Description. **Nutrient canals** may be seen within maxillary sinuses. Nutrient canals are tiny, tubelike passageways through bone, which contain blood vessels and nerves that supply maxillary teeth and interdental areas.

Appearance. On a maxillary periapical image, a nutrient canal appears as a narrow radiolucent band bounded by two thin radiopaque lines (Figure 27-26). The radiopaque lines represent the cortical bone that makes up the walls of the canal.

Inverted Y

Description. The term **inverted Y** refers to the intersection of the maxillary sinus and the nasal cavity as viewed on a dental image.

Appearance. On a maxillary periapical image, the inverted Y appears as a radiopaque upside-down Y formed by the intersection of the lateral wall of the nasal fossa and the anterior border of the maxillary sinus (Figure 27-27). The lateral wall of the nasal cavity and the anterior border of the maxillary sinus are both composed of dense cortical bone and appear as a radiopaque line or band. The inverted Y is located superior to the maxillary canine.

Maxillary Tuberosity

Description. The **maxillary tuberosity** is a rounded prominence of bone that extends posterior to the third molar region (see Figure 27-8). Blood vessels and nerves enter the maxilla in this region and supply posterior teeth.

Appearance. On a maxillary periapical image, the maxillary tuberosity appears as a radiopaque bulge distal to the third molar region (Figure 27-28).

Hamulus

Description. The **hamulus** (also known as the *hamular process*) is a small, hooklike projection of bone extending from the medial pterygoid plate of the sphenoid bone (see

Figure 27-8). The hamulus is located posterior to the maxillary tuberosity region.

Appearance. On a maxillary periapical image, the hamulus appears as a radiopaque hooklike projection posterior to the maxillary tuberosity area (Figure 27-29). The image appearance of the hamulus varies in length, shape, and density.

Zygomatic Process of Maxilla

Description. The **zygomatic process of the maxilla** is a bony projection of the maxilla that articulates with the

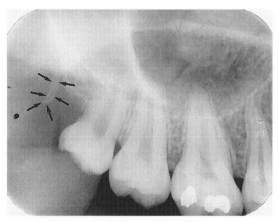

FIGURE 27-29 The hamulus appears as a hooklike radiopacity distal to the maxillary tuberosity area. (From Haring JI, Lind LJ: *Radiographic interpretation for the dental hygienist*, Philadelphia, 1993, Saunders.)

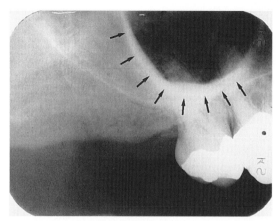

FIGURE 27-31 The zygomatic process of the maxilla appears as a J-shaped or U-shaped radiopacity superior to the maxillary molars. (From Haring JI, Lind LJ: *Radiographic interpretation for the dental hygienist*, Philadelphia, 1993, Saunders.)

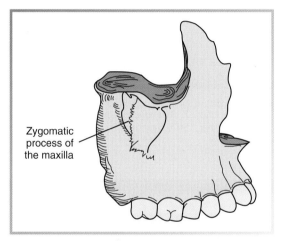

FIGURE 27-30 The zygomatic process of the maxilla is a small portion of the maxilla that articulates with the zygoma.

zygoma, or malar bone (Figure 27-30). The zygomatic process of the maxilla is composed of dense cortical bone.

Appearance. On a maxillary periapical image, the zygomatic process of the maxilla appears as a J-shaped or U-shaped radiopacity located superior to the maxillary first molar region (Figure 27-31).

Zygoma

Description. The **zygoma**, or "cheekbone" (also referred to as the *malar bone* or *zygomatic bone*) articulates with the zygomatic process of the maxilla (Figure 27-32). The zygoma is composed of dense cortical bone.

Appearance. On a maxillary periapical image, the zygoma appears as a diffuse radiopaque band extending posteriorly from the zygomatic process of the maxilla (Figure 27-33).

Bony Landmarks of the Mandible

The mandible, the largest and strongest bone of the face, can be divided into three main parts: the ramus, the body, and the alveolar process (Figure 27-34).

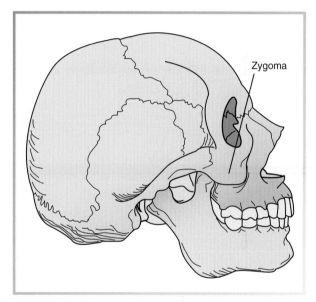

FIGURE 27-32 The zygoma (or cheekbone) articulates with the zygomatic process of the maxilla.

- **Ramus.** The ramus is the vertical portion of the mandible that is found posterior to the third molar. The mandible has two rami (*rami* is the plural of *ramus*), one on each side.
- **Body of mandible.** The body of the mandible is the horizontal, U-shaped portion that extends from ramus to ramus.
- **Alveolar process.** The alveolar process is the portion of the mandible that encases and supports teeth.

This section reviews the bony landmarks that frequently appear in mandibular periapical images.

Genial Tubercles

Description. **Genial tubercles** are tiny bumps of bone that serve as attachment sites for the genioglossus and geniohyoid

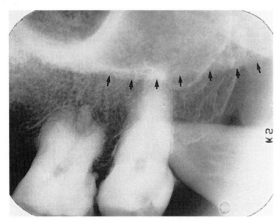

FIGURE 27-33 The zygoma appears as a diffuse radiopaque band that extends distally from the zygomatic process of the maxilla. (From Haring JI, Lind LJ: *Radiographic interpretation for the dental hygienist*, Philadelphia, 1993, Saunders.)

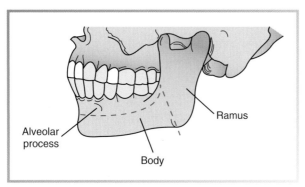

FIGURE 27-34 The mandible.

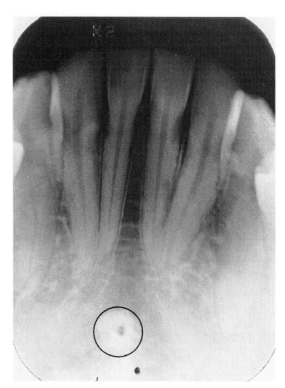

FIGURE 27-35 Genial tubercles appear as a ring-shaped radiopacity. (From Haring JI, Lind LJ: *Radiographic interpretation for the dental hygienist*, Philadelphia, 1993, Saunders.)

muscles (see Figure 27-7). Genial tubercles are located on the lingual aspect of the mandible.

Appearance. On a mandibular periapical image, genial tubercles appear as a ring-shaped radiopacity inferior to the apices of the mandibular incisors (Figure 27-35).

Lingual Foramen

Description. The **lingual foramen** is a tiny opening or hole in bone located on the internal surface of the mandible (see Figure 27-5). The lingual foramen is located near the midline and is surrounded by genial tubercles.

Appearance. On a mandibular periapical image, the lingual foramen appears as a small, radiolucent dot located inferior to the apices of mandibular incisors (Figure 27-36). The lingual foramen is surrounded by genial tubercles, which appear as a radiopaque ring.

Nutrient Canals

Description. As described earlier, nutrient canals are tube-like passageways through bone that contain nerves and blood vessels that supply teeth. Interdental nutrient canals are most often seen in the anterior mandible, a region that typically has thin bone.

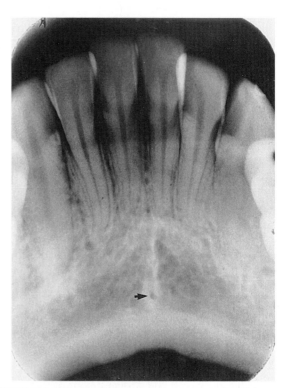

FIGURE 27-36 The lingual foramen appears as a small, radiolucent dot. (From Haring JI, Lind LJ: *Radiographic interpretation for the dental hygienist*, Philadelphia, 1993, Saunders.)

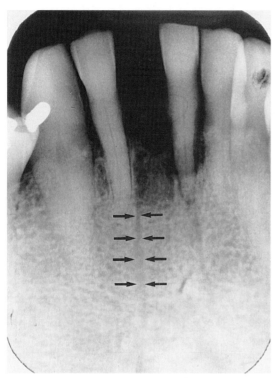

FIGURE 27-37 Nutrient canals appear as thin radiolucent lines. (From Haring JI, Lind LJ: *Radiographic interpretation for the dental hygienist*, Philadelphia, 1993, Saunders.)

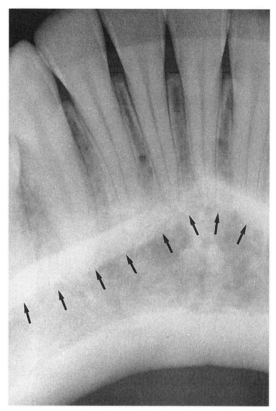

FIGURE 27-38 The mental ridge appears as a radiopaque band in the premolar and incisor region. (From Haring JI, Lind LJ: *Radiographic interpretation for the dental hygienist*, Philadelphia, 1993, Saunders.)

Appearance. On a mandibular periapical image, nutrient canals appear as vertical radiolucent lines (Figure 27-37). On a dental image, nutrient canals are readily seen in areas of thin bone. In the edentulous mandible, nutrient canals may be more prominent.

Mental Ridge

Description. The **mental ridge** is a linear prominence of cortical bone located on the external surface of the anterior portion of the mandible (see Figure 27-6). The mental ridge extends from the premolar region to the midline and slopes slightly upward.

Appearance. On a mandibular periapical image, the mental ridge appears as a thick radiopaque band that extends from the premolar region to the incisor region (Figure 27-38). On a dental image, the mental ridge often appears superimposed over mandibular anterior teeth.

Mental Fossa

Description. The **mental fossa** is a scooped-out, depressed area of bone located on the external surface of the anterior mandible (see Figure 27-6). The mental fossa is located above the mental ridge in the mandibular incisor region.

Appearance. On a mandibular periapical image, the mental fossa appears as a radiolucent area above the mental ridge (Figure 27-39). On a dental image, the appearance of the mental fossa varies and is determined by the thickness of the bone in the anterior region of the mandible.

Mental Foramen

Description. The **mental foramen** is an opening or hole in bone located on the external surface of the mandible in the region of mandibular premolars (see Figure 27-6). Blood vessels and nerves that supply the lower lip exit through the mental foramen.

Appearance. On a mandibular periapical image, the mental foramen appears as a small, ovoid or round radiolucent area located in the apical region of mandibular premolars (Figure 27-40). The mental foramen may be misdiagnosed as a periapical lesion (periapical cyst, granuloma, or abscess) because of its apical location.

Mylohyoid Ridge

Description. The **mylohyoid ridge** is a linear prominence of bone located on the internal surface of the mandible (see Figure 27-5). The mylohyoid ridge extends from the molar region downward and forward toward the lower border of the mandibular symphysis. The mylohyoid ridge serves as an attachment site for a muscle of the same name.

Appearance. On a mandibular periapical image, the mylohyoid ridge appears as a dense radiopaque band that extends downward and forward from the molar region (Figure 27-41). The mylohyoid ridge usually appears most prominently in the molar region and may be superimposed

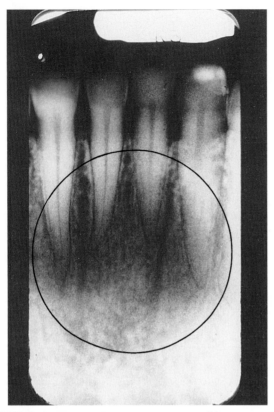

FIGURE 27-39 The mental fossa appears as a radiolucent area above the mental ridge. (From Haring JI, Lind LJ: *Radiographic interpretation for the dental hygienist*, Philadelphia, 1993, Saunders.)

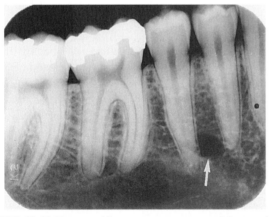

FIGURE 27-40 The mental foramen appears as a radiolucency in the mandibular premolar region. (From Haring JI, Lind LJ: *Radiographic interpretation for the dental hygienist*, Philadelphia, 1993, Saunders.)

over the roots of mandibular teeth. The mylohyoid ridge may appear to be continuous with the internal oblique ridge.

Mandibular Canal

Description. The **mandibular canal** is a tubelike passageway through bone that travels the length of the mandible. The mandibular canal extends from the mandibular foramen to the mental foramen and houses the inferior alveolar nerve and blood vessels.

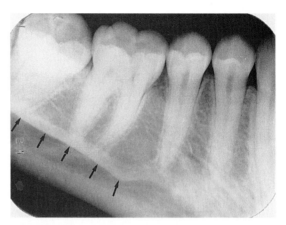

FIGURE 27-41 The mylohyoid ridge appears as a radiopaque band in the mandibular molar region. (From Haring JI, Lind LJ: *Radiographic interpretation for the dental hygienist*, Philadelphia, 1993, Saunders.)

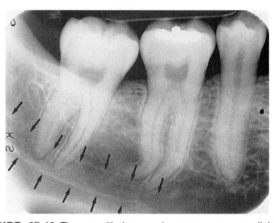

FIGURE 27-42 The mandibular canal appears as a radiolucent band outlined by two thin radiopaque lines. (From Haring JI, Lind LJ: *Radiographic interpretation for the dental hygienist*, Philadelphia, 1993, Saunders.)

Appearance. On a mandibular periapical image, the mandibular canal appears as a radiolucent band (Figure 27-42). The mandibular canal is outlined by two thin radiopaque lines that represent the cortical walls of the canal. The mandibular canal appears below or superimposed over the apices of mandibular molar teeth.

Internal Oblique Ridge

Description. The **internal oblique ridge** (also known as the *internal oblique line*) is a linear prominence of bone located on the internal surface of the mandible that extends downward and forward from the ramus (see Figure 27-5). The internal oblique ridge may end in the region of the mandibular third molar, or it may continue on as the mylohyoid ridge.

Appearance. On a mandibular periapical image, the internal oblique ridge appears as a radiopaque band that extends downward and forward from the ramus (Figure 27-43). Depending on the exposure technique used (bisecting versus paralleling), the internal and external oblique ridges may be superimposed on one another. When the ridges

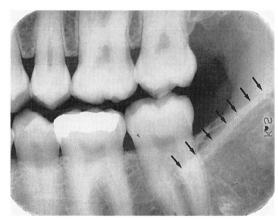

FIGURE 27-43 The internal oblique ridge appears as a radiopaque band. (From Haring JI, Lind LJ: *Radiographic interpretation for the dental hygienist*, Philadelphia, 1993, Saunders.)

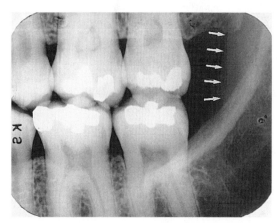

FIGURE 27-45 The external oblique ridge appears as a radiopaque band. (From Haring JI, Lind LJ: *Radiographic interpretation for the dental hygienist*, Philadelphia, 1993, Saunders.)

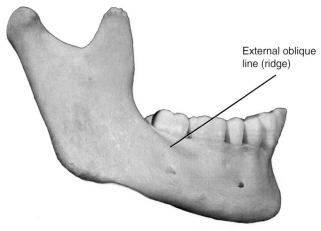

External oblique line (ridge)

FIGURE 27-44 The external oblique line (ridge). (Liebgott B: *The anatomical basis of dentistry*, ed 3, St. Louis, 2011, Mosby).

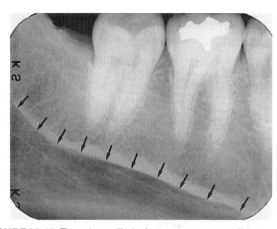

FIGURE 27-46 The submandibular fossa appears as a radiolucent area inferior to the mylohyoid ridge. (From Haring JI, Lind LJ: *Radiographic interpretation for the dental hygienist*, Philadelphia, 1993, Saunders.)

appear separate, the superior radiopaque band is the external oblique ridge, and the inferior radiopaque band is the internal oblique ridge.

External Oblique Ridge

Description. The **external oblique ridge** (also known as the *external oblique line*) is a linear prominence of bone located on the external surface of the body of the mandible (see Figure 27-44). The anterior border of the ramus ends in the external oblique ridge.

Appearance. On a mandibular periapical image, the external oblique ridge appears as a radiopaque band extending downward and forward from the anterior border of the ramus of the mandible (Figure 27-45). The external oblique ridge typically ends in the mandibular third molar region.

Submandibular Fossa

Description. The **submandibular fossa** (also known as the *mandibular fossa* or *submaxillary fossa*) is a scooped-out, depressed area of bone located on the internal surface of the mandible inferior to the mylohyoid ridge (see Figure 27-5).

The submandibular salivary gland is found in the submandibular fossa.

Appearance. On a mandibular periapical image, the submandibular fossa appears as a radiolucent area in the molar region below the mylohyoid ridge (Figure 27-46). Few bony trabeculae are usually seen in the region of the submandibular fossa. On some periapical images, the submandibular fossa may appear as a distinct radiolucency; in others, it may be slightly more radiolucent than the adjacent bone.

Coronoid Process

Description. The **coronoid process** is a marked prominence of bone on the anterior ramus of the mandible (see Figure 27-4). The coronoid process serves as an attachment site for one of the muscles of mastication.

Appearance. The coronoid process is not seen on a mandibular periapical image but does appear on a maxillary molar periapical image. The coronoid process appears as a triangular radiopacity superimposed over, or inferior to, the maxillary tuberosity region (Figure 27-47).

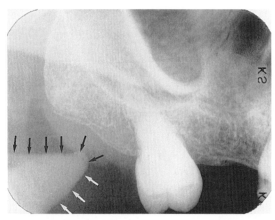

FIGURE 27-47 The coronoid process appears as a triangle-shaped radiopacity. (From Haring JI, Lind LJ: *Radiographic interpretation for the dental hygienist*, Philadelphia, 1993, Saunders.)

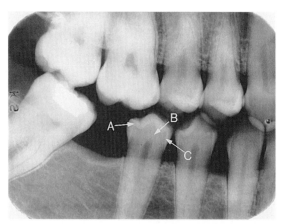

FIGURE 27-49 Tooth structures. **A**, enamel; **B**, dentin; **C**, dentino-enamel junction. (From Haring JI, Lind LJ: *Radiographic interpretation for the dental hygienist*, Philadelphia, 1993, Saunders.)

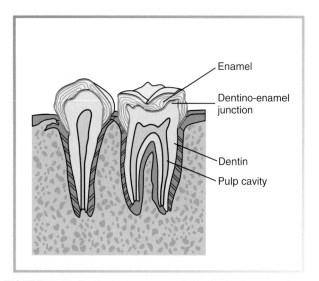

FIGURE 27-48 Tooth structures: enamel, dentin, dentino-enamel junction, and pulp cavity.

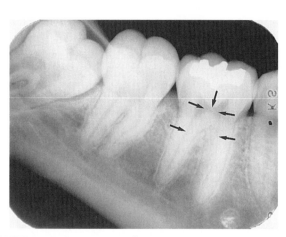

FIGURE 27-50 The pulp cavity. (From Haring JI, Lind LJ: *Radiographic interpretation for the dental hygienist*, Philadelphia, 1993, Saunders.)

NORMAL TOOTH ANATOMY

Tooth Structure

Tooth structures that can be viewed on dental images include the following: enamel, dentin, the dentino-enamel junction, and the pulp cavity (Figure 27-48).

Enamel

Enamel is the densest structure found in the human body. Enamel is the outermost radiopaque layer of the crown of a tooth (Figure 27-49).

Dentin

Dentin is found beneath the enamel layer of a tooth and surrounds the pulp cavity (see Figure 27-49). Dentin appears radiopaque and makes up the majority of the tooth structure. Dentin is not as radiopaque as enamel.

Dentino-Enamel Junction

The **dentino-enamel junction (DEJ)** is the junction between the dentin and the enamel of a tooth. The DEJ appears as a line where the enamel (very radiopaque) meets the dentin (less radiopaque) (see Figure 27-49).

Pulp Cavity

The **pulp cavity** consists of a pulp chamber and pulp canals. It contains blood vessels, nerves, and lymphatics and appears relatively radiolucent on a dental image (Figure 27-50). When viewed on a dental image, the pulp cavity is generally larger in children than in adults because it decreases in size with age due to the formation of secondary dentin. The size and shape of a pulp cavity vary with each tooth.

Supporting Structures

The alveolar process, or alveolar bone, serves as the supporting structure for teeth. The **alveolar bone** is the bone of the maxilla and the mandible that supports and encases the roots

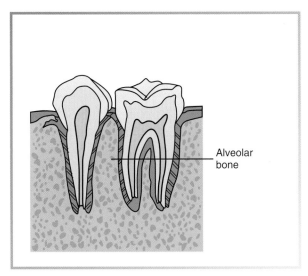

FIGURE 27-51 Alveolar bone.

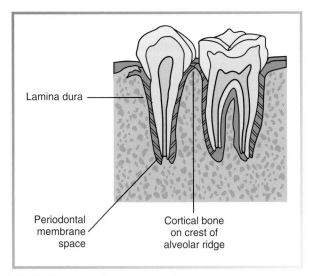

FIGURE 27-52 The alveolar process: lamina dura, alveolar crest, and periodontal ligament space.

of teeth (Figure 27-51). Alveolar bone is composed of dense cortical bone and cancellous bone.

Anatomy of Alveolar Bone

The anatomic landmarks of the alveolar process include the lamina dura, the alveolar crest, and the periodontal ligament space (Figure 27-52).

Lamina Dura

Description. The **lamina dura** is the wall of the tooth socket that surrounds the root of a tooth. The lamina dura is made up of dense cortical bone.

Appearance. On a dental image, the lamina dura appears as a dense radiopaque line that surrounds the root of a tooth (Figure 27-53).

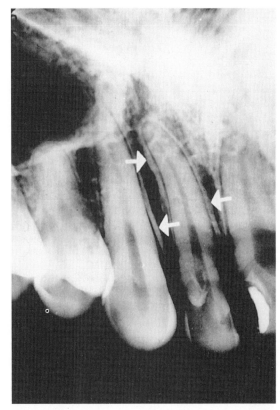

FIGURE 27-53 The lamina dura appears as a dense, thin radiopaque line around the root of a tooth. (From Haring JI, Lind LJ: *Radiographic interpretation for the dental hygienist*, Philadelphia, 1993, Saunders.)

Alveolar Crest

Description. The **alveolar crest** is the most coronal portion of alveolar bone found between teeth. The alveolar crest is made up of dense cortical bone and is continuous with the lamina dura.

Appearance. On a dental image, the alveolar crest appears radiopaque and is typically located 1.5 to 2.0 mm below the junction of the crown and the root surfaces (the cemento-enamel junction) (Figure 27-54).

Periodontal Ligament Space

Description. The **periodontal ligament space (PDL space)** is the space between the root of the tooth and the lamina dura. The PDL space contains connective tissue fibers, blood vessels, and lymphatics.

Appearance. On a dental image, the PDL space appears as a thin radiolucent line around the root of a tooth. In the healthy periodontium, the PDL space appears as a continuous radiolucent line of uniform thickness (Figure 27-55).

Shape and Density of Alveolar Bone

Alveolar bone located between the roots of teeth varies in shape and density.

Anterior Region. Normal alveolar crest located in the anterior region appears pointed and sharp between teeth

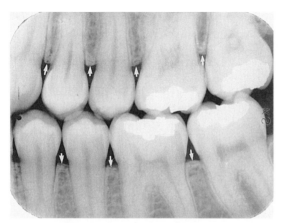

FIGURE 27-54 The alveolar crest typically appears 1.5 to 2.0 mm below the cemento-enamel junction. (From Haring JI, Lind LJ: *Radiographic interpretation for the dental hygienist*, Philadelphia, 1993, Saunders.)

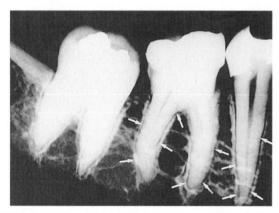

FIGURE 27-55 The periodontal ligament space appears as a thin radiolucent line around the root of the tooth. (From Haring JI, Lind LJ: *Radiographic interpretation for the dental hygienist*, Philadelphia, 1993, Saunders.)

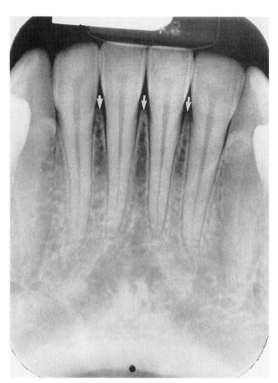

FIGURE 27-56 The anterior alveolar crest normally appears pointed and sharp. (From Haring JI, Lind LJ: *Radiographic interpretation for the dental hygienist*, Philadelphia, 1993, Saunders.)

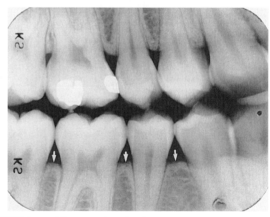

FIGURE 27-57 The posterior alveolar crest normally appears flat and smooth. (From Haring JI, Lind LJ: *Radiographic interpretation for the dental hygienist*, Philadelphia, 1993, Saunders.)

(Figure 27-56). The alveolar crest appears as a dense radiopaque line in the anterior region.

Posterior Region. Normal alveolar crest located in the posterior region appears flat and smooth between teeth (Figure 27-57). The alveolar crest located in the posterior region tends to appear less dense and less radiopaque than the alveolar crest seen in the anterior region.

SUMMARY

- The dental radiographer must have a thorough knowledge of the anatomy of the maxilla and the mandible; each normal anatomic landmark seen on a periapical image corresponds to that seen on the human skull. Knowledge of the anatomy of the maxilla and the mandible as viewed on an image of the human skull enables the dental radiographer to identify the normal anatomy that is found on a periapical image.
- Recognition of normal anatomic landmarks enables the dental radiographer to distinguish between maxillary and mandibular periapical and accurately mount dental images.
- Recognition of normal anatomic landmarks is also necessary for the accurate interpretation of dental images. Knowledge of the normal anatomy seen on periapical images is essential before the dental radiographer can begin to recognize abnormalities (e.g., diseases, lesions).
- Each normal anatomic landmark as viewed on a periapical image is described in this chapter.

BIBLIOGRAPHY

Frommer HH, Savage-Stabulas JJ: Film mounting and radiographic anatomy. In *Radiology for the dental professional*, ed 9, St. Louis, 2011, Mosby.

Haring JI, Lind LJ: Normal anatomy (periapical films). In *Radiographic interpretation for the dental hygienist*, Philadelphia, 1993, Saunders.

Miles DA, Van Dis ML, Jensen CW, Ferretti A: Normal anatomy and film mounting. In *Radiographic imaging for dental auxiliaries*, ed 3, St. Louis, 2009, Saunders.

White SC, Pharaoh MJ: Normal radiographic anatomy. In *Oral radiology: principles of interpretation*, ed 6, St. Louis, 2009, Mosby.

QUIZ QUESTIONS

MATCHING

Match the following terms with the proper definitions:

a. Hole or opening in bone
b. Broad, shallow depression in bone
c. Cavity, recess, or hollow space in bone
d. Passageway through bone
e. Spongelike bone
f. Bony partition that separates two spaces
g. Immovable joint between bones
h. Hard or compact bone

____ 1. Fossa
____ 2. Canal
____ 3. Foramen
____ 4. Sinus
____ 5. Septum
____ 6. Suture
____ 7. Cortical
____ 8. Cancellous

IDENTIFICATION

For questions 9 to 16, refer to Figures 27-58 through 27-65. Identify the normal anatomic landmarks indicated by arrows (or circle) as required.

9. Identify the normal anatomic landmark shown in Figure 27-58.
10. Identify the normal anatomic landmark shown in Figure 27-59.
11. Identify the normal anatomic landmark shown in Figure 27-60.
12. Identify the normal anatomic landmark shown in Figure 27-61.
13. Identify the normal anatomic landmark shown in Figure 27-62.
14. Identify the normal anatomic landmark shown in Figure 27-63.
15. Identify the normal anatomic landmark shown in Figure 27-64.
16. Identify the normal anatomic landmark shown in Figure 27-65.

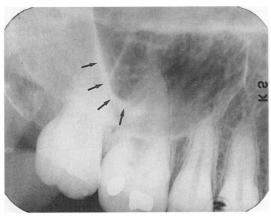

FIGURE 27-58

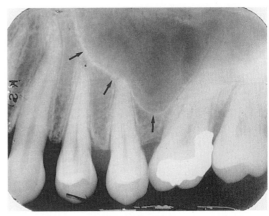

FIGURE 27-59

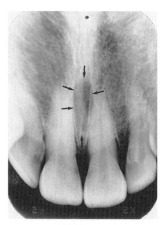

FIGURE 27-60

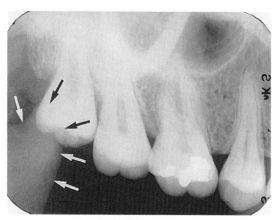

FIGURE 27-61

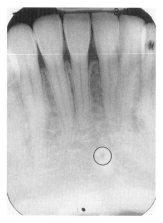

FIGURE 27-62

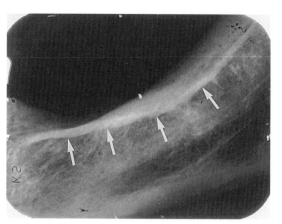

FIGURE 27-63

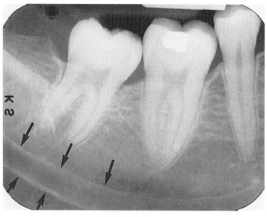

FIGURE 27-64

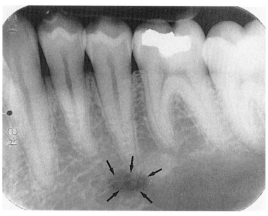

FIGURE 27-65

chapter 28

Film Mounting and Viewing

OUTLINE

FILM MOUNTING
    Basic Concepts
    Normal Anatomy and Film Mounting
    Film Mounting Methods
    Step-by-Step Procedure

FILM VIEWING
    Basic Concepts
    Step-by-Step Procedure

LEARNING OBJECTIVES

After completion of this chapter, the student will be able to do the following:

- Define the key terms associated with film mounting and viewing
- List the individuals who are qualified to mount and view dental radiographs
- Describe when and where films are mounted
- List five reasons to use a film mount
- Describe what information is placed on a film mount
- Discuss the importance of normal anatomy in film mounting
- Describe how the identification dot is used to determine film orientation
- List and describe two methods of film mounting and identify the preferred method
- List and describe the step-by-step procedures for film mounting

- List and describe the necessary equipment for film viewing
- Discuss the importance of masking extraneous viewbox light seen around a film mount
- Describe optimal viewing conditions, as well as when and where images should be viewed
- Explain the importance of examining images in an established viewing sequence
- List and describe the step-by-step procedures for film viewing
- Explain why multiple viewings of dental images are necessary, and list the areas, diseases, and abnormalities that must be included in the examinations

KEY TERMS

Anatomic order	Identification dot	Mount
Film mount	Interpretation	Viewbox
Film mounting	Labial mounting	Viewing
Film viewing	Lingual mounting	

Film mounting is an essential step in the interpretation of dental radiographs. The dental radiographer must be able to mount dental radiographs in correct anatomic order. To mount dental radiographs properly, the radiographer must have a thorough knowledge of the normal anatomy of the maxilla, the mandible, and related structures (see Chapter 27). Film viewing is also essential in the interpretation of dental radiographs; the dental radiographer must understand the importance of examining films under optimal viewing conditions.

The purpose of this chapter is to present the basic concepts of film mounting and film viewing and to describe the step-by-step procedures that must be followed to prepare for the interpretation of radiographs.

FILM MOUNTING

Mounted radiographs, or radiographs placed in a film holder in anatomic order, are invaluable to the dental professional. Compared with individual films, a series of mounted radiographs can be viewed more efficiently and are easier to interpret.

Basic Concepts

The term **mount** can be defined as "to place in an appropriate setting, as for display or study." In dental radiography, **film mounting** is the placement of radiographs in a supporting structure or holder.

What Is a Film Mount?

A **film mount** is a cardboard, plastic, or vinyl holder that is used to support and arrange dental radiographs in anatomic order (Figure 28-1). *Anatomic order* refers to how teeth are arranged within the dental arches. Each film mount has a number of windows or frames in which the individual radiographs are placed, or "mounted." A film mount may be opaque or clear (Figure 28-2). An opaque film mount is preferred because it masks the light around each radiograph. Subtle changes in density and contrast are easier to detect when extraneous light is eliminated. To minimize extraneous viewbox light, each window of a film mount should contain a radiograph. When all the windows are not filled with

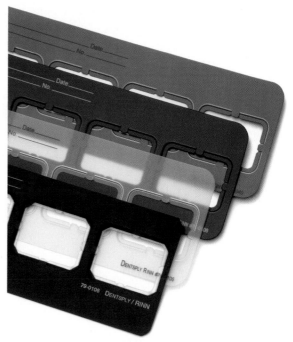

FIGURE 28-1 Examples of various film mounts. (Courtesy of Rinn Corporation, Elgin, IL.)

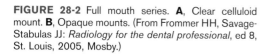
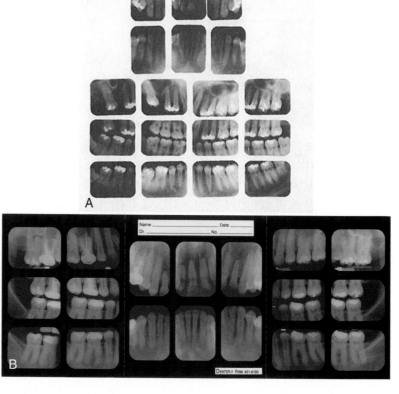

FIGURE 28-2 Full mouth series. **A,** Clear celluloid mount. **B,** Opaque mounts. (From Frommer HH, Savage-Stabulas JJ: *Radiology for the dental professional*, ed 8, St. Louis, 2005, Mosby.)

radiographs, black opaque paper can be placed in the unused frames.

Film mounts are commercially available in many sizes and configurations and accommodate any number of films; mounts are available for single films, bite-wing films, a complete mouth radiographic series (CMRS) of films, and countless other combinations of films (Figure 28-3). The overall size and shape of the film mounts are designed to fit a variety of viewboxes found in the dental office; the size of the film mount should correspond to the size of the viewbox.

Who Mounts Films?

Any trained dental professional (dentist, dental hygienist, dental assistant) with knowledge of the normal anatomic landmarks of the maxilla, the mandible, and related structures is qualified to mount dental radiographs. In most dental offices, mounting films is the responsibility of the dental radiographer.

When and Where Are Films Mounted?

The dental radiographer should always mount films immediately after processing. Films should be mounted in an area designated for film mounting. This area should consist of a clean, dry, light-colored work surface in front of an illuminator or viewbox.

Why Use a Film Mount?

The use of a film mount is strongly recommended for the following reasons:

- Mounted radiographs are quicker and easier to view and interpret.
- Mounted radiographs are easily stored in the patient record and are readily accessible for interpretation.
- Film mounts decrease the chances of error in determining the patient's right and left sides because each film is mounted in anatomic order.
- Film mounts decrease the handling of individual films and prevent damage to the emulsion (e.g., fingerprint marks and scratches).
- Film mounts mask illumination immediately adjacent to individual radiographs and aid in interpretation.

What Information Is Placed on a Film Mount?

The dental radiographer should label the film mount before the films are mounted. A special marking pencil designed to write on paper, plastic, or vinyl can be used to label film mounts. Radiographs are easily identified when the film mount has been clearly and legibly labeled with the following information:

- Patient's full name
- Date of exposure
- Dentist's name
- Radiographer's name

The patient's name and date of exposure are essential, the dentist's name is useful if the radiographs are sent to a third

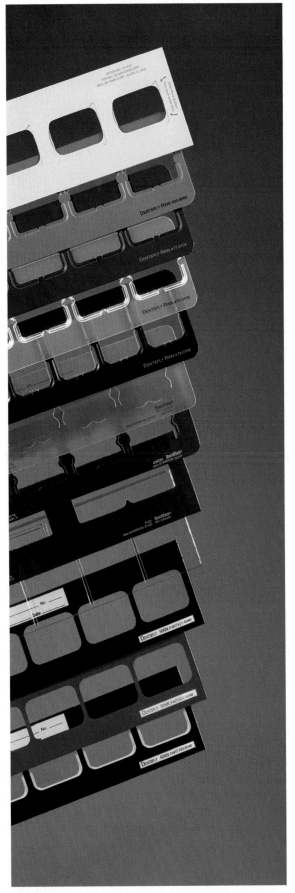

FIGURE 28-3 A variety of film mounts are available in many sizes and film combinations. (Courtesy of Dentsply Rinn, Elgin, Il.)

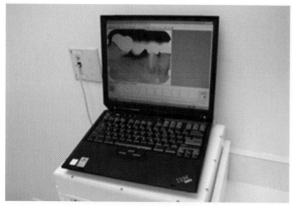

FIGURE 28-4 A digital image of the mandibular right periapical region in a mount as seen on a computer monitor.

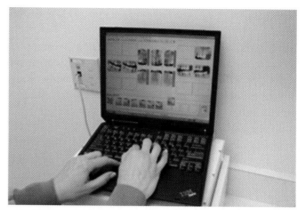

FIGURE 28-6 A full mouth series of radiographs exposed using digital imaging. Each image is placed in the appropriate window on the mount, arranged in anatomic order.

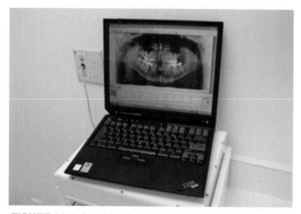

FIGURE 28-5 A panoramic image viewed on a laptop monitor.

TABLE 28-1	Landmarks Distinguishing Maxillary from Mandibular Periapical Images	
Area	**Maxillary Landmarks**	**Mandibular Landmarks**
Incisor	Incisive foramen	Mental ridge
	Median palatal suture	Mental fossa
	Nasal cavity	Lingual foramen
	Inferior nasal conchae	Genial tubercles
	Anterior nasal spine	Nutrient canals
Canine	Lateral fossa	
	Inverted Y	
Premolar	Maxillary sinus	Mental foramen
		Mylohyoid ridge
Molar	Maxillary sinus	External oblique ridge
	Maxillary tuberosity	Internal oblique ridge
	Hamulus	Submandibular fossa
	Zygomatic process of maxilla	Mandibular canal
	Zygoma	
	Coronoid process of mandible	

party (e.g., insurance company), and the radiographer's name is important if any questions should arise about the exposure of the images.

Are Mounts Used with Digital Imaging?

Similar to conventional radiography, digital images observed on the computer monitor must also be mounted correctly in anatomic order for proper viewing and interpretation. Most digital imaging software allows the dental radiographer to choose the appropriate-size mount, whether it be one periapical image, four bite-wing images, a full mouth series, or a panoramic image (Figures 28-4 and 28-5). For example, with a full mouth series of radiographs, the dental radiographer must "click and drag" each image to the correct corresponding window or frame on the mount on the computer monitor screen (Figure 28-6).

The images should be saved with the patient's full name and date of exposure. Digital systems vary from each manufacturer, but information regarding the name of the radiographer, amount of radiation the patient received during exposure, and the dentist's name may also be recorded. Once the mounting has been completed and verified, the images are saved in the patient's electronic file.

Normal Anatomy and Film Mounting

As stressed in Chapter 27, knowledge of normal anatomy is necessary to mount dental radiographs properly. The dental radiographer must be familiar with the characteristic anatomic landmarks seen in each region of the jaws. Identification of landmarks aids in distinguishing maxillary periapical images from mandibular periapical images (Table 28-1).

Film Mounting Methods

Two methods are used to mount films: (1) labial and (2) lingual. Both methods rely on identification of the embossed

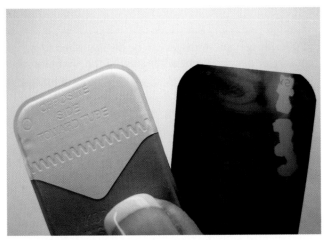

FIGURE 28-7 The dot on the packet indicates the relative location of the embossed identifying dot on the radiograph. (Photo courtesy of Allyson Bowcutt.)

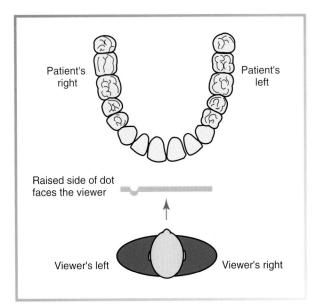

FIGURE 28-8 With the labial mounting method, the radiographs are viewed as if the dental radiographer were looking directly at the patient.

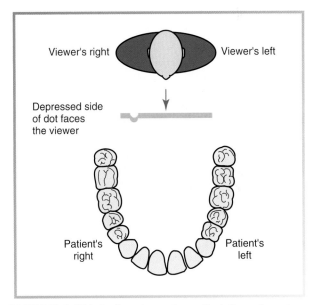

FIGURE 28-9 With the lingual mounting method, the radiographs are viewed as if the dental radiographer were inside the patient's mouth and looking out.

dot found on the film. As described in Chapter 7, a small, raised bump, known as the **identification dot**, is seen in one corner of each intraoral film packet; the dot on the packet indicates the location of the embossed identification dot on the radiograph (Figure 28-7). The film is positioned in the packet such that the raised side of the dot faces the x-ray beam during exposure.

The identification dot is used to determine film orientation (i.e., determining the patient's right and left sides). After the films are processed, they should be placed in the film mount so that all the embossed dots are either raised (labial mounting) or depressed (lingual mounting); all the embossed dots must face in the same direction. The dental radiographer can then distinguish between the right and left sides of the patient. Either labial or lingual mounting can be used.

Labial Mounting

Labial mounting is the preferred method of mounting dental radiographs and is recommended by the American Dental Association. In the **labial mounting** method, radiographs are placed in the film mount with the *raised* (convex) side of the identification dot *facing the viewer* (dental radiographer). The radiographs are then viewed from the labial aspect (thus the term *labial mounting*). With this method, the radiographs are viewed as if the viewer is looking directly at the patient; the patient's left side is on the viewer's right, and the patient's right side is on the viewer's left (Figure 28-8). Images of teeth are mounted in anatomic order and have the same relationship to the viewer as they do when facing the patient.

Lingual Mounting

Lingual mounting can be used as an alternative method. Although some practitioners still use lingual mounting, this system of film mounting is not recommended. In the **lingual mounting** method, radiographs are placed in the film mount with the *depressed* (concave) side of the identification dot

facing the viewer. The dental radiographer then views the radiographs from the lingual aspect (thus the term *lingual mounting*). With this method, the radiographs are viewed as if the dental radiographer is inside the patient's mouth and looking out; the patient's left side is on the viewer's left, and the patient's right side is on the viewer's right (Figure 28-9).

Step-by-Step Procedure

The dental radiographer in training can use the steps for film mounting listed in Procedure 28-1. As the mounting skills of the radiographer improve, simpler and faster techniques may be used.

PROCEDURE 28-1   Mounting Dental Radiographs

1. Prepare for film mounting by placing a clean, light-colored paper towel over the work surface in front of the viewbox.
2. Turn on the viewbox.
3. Label and date the film mount (Figure 28-10).
4. Wash and dry your hands.
5. Examine each radiograph, identify the embossed dot, and then place each radiograph on the work surface with the raised side of the dot facing up (for labial mounting, as recommended by the American Dental Association). All radiographs must be mounted with the raised side of the dot facing in the same direction. Hold radiographs by the edges only (Figure 28-11).
6. Sort the radiographs into three groups: bite-wings, anterior periapicals, and posterior periapicals. Bite-wing images can be distinguished from periapical images because the crowns of both maxillary and mandibular teeth are seen on the image (Figure 28-12).

Anterior periapical images can be distinguished from posterior periapical images because of the orientation of the film: in anterior periapical images, the long axis of the film is oriented vertically, and in posterior periapical images, the long axis is oriented horizontally (Figure 28-13).

7. Arrange the radiographs on the work surface in anatomic order. The normal anatomic landmarks can be used to distinguish maxillary images from mandibular images. In addition, all maxillary radiographs must be oriented with the roots of teeth pointing upward, and all mandibular radiographs must be oriented with the roots pointing downward (Figure 28-14). The order of teeth can be used to distinguish the right side from the left side (Figure 28-15).
8. Place each film in the corresponding frame of the film mount, and secure it (Figure 28-16).
   The following order for film mounting is suggested:
   a. Bite-wings
   b. Maxillary anterior periapicals
   c. Mandibular anterior periapicals
   d. Maxillary posterior periapicals
   e. Mandibular posterior periapicals
9. Check radiographs by verifying the following:
   a. All embossed dots are oriented correctly.
   b. All films are properly arranged in anatomic order.
   c. All films are mounted securely.
   d. The film mount is properly labeled and dated.

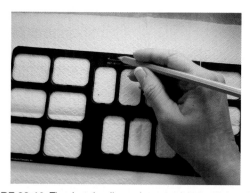

FIGURE 28-10 The dental radiographer must label and date the film mount before mounting the films. (Photo courtesy of Allyson Bowcutt.)

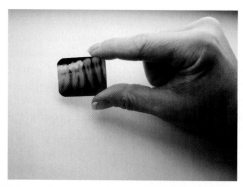

FIGURE 28-11 The dental radiographer should hold radiographs by the edges only. (Photo courtesy of Allyson Bowcutt.)

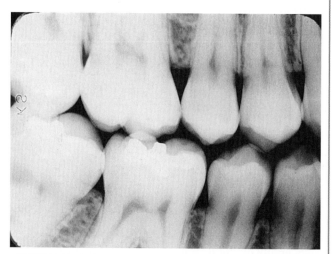

FIGURE 28-12 A bite-wing image shows the crowns of both maxillary and mandibular teeth on one film.

PROCEDURE 28-1 Mounting Dental Radiographs—cont'd

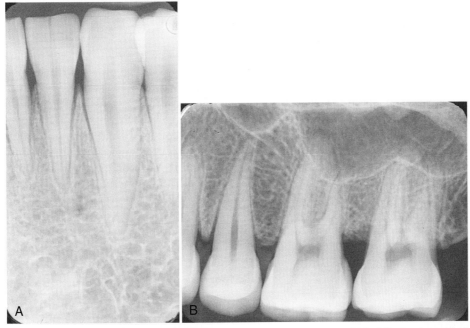

FIGURE 28-13 A, An anterior periapical film is oriented vertically. **B,** A posterior periapical film is oriented horizontally.

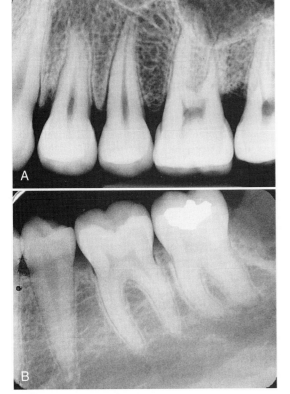

FIGURE 28-14 A, A maxillary periapical film is mounted with the roots pointing upward. **B,** A mandibular periapical film is mounted with the roots pointing downward.

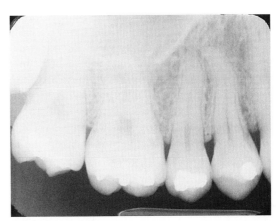

FIGURE 28-15 The order of teeth can be used to distinguish right from left; premolars are located in front of molars; therefore, this is a maxillary right periapical image.

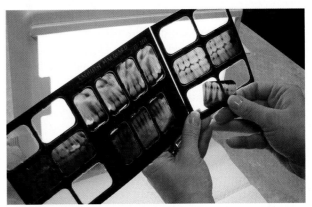

FIGURE 28-16 After the films have been arranged in proper order, the dental radiographer can place each film in the corresponding frame of the film mount.

HELPFUL HINTS

For mounting radiographs:

- **DO** master the normal anatomy of the maxilla, the mandible, and adjacent structures. A working knowledge of normal anatomy is necessary to correctly mount films.
- **DO** label and date the film mount before mounting the films; always include the patient's full name, the date of exposure, the dentist's name, and the radiographer's name.
- **DO** mount films immediately after processing.
- **DO** mount radiographs in a designated area; use a light-colored working surface in front of a viewbox.
- **DO** use an opaque film mount to block out extraneous light around each film.
- **DO** use clean dry hands to mount radiographs, and hold each radiograph by the edges only.
- **DO** identify the embossed dot on each film; always mount radiographs with the raised side of the dot facing the same direction. For labial mounting, all the raised dots must face the viewer.
- **DO** sort the radiographs before mounting them.
- **DO** use normal anatomic landmarks to distinguish maxillary images from mandibular images.
- **DO** use the order of teeth to distinguish the right side from the left side.
- **DO** use a definite order for mounting films. For example, begin with bite-wing images, then mount maxillary anterior periapical films, proceed to mandibular anterior periapical films, and then finish with maxillary posterior periapical films and mandibular posterior periapical films.
- **DO** mount bite-wing radiographs with the curve of Spee (occlusal plane between maxillary and mandibular teeth) directed upward toward the distal.
- **DO** recognize the differences between maxillary and mandibular teeth (e.g., maxillary anterior teeth have larger crowns and longer roots than do mandibular anterior teeth).
- **DO** remember that most mandibular molars have two roots, whereas most maxillary molars have three.
- **DO** recognize that most roots curve toward the distal.
- **DO** verify the following points after mounting the radiographs: all the embossed dots are oriented correctly, the radiographs are arranged in anatomic order, the radiographs are mounted securely, and the film mount is labeled and dated.
- **DO** place the mounted radiographs in the patient's file as soon as possible to eliminate the possibility of loss or mix-up.

FILM VIEWING

Film viewing is essential in the interpretation of dental radiographs. The dental radiographer must be knowledgeable about optimal film viewing conditions and the recommended evaluation sequence for film viewing.

Basic Concepts

The term **viewing** means "examining or inspecting." In dental radiography, **film viewing** is the examination of dental radiographs.

Who Views Films?

Any trained dental professional (dentist, dental hygienist, dental assistant) with knowledge of the normal anatomic landmarks of the maxilla, the mandible, and related structures is qualified to view dental radiographs. Although all members of the dental team may interpret dental radiographs, it is the responsibility of the dentist to establish a final or definitive interpretation and diagnosis. **Interpretation**, or the explanation of what is viewed on a dental radiograph, is discussed in Chapter 30.

What Equipment Is Required for Film Viewing?

An adequate light source and magnification are required for optimal film viewing; both a viewbox and a magnifying glass are necessary.

- *Light source:* A light source known as the **viewbox**, or *illuminator* (see Chapter 10), is required to view dental radiographs accurately and assist in the interpretation of images (Figure 28-17). The viewing area of the illuminator should be large enough to accommodate a variety of mounted films as well as unmounted extra-oral films. The light from the viewbox should be of uniform intensity and evenly diffused. If the screen of the viewbox is not completely covered by the mounted radiographs, the harsh light around the mounted films must be masked to reduce glare and intensify the detail and contrast of the radiographic images (Figure 28-18).
- *Magnification:* The use of a pocket-sized magnifying glass is useful in interpretation. Magnification aids the viewer in evaluating slight changes in density and contrast in radiographic images (Figure 28-19).

When and Where Are Films Viewed?

The dental radiographer should view radiographs immediately after mounting. Immediate film viewing is necessary to verify the correct arrangement of the images in the mount.

Films are best viewed by the dental radiographer on a viewbox in a room with dimmed lighting. When interpreting dental radiographs, an area free of distractions with subdued lighting provides optimal conditions for film viewing. Because such viewing conditions are typically present only in a medical facility, most films are examined on the viewbox at chairside in the dental setting.

Step-by-Step Procedure

Mounted radiographs must be viewed in sequential order. The dental radiographer must have an established viewing sequence to prevent errors in interpretation. The steps shown in Procedure 28-2 can be used to examine a CMRS of dental radiographs (Figure 28-20).

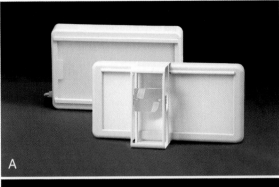

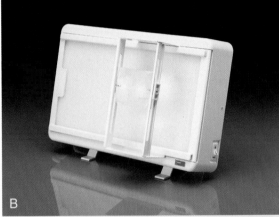

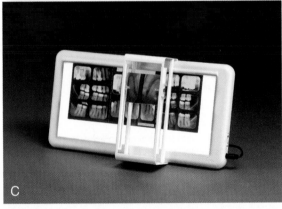

FIGURE 28-17 Examples of various viewboxes. (Courtesy of Rinn Corporation, Elgin, IL.)

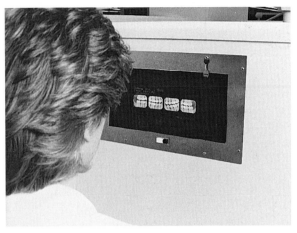

FIGURE 28-18 Extraneous light should be masked to reduce glare and intensify the contrast of the radiographic image. (From Haring JL, Lind LJ: *Radiographic interpretation for the dental hygienist*, Philadelphia, 1993, Saunders.)

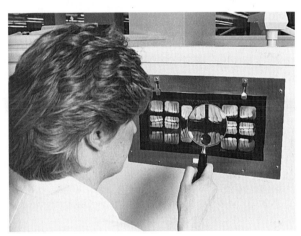

FIGURE 28-19 A magnifying glass aids the viewer in the evaluation of subtle changes in density and contrast. (From Haring JL, Lind LJ: *Radiographic interpretation for the dental hygienist*, Philadelphia, 1993, Saunders.)

The dental radiographer must use this recommended viewing sequence to examine films for each of the following:

- Unerupted, missing, and impacted teeth
- Dental caries and the size and shape of the pulp cavities
- Bony changes, the level of alveolar bone, and calculus
- Roots and periapical areas
- All areas not previously examined (e.g., remaining areas of the jaws, sinuses)

Many examinations of dental radiographs are necessary to check for all the problems listed. For example, the dental radiographer should first view the images quickly for evidence of unerupted, bony, or impacted teeth. Next, the examination sequence should be repeated for caries, pulp size, and pulp shape. The sequence must be repeated as many times as necessary to evaluate all surfaces of teeth and supporting structures for evidence of disease and abnormalities.

After film viewing, the dental professional must note any findings in the patient record. A standard diagram is included in the patient record and can be used to record significant findings (Figure 28-21). Although all dental professionals may note significant findings, it is important to remember that the final interpretation and diagnosis are the responsibility of the dentist.

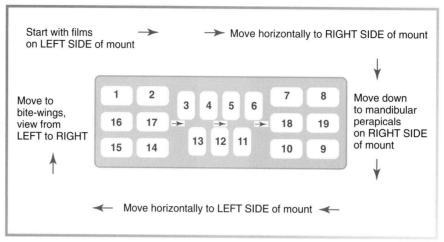

FIGURE 28-20 The dental radiographer must use a definite order for viewing radiographs. The sequence illustrated here is recommended.

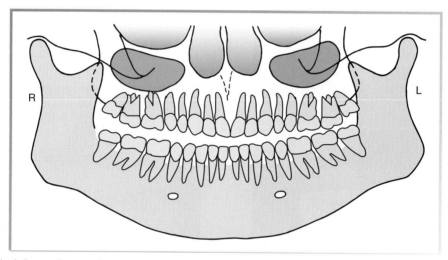

FIGURE 28-21 Standard diagram for recording radiologic findings. This one is used for panoramic and intraoral radiographs, but a similar arrangement can be used for other images. In the form of rubber stamps, these diagrams can be placed anywhere in the patient's notes.

PROCEDURE 28-2 Viewing Mounted Radiographs

1. Begin with maxillary teeth on the right side (maxillary periapical films on the upper left side of the film mount).
2. Move horizontally across to maxillary teeth on the left (maxillary periapical films on the upper right side of the mount).
3. Move down to mandibular teeth on the left side (mandibular periapical films on the lower right side of the mount).
4. Move horizontally across to mandibular teeth on the right (mandibular periapical films on the lower left side of the mount).
5. Move up to bite-wing films. View bite-wings on the left side of the mount, and then move to bite-wings on the right side of the mount.

HELPFUL HINTS

For viewing radiographs:

- **DO** use a viewbox to examine radiographs; avoid holding mounted films "up to the room light" to view.
- **DO** block out the harsh light on a viewbox that occurs around the edges of the film mount; harsh light must be masked to reduce glare.
- **DO** use a magnifying glass to evaluate slight changes in density and contrast in radiographic images.
- **DO** view films immediately after mounting.
- **DO** view films under optimal viewing conditions whenever possible; use an area free of distractions with dimmed lighting.
- **DO** use a definite order for film viewing. To view a CMRS, start with the films on the upper left side of the mount, move horizontally to the upper right, down to the lower right, across the lower left, up to the bite-wings, and then view the bite-wings from left to right.

- ▪ **DO** examine radiographs using the recommended viewing sequence as many times as necessary to evaluate them for (1) unerupted, impacted, and missing teeth; (2) dental caries, pulp size, and pulp shape; (3) bony changes, level of alveolar bone, and calculus; (4) roots and periapical areas; and (5) all areas not previously examined.
- ▪ **DO** record all radiographic findings in the patient record.

SUMMARY

- Film mounting is the placement of radiographs in a supporting structure or holder.
- A film mount is a plastic or cardboard holder used to arrange radiographs in anatomic order (i.e., the order in which teeth are arranged in the dental arches).
- Any trained dental professional with knowledge of normal anatomy is qualified to mount dental radiographs. In most offices, the dental radiographer is responsible for the mounting of films.
- Dental radiographs should always be mounted immediately after processing in an area designated for film mounting.
- Mounted radiographs are quicker and easier to view and interpret and are more easily stored in the patient record. Mounted radiographs also decrease the chances of error in determining the patient's right and left sides, and they decrease the handling of films.
- A film mount should be labeled before mounting the films. The label includes patient's full name, date of exposure, dentist's name, and radiographer's name.
- Digital images should also be mounted correctly on the computer monitor and properly labeled with patient's name and date of exposure. The images are saved under the electronic file for each patient.
- The two methods of mounting radiographs based on the orientation of the embossed dot are labial mounting and lingual mounting. The labial mounting method is recommended by the American Dental Association.
- After films are mounted, the following must be verified: all embossed dots are oriented correctly, all films are arranged in anatomic order, all films are mounted securely, and the film mount is properly labeled and dated.
- Film viewing is the examination of radiographs. Films are best viewed on a viewbox (light source) in a room with dimmed lighting. Radiographs can be viewed by any trained dental professional and should be viewed immediately after mounting.
- Radiographs should be viewed in a sequential order as many times as necessary and should be examined for (1) unerupted, impacted, and missing teeth; (2) dental caries, pulp size, and pulp shape; (3) bony changes, level of alveolar bone, and calculus; (4) roots and periapical areas; and (5) all areas not previously examined.
- After film viewing, all significant findings must be noted in the patient record.

BIBLIOGRAPHY

Frommer HH, Savage-Stabulas JJ: Film mounting and radiographic anatomy. In *Radiology for the dental professional*, ed 9, St. Louis, 2011, Mosby.

Haring JI, Lind LJ: The importance of dental radiographs and interpretation. In *Radiographic interpretation for the dental hygienist*, Philadelphia, 1993, Saunders.

Johnson ON, Thomson EM: Identification of anatomical landmarks for mounting radiographs. In *Essentials of dental radiography for dental assistants and hygienists*, ed 6, Upper Saddle River, NJ, 2007, Pearson.

Miles DA, Van Dis ML, Razmus TF: Radiographic processing and processing quality assurance. In *Basic principles of oral and maxillofacial radiology*, Philadelphia, 1992, Saunders.

Miles DA, Van Dis ML, Williamson GF, Jensen CW: Film processing and quality assurance. In *Radiographic imaging for the dental team*, ed 4, St. Louis, Saunders, 2009.

White SC, Pharoah MJ: Processing x-ray film. In *Oral radiology: principles of interpretation*, ed 6, St. Louis, 2009, Mosby.

QUIZ QUESTIONS

TRUE OR FALSE

____ 1. *Anatomic order* refers to how teeth are arranged in the dental arches.

____ 2. A clear film mount is preferred (instead of an opaque film mount) for better interpretation of radiographs.

____ 3. Only the dentist is qualified to mount dental radiographs.

____ 4. Films may be mounted at any time after processing.

____ 5. Mounted films are quicker and easier to view and interpret.

____ 6. Mounted films decrease the chances of error in distinguishing the patient's right and left sides.

____ 7. Film mounts decrease the handling of individual films and prevent damage to the emulsion.

____ 8. In the labial film mounting method, all the embossed identification dots are placed in the film mount with the raised (convex) side facing the viewer.

____ 9. The lingual mounting method is widely used and is recommended by the American Dental Association.

____ 10. Bite-wing radiographs must be mounted with the curve of Spee directed downward toward the distal.

____ **11.** *Film viewing* refers to the placing of films in a supporting structure.

____ **12.** Although all members of the dental team may view films, it is the responsibility of the dentist to establish a final, or definitive, interpretation and diagnosis.

____ **13.** Mounted radiographs may be viewed by holding the film mount up to the room light.

____ **14.** If the viewbox screen is not completely covered by the mounted radiographs, the harsh light around the mounted films must be masked to reduce glare and for better interpretation.

____ **15.** When interpreting dental radiographs, an area free of distractions and with dimmed room lighting provides optimal viewing conditions.

____ **16.** Optimal viewing conditions are typically present in the dental setting.

____ **17.** Mounted radiographs must be viewed in an established sequence to prevent errors in interpretation.

____ **18.** The dental radiographer must examine mounted radiographs many times to check for the presence of disease and abnormalities.

____ **19.** After film viewing, all positive findings must be noted in the patient record.

____ **20.** A viewbox is not necessary to examine dental radiographs.

SHORT ANSWER

21. List five reasons for using a film mount.

22. List and describe the two methods of film mounting.

23. Describe the step-by-step procedure for film mounting.

24. List and describe the necessary pieces of equipment for film viewing.

25. Describe the step-by-step procedure for film viewing.

chapter 29

Normal Anatomy: Panoramic Images

OUTLINE

NORMAL ANATOMIC LANDMARKS
    Bony Landmarks of Maxilla and Surrounding Structures
    Bony Landmarks of Mandible and Surrounding
      Structures

AIR SPACES SEEN ON PANORAMIC IMAGES
SOFT TISSUES SEEN ON PANORAMIC IMAGES

LEARNING OBJECTIVES

After completion of this chapter, the student will be able to do the following:

- Define the key terms associated with normal anatomy on panoramic images
- Identify and describe the bony landmarks of the maxilla and surrounding structures as viewed on the panoramic image

- Identify and describe the bony landmarks of the mandible and surrounding structures as viewed on the panoramic image
- Identify air spaces as viewed on the panoramic image
- Identify soft tissues as viewed on the panoramic image

KEY TERMS

Angle of mandible	Inferior border of mandible	Mental fossa
Anterior nasal spine	Infraorbital foramen	Mental ridge
Articular eminence	Internal oblique ridge	Mylohyoid ridge
Coronoid notch	Lateral pterygoid plate	Nasal cavity
Coronoid process	Lingual foramen	Nasal septum
Ear	Lingula	Nasopharyngeal air space
External auditory meatus	Lipline	Orbit
External oblique ridge	Mandibular canal	Palatoglossal air space
Genial tubercles	Mandibular condyle	Pterygomaxillary fissure
Glenoid fossa	Mandibular foramen	Soft palate and uvula
Glossopharyngeal air space	Mastoid process	Styloid process
Hamulus	Maxillary sinus	Tongue
Hard palate	Maxillary tuberosity	Zygoma
Incisive canal	Mental foramen	Zygomatic process of maxilla
Incisive foramen		

A panoramic image allows the dental professional to view large areas of the mandible and the maxilla on a single projection. Just as dental professionals must be able to recognize normal anatomic landmarks on periapical images, they must also be able to recognize normal anatomic structures viewed on panoramic images. The recognition of landmarks enables dental professionals to interpret panoramic images accurately. Without a working knowledge of anatomy, normal anatomic structures may be mistaken for pathologic conditions.

To interpret the panoramic image and identify normal anatomic landmarks, dental professionals must have thorough knowledge of the anatomy of the maxilla and the mandible. Each normal anatomic landmark seen on a panoramic image corresponds to what is seen on the human skull. If dental professionals are familiar with the anatomy of the human skull, they will be able to identify normal anatomy viewed on a panoramic image.

The purpose of this chapter is to describe the normal anatomy of the maxilla and the mandible as viewed on a panoramic image. In addition to the normal anatomic landmarks, air space images and soft tissue images are also described in this chapter.

NORMAL ANATOMIC LANDMARKS

Bony Landmarks of Maxilla and Surrounding Structures

The maxilla forms the floor of the orbit of the eyes, the sides and floor of the nasal cavity, and the hard palate. The lower border of the maxilla supports maxillary teeth. This section reviews the bony landmarks of the maxilla and surrounding structures that can be viewed on a panoramic image.

Each of the following bony landmarks of the maxilla and surrounding structures is identified on Figure 29-1.

Mastoid Process

Description. The **mastoid process** is a marked prominence of bone located posterior and inferior to the temporomandibular joint (TMJ). The mastoid process is part of the temporal bone.

Appearance. On a panoramic image, the mastoid process appears as a rounded *radiopacity* located posterior and

inferior to the TMJ area. The mastoid process is *not* seen on periapical images.

Styloid Process

Description. The **styloid process** is a long, pointed, and sharp projection of bone that extends downward from the inferior surface of the temporal bone. The styloid process is located anterior to the mastoid process.

Appearance. On a panoramic image, the styloid process appears as a long *radiopaque* spine that extends from the temporal bone anterior to the mastoid process. The styloid process is *not* seen on periapical images.

External Auditory Meatus

Description. The **external auditory meatus** (also known as the *external acoustic meatus*) is a hole, or opening, in the temporal bone located superior and anterior to the mastoid process.

Appearance. On a panoramic image, the external auditory meatus appears as a round or ovoid *radiolucency* anterior and superior to the mastoid process. The external auditory meatus is *not* seen on periapical images.

Glenoid Fossa

Description. The **glenoid fossa** (also known as the *mandibular fossa*) is a concave, depressed area of the temporal bone. The mandibular condyle rests in the glenoid fossa. The glenoid fossa is located anterior to the mastoid process and the external auditory meatus.

Appearance. On a panoramic image, the glenoid fossa appears as a concave *radiopacity* superior to the mandibular

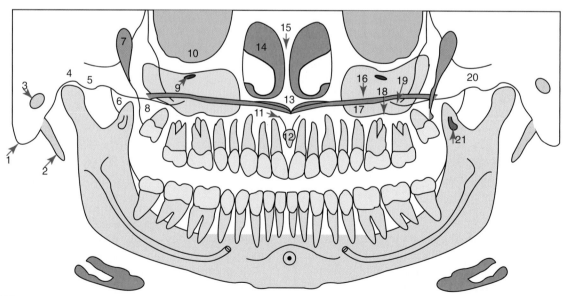

FIGURE 29-1 Normal anatomic landmarks of the maxilla and surrounding structures: **1**, mastoid process; **2**, styloid process; **3**, external auditory meatus; **4**, glenoid fossa; **5**, articular eminence; **6**, lateral pterygoid plate; **7**, pterygomaxillary fissure; **8**, maxillary tuberosity; **9**, infraorbital foramen; **10**, orbit; **11**, incisive canal; **12**, incisive foramen; **13**, anterior nasal spine; **14**, nasal cavity and conchae; **15**, nasal septum; **16**, hard palate; **17**, maxillary sinus; **18**, floor of maxillary sinus; **19**, zygomatic process of maxilla; **20**, zygomatic arch; **21**, hamulus. (Modified from Dental Auxiliary Education Projects: *Normal radiographic landmarks*, New York, Teachers College Press, 1982 by Teachers College, Columbia University. All rights reserved.)

condyle. The glenoid fossa is *not* seen on periapical images.

Articular Eminence

Description. The **articular eminence** (also known as the *articular tubercle*) is a rounded projection of the temporal bone located anterior to the glenoid fossa.

Appearance. On a panoramic image, the articular eminence appears as a rounded *radiopaque* projection of the bone located anterior to the glenoid fossa. The articular eminence is *not* seen on periapical images.

Lateral Pterygoid Plate

Description. The **lateral pterygoid plate** is a wing-shaped bony projection of the sphenoid bone located distal to the maxillary tuberosity region.

Appearance. On a panoramic image, the lateral pterygoid plate appears as a *radiopaque* projection of bone distal to the maxillary tuberosity region. The lateral pterygoid plate is *not* seen on periapical images.

Pterygomaxillary Fissure

Description. The **pterygomaxillary fissure** is a narrow space or cleft that separates the lateral pterygoid plate and the maxilla.

Appearance. On a panoramic image, the pterygomaxillary fissure appears as a *radiolucent* area between the lateral pterygoid plate and the maxilla. The zygoma is often superimposed on this region and obscures the pterygomaxillary fissure. The pterygomaxillary fissure is *not* seen on periapical images.

Maxillary Tuberosity

Description. The **maxillary tuberosity** is a rounded prominence of bone that extends posterior to the third molar region.

Appearance. On a panoramic image, the maxillary tuberosity appears as a *radiopaque* bulge distal to the third molar region.

Infraorbital Foramen

Description. The **infraorbital foramen** is a hole, or opening, in bone inferior to the border of the orbit.

Appearance. On a panoramic image, the infraorbital foramen appears as a round or ovoid *radiolucency* inferior to the orbit. The infraorbital foramen may be superimposed over the maxillary sinus. The infraorbital foramen is *not* seen on periapical images.

Orbit

Description. The **orbit** is the bony cavity that contains the eyeball.

Appearance. On a panoramic image, the orbit appears as a round *radiolucent* compartment with radiopaque borders located superior to the maxillary sinuses. On most panoramic images, only the inferior border of the orbit is visible, where it appears as a radiopaque line.

Incisive Canal

Description. The **incisive canal** (also known as the *nasopalatine canal*) is a passageway through bone, that extends from the superior foramina of the incisive canal (located on the floor of the nasal cavity) to the incisive foramen (located on the anterior hard palate).

Appearance. On a panoramic image, the incisive canal appears as a tubelike *radiolucent* area with radiopaque borders. The incisive canal is located between the maxillary central incisors.

Incisive Foramen

Description. The **incisive foramen** (also known as the *nasopalatine foramen*) is an opening, or hole, in bone that is located at the midline of the anterior portion of the hard palate directly posterior to the maxillary central incisors.

Appearance. On a panoramic image, the incisive foramen appears as a small, ovoid or round *radiolucency* located between the roots of the maxillary central incisors.

Anterior Nasal Spine

Description. The **anterior nasal spine** is a sharp bony projection of the maxilla located at the anterior–inferior portion of the nasal cavity.

Appearance. On a panoramic image, the anterior nasal spine appears as a V-shaped *radiopaque* area located at the intersection of the floor of the nasal cavity and the nasal septum.

Nasal Cavity

Description. The **nasal cavity** (also known as the *nasal fossa*) is a pear-shaped compartment of bone located superior to the maxilla.

Appearance. On a panoramic image, the nasal cavity appears as a large *radiolucent* area superior to the maxillary incisors.

Nasal Septum

Description. The **nasal septum** is a vertical bony wall or partition that divides the nasal cavity into the right and left nasal fossae.

Appearance. On a panoramic image, the nasal septum appears as a vertical *radiopaque* partition that divides the nasal cavity.

Hard Palate

Description. The **hard palate** is the bony wall that separates the nasal cavity from the oral cavity.

Appearance. On a panoramic image, the hard palate appears as a horizontal *radiopaque* band superior to the apices of maxillary teeth.

Maxillary Sinus and Floor of Maxillary Sinus

Description. The **maxillary sinuses** are paired cavities or compartments of bone that are located within the maxilla, superior to maxillary posterior teeth.

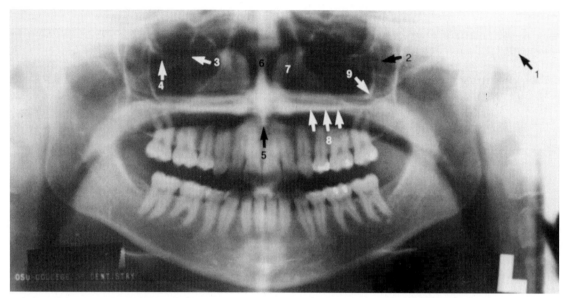

FIGURE 29-2 Normal anatomic landmarks of the maxilla and surrounding structures seen on panoramic images: **1**, external auditory meatus; **2**, pterygomaxillary fissure; **3**, infraorbital foramen; **4**, orbit; **5**, anterior nasal spine; **6**, nasal septum; **7**, nasal conchae; **8**, hard palate; **9**, zygomatic process of maxilla. (From Haring JI, Lind LJ: *Radiographic interpretation for the dental hygienist*, Philadelphia, 1993, Saunders.)

Appearance. On a panoramic image, the maxillary sinuses appear as paired *radiolucent* areas located superior to the apices of maxillary premolars and molars. The floor of the **maxillary sinus** is composed of dense cortical bone and appears as a *radiopaque* line.

Zygomatic Process of Maxilla

Description. The **zygomatic process of the maxilla** is a bony projection of the maxilla, that articulates with the zygoma, or malar bone (cheekbone).

Appearance. On a panoramic image, the zygomatic process of the maxilla appears as a J- or U-shaped *radiopacity* located superior to the maxillary first molar region.

Zygoma

Description. The **zygoma** (also known as the *malar bone* or *zygomatic bone*) is the cheekbone, and it articulates with the zygomatic process of the maxilla.

Appearance. On a panoramic image, the zygoma appears as a *radiopaque* band that extends posteriorly from the zygomatic process of the maxilla.

Hamulus

Description. The **hamulus** (also known as the *hamular process*) is a small, hooklike projection of bone that extends from the medial pterygoid plate of the sphenoid bone. The hamulus is located posterior to the maxillary tuberosity.

Appearance. On a panoramic image, the hamulus appears as a *radiopaque* hooklike projection posterior to the maxillary tuberosity area.

Figures 29-2, 29-3, and 29-4 illustrate the normal anatomic landmarks of the maxilla and surrounding structures that can be viewed on a panoramic image.

Bony Landmarks of Mandible and Surrounding Structures

This section reviews the bony landmarks of the mandible and surrounding structures that can be viewed on a panoramic image. Each of the following bony landmarks of the mandible and surrounding structures is identified on Figure 29-5.

Mandibular Condyle

Description. The **mandibular condyle** is a rounded projection of bone extending from the posterior superior border of the ramus of the mandible. The mandibular condyle articulates with the glenoid fossa of the temporal bone.

Appearance. On a panoramic image, the mandibular condyle appears as a bony, rounded *radiopaque* projection extending from the posterior border of the ramus of the mandible. The mandibular condyle is *not* seen on periapical images.

Coronoid Notch

Description. The **coronoid notch** is a scooped-out concavity of bone located distal to the coronoid process of the mandible.

Appearance. On a panoramic image, the coronoid notch appears as a *radiopaque* concavity located distal to the coronoid process on the superior border of the ramus. The coronoid notch is *not* seen on periapical images.

Coronoid Process

Description. The **coronoid process** is a marked prominence of bone found on the anterior–superior ramus of the mandible.

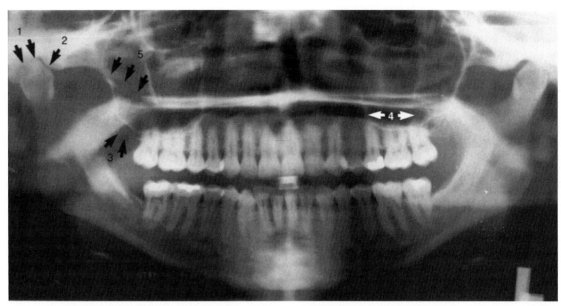

FIGURE 29-3 Normal anatomic landmarks of the maxilla and surrounding structures seen on panoramic images: **1**, glenoid fossa; **2**, articular eminence; **3**, maxillary tuberosity; **4**, maxillary sinus; **5**, zygoma. (From Haring JI, Lind LJ: *Radiographic interpretation for the dental hygienist*, Philadelphia, 1993, Saunders.)

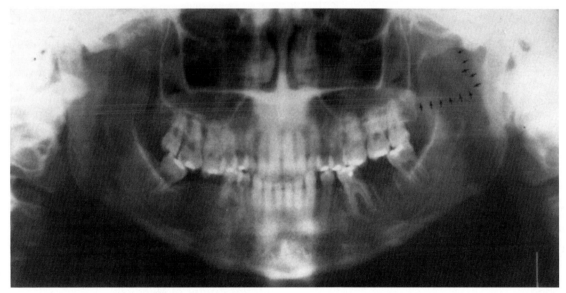

FIGURE 29-4 Lateral pterygoid plate. (From Haring JI, Lind LJ: *Radiographic interpretation for the dental hygienist*, Philadelphia, 1993, Saunders.)

Appearance. On a panoramic image, the coronoid process appears as a triangular *radiopacity* posterior to the maxillary tuberosity region.

Mandibular Foramen

Description. The **mandibular foramen** is a round or ovoid hole in bone on the lingual aspect of the ramus of the mandible.

Appearance. On a panoramic image, the mandibular foramen appears as a round or ovoid *radiolucency* centered within the ramus of the mandible. The mandibular foramen is *not* seen on periapical images.

Lingula

Description. The **lingula** is a small, tongue-shaped projection of bone seen adjacent to the mandibular foramen.

Appearance. On a panoramic image, the lingula appears as an indistinct *radiopacity* anterior to the mandibular foramen. The lingula is *not* seen on periapical images.

Mandibular Canal

Description. The **mandibular canal** is a tubelike passageway through bone, that travels the length of the mandible. The mandibular canal extends from the mandibular foramen

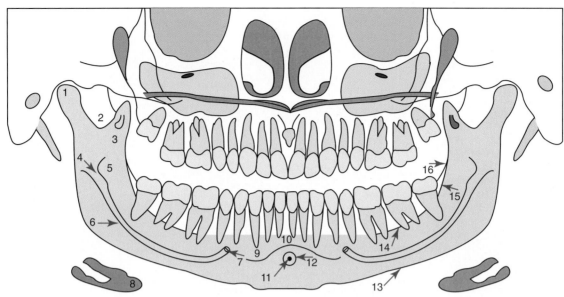

FIGURE 29-5 Normal anatomic landmarks of the mandible and surrounding structures: **1**, condyle; **2**, coronoid notch; **3**, coronoid process; **4**, mandibular foramen; **5**, lingula; **6**, mandibular canal; **7**, mental foramen; **8**, hyoid bone; **9**, mental ridge; **10**, mental fossa; **11**, lingual foramen; **12**, genial tubercles; **13**, inferior border of mandible; **14**, mylohyoid ridge; **15**, internal oblique ridge; **16**, external oblique ridge. (Modified from Dental Auxiliary Education Project: *Normal radiographic landmarks*, New York, Teachers College Press, 1982 by Teachers College, Columbia University. All rights reserved.)

to the mental foramen and houses the inferior alveolar nerve and blood vessels.

Appearance. On a panoramic image, the mandibular canal appears as a *radiolucent* band outlined by two thin radiopaque lines representing the cortical walls of the canal.

Mental Foramen

Description. The **mental foramen** is an opening or hole in bone located on the external surface of the mandible in the region of the mandibular premolars.

Appearance. On a panoramic image, the mental foramen appears as a small, ovoid or round *radiolucency* located in the apical region of the mandibular premolars.

Mental Ridge

Description. The **mental ridge** is a linear prominence of cortical bone located on the external surface of the anterior portion of the mandible that extends from the premolar region to the midline.

Appearance. On a panoramic image, the mental ridge appears as a thick *radiopaque* band that extends from the mandibular premolar region to the incisor region.

Mental Fossa

Description. The **mental fossa** is a scooped-out depressed area of bone located on the external surface of the anterior mandible above the mental ridge in the mandibular incisor region.

Appearance. On a panoramic image, the mental fossa appears as a *radiolucent* area above the mental ridge.

Lingual Foramen

Description. The **lingual foramen** is a tiny opening, or hole, in bone located on the internal surface of the mandible near the midline.

Appearance. On a panoramic image, the lingual foramen appears as a small *radiolucent* dot located inferior to the apices of the mandibular incisors.

Genial Tubercles

Description. **Genial tubercles** are tiny bumps of bone that are located on the lingual aspect of the mandible.

Appearance. On a panoramic image, genial tubercles appear as a ring-shaped *radiopacity* surrounding the lingual foramen.

Inferior Border of Mandible

Description. The **inferior border of the mandible** is a linear prominence of cortical bone that defines the lower border of the mandible.

Appearance. On a panoramic image, the inferior border of the mandible appears as a dense *radiopaque* band that outlines the lower border of the mandible.

Mylohyoid Ridge

Description. The **mylohyoid ridge** is a linear prominence of bone located on the internal surface of the mandible that extends from the molar region downward and forward toward the lower border of the mandibular symphysis.

Appearance. On a panoramic image, the mylohyoid ridge appears as a dense *radiopaque* band that extends downward and forward from the molar region.

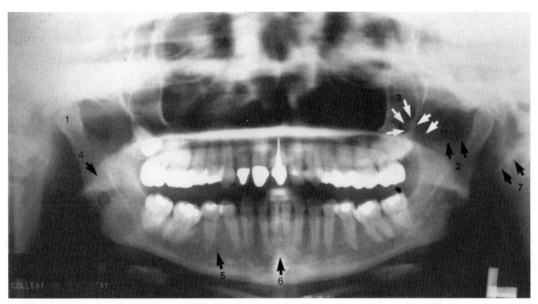

FIGURE 29-6 Normal anatomic landmarks of the mandible and surrounding structures seen on panoramic images: **1**, condyle; **2**, coronoid notch; **3**, coronoid process; **4**, mandibular foramen; **5**, mental foramen; **6**, genial tubercles; **7**, styloid process. (From Haring JI, Lind LJ: *Radiographic interpretation for the dental hygienist*, Philadelphia, 1993, Saunders.)

Internal Oblique Ridge

Description. The **internal oblique ridge** is a linear prominence of bone located on the internal surface of the mandible that extends downward and forward from the ramus.

Appearance. On a panoramic image, the internal oblique ridge appears as a dense *radiopaque* band that extends downward and forward from the ramus.

External Oblique Ridge

Description. The **external oblique ridge** is a linear prominence of bone located on the external surface of the body of the mandible.

Appearance. On a panoramic image, the external oblique ridge appears as a dense *radiopaque* band that extends downward and forward from the anterior border of the ramus of the mandible.

Angle of Mandible

Description. The **angle** is the area of the mandible where the body of the mandible meets the ramus.

Appearance. On a panoramic image, the angle of the mandible appears as a *radiopaque* bony structure where the ramus joins the body of the mandible.

Figures 29-6, 29-7, and 29-8 illustrate the normal anatomic landmarks of the mandible and surrounding structures that can be viewed on a panoramic projection.

AIR SPACES SEEN ON PANORAMIC IMAGES

This section reviews air space images that can be seen on a panoramic image. Each of the following air space images is identified on Figure 29-9.

Palatoglossal Air Space

Description. The term **palatoglossal air space** refers to the space between the palate (*palato*) and the tongue (*glossal*).

Appearance. On a panoramic image, the palatoglossal air space appears as a horizontal *radiolucent* band located superior to the apices of maxillary teeth.

Nasopharyngeal Air Space

Description. The term **nasopharyngeal air space** refers to the portion of the pharynx (*pharyngeal*) that is located posterior to the nasal cavity (*naso*).

Appearance. On a panoramic image, the nasopharyngeal air space appears as a diagonal *radiolucency* located superior to the radiopaque shadow of the soft palate and the uvula.

Glossopharyngeal Air Space

Description. The term **glossopharyngeal air space** refers to the portion of the pharynx (*pharyngeal*) that is located posterior to the tongue (*glosso*) and the oral cavity.

Appearance. On a panoramic image, the glossopharyngeal air space appears as a vertical *radiolucent* band superimposed over the ramus of the mandible. The glossopharyngeal air space is continuous with the nasopharyngeal air space superiorly and the palatoglossal air space inferiorly.

Figure 29-10 shows air spaces that can be viewed on a panoramic image.

SOFT TISSUES SEEN ON PANORAMIC IMAGES

This section describes soft tissues that can be seen on a panoramic image. Each of the following soft tissues is labeled on Figure 29-11.

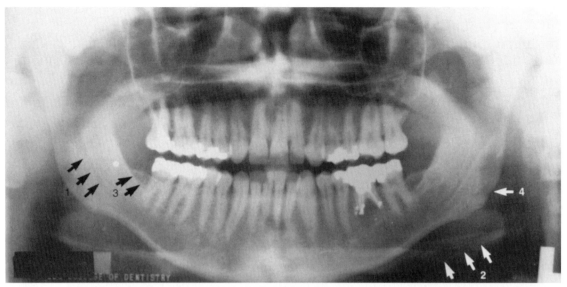

FIGURE 29-7 Normal anatomic landmarks of the mandible and surrounding structures seen on panoramic images: **1**, mandibular canal; **2**, hyoid; **3**, internal oblique ridge; **4**, angle of mandible. (From Haring JI, Lind LJ: *Radiographic interpretation for the dental hygienist*, Philadelphia, 1993, Saunders.)

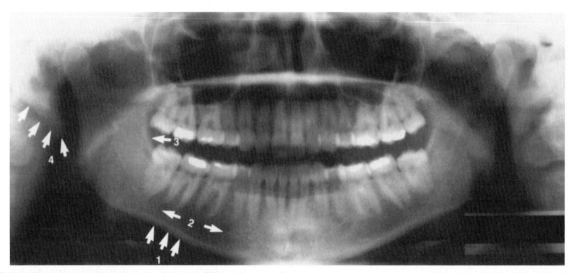

FIGURE 29-8 Normal anatomic landmarks of the mandible and surrounding structures as seen on panoramic images: **1**, inferior border of mandible; **2**, submandibular fossa; **3**, external oblique ridge; **4**, soft tissue of ear. (From Haring JI, Lind LJ: *Radiographic interpretation for the dental hygienist*, Philadelphia, 1993, Saunders.)

Tongue

Description. The **tongue** is a movable muscular organ attached to the floor of the mouth.

Appearance. On a panoramic image, the tongue appears as a *radiopaque* area superimposed over maxillary posterior teeth.

Soft Palate and Uvula

Description. The **soft palate** and the **uvula** form a muscular curtain that separates the oral cavity from the nasal cavity.

Appearance. On a panoramic image, the soft palate and the uvula appear as a diagonal *radiopacity* projecting posteriorly and inferiorly from the maxillary tuberosity region.

Lipline

Description. The **lipline** is formed by the positioning of the patient's lips.

Appearance. On a panoramic image, the lipline is seen in the region of anterior teeth. Areas of teeth not covered by the lips appear more *radiolucent*; areas covered by the lips appear more *radiopaque*.

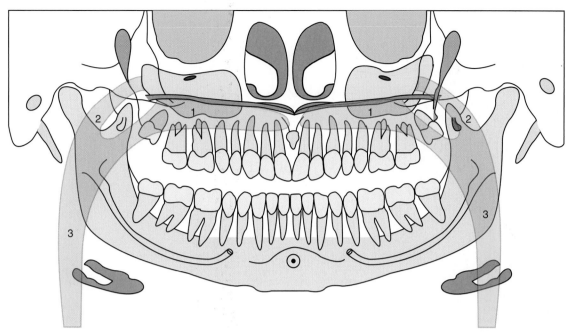

FIGURE 29-9 Air spaces seen on panoramic images: **1**, palatoglossal air space; **2**, nasopharyngeal air space; **3**, glossopharyngeal air space. (Modified from Dental Auxiliary Education Project: *Normal radiographic landmarks*, New York, Teachers College Press, 1982 by Teachers College, Columbia University. All rights reserved.)

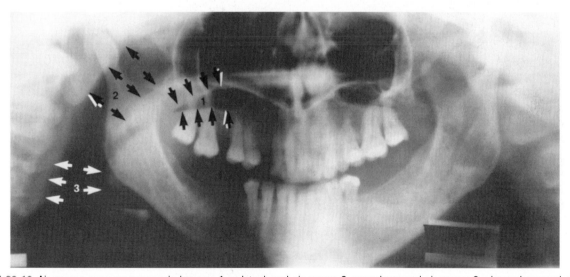

FIGURE 29-10 Air spaces seen on panoramic images: **1**, palatoglossal air space; **2**, nasopharyngeal air space; **3**, glossopharyngeal air space. (From Haring JI, Lind LJ: *Radiographic interpretation for the dental hygienist*, Philadelphia, 1993, Saunders.)

Ear

Appearance. On a panoramic image, the **ear** appears as a *radiopaque* shadow that projects anteriorly and inferiorly from the mastoid process. The ear is seen superimposed over the styloid process.

Figure 29-12 shows soft tissues that can be seen on a panoramic image.

SUMMARY

- The panoramic image allows the dental professional to view a large area of the maxilla and the mandible on a single projection.
- Knowledge of normal anatomic landmarks is necessary to interpret panoramic images; each normal anatomic landmark seen on a panoramic image corresponds to that seen

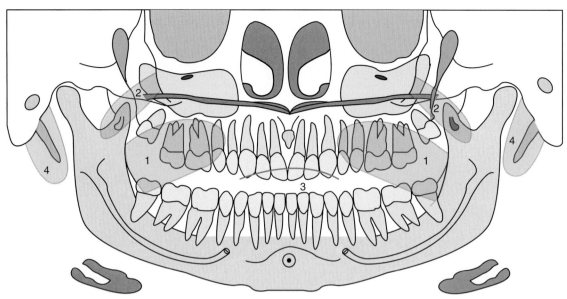

FIGURE 29-11 Soft tissues seen on panoramic images: **1**, tongue; **2**, soft palate and uvula; **3**, lipline; **4**, ear. (Modified from Dental Auxiliary Education Project: *Normal radiographic landmarks*, New York, Teachers College Press, 1982 by Teachers College, Columbia University. All rights reserved.)

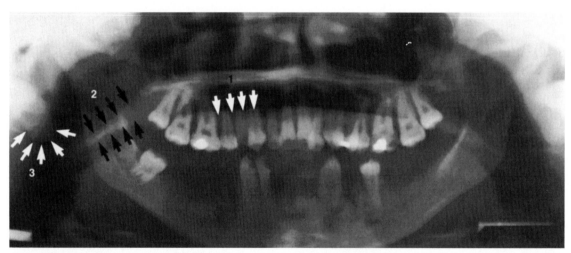

FIGURE 29-12 Soft tissues seen on panoramic images: **1**, tongue; **2**, soft palate and uvula; **3**, ear. (From Haring JI, Lind LJ: *Radiographic interpretation for the dental hygienist*, Philadelphia, 1993, Saunders.)

on a human skull. Knowledge of the anatomy of the maxilla, the mandible, and adjacent bones as viewed on the human skull enables the dental radiographer to identify normal anatomy seen on a panoramic image.

- Knowledge of air spaces and soft tissues is necessary to interpret panoramic images.
- All anatomic landmarks, air spaces, and soft tissues viewed on a panoramic image are described in this chapter.

BIBLIOGRAPHY

Haring JI, Lind LJ: Normal anatomy (panoramic films). In *Radiographic interpretation for the dental hygienist*, Philadelphia, 1993, Saunders.

White SC, Pharoah MJ: Panoramic radiography. In *Oral radiology: principles of interpretation*, ed 6, St. Louis, 2009, Mosby.

QUIZ QUESTIONS

IDENTIFICATION

___ **1.** Identify the normal anatomic landmarks labeled 1 to 15 in Figure 29-13.

___ **2.** Identify the normal anatomic landmarks labeled 1 to 16 in Figure 29-14.

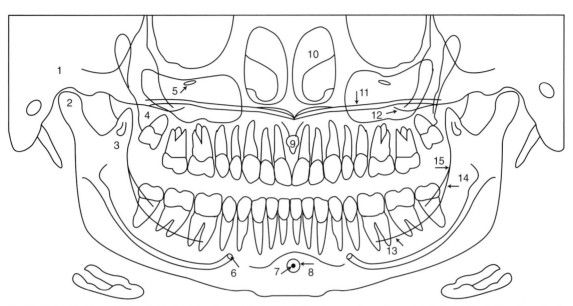

FIGURE 29-13 (From Haring JI, Lind LJ: *Radiographic interpretation for the dental hygienist*, Philadelphia, 1993, Saunders.)

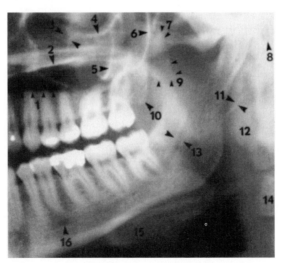

FIGURE 29-14 (From Haring JI, Lind LJ: *Radiographic interpretation for the dental hygienist*, Philadelphia, 1993, Saunders.)

part VII

Image Interpretation Basics

Chapter 30 Introduction to Image Interpretation, 369

Chapter 31 Descriptive Terminology, 372

Chapter 32 Identification of Restorations, Dental Materials, and Foreign
            Objects, 383

Chapter 33 Interpretation of Dental Caries, 402

Chapter 34 Interpretation of Periodontal Disease, 412

Chapter 35 Interpretation of Trauma, and Pulpal and Periapical Lesions, 426

Introduction to Image Interpretation

OUTLINE

BASIC CONCEPTS
>   Interpretation Terminology
>   Importance of Interpretation

GUIDELINES
>   Who Interprets Images?
>   Interpretation versus Diagnosis
>   When and Where Are Images Interpreted?
>   Interpretation and Patient Education

LEARNING OBJECTIVES

After completion of this chapter, the student will be able to do the following:
- Define the key terms associated with interpreting images
- Summarize the importance of the interpretation of images
- Define the roles of the dentist and the dental auxiliary in the interpretation of dental images
- Discuss the difference between interpretation and diagnosis
- Describe who is able to interpret dental images
- Describe when and where dental images are interpreted
- Describe how interpretation can be used to educate the dental patient about the importance and use of dental images

KEY TERMS

Diagnosis
Interpret
Interpretation
Interpretation, image

Image interpretation is an essential part of the diagnostic process. The ability to evaluate and recognize what is revealed by a dental image enables the dental professional to play a vital role in the detection of those diseases, lesions, and conditions of jaws which cannot be identified clinically. The chapters in this part of the text present an overview of interpretation topics. Detailed information on interpretation is beyond the scope of this text.

The purpose of this chapter is to present the basic concepts of image interpretation and to review interpretation guidelines.

BASIC CONCEPTS

An explanation of what is viewed on a dental image, or interpretation, is an important component of patient care. Before the dental radiographer can inspect dental images adequately, a thorough understanding of the terminology and importance of interpretation is necessary.

Interpretation Terminology

Before discussion of the principles of interpretation, an explanation of basic terms is provided below:

Interpret: To offer an explanation.

Interpretation: An explanation.

Image interpretation: An explanation of what is viewed on a dental image; the ability to read what is revealed by a dental image.

Diagnosis: The identification of a disease by examination or analysis. In the dental setting, the dentist is responsible for establishing a diagnosis. Other members of the dental team are restricted by law from providing a diagnosis.

Importance of Interpretation

In addition to understanding the importance of dental images, the dental radiographer must also understand the importance of interpretation. As described in Chapter 11, dental images are essential for diagnostic purposes. *All* dental images must be carefully reviewed and interpreted. A great deal of information about teeth and supporting bone is obtained from interpretation. Consequently, image interpretation is of paramount importance to the dental professional. As mentioned above, image interpretation enables the dental professional to play a vital role in the detection of those diseases, lesions, and conditions of teeth and jaws which cannot be identified clinically.

GUIDELINES

The dental radiographer must know who can interpret dental images, the difference between interpretation and diagnosis, when and where images are interpreted, and how to use interpretation to educate the dental patient.

Who Interprets Images?

Training is necessary to interpret dental images. Any dental professional with training in interpretation can examine images. Both the dentist and the dental hygienist are trained to interpret dental images; dental and dental hygiene curricula include instruction in image interpretation. The dental assistant, however, may or may not be trained in the interpretation of dental images. The amount and scope of training in dental radiography dictate whether the dental assistant can perform image interpretation.

The dental radiographer plays an important role in the preliminary interpretation of dental images. The dental radiographer acts as an additional pair of eyes examining the images, and can direct the attention of the dentist to any areas of question or concern. To interpret images, the dental radiographer must be confident in the identification and recognition of the following:

- Normal anatomy (see Chapters 27 and 29)
- Dental restorations, dental materials, and foreign objects (see Chapter 32)
- Dental caries (see Chapter 33)
- Periodontal disease (see Chapter 34)
- Trauma, pulpal lesions and periapical lesions (see Chapter 35)

Interpretation versus Diagnosis

In the dental setting, the terms *interpretation* and *diagnosis* are often confused; it is important to note that these terms have very different meanings and should not be used synonymously. *Interpretation* refers to an explanation of what is viewed on a dental image, whereas *diagnosis* refers to the identification of disease by examination or analysis. In dentistry, a diagnosis is made by the dentist after a thorough review of the medical history, dental history, clinical examination, radiographic examination, and clinical or laboratory tests.

Although any dental professional with training in interpretation may examine dental images, the final interpretation and diagnosis are the responsibilities of the dentist. Dental hygienists and dental assistants are restricted by law from rendering a diagnosis.

When and Where Are Images Interpreted?

It is essential to remember that dental images are taken to benefit the patient. To benefit the patient optimally, dental images must be taken at the beginning of the dental appointment, mounted, interpreted, and then used for diagnostic, therapeutic, and educational purposes. Ideally, dental images should be reviewed and interpreted immediately after mounting them in the presence of the patient. If any suspicious or questionable areas are seen on the images, the patient can be examined by the dentist or dental hygienist to obtain additional information or to confirm the suspected problem. If the patient were not present during the interpretation of dental images, much needed clinical information would be unavailable.

Digital images are typically viewed by the dental professional on a computer monitor in the operatory. Dental radiographs are usually examined on the viewbox in the operatory and are best interpreted in a room with dimmed lighting, as described in Chapter 28.

Interpretation and Patient Education

Interpretation of dental images can be used as an educational tool in the professional setting. In addition to providing a preliminary interpretation, the dental radiographer can educate the patient by identifying and discussing what is normally found on a dental image. Then the dentist can focus on specific problems or areas of concern. In this manner, all members of the dental team can work together using interpretation to educate patients about the importance and use of dental images.

SUMMARY

- Image interpretation is an explanation of what is viewed on a dental image, or the ability to read what is revealed by a dental radiographic image.
- Image interpretation is an important component of patient care and enables the dental professional to detect diseases, lesions, and conditions that cannot be identified clinically.
- Any dental professional with training in interpretation can examine images. To interpret dental images, the dental radiographer must be confident in the identification and recognition of normal anatomy; restorations, dental materials, and foreign objects; dental caries; periodontal disease; traumatic injuries; and periapical lesions.
- Although any dental professional with training in interpretation may examine dental images, final interpretation and diagnosis are the responsibilities of the dentist.
- Dental auxiliaries are restricted by law from providing a diagnosis but can facilitate patient care by performing a preliminary image interpretation.
- Dental radiographic examination should take place at the beginning of the appointment, and dental images should be interpreted in the presence of the patient.

- The dental professional can use interpretation to educate patients about the importance and use of dental images.

BIBLIOGRAPHY

Haring JI, Lind LJ: The importance of dental radiographs and interpretation. In *Radiographic interpretation for the dental hygienist*, Philadelphia, 1993, Saunders.

Johnson ON, Thomson EM: Preliminary interpretation of the radiographs. In *Essentials of dental radiography for dental assistants and hygienists*, ed 8, Upper Saddle River, 2007, NJ, Pearson.

Miles DA, Van Dis ML, Williamson GF, Jensen CW: Interpretation: normal versus abnormal and common radiographic presentation of lesions. In *Radiographic imaging for the dental team*, ed 4, St. Louis, 2009, Saunders.

White SC, Pharoah MJ: Principles of image interpretation. In *Oral radiology: principles of interpretation*, ed 6, St. Louis, 2009, Mosby.

QUIZ QUESTIONS

SHORT ANSWER

1. Summarize the importance of image interpretation.
2. Define the roles of each member of the dental team in the interpretation of dental images.
3. Discuss the difference between interpretation and diagnosis.
4. List the members of the dental team who may interpret dental images.
5. Describe when and where dental images are interpreted.
6. Describe how interpretation can be used to educate the patient about the importance and use of dental images.

TRUE OR FALSE

___ 7. All images must be carefully reviewed and interpreted.
___ 8. Any dental professional with training in interpretation can examine images.
___ 9. The amount and scope of training received dictate whether the dental assistant can perform image interpretation.
___ 10. The terms *interpretation* and *diagnosis* can be used synonymously.
___ 11. Any dental professional can provide a diagnosis.
___ 12. Dental images should not be interpreted in the presence of the patient.
___ 13. No specific guidelines exist regarding when and where dental images should be interpreted.
___ 14. The dental radiographer can educate the patient by identifying and discussing what is normally found on a dental image.
___ 15. All members of the dental team can work together using interpretation to educate patients about the importance and use of dental images.

chapter 31

Descriptive Terminology

OUTLINE

DEFINITION AND USES
What Is Descriptive Terminology?
Why Use Descriptive Terminology?
Descriptive Terminology versus Diagnosis

REVIEW OF BASIC TERMS
Radiograph/Dental Image versus X-Ray
Radiolucent versus Radiopaque
Terms Used to Describe Radiolucent Lesions
Terms Used to Describe Radiopaque Lesions

LEARNING OBJECTIVES

After completion of this chapter, the student will be able to do the following:

- Identify the categories of information that should be documented for all lesions viewed on dental images
- Define descriptive terminology and describe why the dental professional should use descriptive terms
- Define the terms dental image, radiograph, x-ray, radiolucent, and radiopaque
- Distinguish the terms radiograph, dental image, and x-ray
- Distinguish the terms radiolucent and radiopaque
- Define the terms unilocular and multilocular

- Define the terms periapical, inter-radicular, edentulous zone, pericoronal, and alveolar bone loss
- Identify radiolucent lesions on a dental image in terms of appearance, location, and size
- Define the terms focal opacity, target lesion, multifocal confluent pattern, irregular/ill-defined opacity, ground glass opacity, mixed lucent–opaque lesion, and soft tissue opacity
- Identify radiopaque lesions on a dental image in terms of appearance, location, and size

KEY TERMS

Alveolar bone loss
Edentulous zone
Expansile
Dental image
Focal opacity
Ground glass
Inter-radicular

Irregular
Mixed lucent–opaque
Multifocal confluent
Multilocular
Periapical
Pericoronal
Radiograph

Radiolucent
Radiopaque
Soft tissue opacity
Target lesion
Unilocular corticated
Unilocular noncorticated
X-ray

Interpretation, as defined in Chapter 30, is the ability to read what is revealed by a dental image. To interpret dental images, the dental professional must be able to describe what is observed in accurate and succinct terms. A working knowledge of *descriptive terminology* is important for communication and documentation and is essential in interpretation.

DEFINITION AND USES

What Is Descriptive Terminology?

In dental imaging, a number of different terms can be used to describe the appearance, location, and size of a lesion; these terms represent what is called *descriptive terminology*. This information should be documented for all lesions viewed on dental images.

Why Use Descriptive Terminology?

Descriptive terminology allows dental professionals to describe and discuss what is seen on a dental image intelligently and to communicate using a common language. Communication among dental professionals about dental image findings takes place each time a case is discussed or when a patient is referred to a specialist for evaluation. The use of descriptive terminology eliminates the chance for miscommunication among dental professionals.

Descriptive terminology also allows the dental professional to document what is seen on a dental image in the patient record in terms of appearance, location, and size. Documentation of what is viewed on dental images is essential for legal purposes. A written description of what is viewed indicates that a qualified dental professional interpreted the dental image. If no notation of interpretation is included in the patient record, no legal documentation can be made that the dental images were reviewed.

Descriptive Terminology versus Diagnosis

Is describing a lesion the same as making a diagnosis? Descriptive terminology allows the dental professional to describe what is seen on a dental image *without* implying a diagnosis. It is important to note that it is extremely difficult, if not impossible, to make a diagnosis from a dental image alone. The patient's medical and dental histories, clinical findings, signs and symptoms, laboratory tests, and biopsy results all contribute to aiding the dentist to make a definitive diagnosis.

REVIEW OF BASIC TERMS

The use of descriptive terminology requires that the dental professional have a basic understanding of five general terms: *radiograph*, *dental image*, *x-ray*, *radiolucent*, and *radiopaque*.

Radiograph/Dental Image versus X-ray

The terms *radiograph* and *x-ray* are often used interchangeably by dental professionals, but it is important to note that these two terms have distinct and different meanings.

A **radiograph** is defined (as in Chapter 1) as a two-dimensional representation of a three-dimensional object. When using film, a radiograph is an image that is produced by exposing the film to x-rays and then processing the film so that a negative is produced. In older literature, a radiograph may also be called an *x-ray film*, "radiogram," "roentgenogram," or "roentgenograph." The terms *radiograph* and *x-ray* are **not** synonymous. A radiograph refers to the actual *film* exposed, and an x-ray refers to the *beam of energy*, or radiation. Therefore, the dental professional should not refer to a radiograph as an "x-ray" but rather an "x-ray film." An **x-ray**, or *roentgen ray*, is a beam of energy that has the power to penetrate substances and to record shadow images on receptors.

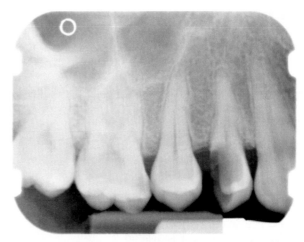

FIGURE 31-1 Dental caries appears radiolucent on a dental image.

With the use of digital radiography, no film is utilized so the term *radiograph* is not pertinent. Instead the term *digital image* is used and refers to an image composed of pixels (refer to Chapter 25 for details). A digital image is diagnostically equivalent to film-based imaging. In this text, the term ***dental image*** is used to describe what is viewed on radiographs and/or on digital images.

Radiolucent versus Radiopaque

The terms *radiolucent* and *radiopaque* are used to describe the appearances of all the structures seen on a dental image. A dental image appears radiolucent (black or dark) where the tissues are soft or thin, and it appears radiopaque (white or light) where the tissues are thick or dense. Most structures do not exhibit uniform thickness and therefore appear gray instead of black or white.

Radiolucent refers to that portion of a processed dental image that is dark or black. Radiolucent structures lack density and permit the passage of the x-ray beam with little or no resistance.

Dental caries appears radiolucent because the area of tooth with dental caries is less dense than surrounding structures and therefore readily permits the passage of the x-ray beam (Figure 31-1). Consequently, most of the energy of the x-ray beam freely passes through the area of dental caries to the recording surface of the receptor, resulting in a dark or radiolucent area on the dental image (Figure 31-2). Other radiolucent structures include air spaces, soft tissues, dental pulp, and the periodontal ligament space.

Radiopaque refers to that portion of a dental image that appears light or white. Radiopaque structures are dense and absorb or resist the passage of the x-ray beam.

A metallic restoration appears radiopaque because it is very dense and absorbs the radiation (Figure 31-3). As a result, very little, if any, radiation reaches the surface of the receptor, which results in a white or radiopaque area on the dental image (see Figure 31-2). Examples of other radiopaque structures include enamel, dentin, and bone.

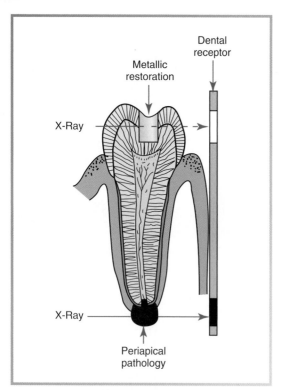

FIGURE 31-2 This diagram shows variations of x-ray absorption in a tooth with an amalgam restoration and a periapical lesion. The amalgam restoration absorbs the x-ray beam. The x-ray beam does not reach the receptor surface, and a white or radiopaque area results. The lesion at the apex of the tooth lacks density and is easily penetrated by the x-ray beam. The beam reaches the receptor and results in a dark or radiolucent area.

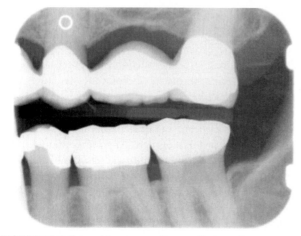

FIGURE 31-3 Two gold crowns on the mandibular molars appear radiopaque on a dental image.

Terms Used to Describe Radiolucent Lesions

A number of terms can be used to describe lesions found on dental images. A lesion that appears radiolucent permits the passage of the x-ray beam and represents destruction of bone or a space-occupying entity within the bones of the jaws. Radiolucent lesions may be described in terms of appearance, location, and size.

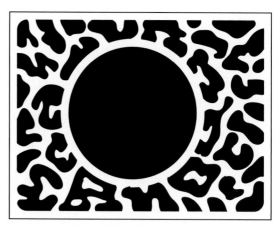

FIGURE 31-4 Unilocular radiolucent lesion with corticated borders. (Modified from Eversole LR: *Clinical outline of oral pathology: diagnosis and treatment*, ed 2, Philadelphia, 1984, Lea and Febiger.)

Appearance

The appearance of most radiolucent lesions can be classified as either unilocular or multilocular. Other radiolucent classifications include a "moth-eaten" pattern, a multifocal pattern, or a widened periodontal ligament space. Box 31-1 lists examples of radiolucent lesions in each of these categories.

Unilocular Radiolucent Lesions. The term *unilocular* is derived from two Latin words, *uni* ("one") and *loculus* ("small space" or "compartment") and refers to a radiolucent lesion that exhibits one compartment. Unilocular lesions tend to be small and nonexpansile and have borders that may appear corticated or noncorticated on the dental image.

Unilocular Lesion—Corticated Borders. The term *corticated* comes from the Latin *cortex* ("an outer layer") and refers to the outer layer or border of a radiolucent lesion. A unilocular radiolucent lesion with corticated borders exhibits a thin, well-demarcated radiopaque rim of bone at the periphery (Figure 31-4). A **unilocular corticated** lesion is usually indicative of a benign, slow-growing process.

Unilocular Lesion—Noncorticated Borders. A unilocular lesion with noncorticated borders does *not* exhibit a thin radiopaque rim of bone at the periphery (Figure 31-5). Instead, the periphery of a **unilocular noncorticated** lesion appears fuzzy or poorly defined. Radiolucencies with ill-defined or irregular margins may represent either a benign process or a malignant process.

Multilocular Radiolucent Lesions. The term **multilocular** refers to a lesion that exhibits multiple radiolucent compartments (Figure 31-6). A lesion with multiple compartments is larger than a lesion with one compartment; therefore, by definition, a multilocular lesion is larger than a unilocular lesion. Multilocular lesions typically exhibit well-defined, corticated margins. Multilocular radiolucent lesions are frequently **expansile** and tend to displace the buccal and lingual plates of bone.

Multilocular lesions are typically benign lesions with aggressive growth potential. As a general rule, most multilocular lesions represent a reactive or neoplastic process. The

BOX 31-1 Radiolucent Lesions of the Jaws

Unilocular Radiolucencies
Periapical cyst
Periapical granuloma
Periapical abscess
Periapical cemental dysplasia*†
Incisive canal cyst
Traumatic bone cyst
Residual bone cyst
Lateral periodontal cyst
Odontogenic keratocyst*
Primordial cyst
Osteoporotic bone marrow defect
Dentigerous cyst
Static bone cyst
Ameloblastoma*
Adenomatoid odontogenic tumor†
Calcifying epithelial odontogenic tumor*†
Ameloblastic fibroma*
Central giant cell granuloma*

Multilocular Radiolucencies
Odontogenic keratocyst*
Ameloblastoma*
Central giant cell granuloma*
Botryoid odontogenic cyst
Aneursymal bone cyst
Cherubism*
Hyperparathyroidism

Myxoma
Central neurogenic neoplasms
Ameloblastic fibroma*
Calcifying epithelial odontogenic tumor*†

"Moth-Eaten" Radiolucencies
Osteomyelitis
Metastatic carcinoma†
Osteosarcoma*†
Chondrosarcoma*†
Ewing's sarcoma
Lymphoma
Burkitt's lymphoma
Fibrosarcoma
Multiple myeloma*

Widened Periodontal Ligament Space
Scleroderma
Osteosarcoma*
Periodontal inflammation
Endodontic inflammation

Multifocal Radiolucencies
Basal cell nevus syndrome
Histiocytosis X
Multiple myeloma*
Cherubism*†
Periapical cemental dysplasia*†

*Indicates the lesion may exhibit more than one radiolucent appearance.
†Indicates the lesion may also appear with a radiopaque component.

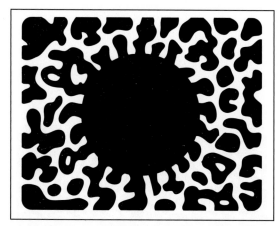

FIGURE 31-5 Unilocular radiolucent lesion with noncorticated borders. (Modified from Eversole LR: *Clinical outline of oral pathology: diagnosis and treatment*, ed 2, Philadelphia, 1984, Lea and Febiger.)

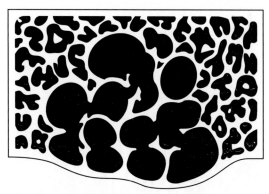

FIGURE 31-6 Multilocular radiolucent lesion. (Modified from Eversole LR: *Clinical outline of oral pathology: diagnosis and treatment*, ed 2, Philadelphia, 1984, Lea and Febiger.)

odontogenic keratocyst, ameloblastoma, and the central giant cell granuloma are examples of multilocular radiolucencies viewed on dental images.

Location

In addition to appearance, radiolucent lesions can also be described in terms of location. The location of a lesion is important for communication and documentation purposes. A radiolucent lesion may appear in a periapical, interradicular, edentulous, or pericoronal location. A radiolucent lesion may also appear as alveolar bone loss. Box 31-2 lists examples of radiolucent lesions and their most likely locations.

Periapical Location. The term **periapical** refers to the area around the apex of a tooth (Figure 31-7). It is derived from

BOX 31-2 Locations of Radiolucent Lesions

Periapical Radiolucencies
Periapical cyst
Periapical granuloma
Periapical abscess
Periapical cemento-osseous dysplasia*†
Incisive canal cyst
Traumatic bone cyst*
Residual cyst*
Odontogenic keratocyst*
Central giant cell granuloma

Inter-radicular Radiolucencies
Lateral periodontal cyst
Residual cyst*
Odontogenic keratocyst*
Primordial cyst*
Traumatic bone cyst*
Botryoid odontogenic cyst

Edentulous Zone
Periapical cyst‡
Periapical granuloma‡
Periapical abscess‡
Periapical cemental dysplasia*†‡
Incisive canal cyst‡
Residual cyst‡
Odontogenic keratocyst*
Central giant cell granuloma*
Primordial cyst*
Ameloblastoma*
Calcifying epithelial odontogenic tumor*†
Static bone cyst

Pericoronal Radiolucencies
Dentigerous cyst
Odontogenic keratocyst*
Ameloblastoma*
Adenomatoid odontogenic tumor†
Calcifying epithelial odontogenic tumor†*

Alveolar Bone Loss
Periodontitis
Histiocytosis X
Cyclic neutropenia
Leukemia

No Specific Location
Multiple myeloma
Cherubism
Myxoma
Osteosarcoma†
Osteomyelitis
Metastatic carcinoma†
Chondrosarcoma†
Ewing's sarcoma
Lymphoma
Burkitt's lymphoma
Fibrosarcoma
Multiple myeloma
Osteoporotic bone marrow defect
Ameloblastic fibroma
Aneurysmal bone cyst
Hyperparathyroidism

*Indicates the lesion may exhibit more than one location.
†Indicates the lesion may also appear with a radiopaque component.
‡Indicates this location is possible, after extraction of a related tooth.

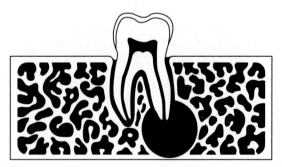

FIGURE 31-7 Unilocular corticated radiolucent lesion in periapical location. (Modified from Eversole LR: *Clinical outline of oral pathology: diagnosis and treatment,* ed 2, Philadelphia, 1984, Lea and Febiger.)

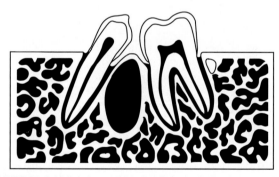

FIGURE 31-8 Unilocular corticated radiolucent lesion in inter-radicular location. (Modified from Eversole LR: *Clinical outline of oral pathology: diagnosis and treatment,* ed 2, Philadelphia, 1984, Lea and Febiger.)

the Greek word *peri* ("around") and the Latin word *apex,* referring, in this case, to the terminal end of a tooth root. An example of a common periapical radiolucency is a periapical cyst seen secondary to pulpal necrosis.

Inter-Radicular Location. The term **inter-radicular** refers to the area between the roots of adjacent teeth (Figure 31-8).

The term *inter* is Latin for "between," and *radicular* means "pertaining to a root." An example of a radiolucent lesion that the radiographer would expect to find in an inter-radicular location is the lateral periodontal cyst.

Edentulous Zone. **Edentulous zone** refers to an area without teeth (Figure 31-9). (*Edentulous* means "without teeth.") A variety of radiolucent lesions may occur in an edentulous zone.

Pericoronal Location. The term **pericoronal** refers to the area around the crown of an impacted tooth (Figure 31-10). It is derived from the Greek word *peri* ("around,") and *corona* is Latin for "crown." A dentigerous cyst is an example of a radiolucent lesion seen in a pericoronal location.

Alveolar Bone Loss. **Alveolar bone loss** refers to loss of maxillary or mandibular bone that surrounds and supports the teeth (Figure 31-11). Alveolar bone loss appears radiolucent. Alveolar bone loss is seen not only with periodontal disease but also with systemic illnesses, such as diabetes, histiocytosis X, and leukemia. Malignant neoplasms may also cause alveolar bone loss.

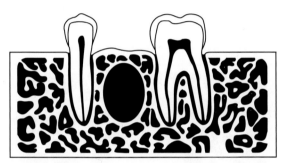

FIGURE 31-9 Unilocular corticated radiolucent lesion in edentulous zone. (Modified from Eversole LR: *Clinical outline of oral pathology: diagnosis and treatment*, ed 2, Philadelphia, 1984, Lea and Febiger.)

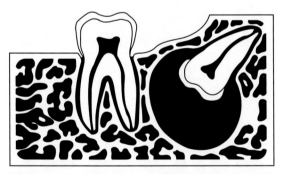

FIGURE 31-10 Unilocular corticated radiolucent lesion located in pericoronal location. (Modified from Eversole LR: *Clinical outline of oral pathology: diagnosis and treatment*, ed 2, Philadelphia, 1984, Lea and Febiger.)

Size

Radiolucent lesions viewed on a dental image can vary in size from several millimeters in diameter to several centimeters in diameter. Often the size of a lesion dictates the type of treatment necessary. Documentation of the size of a lesion is important for treatment considerations as well as for future comparisons. Radiolucent lesions can be easily measured on a dental image with a millimeter ruler. Figure 31-12 illustrates some common items and their respective sizes for comparison purposes.

Terms Used to Describe Radiopaque Lesions

A number of terms can be used to describe radiopaque lesions, which resist the passage of the x-ray beam and represent osseous tissue, cartilage, enamel, dentin, and cementum. Radiopaque lesions can also be described in terms of appearance, location, and size.

Appearance

The appearance of a radiopaque lesion can be described using one of the following terms: *focal opacity, target lesion, multifocal confluent, irregular, ground glass,* or *mixed lucent-opaque.* Radiopaque lesions occur not only in bone but in soft tissue as well. A radiopaque lesion located in soft tissue can be described as a "soft tissue radiopacity." Box 31-3 lists examples of radiopaque lesions of the jaw.

Focal Opacity. The term **focal opacity** refers to a well-defined, localized radiopaque lesion on a dental image (Figure 31-13). Condensing osteitis is an example of a radiopaque lesion that can be described as a focal opacity.

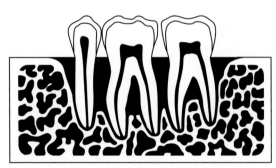

FIGURE 31-11 Radiolucent area caused by alveolar bone loss. (Modified from Eversole LR: *Clinical outline of oral pathology: diagnosis and treatment*, ed 2, Philadelphia, 1984, Lea and Febiger.)

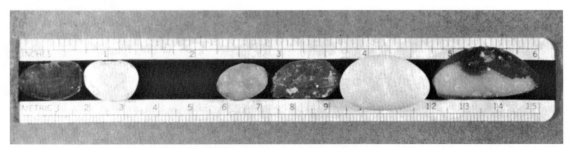

FIGURE 31-12 Beans and nuts used to illustrate the sizes of lesions.

BOX 31-3   Radiopaque Lesions of the Jaws

Focal Opacities
Periapical cemento-osseous dysplasia*
Condensing osteitis
Sclerotic bone

Target Lesions
Benign cementoblastoma
Complex odontoma

Multifocal Confluent Radiopacities
Osteitis deformans
Florid osseous dysplasia
Gardner's syndrome

Mixed Lucent–Opaque Lesions
Adenomatoid odontogenic tumor
Calcifying epithelial odontogenic tumor
Ameloblastic fibroma
Ameloblastic fibro-odontoma
Compound odontoma
Ossifying/cementifying fibroma
Periapical cemental dysplasia
Calcifying and keratinizing epithelial odontogenic cyst

Irregular Radiopacities
Osteosarcoma*
Chondrosarcoma*
Metastatic carcinoma*

Soft Tissue Radiopacities
Sialolithiasis
Calcified lymph nodes
Foreign bodies
Myositis ossificans

Ground-Glass Radiopacities
Fibrous dysplasia
Osteitis deformans
Osteopetrosis
Hyperparathyroidism

*Indicates the lesion may also appear with a radiolucent component.

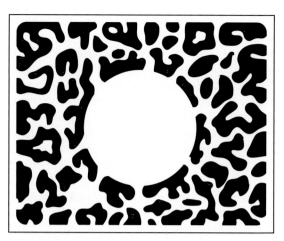

FIGURE 31-13 Focal opacity. (Modified from Eversole LR: *Clinical outline of oral pathology: diagnosis and treatment*, ed 2, Philadelphia, 1984, Lea and Febiger.)

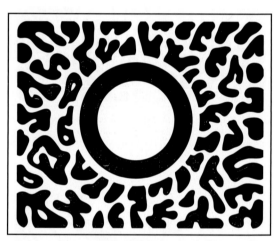

FIGURE 31-14 Target lesion. (Modified from Eversole LR: *Clinical outline of oral pathology: diagnosis and treatment*, ed 2, Philadelphia, 1984, Lea and Febiger.)

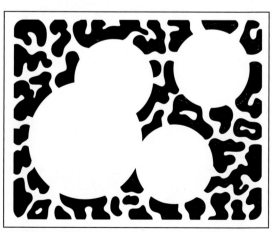

FIGURE 31-15 Multifocal confluent radiopacity. (Modified from Eversole LR: *Clinical outline of oral pathology: diagnosis and treatment*, ed 2, Philadelphia, 1984, Lea and Febiger.)

Target Lesion. The term **target lesion** refers to a well-defined, localized radiopaque area surrounded by a uniform radiolucent halo (Figure 31-14). A benign cementoblastoma is an example of a radiopacity that can be described as a target lesion.

Multifocal Confluent Pattern. A **multifocal confluent** radiopaque pattern can be described as multiple radiopacities that appear to overlap or flow together (Figure 31-15). Diseases such as osteitis deformans and florid osseous dysplasia exhibit a multifocal confluent radiopaque pattern. Multifocal confluent radiopacities that involve multiple quadrants of the jaws usually represent benign fibro-osseous disorders.

Irregular/Ill-Defined Opacity. A radiopacity may exhibit an irregular, poorly defined pattern (Figure 31-16). **Irregular**

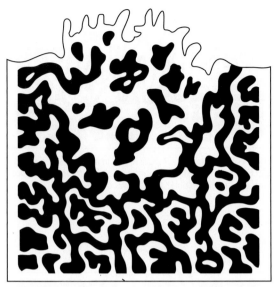

FIGURE 31-16 Irregular ill-defined radiopaque pattern. (Modified from Eversole LR: *Clinical outline of oral pathology: diagnosis and treatment*, ed 2, Philadelphia, 1984, Lea and Febiger.)

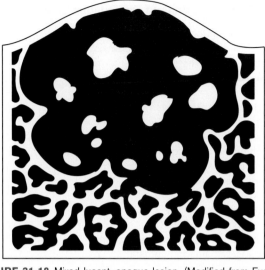

FIGURE 31-18 Mixed lucent–opaque lesion. (Modified from Eversole LR: *Clinical outline of oral pathology: diagnosis and treatment*, ed 2, Philadelphia, 1984, Lea and Febiger.)

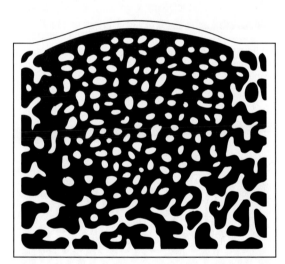

FIGURE 31-17 Ground-glass radiopacity. (Modified from Eversole LR: *Clinical outline of oral pathology: diagnosis and treatment*, ed 2, Philadelphia, 1984, Lea and Febiger.)

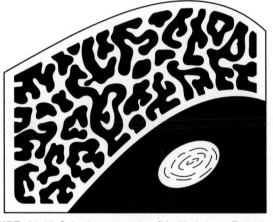

FIGURE 31-19 Soft tissue opacity. (Modified from Eversole LR: *Clinical outline of oral pathology: diagnosis and treatment*, ed 2, Philadelphia, 1984, Lea and Febiger.)

radiopacities may represent a malignant condition. Examples of irregular, ill-defined radiopaque lesions include osteosarcoma and chondrosarcoma.

Ground-Glass Opacity. A **ground-glass** appearance of bone can be described as a granular or pebbled radiopacity that resembles pulverized glass (Figure 31-17). A ground-glass radiopacity is often said to resemble the appearance or texture of an orange peel. Diseases such as fibrous dysplasia, osteitis deformans, and osteopetrosis may exhibit a ground-glass or orange-peel appearance.

Mixed Lucent–Opaque Lesion. A **mixed lucent–opaque** lesion exhibits both radiopaque and radiolucent components (Figure 31-18). Mixed lucent–opaque lesions often represent calcifying tumors. Many such tumors appear as a radiolucent area with central opaque flecks or calcifications. With time, as the mineralization progresses, the lesion becomes predominantly radiolucent with radiopaque flecks. An example of a mixed lucent–opaque lesion is a compound odontoma.

Soft Tissue Opacity. A **soft tissue opacity** appears as a well-defined, radiopaque area located in soft tissue (Figure 31-19). A *sialolith* (salivary stone) or a calcified lymph node is an example of a soft tissue opacity.

Location

As with radiolucent lesions, radiopaque lesions can also be described in terms of location. The location of a lesion is important for communication and documentation purposes. Radiopaque lesions may appear in the same locations as radiolucent lesions: in periapical, inter-radicular, edentulous, or pericoronal locations. Box 31-4 lists examples of radiopaque lesions and their most common locations.

BOX 31-4   Locations of Radiopaque Lesions

Periapical Radiopacities
Periapical cemento-osseous dysplasia*
Condensing osteitis
Benign cementoblastoma

Inter-radicular Radiopacities
Sclerotic bone
Calcifying and keratinizing epithelial odontogenic cyst*
Adenomatoid odontogenic tumor*†
Compound odontoma†
Ossifying/cementifying fibroma*

Edentulous Zone
Complex odontoma
Calcifying epithelial odontogenic tumor*†
Ossifying/cementifying fibroma*†

Pericoronal Radiopacities
Adenomatoid odontogenic tumor*†
Calcifying epithelial odontogenic tumor*†
Ameloblastic fibro-odontoma
Compound odontoma†

Multifocal Radiopacities
Osteitis deformans
Florid osseous dysplasia
Gardner's syndrome
Fibrous dysplasia
Osteopetrosis

No Specific Location
Osteosarcoma*
Chondrosarcoma*
Metastatic carcinoma*

*Indicates the lesion may also appear with a radiolucent component.
†Indicates the lesion may exhibit more than one location.

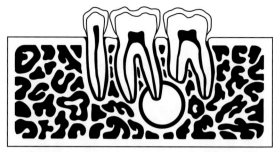

FIGURE 31-20 Radiopaque target lesion in a periapical location. (Modified from Eversole LR: *Clinical outline of oral pathology: diagnosis and treatment*, ed 2, Philadelphia, 1984, Lea and Febiger.)

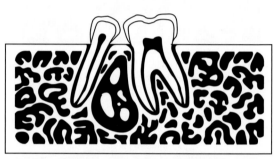

FIGURE 31-21 Mixed lucent–opaque lesion in inter-radicular location. (Modified from Eversole LR: *Clinical outline of oral pathology: diagnosis and treatment*, ed 2, Philadelphia, 1984, Lea and Febiger.)

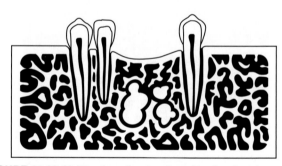

FIGURE 31-22 Multifocal confluent radiopacities in edentulous zone. (Modified from Eversole LR: *Clinical outline of oral pathology: diagnosis and treatment*, ed 2, Philadelphia, 1984, Lea and Febiger.)

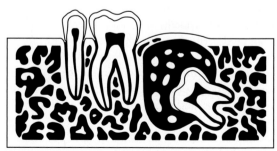

FIGURE 31-23 Mixed lucent–opaque lesion in pericoronal location. (Modified from Eversole LR: *Clinical outline of oral pathology: diagnosis and treatment*, ed 2, Philadelphia, 1984, Lea and Febiger.)

Periapical Location. The term *periapical* refers to the area around the apex of a tooth (Figure 31-20). An example of a periapical radiopacity is benign cementoblastoma.

Inter-Radicular Location. The term *inter-radicular* refers to the area between the roots of adjacent teeth (Figure 31-21). An example of a radiopaque lesion that the radiographer would expect to find in an inter-radicular location is sclerotic bone.

Edentulous Zone. The term *edentulous zone* refers to an area without teeth; an example of a radiopaque lesion in an edentulous zone is complex odontoma (Figure 31-22). A variety of radiopaque lesions may occur in an edentulous zone.

Pericoronal Location. The term *pericoronal* refers to the area around the crown of an impacted tooth (Figure 31-23). An adenomatoid odontogenic tumor is an example of a mixed lucent–opaque lesion seen in a pericoronal location.

Size

Radiopaque lesions can vary in size from several millimeters to several centimeters in diameter and can be easily measured on a dental image with a ruler. Documentation of the size of a lesion is important for treatment decisions as well as for comparative purposes.

SUMMARY

- To interpret dental images, the dental professional must be able to accurately describe what is seen.
- The use of descriptive terminology allows the dental professional to describe and discuss what is seen on a dental image intelligently.
- Descriptive terminology is important for communication and documentation purposes.
- To communicate with other professionals as well as patients, the dental professional must be familiar with the basic terminology used in dental imaging. The dental professional should be familiar with the definitions and use of general terms such as *radiograph*, *dental image*, *x-ray*, *radiolucent*, and *radiopaque*.
- The term *radiograph* refers to the actual receptor exposed; the term *x-ray* refers to the beam of energy or radiation. These two terms should not be used interchangeably.
- The term *radiolucent* describes areas of a dental image that appear dark or black. Radiolucent structures lack density and permit the passage of the x-ray beam. Air spaces and soft tissues appear radiolucent.
- The term *radiopaque* describes areas of a dental image that appear light or white. Radiopaque structures are dense and resist the passage of the x-ray beam. Enamel, dentin, and bone appear radiopaque.

- All lesions viewed on a dental image should be documented and described in terms of appearance, location, and size.
- To play an important role in the interpretation of dental images, dental professionals must have a working knowledge of key terms to be able to describe the appearance, location, and size of radiolucent and radiopaque lesions.

BIBLIOGRAPHY

Eversole LR: Radiolucent lesions of the jaws. In *Clinical outline of oral pathology: diagnosis and treatment*, ed 3, Philadelphia, 1992, Lea & Febiger.

Eversole LR: Radiopaque lesions of the jaws. In *Clinical outline of oral pathology: diagnosis and treatment*, ed 3, Philadelphia, 1992, Lea & Febiger.

Rubar JS: Survey of dental radiographic terms. *Oral Surg Oral Med Oral Pathol* 69:530–531, 1990.

White SC, Pharoah MJ: Benign tumors of the jaws. In *Oral radiology principles and interpretation*, ed 6, St. Louis, 2009, Mosby.

White SC, Pharoah MJ: Cysts and cystlike lesions of the jaws. In *Oral radiology: principles and interpretation*, ed 6, St. Louis, 2009, Mosby.

Wood NK, Goaz PW: Generalized radiopacities. In *Differential diagnosis of oral lesions*, ed 5, St. Louis, 1997, Mosby.

Wood NK, Goaz PW: Multilocular radiolucencies. In *Differential diagnosis of oral lesions*, ed 5, St. Louis, 1997, Mosby.

Wood NK, Goaz PW: Periapical radiolucencies. In *Differential diagnosis of oral lesions*, ed 5, St. Louis, 1997, Mosby.

Wood NK, Goaz PW: Periapical radiopacities. In *Differential diagnosis of oral lesions*, ed 5, St. Louis, 1997, Mosby.

Wood NK, Goaz PW: Pericoronal radiolucencies. In *Differential diagnosis of oral lesions*, ed 5, St. Louis, 1997, Mosby.

QUIZ QUESTIONS

SHORT ANSWER

1. Describe the lesion illustrated in Figure 31-24 in terms of the following:
   a. Appearance: _____
   b. Location: _____
   c. Size: _____
2. Describe the lesion illustrated in Figure 31-25 in terms of the following:
   a. Appearance: _____
   b. Location: _____
   c. Size: _____
3. Describe the lesion illustrated in Figure 31-26 in terms of the following:
   a. Appearance: _____
   b. Location: _____
   c. Size: _____

MATCHING

Match the following terms with the proper definitions:

___ **4.** Ground glass
___ **5.** Inter-radicular
___ **6.** Radiopaque
___ **7.** Pericoronal
___ **8.** Corticated
___ **9.** Target lesion
___ **10.** Periapical

a. Location of a lesion surrounding the crown of an impacted tooth.
b. Location of a lesion between the roots of adjacent teeth.
c. Location of a lesion surrounding the apex of a tooth.
d. Descriptive term for a radiopaque lesion that resembles an orange peel or has a granular appearance.
e. Descriptive term for structures that are dense and absorb or resist the passage of the x-ray beam.
f. Descriptive term for the periphery of a lesion surrounded by dense cortical bone.

g. Descriptive term for a radiopaque lesion that exhibits a well-demarcated localized area with a surrounding radiolucent ring.

h. Descriptive term for structures that lack density and permit the passage of the x-ray beam with little or no resistance.

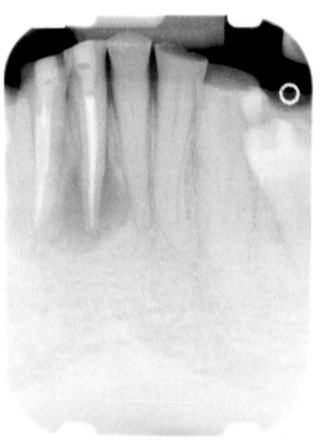

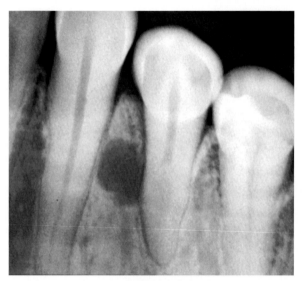

FIGURE 31-24

FIGURE 31-25

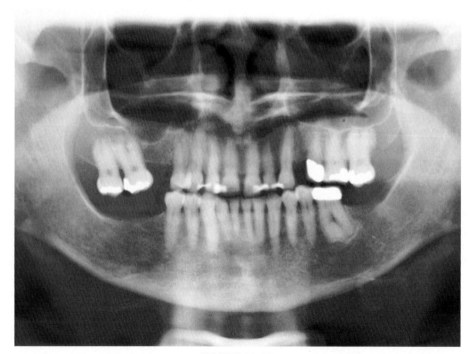

FIGURE 31-26

chapter 32

Identification of Restorations, Dental Materials, and Foreign Objects

OUTLINE

IDENTIFICATION OF RESTORATIONS
    Amalgam Restorations
    Gold Restorations
    Stainless Steel and Chrome Crowns
    Post and Core Restorations
    Porcelain Restorations
    Composite Restorations
    Acrylic Restorations

IDENTIFICATION OF MATERIALS USED IN DENTISTRY
    Materials Used in Restorative Dentistry
    Materials Used in Endodontics
    Materials Used in Prosthodontics
    Materials Used in Orthodontics
    Materials Used in Oral Surgery
IDENTIFICATION OF MISCELLANEOUS OBJECTS
    Jewelry
    Eyeglasses and Napkin Chain

LEARNING OBJECTIVES

After completion of this chapter, the student will be able to do the following:

- Define the key terms associated with identifying restorations, materials, and foreign objects on dental images
- Discuss the importance of interpreting dental images while the patient is present
- On dental images, identify and describe the appearance of the following restorations: amalgam, gold, stainless steel and chrome, post and core, porcelain, porcelain-fused-to-metal, composite, and acrylic

- On dental images, identify and describe the appearance of the following dental materials and devices: base materials, metallic pins, gutta percha, silver points, removable partial dentures, complete dentures, orthodontic bands, brackets and wires, fixed retainers, implants, suture wires, splints, and stabilizing arches and wires
- On dental images, identify and describe the appearance of the following miscellaneous objects: jewelry, eyeglasses, and patient napkin chains

KEY TERMS

Amalgam	Gutta percha	Radiolucent
Diatoric	Metallic restoration	Radiopaque
Ghost image	Nonmetallic restoration	

Dental images are an important diagnostic tool that enables the practitioner to view dental restorations and dental materials. Dental images are also useful in identifying and locating foreign objects. Some restorations, materials, and foreign objects are easily identified on dental images; others are not. On dental images, the appearances of restorations, materials, and foreign objects vary, depending on the thickness of the material, density, and atomic number. Some restorations, materials, and foreign objects may be identified by the degree of radiopacity present, outline, contour, or size; others require additional clinical information.

The dental professional should interpret all dental images while the patient is present. If questions arise as to what is seen on a dental image concerning dental restorations, dental materials, or foreign objects, clinical examination of the patient can be done to obtain additional information or to verify what is seen. When dental images are interpreted without the patient present, some important clinical information is not available.

The purpose of this chapter is to review common dental restorations, dental materials, and foreign objects that may be seen on dental images.

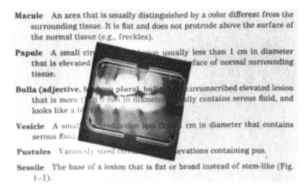

Macule   An area that is usually distinguished by a color different from the surrounding tissue. It is flat and does not protrude above the surface of the normal tissue (e.g., freckles).

Papule   A small cir—— ——on usually less than 1 cm in diameter that is elevated ——face of normal surrounding tissue.

Bulla (adjective, b—— plural, bull——circumscribed elevated lesion that is more ——6 mm in diameter—lly contains serous fluid, and looks like a b——

Vesicle   A smal—— ——sion less th—— cm in diameter that contains serous fluid——

Pustules   Variously sized circ—— ——evations containing pus.

Sessile   The base of a lesion that is flat or broad instead of stem-like (Fig. 1–1).

FIGURE 32-1 When a radiograph with a metallic restoration is placed on a printed page, the print can be easily seen.

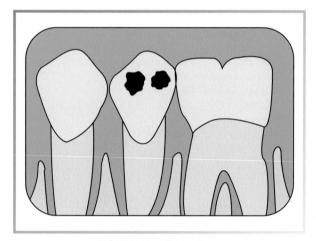

FIGURE 32-2 Pit amalgam.

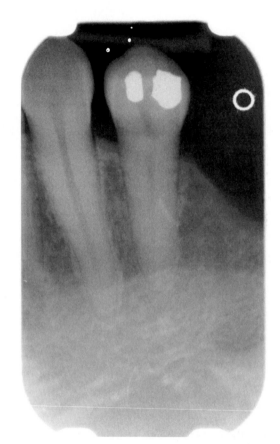

FIGURE 32-3 Two pit amalgams are seen in a mandibular premolar.

IDENTIFICATION OF RESTORATIONS

A variety of common restorative materials, including amalgam, gold, stainless steel, porcelain, composite, and acrylic, can be identified on dental images.

Metallic restorations (e.g., amalgam, gold) absorb x-rays, and as a result, very little (if any) radiation comes in contact with the receptor. Consequently, that area of the receptor remains unexposed, and the metallic restorations appear completely radiopaque (light or white) on a dental image. To illustrate this concept, place a processed film with an amalgam restoration on a printed page. The underlying print can be easily read through the radiopaque area on the film (Figure 32-1).

Nonmetallic restorations (e.g., porcelain, composite, acrylic) may vary in appearance from radiolucent (dark or black) to slightly radiopaque, depending on the density of the material. Of the nonmetallic restorations, porcelain is the most dense and least radiolucent, and acrylic is the least dense and most radiolucent.

Amalgam Restorations

Amalgam is the most common restorative material used in dentistry. Amalgam absorbs the x-ray beam and prevents

x-rays from reaching the receptor; consequently, amalgam appears completely radiopaque on a dental image. Amalgam may be seen in a variety of shapes, sizes, and locations on a dental image.

One-Surface Amalgam Restorations

One-surface amalgam restorations ("pit amalgams") appear as distinct, small, round or ovoid radiopacities (Figures 32-2 and 32-3). One-surface amalgams may be seen on the buccal, lingual, or occlusal surfaces of teeth. Larger two-surface and multi-surface amalgam restorations also appear radiopaque and are characterized by their irregular outlines or borders (Figures 32-4 and 32-5). Multi-surface amalgam restorations may involve any tooth surface.

Amalgam Overhangs

Amalgam overhangs can be described as extensions of amalgam seen beyond the crown portion of a tooth in the interproximal region. An amalgam overhang results from improper band placement around a tooth before condensing the amalgam restoration. Amalgam overhangs can be easily visualized on a dental image and appear radiopaque (Figures 32-6 and 32-7). An amalgam overhang disrupts the natural cleansing contours of the tooth, traps food and plaque, and contributes to bone loss. To prevent destruction of interproximal bone, amalgam overhangs must be removed.

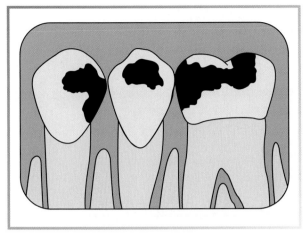

FIGURE 32-4 Multi-surface amalgam.

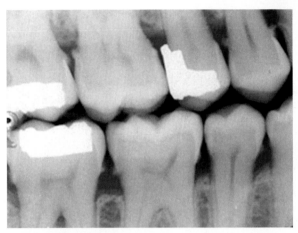

FIGURE 32-7 Amalgam overhang seen on the maxillary second premolar.

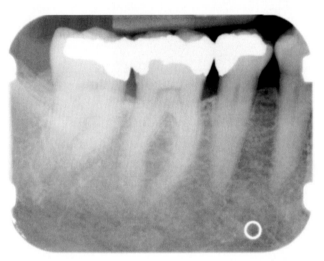

FIGURE 32-5 Three multi-surface amalgam restorations. Note the irregular outlines.

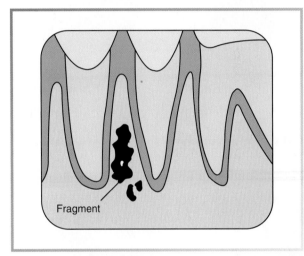

FIGURE 32-8 Amalgam fragments.

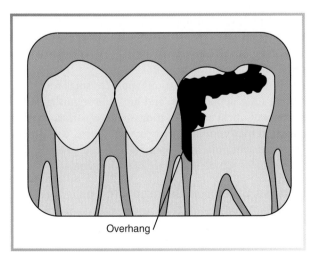

FIGURE 32-6 Amalgam overhang.

Amalgam Fragments

Fragments of amalgam may be inadvertently embedded in adjacent soft tissue during restoration of a tooth. Amalgam fragments or scraps vary in size and shape and appear radiographically as dense radiopacities with irregular borders on a dental image (Figures 32-8 and 32-9). Amalgam fragments may be seen in any location where soft tissue is present. If amalgam fragments are displaced into soft tissue during the placement or removal of an amalgam restoration or during the extraction of a tooth with an amalgam restoration present, a permanent area of pigmentation, known as an amalgam tattoo, may occur (Figure 32-10). Amalgam tattoos may be seen clinically and radiographically.

Gold Restorations

It is not always possible to differentiate one metallic restoration from another on a dental image; however, an educated guess is often possible if the shape and size of the restoration are considered. Both gold and amalgam appear equally

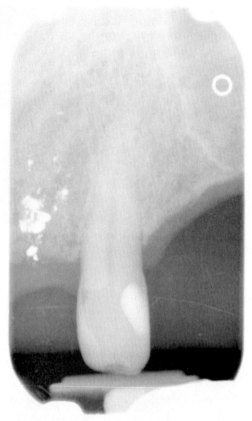

FIGURE 32-9 Amalgam fragment seen in soft tissue near the maxillary canine.

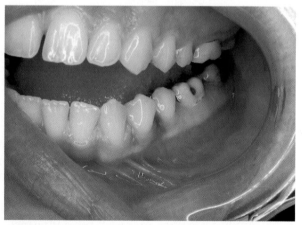

FIGURE 32-10 Amalgam tattoo seen by the bluish pigmentation of the gingiva. (From Ibsen OAC, Phelan JA: *Oral pathology for the dental hygienist*, ed 5, St. Louis, 2009, Saunders.)

radiopaque on a dental image. A large radiopaque restoration with smooth borders is most likely gold. Gold restorations appear completely radiopaque and, unlike amalgam restorations, exhibit a smooth marginal outline (Figures 32-11 and 32-12). If dental images are interpreted with the patient present, examination of the patient can help obtain additional information about the material—gold versus amalgam—or to verify what is seen.

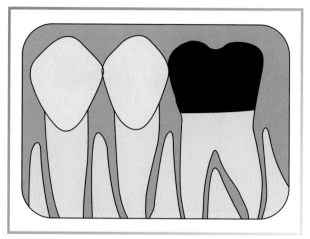

FIGURE 32-11 Gold crown.

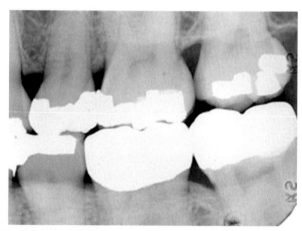

FIGURE 32-12 Two gold crowns seen on mandibular molars. Note the smooth outline and contour.

Gold Crowns and Bridges

Gold crowns and bridges appear as large radiopaque restorations with smooth contours and regular borders (Figure 32-13). Similarly, gold inlays and onlays exhibit marginal outlines that appear smooth and regular (Figures 32-14 and 32-15).

Gold Foil Restorations

One-surface gold foil restorations appear as small round radiopacities on a dental image and are indistinguishable from one-surface amalgam restorations. A two-surface gold foil restoration may appear similar to a gold inlay, with smooth, regular marginal outlines, or may exhibit slightly irregular margins and resemble a two-surface amalgam.

Stainless Steel and Chrome Crowns

Stainless steel and chrome crowns are prefabricated restorations that are usually used as interim or temporary restorations. These crowns are thin and do not absorb dental x-rays to the extent that amalgam, gold, and other cast metals do.

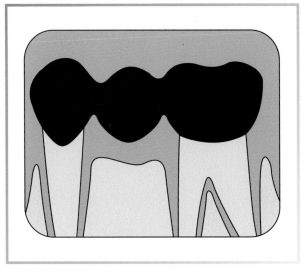

FIGURE 32-13 Gold bridge.

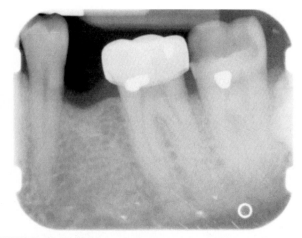

FIGURE 32-16 Stainless steel crown seen on the mandibular first molar.

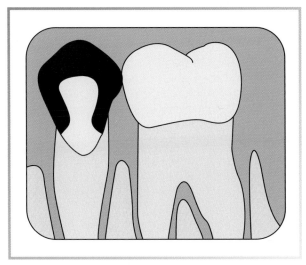

FIGURE 32-14 Gold onlay.

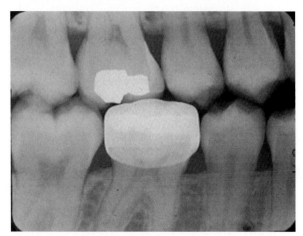

FIGURE 32-17 Stainless steel crown seen on the mandibular first molar. Note the area that appears "see-through."

As a result, both stainless steel and chrome crowns appear radiopaque, but not as densely radiopaque as amalgam or gold.

Stainless steel and chrome crowns appear radiopaque on a dental image. Because these crowns are prefabricated, their outlines and margins appear very smooth and regular. Often these crowns are not contoured properly to the cervical portion of the tooth and thus do not appear to fit the tooth well (Figure 32-16). Restorations that are not contoured with the shape of the tooth may cause periodontal problems ranging from food impaction to gingival bleeding or possible bone loss. Because stainless steel and chrome crowns are thin, some areas may appear "see-through" on the dental image (Figures 32-17 and 32-18).

Post and Core Restorations

Post and core restorations can be seen in teeth treated with endodontic therapy. The post and core restoration is cast metal and appears as radiodense as amalgam or gold. Post and core restorations appear radiopaque on a dental image.

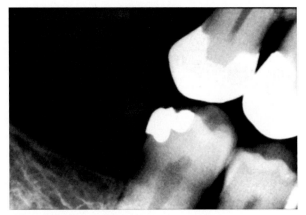

FIGURE 32-15 Gold onlays seen on maxillary premolars. Note the distinct outline and contours.

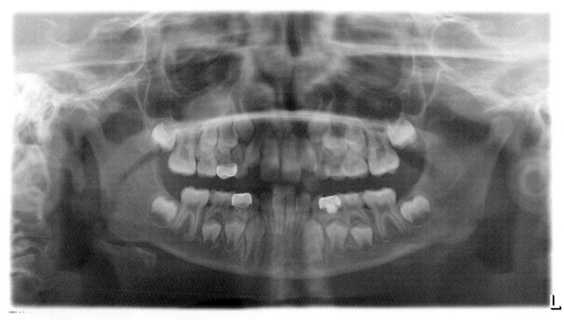

FIGURE 32-18 Stainless steel crowns visible on primary teeth *B*, *L*, and *S* on this panoramic image. (Courtesy of Cary Pediatric Dentistry, Cary, NC.)

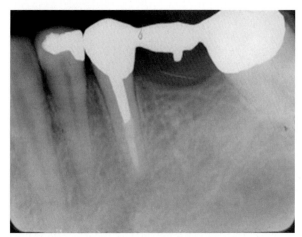

FIGURE 32-19 Post and core restoration seen on the mandibular second premolar.

The core portion of the restoration resembles the prepared portion of a tooth crown, and the post portion extends into the pulp canal (Figure 32-19).

Porcelain Restorations

A porcelain restoration appears radiopaque on a dental image. Unlike metallic restorations, which appear totally radiopaque, porcelain restorations are slightly radiopaque and resemble the radiodensity of dentin.

All-Porcelain Crowns

All-porcelain crowns appear slightly radiopaque on a dental image (Figure 32-20). A thin radiopaque line outlining the

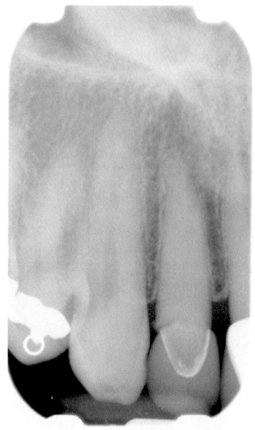

FIGURE 32-20 Porcelain crown seen on the maxillary lateral incisor. Note the outline of the tooth preparation covered with radiopaque cement.

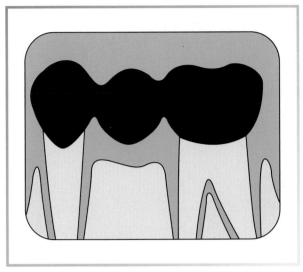

FIGURE 32-13 Gold bridge.

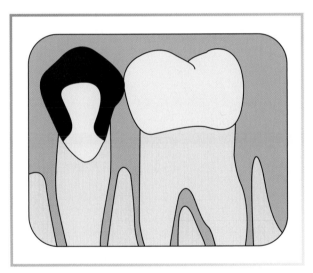

FIGURE 32-14 Gold onlay.

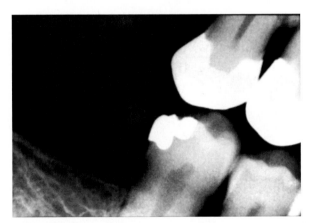

FIGURE 32-15 Gold onlays seen on maxillary premolars. Note the distinct outline and contours.

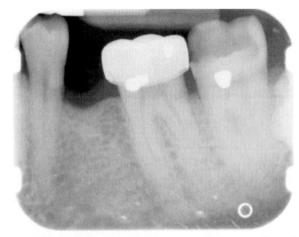

FIGURE 32-16 Stainless steel crown seen on the mandibular first molar.

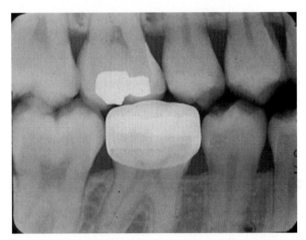

FIGURE 32-17 Stainless steel crown seen on the mandibular first molar. Note the area that appears "see-through."

As a result, both stainless steel and chrome crowns appear radiopaque, but not as densely radiopaque as amalgam or gold.

Stainless steel and chrome crowns appear radiopaque on a dental image. Because these crowns are prefabricated, their outlines and margins appear very smooth and regular. Often these crowns are not contoured properly to the cervical portion of the tooth and thus do not appear to fit the tooth well (Figure 32-16). Restorations that are not contoured with the shape of the tooth may cause periodontal problems ranging from food impaction to gingival bleeding or possible bone loss. Because stainless steel and chrome crowns are thin, some areas may appear "see-through" on the dental image (Figures 32-17 and 32-18).

Post and Core Restorations

Post and core restorations can be seen in teeth treated with endodontic therapy. The post and core restoration is cast metal and appears as radiodense as amalgam or gold. Post and core restorations appear radiopaque on a dental image.

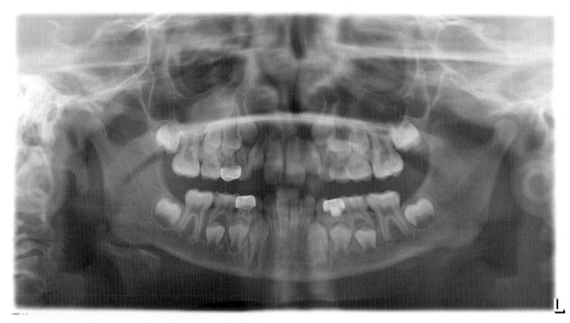

FIGURE 32-18 Stainless steel crowns visible on primary teeth *B*, *L*, and *S* on this panoramic image. (Courtesy of Cary Pediatric Dentistry, Cary, NC.)

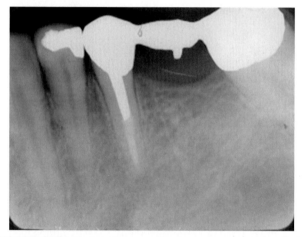

FIGURE 32-19 Post and core restoration seen on the mandibular second premolar.

The core portion of the restoration resembles the prepared portion of a tooth crown, and the post portion extends into the pulp canal (Figure 32-19).

Porcelain Restorations

A porcelain restoration appears radiopaque on a dental image. Unlike metallic restorations, which appear totally radiopaque, porcelain restorations are slightly radiopaque and resemble the radiodensity of dentin.

All-Porcelain Crowns

All-porcelain crowns appear slightly radiopaque on a dental image (Figure 32-20). A thin radiopaque line outlining the

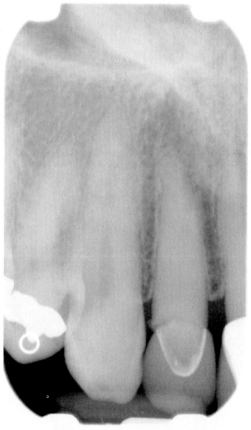

FIGURE 32-20 Porcelain crown seen on the maxillary lateral incisor. Note the outline of the tooth preparation covered with radiopaque cement.

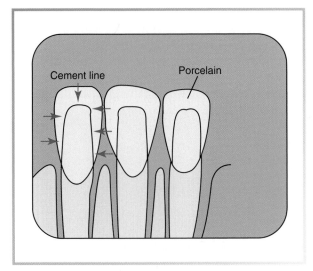

FIGURE 32-21 Porcelain crown.

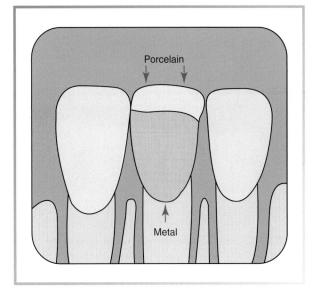

FIGURE 32-23 Porcelain-fused-to-metal crown.

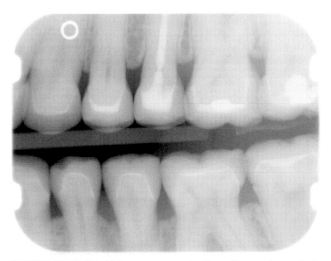

FIGURE 32-22 Porcelain crowns seen in all maxillary and mandibular teeth on this bite-wing image.

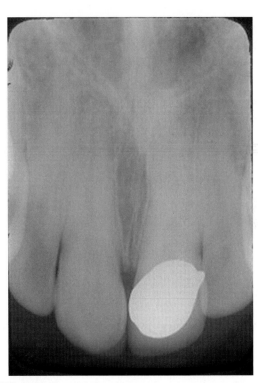

FIGURE 32-24 Porcelain-fused-to-metal crown seen on the maxillary central incisor.

prepared tooth may be evident through the slightly radiopaque porcelain crown (Figures 32-21 and 32-22). This thin line represents cement. The radiodensity of an all-porcelain bridge appears identical to that of the all-porcelain crown.

Porcelain-Fused-to-Metal Crown

When viewed on a dental image, a porcelain-fused-to-metal crown has two components. The metal component appears *completely* radiopaque, and the porcelain component appears *slightly* radiopaque (Figures 32-23 and 32-24). The radiodensities of a porcelain-fused-to-metal bridge appear identical to that seen in the porcelain-fused-to-metal crown (Figure 32-25).

Composite Restorations

When viewed on a dental image, a composite restoration may vary in appearance from radiolucent to slightly radiopaque,

depending on the composition of the composite material (Figures 32-26 and 32-27). Some manufacturers of composite materials add radiopaque particles to their products to help the viewer differentiate a composite restoration from dental caries (which appears radiolucent) on a dental image.

Should there be any confusion between a composite restoration and dental caries, a careful visual and digital examination of the tooth in question enables the clinician to distinguish between the two.

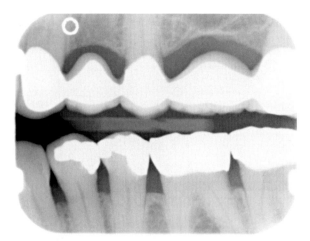

FIGURE 32-25 Porcelain-fused-to-metal bridge seen in the maxillary arch.

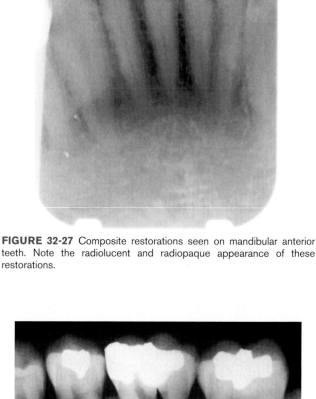

FIGURE 32-27 Composite restorations seen on mandibular anterior teeth. Note the radiolucent and radiopaque appearance of these restorations.

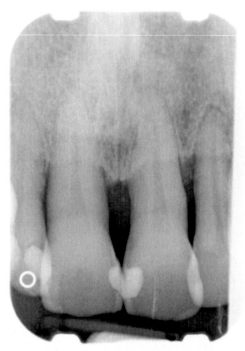

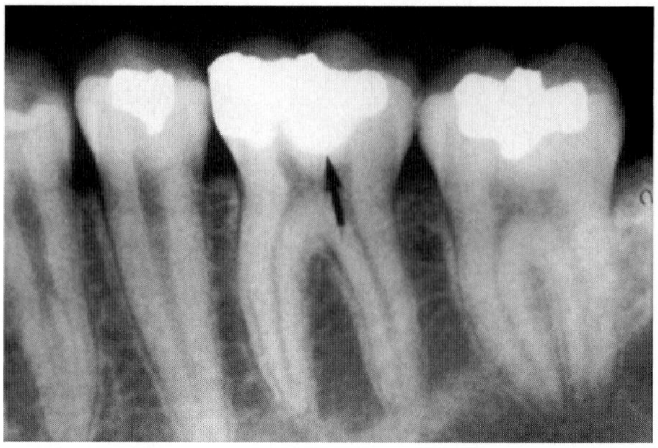

FIGURE 32-26 Composite restorations seen on maxillary anterior teeth.

FIGURE 32-28 Base material seen under an amalgam restoration on a mandibular first molar.

Acrylic Restorations

Acrylic resin restorations are often used as an interim, or temporary, crown or filling. Of all the nonmetallic restorations, acrylic is the least dense and appears radiolucent or barely visible on a dental image.

IDENTIFICATION OF MATERIALS USED IN DENTISTRY

A number of materials are used in dentistry for a variety of reasons, each specific to the specialty that requires the material. Practitioners in restorative dentistry, endodontics, prosthodontics, orthodontics, and oral surgery all use materials that can be identified on dental images.

Materials Used in Restorative Dentistry

Base Materials

Base materials, which include zinc phosphate cement and zinc oxide–eugenol paste, are used as cavity liners to protect the pulp of the tooth. Base materials are placed on the floor of a cavity preparation. A restorative material, such as amalgam, is then placed over the base material. A base material appears radiopaque. Compared with amalgam, the base material appears less radiodense (Figure 32-28).

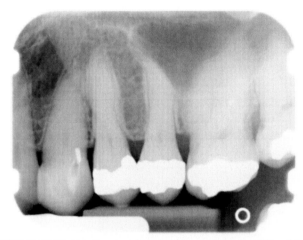

FIGURE 32-29 Metallic pin enhancing the retention capability of the composite restoration seen in this maxillary canine.

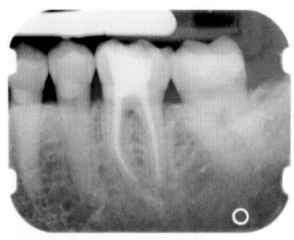

FIGURE 32-31 Gutta percha seen in the pulp canal of a mandibular first molar.

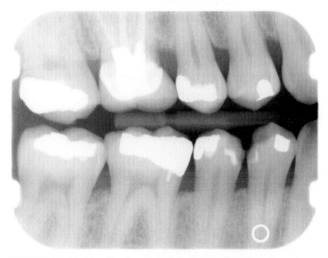

FIGURE 32-30 Metallic pin used to give strength to the restoration on the mandibular first molar.

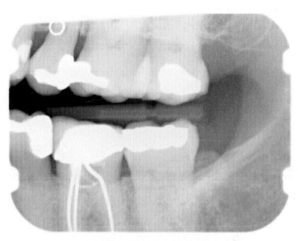

FIGURE 32-32 Silver point seen in the pulp canal underneath a porcelain-fused-to-metal crown on the mandibular first molar.

Metallic Pins

Metallic pins, used to enhance the retention of amalgam or composite, appear as cylindrical or screw-shaped radiopacities on a dental image (Figures 32-29 and 32-30).

Materials Used in Endodontics

Gutta Percha

Gutta percha is a claylike material used in endodontic therapy to fill the canals of the pulp. Gutta percha appears radiopaque, similar in density to that of base materials (Figure 32-31). When compared with metallic restorations, gutta percha appears less radiodense.

Silver Points

Silver points are also used in endodontic therapy to fill the canals of the pulp. Silver points appear highly radiopaque, similar to other metallic materials. Silver points appear more radiodense than does gutta percha (Figure 32-32).

Materials Used in Prosthodontics

Complete and removable partial dentures are common and may be occasionally observed on dental images. The appearances of complete and removable partial dentures vary, depending on the base materials and type of denture teeth used.

Patients should be instructed to remove all complete and partial dentures before dental images are taken. If not removed, complete and partial dentures may obscure important information concerning adjacent teeth and underlying bone.

Complete Dentures

A complete denture consists of two component parts: (1) a base material and (2) denture teeth. The typical denture base material is composed of acrylic and appears as a very faint radiopacity on a dental image or, in some cases, may not be seen at all. Denture teeth may be composed of porcelain or

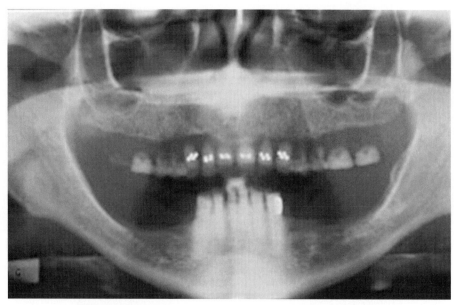

FIGURE 32-33 Diatorics seen on the teeth of the maxillary denture.

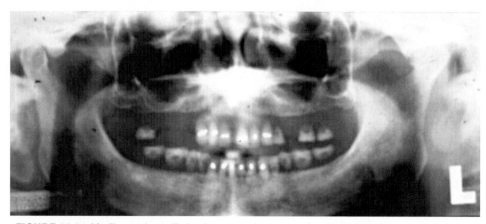

FIGURE 32-34 Maxillary and mandibular denture teeth appear to be "floating" in this panoramic image.

acrylic and vary in appearance. Porcelain denture teeth appear radiopaque and resemble the radiodensity of dentin. Anterior porcelain denture teeth include one or two metal retention pins, or **diatorics**. On a dental image, diatorics appear as tiny, dense radiopacities superimposed over the radiopaque porcelain denture teeth (Figure 32-33). Posterior porcelain denture teeth also appear radiopaque but do not contain diatorics. Acrylic (plastic) denture teeth lack density and appear faintly radiopaque or radiolucent on a dental image.

A complete denture that is not removed before the exposure of a dental image gives the illusion of rootless, or "floating," teeth (Figure 32-34).

Removable Partial Dentures

A removable partial denture can be constructed from a variety of base materials, including cast metal, a combination of cast metal and acrylic, and all acrylic. The removable partial denture constructed of cast metal appears densely radiopaque on a dental image. The size and shape of the radiopacity depend on the design of the metal framework of the partial denture. A removable partial denture constructed of a metal base with acrylic saddles appears densely radiopaque where metal is present and slightly radiopaque in the areas of acrylic. A removable partial denture base constructed totally of acrylic is usually seen with wrought-metal clasps. The acrylic base appears slightly radiopaque or radiolucent on a dental image. The metal clasps appear radiopaque and are seen resting on abutment teeth.

Teeth in a removable partial denture may be composed of acrylic or porcelain. Porcelain teeth appear radiopaque and resemble the radiodensity of dentin. Acrylic teeth appear faintly radiopaque or radiolucent (Figure 32-35).

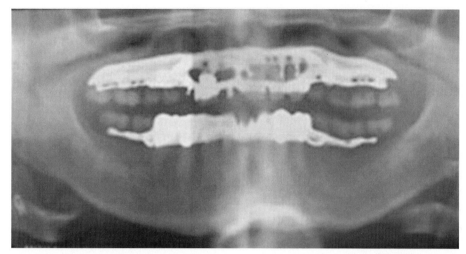

FIGURE 32-35 Metal framework of both partial dentures as well as porcelain teeth in the posterior quadrants of both arches visible in this panoramic image.

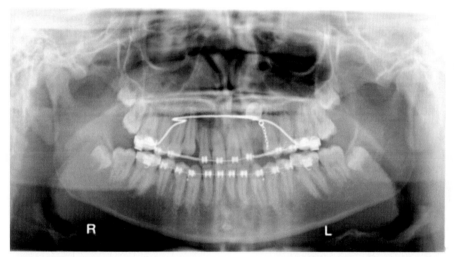

FIGURE 32-36 Orthodontic appliances that aid in the proper eruption of the maxillary canines.

Materials Used in Orthodontics

Orthodontic bands, brackets, and wires may be observed on dental images. Each of these orthodontic materials has a characteristic radiopaque appearance (Figures 32-36, 32-37, and 32-38). Fixed orthodontic retainers may also be observed on dental images and have an equally characteristic appearance (Figure 32-39).

Materials Used in Oral Surgery

Implants are being used in oral surgery with increased frequency. The appearances of the numerous endosteal implants that are currently used vary, depending on their shapes and designs. The endosteal implant is made of a metallic material and appears radiopaque on a dental image (Figures 32-40, 32-41, and 32-42).

Suture wires, metallic splints and plates, bone screws, and stabilizing arches are used in oral surgery to stabilize fractures of the maxilla and the mandible. Suture wires appear as thin radiopaque lines. Metallic splints, plates, fixation screws, and stabilizing arches also appear radiopaque; their characteristic shapes and sizes may vary (Figures 32-43 and 32-44).

IDENTIFICATION OF MISCELLANEOUS OBJECTS

A number of miscellaneous objects, including jewelry, eyeglasses, and napkin chains, can be viewed on dental images. Such objects may obscure important diagnostic information. Some miscellaneous objects may be seen on intraoral images; others may be noted on extraoral images.

To avoid nondiagnostic images, patients should be instructed to remove earrings, necklaces, nose jewelry, eyeglasses, and napkin chains before exposure of extraoral images. In the case of intraoral images, patients should be

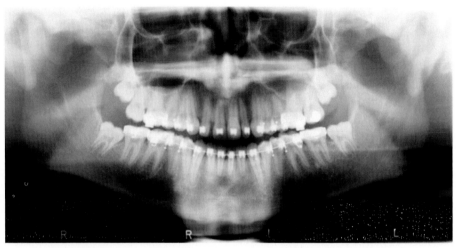

FIGURE 32-37 Orthodontic bands easily recognizable on this panoramic image.

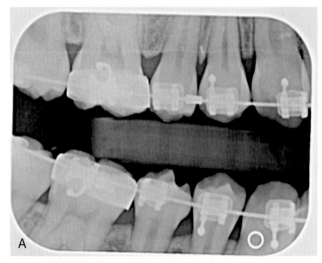

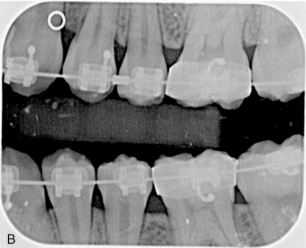

FIGURE 32-38 A, B, Orthodontic appliances easily recognizable on bite-wing images. (Courtesy of Cary Pediatric Dentistry, Cary, NC.)

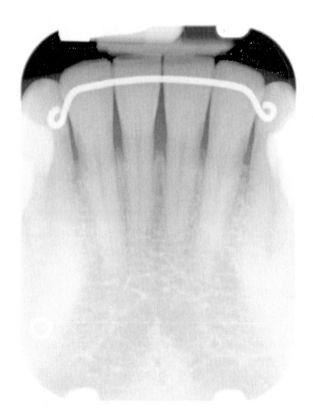

FIGURE 32-39 Fixed orthodontic retainer seen in the mandibular anterior region.

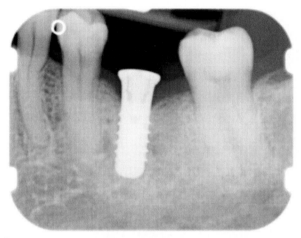

FIGURE 32-40 Implant placed in the area of the mandibular left first molar.

instructed to remove eyeglasses and nose jewelry, if necessary.

Jewelry

Earrings most often appear on extraoral images. Metal earrings appear as dense radiopacities on a dental image; the size and shape of the radiopacity correspond to the size and shape of the earring (Figures 32-45 and 32-46). Plastic earrings with metallic posts and backings or metal clips can also be seen on dental images; the metallic portions appear as dense radiopacities. A radiodense object, such as a metal earring, causes an artifact, known as a **ghost image**, on panoramic images (see Chapter 22). Ghost images can obscure important information about teeth and bones and render the image nondiagnostic (Figure 32-47).

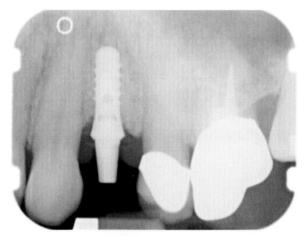

FIGURE 32-41 Implant placed in the area of the maxillary left first premolar.

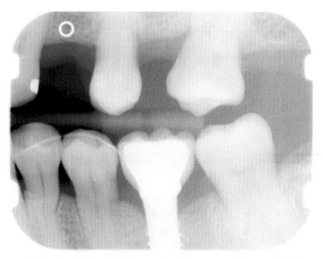

FIGURE 32-42 An implant is placed in the area of the mandibular left first molar.

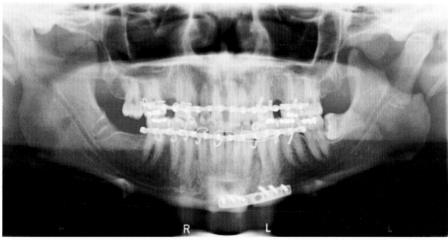

FIGURE 32-43 Stabilizing arches and wires seen on a panoramic image from a patient with a mandibular fracture.

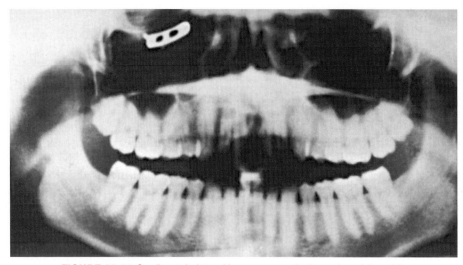

FIGURE 32-44 Small metal plate with screws seen in the region of the orbit.

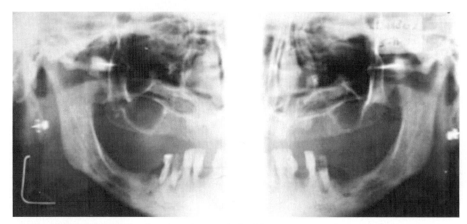

FIGURE 32-45 Small post earrings and ghost images seen on a panoramic image.

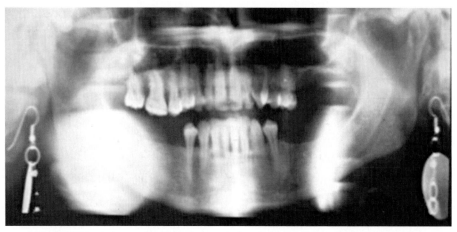

FIGURE 32-46 Large metallic earrings and ghost images seen on a panoramic image.

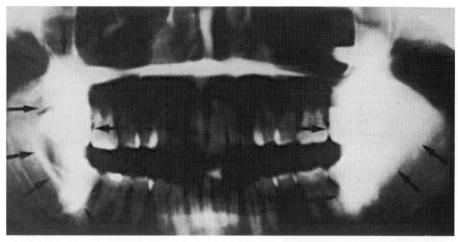

FIGURE 32-47 Note the loss of diagnostic information that results from the ghost images of the large metallic earrings.

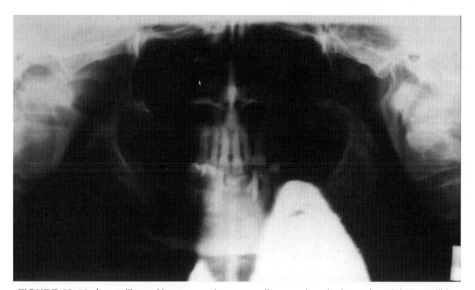

FIGURE 32-48 A metallic necklace appearing as a radiopaque loop in the region of the mandible.

A necklace may also appear on an extraoral image as a radiopacity that corresponds in shape and size to the jewelry (Figure 32-48). Nose jewelry (small studs or hoop earrings worn on the nose) may be seen on extraoral as well as intraoral images (e.g., maxillary anterior periapical images). This type of jewelry appears as a radiopacity on a dental image and corresponds in size and shape to the object it represents (Figure 32-49).

Eyeglasses and Napkin Chain

Eyeglasses may be seen on extraoral and intraoral images. Most eyeglasses have some metal components in their frames. The metal portion of the frames appears as a radiopacity on a dental image (Figure 32-50).

The napkin chain, similar to a necklace, may be seen on an extraoral image. If the napkin chain is in the path of the x-ray beam, a radiopacity resembling the napkin chain will be seen on the image.

SUMMARY

- Dental restorations, dental materials, and foreign objects can be seen and evaluated on extraoral and intraoral images.
- The appearances of restorations, materials, and foreign objects vary, depending on material composition, density, and thickness. The appearances of restorations and materials can range from completely radiopaque to totally radiolucent.

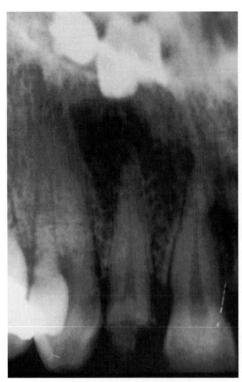

FIGURE 32-49 Nose jewelry.

- Some restorations and objects are easily identified on dental images; others may require additional clinical information. Dental images play an important role in the evaluation of dental restorations, materials, and objects.
- It is important that the dental professional interpret dental images with the patient present. Without the patient present, important clinical information is not available.
- With the patient present, if a question arises about what is seen on a dental image, a clinical examination can provide additional information or verify what is seen.

BIBLIOGRAPHY

Frommer HH, Savage-Stabulas JJ: Film mounting and radiographic anatomy. In *Radiology for the dental professional*, ed 9, St. Louis, 2011, Mosby.

Langlais RP: *Exercises in oral radiology and interpretation*, ed 4, St. Louis, 2004, Saunders.

White SC, Pharoah MJ: Normal radiographic anatomy. In *Oral radiology: principles and interpretation*, ed 6, St. Louis, 2009, Mosby.

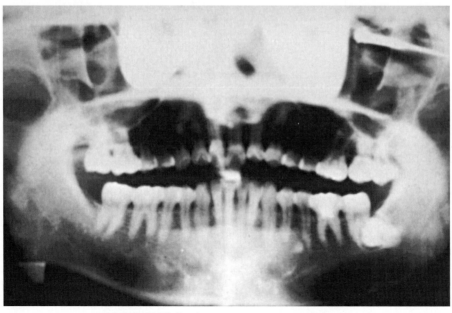

FIGURE 32-50 Eyeglasses seen on a panoramic image.

QUIZ QUESTIONS

IDENTIFICATION

___ **1.** Identify in the image the restorative material used in the pulp canal of the maxillary first molar (Figure 32-51).

_____

___ **2.** Identify the restorative material seen in each tooth of this dental image (Figure 32-52).

_____

___ **3.** Identify the restorative material used to fabricate this bridge (Figure 32-53).

_____

___ **4.** Identify in the image the restorative material used in the maxillary anterior region (Figure 32-54).

_____

___ **5.** Identify in the image the restoration present in the area of the mandibular first molar (Figure 32-55).

_____

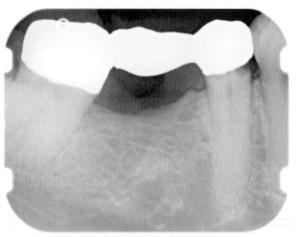

FIGURE 32-53

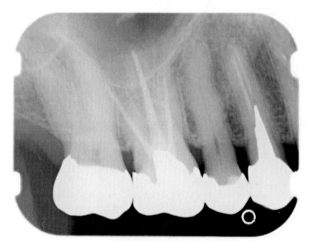

FIGURE 32-51

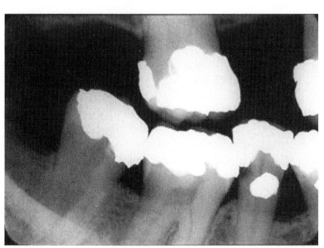

FIGURE 32-52

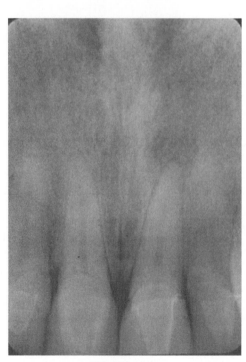

FIGURE 32-54

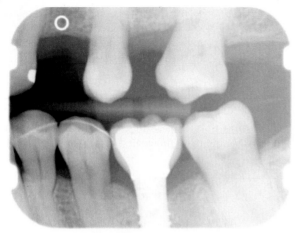

FIGURE 32-55

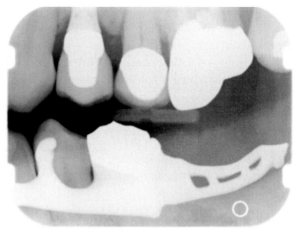

FIGURE 32-56

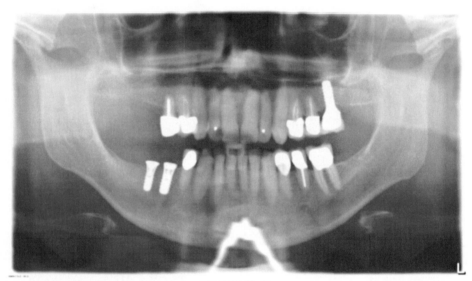

FIGURE 32-57

___ **6.** Identify in the image the large radiopacity seen in the posterior mandible (Figure 32-56).

_____

___ **7.** Identify the radiopacity, which is seen in the middle of this panoramic image, obscuring the border of the mandible (Figure 32-57).

_____

___ **8.** Explain why the maxillary teeth in this dental image appear to be "floating" (Figure 32-58).

_____

MULTIPLE CHOICE

___ **9.** Rank the following restorative materials from most radiopaque (1) to least radiopaque or radiolucent (4).
___ gutta percha
___ acrylic restorations
___ amalgam
___ stainless steel crown

___ **10.** Which of the following appear equally radiopaque on a dental image?
  a. gold crowns and amalgam
  b. gold crowns and porcelain crowns
  c. gutta percha and silver points
  d. gold crowns and stainless steel crowns

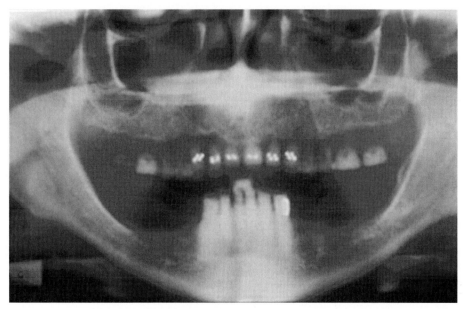

FIGURE 32-58

____ **11.** Which of the following is most radiopaque?
  a. amalgam
  b. porcelain
  c. composite
  d. acrylic

____ **12.** Which of the following is least radiopaque?
  a. amalgam
  b. porcelain
  c. stainless steel
  d. acrylic

____ **13.** Which of the following describes how gold can be distinguished from amalgam on a dental image?
  a. Gold appears more radiopaque than does amalgam.
  b. Gold appears more radiolucent than does amalgam.
  c. Gold margins are smooth and regular.
  d. Amalgam margins are smooth and regular.

SHORT ANSWER

____ **14.** Describe the difference between a gold crown and a stainless steel crown as viewed on a dental image.

_____

____ **15.** Describe the difference between gutta percha and silver points as viewed on a dental image.

_____

____ **16.** Discuss the importance of interpreting dental images with the patient present.

_____

chapter 33

Interpretation of Dental Caries

OUTLINE

DESCRIPTION OF CARIES
DETECTION OF CARIES
    Clinical Examination
    Dental Image Examination
INTERPRETATION OF CARIES ON DENTAL IMAGES
    Interpretation Tips
    Factors Influencing Caries Interpretation

CLASSIFICATION OF CARIES ON DENTAL IMAGES
    Interproximal Caries
    Occlusal Caries
    Buccal and Lingual Caries
    Root Surface Caries
    Recurrent Caries
    Rampant Caries

LEARNING OBJECTIVES

After completion of this chapter, the student will be able to do the following:

- Define the key terms associated with the interpretation of dental caries
- Describe dental caries
- Explain why caries appears radiolucent on a dental image
- Discuss interpretation tips for evaluating caries on a dental image
- Discuss the factors that may influence the image interpretation of dental caries
- Detail the classification of caries on dental images

- On a dental image, identify and describe the appearance of the following: incipient, moderate, advanced, and severe interproximal caries
- On a dental image, identify and describe the appearance of the following: incipient, moderate, and severe occlusal caries
- On a dental image, identify and describe the appearance of the following: buccal, lingual, root surface, recurrent, and rampant caries

KEY TERMS

Caries
Caries, buccal
Caries, interproximal
Caries, interproximal advanced
Caries, interproximal incipient
Caries, interproximal moderate
Caries, interproximal severe
Caries, lingual

Caries, occlusal
Caries, occlusal incipient
Caries, occlusal moderate
Caries, occlusal severe
Caries, rampant
Caries, recurrent
Caries, root surface

Cavitation
Cavity
Incipient
Interproximal
Occlusal
Radiolucent
Rampant

In the practice of dentistry, caries is probably the most frequent reason for obtaining dental images. The dental radiographer must be confident about the identification and recognition of caries as viewed on a dental image. An overview of the interpretation of caries is presented in this chapter. Detailed information about dental caries, however, is beyond the scope of this text. The purpose of this chapter is to describe dental caries and to describe caries detection. In addition, interpretation tips and factors that influence caries interpretation are presented, and an introduction to the classification of caries on dental images is included.

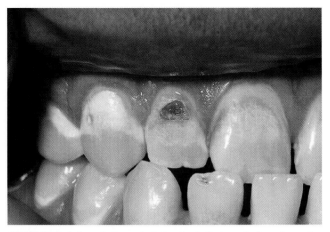

FIGURE 33-1 A cavitation—a hole in a tooth that results from the caries process.

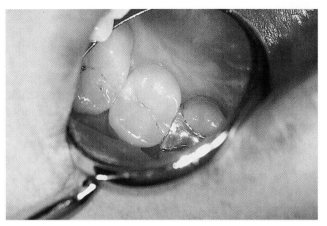

FIGURE 33-2 Discoloration on the distal of the maxillary first premolar that represents dental caries.

DESCRIPTION OF CARIES

Dental **caries,** or tooth decay, is the localized destruction of teeth by microorganisms. Normal mineralized tooth structure (enamel, dentin, cementum) is altered and destroyed by dental caries. The term *caries* comes from the Latin *cariosus,* which means "rottenness" and literally refers to the "rotting of the teeth." A carious lesion, or an area of tooth decay, is often referred to as a **cavity.** In dentistry, the term *cavity* refers to **cavitation,** or hole, in a tooth that is the result of the caries process (Figure 33-1).

DETECTION OF CARIES

To detect dental caries, careful clinical examination and careful interpretation are both necessary. A dental examination for caries cannot be considered complete without dental images. Dental images enable the dental professional to identify carious lesions that are not visible clinically. In addition, dental images allow the dental professional to evaluate the extent and severity of carious lesions.

Clinical Examination

Some carious lesions can be detected by simply looking into the mouth, and some cannot. All teeth must be examined clinically for dental caries with a mirror and an explorer. The mirror can be used to reflect light, to allow indirect vision, and to retract the tongue. The explorer can be used as a tactile device to detect the presence of any changes in consistency (e.g., "catches" or "tug-back") in the pits, grooves, and fissures of teeth.

A number of color changes may be seen in teeth with dental caries. Occlusal surfaces may show dark staining in the fissures, pits, and grooves or may show an obvious cavitation.

Smooth surfaces may exhibit a chalky white spot, or opacity, indicating demineralization. An interproximal ridge overlying a carious lesion may also appear discolored.

While some teeth with dental caries exhibit a discolored area or a cavitation (Figure 33-2), others have no visible changes. In addition, caries that occur between teeth may be difficult or impossible to detect clinically. In such cases, dental images play an important role. It is important to remember that a clinical examination alone is not adequate to detect dental caries; the clinical examination must be used in conjunction with the exposure of dental images.

Dental Image Examination

Dental images are useful in the detection of caries because of the nature of this disease process. Demineralization and destruction of hard tooth structures result in loss of tooth density in the area of the lesion. Decreased density allows greater penetration of x-rays in the carious area, so the carious lesion appears **radiolucent** (dark or black) on a dental image. Dental caries is the most frequently encountered radiolucent lesion on dental images.

The bite-wing image is the image of choice for the evaluation of caries because it provides the dental professional with diagnostic information that cannot be obtained from any other source. A periapical image using the paralleling technique can also be used for the evaluation of dental caries.

INTERPRETATION OF CARIES ON DENTAL IMAGES

To recognize caries on a dental image, the dental professional must be confident in the use of interpretation methods and must be able to identify factors that influence the interpretation of caries.

Interpretation Tips

As reviewed in Chapter 28, proper mounting and viewing techniques are essential in the interpretation of dental images, especially the evaluation of dental caries. With film, all images must be properly mounted before image interpretation. Mounted films should be viewed in a room with subdued lighting that is free of distractions. An illuminator or viewbox is required for accurate viewing and interpretation of images. If the screen of the viewbox is not completely covered by the mounted radiographs, the harsh light around must be masked to reduce glare and intensify the detail and contrast of the radiographic images. The use of a pocket-sized magnifying glass is helpful in evaluating the radiographic appearance of dental caries and can be used to detect slight changes in density and contrast in radiographic images.

With digital images, all exposures should be properly displayed on the computer screen before interpretation. Individual images may be enlarged to full screen to view in detail the presence or absence of dental caries. Dental images should be viewed in the presence of the patient (see Chapter 28).

Factors Influencing Caries Interpretation

A number of factors can influence the interpretation of dental caries on dental images. Images must be of diagnostic quality to allow accurate evaluation of dental caries. As described in Chapter 20, errors in technique may result in nondiagnostic images. For example, a bite-wing image used to detect dental caries must be free of overlapped contacts. Improper horizontal angulation causes overlapped contact areas and makes it impossible to identify dental caries in the interproximal regions.

As discussed in Chapter 20, errors in exposure may also result in nondiagnostic images. For example, a dental image used to detect dental caries must have proper contrast and density. Incorrect exposure factors result in images that are too dark or too light and thus useless in the detection of caries.

CLASSIFICATION OF CARIES ON DENTAL IMAGES

The appearance of caries on dental images can be classified according to the location of the caries on the tooth. Caries that involves interproximal, occlusal, buccal, lingual, and root surfaces may be seen on a dental image. In addition, recurrent and rampant caries may also be viewed on dental images.

Interproximal Caries

The term **interproximal** means "between two adjacent surfaces." Caries found between two teeth is termed **interproximal caries** (Figure 33-3). On a dental image, interproximal caries is typically seen at or just below (apical to) the contact point (Figure 33-4). This area is difficult, if not impossible, to examine clinically with an explorer.

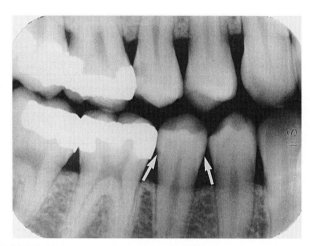

FIGURE 33-3 Interproximal caries found at or just below the contact area. (From Haring JI, Lind LJ: *Radiographic interpretation for the dental hygienist*, Philadelphia, 1993, Saunders.)

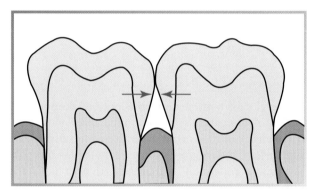

FIGURE 33-4 Caries found at or just below the contact area. (From Haring JI, Lind LJ: *Radiographic interpretation for the dental hygienist*, Philadelphia, 1993, Saunders.)

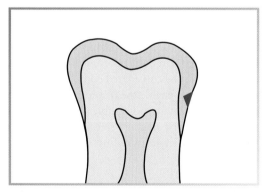

FIGURE 33-5 Caries confined to enamel, exhibiting a triangular configuration. (From Haring JI, Lind LJ: *Radiographic interpretation for the dental hygienist*, Philadelphia, 1993, Saunders.)

As the caries progresses inward through the enamel of the tooth, it assumes a triangular configuration; the apex (or point) of the triangle is seen at the dentino-enamel junction (DEJ) (Figure 33-5). As the caries reaches the DEJ, it spreads laterally and continues into dentin. Another triangular configuration is seen in dentin; this time the base of the triangle

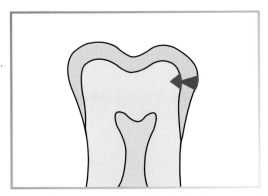

FIGURE 33-6 Caries that has reached the dentino-enamel junction (DEJ) and has spread along the DEJ, resulting in another triangular configuration. (From Haring JI, Lind LJ: *Radiographic interpretation for the dental hygienist*, Philadelphia, 1993, Saunders.)

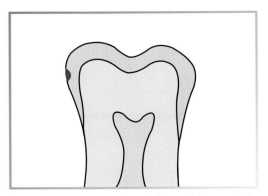

FIGURE 33-7 An incipient carious lesion, which extends less than halfway through enamel. (From Haring JI, Lind LJ: *Radiographic interpretation for the dental hygienist*, Philadelphia, 1993, Saunders.)

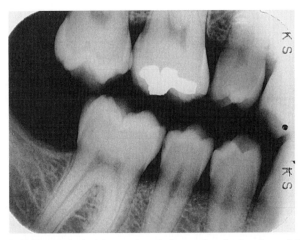

FIGURE 33-8 An incipient carious lesion on the distal surface of the mandibular second premolar. (From Haring JI, Lind LJ: *Radiographic interpretation for the dental hygienist*, Philadelphia, 1993, Saunders.)

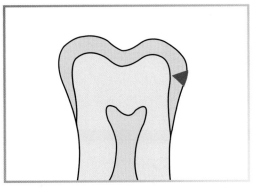

FIGURE 33-9 A moderate carious lesion, which extends more than halfway through enamel but does not involve the dentino-enamel junction (DEJ). (From Haring JI, Lind LJ: *Radiographic interpretation for the dental hygienist*, Philadelphia, 1993, Saunders.)

is along the DEJ, and the apex is pointed toward the pulp chamber (Figure 33-6).

Interproximal caries can be classified according to the depth of penetration of the lesion through enamel and dentin. Interproximal carious lesions can be classified as incipient, moderate, advanced, and severe.

Incipient Interproximal Caries

Incipient interproximal caries extends less than halfway through the thickness of enamel (Figures 33-7 and 33-8). The term **incipient** means "beginning to exist or appear." An incipient, or class I, lesion is seen *only* in enamel.

Moderate Interproximal Caries

Moderate interproximal caries extends more than halfway through the thickness of enamel but does not involve the DEJ (Figures 33-9 and 33-10). A moderate, or class II, lesion is seen *only* in enamel.

Advanced Interproximal Caries

Advanced interproximal caries extends to or through the DEJ and into dentin but does not extend through dentin more than half the distance toward the pulp (Figures 33-11 and 33-12).

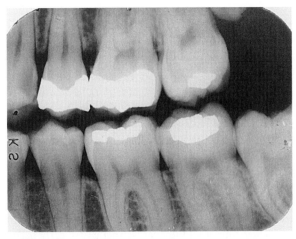

FIGURE 33-10 A moderate carious lesion on the distal surface of the mandibular second premolar. (From Haring JI, Lind LJ: *Radiographic interpretation for the dental hygienist*, Philadelphia, 1993, Saunders.)

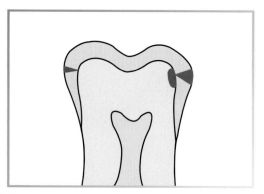

FIGURE 33-11 An advanced carious lesion, which extends through enamel and to or through the dentino-enamel junction (DEJ) but does not extend through dentin more than half the distance to the pulp chamber. (From Haring JI, Lind LJ: *Radiographic interpretation for the dental hygienist*, Philadelphia, 1993, Saunders.)

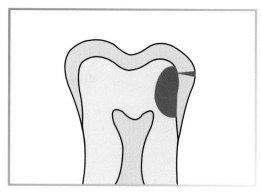

FIGURE 33-13 A severe carious lesion, which extends through enamel and dentin more than half the distance to the pulp chamber. (From Haring JI, Lind LJ: *Radiographic interpretation for the dental hygienist*, Philadelphia, 1993, Saunders.)

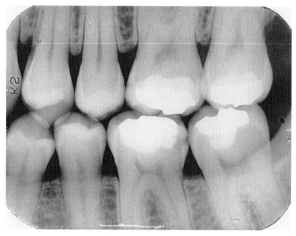

FIGURE 33-12 An advanced carious lesion, which extends through the dentino-enamel junction (DEJ) and into dentin, seen on the distal surface of the mandibular first molar. (From Haring JI, Lind LJ: *Radiographic interpretation for the dental hygienist*, Philadelphia, 1993, Saunders.)

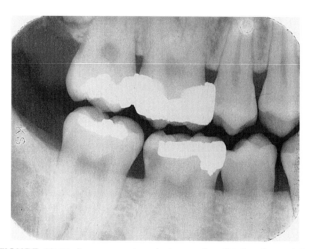

FIGURE 33-14 A severe carious lesion on the distal surface of the mandibular first molar. (From Haring JI, Lind LJ: *Radiographic interpretation for the dental hygienist*, Philadelphia, 1993, Saunders.)

An advanced, or class III, lesion affects *both* enamel and dentin.

Severe Interproximal Caries

Severe interproximal caries extends through enamel, through dentin, and more than half the distance toward the pulp (Figures 33-13 and 33-14). A severe, or class IV, lesion involves *both* enamel and dentin and may appear clinically as a cavitation in the tooth.

Occlusal Caries

The term **occlusal** refers to the chewing surfaces of teeth. Caries that involves the chewing surfaces of posterior teeth is termed **occlusal caries**. A thorough clinical examination with the mirror, explorer, and light is the method of choice for the detection of occlusal caries. Because of the superimposition of the dense buccal and lingual enamel cusps, early occlusal caries is difficult to see on a dental image. Consequently, occlusal caries is not seen on a dental image until involvement

of the DEJ occurs. Occlusal carious lesions can be classified as incipient, moderate, or severe.

Incipient Occlusal Caries

Incipient occlusal caries cannot be seen on a dental image and must be detected clinically with an explorer.

Moderate Occlusal Caries

Moderate occlusal caries extends into dentin and appears as a very thin radiolucent line (Figures 33-15 and 33-16). The radiolucency is located under the enamel of the occlusal surface of the tooth. On a dental image, little, if any, change is noted in enamel.

Severe Occlusal Caries

Severe occlusal caries extends into dentin and appears as a large radiolucency (Figures 33-17 and 33-18). The radiolucency extends under the enamel of the occlusal surface of the tooth. Severe occlusal caries is apparent clinically and appears as a cavitation in the tooth.

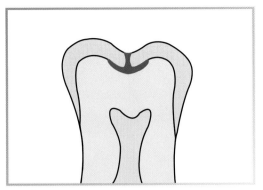

FIGURE 33-15 A moderate occlusal carious lesion, which extends through enamel and into dentin along the dentino-enamel junction (DEJ). (From Haring JI, Lind LJ: *Radiographic interpretation for the dental hygienist*, Philadelphia, 1993, Saunders.)

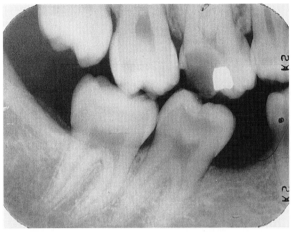

FIGURE 33-18 A severe occlusal carious lesion seen as a large radiolucency in dentin on the mandibular first molar. (From Haring JI, Lind LJ: *Radiographic interpretation for the dental hygienist*, Philadelphia, 1993, Saunders.)

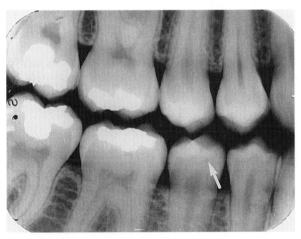

FIGURE 33-16 Occlusal caries, which appears as a tiny radiolucency just below the dentino-enamel junction (DEJ) on the mandibular second premolar. (From Haring JI, Lind LJ: *Radiographic interpretation for the dental hygienist*, Philadelphia, 1993, Saunders.)

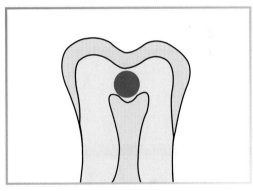

FIGURE 33-19 Buccal or lingual caries seen as a round radiolucency on molars. (From Haring JI, Lind LJ: *Radiographic interpretation for the dental hygienist*, Philadelphia, 1993, Saunders.)

Buccal and Lingual Caries

As the names suggest, **buccal caries** involves the buccal tooth surface, whereas **lingual caries** involves the lingual tooth surface. Because of the superimposition of the densities of normal tooth structure, buccal and lingual caries are difficult to detect on a dental image and are best detected clinically. When viewed on a dental image, caries that involves the buccal or lingual surface appears as a small, circular radiolucent area (Figures 33-19 and 33-20). To determine the location of the lesion, clinical examination with an explorer is necessary.

Root Surface Caries

Root surface caries involves only the roots of teeth. The cementum and dentin located just below the cervical region of the tooth are involved (Figures 33-21 and 33-22). No involvement of enamel occurs. Bone loss and corresponding gingival recession precede the caries process and result in exposed root surfaces.

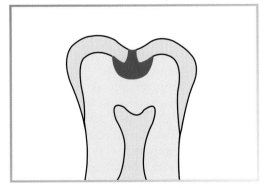

FIGURE 33-17 Severe occlusal caries, which extends through enamel and into dentin beyond the dentino-enamel junction (DEJ). (From Haring JI, Lind LJ: *Radiographic interpretation for the dental hygienist*, Philadelphia, 1993, Saunders.)

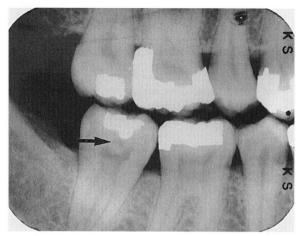

FIGURE 33-20 Buccal caries seen as a small, circular radiolucency on the mandibular second molar. (From Haring JI, Lind LJ: *Radiographic interpretation for the dental hygienist*, Philadelphia, 1993, Saunders.)

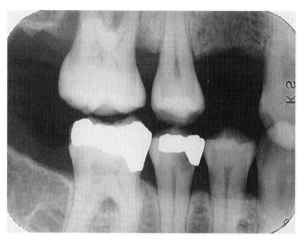

FIGURE 33-23 Recurrent caries seen as a radiolucency below a two-surface amalgam restoration on the mandibular second premolar. (From Haring JI, Lind LJ: *Radiographic interpretation for the dental hygienist*, Philadelphia, 1993, Saunders.)

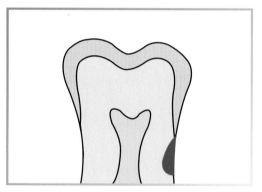

FIGURE 33-21 Root caries involving only cementum and dentin, not enamel. (From Haring JI, Lind LJ: *Radiographic interpretation for the dental hygienist*, Philadelphia, 1993, Saunders.)

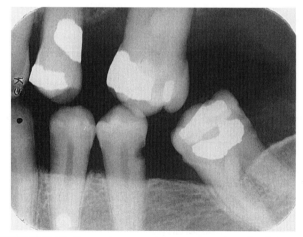

FIGURE 33-22 Root caries appearing as a crater-shaped radiolucency just below the cemento-enamel junction (CEJ) on the mandibular second premolar. (From Haring JI, Lind LJ: *Radiographic interpretation for the dental hygienist*, Philadelphia, 1993, Saunders.)

Clinically, root surface caries is easily detected on exposed root surfaces. The most common locations include the exposed roots of mandibular premolar and molar areas. On a dental image, root surface caries appears as a cupped-out or crater-shaped radiolucency just below the cemento-enamel junction (CEJ). Early lesions may be difficult to detect on a dental image.

Recurrent Caries

Secondary caries, or **recurrent caries**, occurs adjacent to a pre-existing restoration. Caries occurs in this region because of inadequate cavity preparation, defective margins, or incomplete removal of caries before placement of the restoration material. On a dental image, recurrent caries appears as a radiolucent area just beneath a restoration (Figure 33-23). Recurrent caries occurs most often beneath the interproximal margins of a restoration.

Rampant Caries

The term **rampant** means "growing or spreading unchecked." Rampant caries is advanced and severe caries that affects numerous teeth (Figure 33-24). **Rampant caries** is typically seen in children with poor dietary habits or in adults with decreased salivary flow.

SUMMARY

- Dental caries is a destructive process that causes decalcification of enamel, destruction of enamel and dentin, and cavitation of teeth.
- To detect dental caries, careful clinical examination and interpretation are necessary.
- Dental images allow the dental professional to identify carious lesions that are not visible clinically.
- Caries appears radiolucent on a dental image. Of all the radiolucent lesions that can be seen on a dental image, dental caries is the most frequently seen.

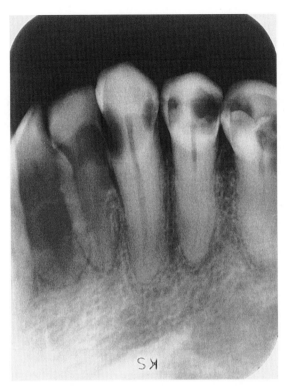

FIGURE 33-24 Rampant caries. (From Haring JI, Lind LJ: *Radiographic interpretation for the dental hygienist*, Philadelphia, 1993, Saunders.)

- On a dental image, the appearance of interproximal caries can be classified as incipient, moderate, advanced, or severe, depending on the amount of enamel and dentin involved in the caries process.
- On a dental image, the appearance of occlusal caries can be classified as moderate or severe, depending on the amount of enamel and dentin involved in the caries process.
- Buccal and lingual carious lesions are difficult to detect on dental images because of the superimposition of normal tooth structure. Instead, these lesions are best detected clinically.
- Root surface caries involves cementum and dentin and is easily detected clinically. On a dental image, root surface caries appears as a cupped-out radiolucency below the cemento-enamel junction.
- On a dental image, other appearances of dental caries include recurrent caries, which appears as a radiolucency adjacent to an existing restoration, and rampant caries, which affects numerous teeth.

BIBLIOGRAPHY

Frommer HH, Savage-Stabulas JJ: Caries and periodontal disease. In *Radiology for the dental professional*, ed 9, St. Louis, 2011, Mosby.

Haring JI, Lind LJ: Dental caries. In *Radiographic interpretation for the dental hygienist*, Philadelphia, 1993, Saunders.

Johnson ON, McNally MA, Essay CE: Preliminary interpretation of the radiographs. In *Essentials of dental radiography for dental assistants and hygienists*, ed 8, Upper Saddle River, NJ, 2007, Pearson Education, Inc.

Miles DA, Van Dis ML, Jensen CW, Williamson GF: Interpretation: normal versus abnormal and common radiographic presentation of lesions. In *Radiographic imaging for the dental team*, ed 4, Philadelphia, 2009, Saunders.

White SC, Pharoah MJ: Dental caries. In *Oral radiology: principles of interpretation*, ed 6, St. Louis, 2009, Mosby.

- The dental professional must be confident in the use of interpretation methods to identify dental caries and to recognize factors that influence caries interpretation (e.g., errors in technique and exposure).
- Dental caries may involve any surface of the tooth crown or root. The appearance of dental caries can be classified according to the location of the caries on the tooth. Caries involving interproximal, occlusal, buccal, lingual, and root surfaces may be seen on dental images.

QUIZ QUESTIONS

IDENTIFICATION

For questions 1 to 5, refer to Figures 33-25 through 33-29. On each dental image, identify the classification of the carious lesion shown.

1. _____

2. _____

3. _____

4. _____

5. _____

MATCHING

For questions 6 to 12, match the classification of caries with the appropriate description.

a. Caries that extends more than halfway through enamel but does not involve the dentino-enamel junction (DEJ)

b. Caries that extends to or through the DEJ but does not extend more than half the distance to the pulp

c. Caries that cannot be seen on an image

d. Caries that extends through enamel, through dentin, and more than half the distance to the pulp

e. Caries that extends less than halfway through enamel

f. Caries seen as a large radiolucency in dentin under the enamel of the chewing surfaces of teeth

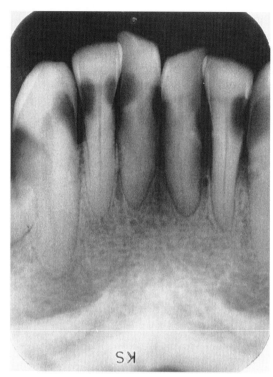

FIGURE 33-25 (From Haring JI, Lind LJ: *Radiographic interpretation for the dental hygienist*, Philadelphia, 1993, Saunders.)

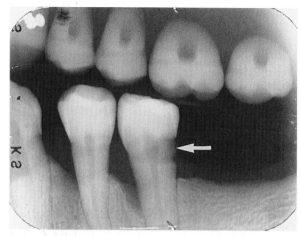

FIGURE 33-27 (From Haring JI, Lind LJ: *Radiographic interpretation for the dental hygienist*, Philadelphia, 1993, Saunders.)

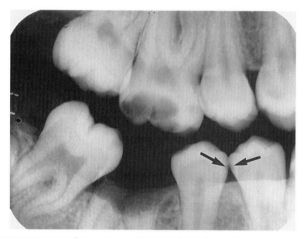

FIGURE 33-26 (From Haring JI, Lind LJ: *Radiographic interpretation for the dental hygienist*, Philadelphia, 1993, Saunders.)

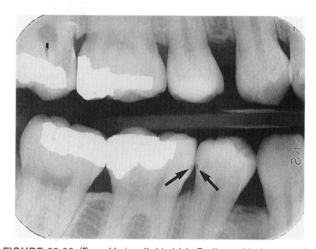

FIGURE 33-28 (From Haring JI, Lind LJ: *Radiographic interpretation for the dental hygienist*, Philadelphia, 1993, Saunders.)

g. Caries seen as a thin radiolucent line in dentin under the enamel of the chewing surfaces of teeth
h. None of the above
___ 6. Incipient interproximal
___ 7. Moderate interproximal
___ 8. Advanced interproximal
___ 9. Severe interproximal
___ 10. Incipient occlusal
___ 11. Moderate occlusal
___ 12. Severe occlusal

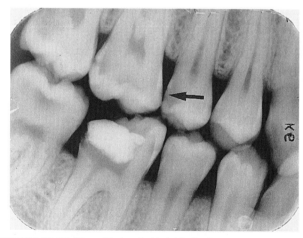

FIGURE 33-29 (From Haring JI, Lind LJ: *Radiographic interpretation for the dental hygienist*, Philadelphia, 1993, Saunders.)

SHORT ANSWER

13. Describe dental caries.

14. Explain why caries appears radiolucent on a dental image.

15. List the classifications of interproximal caries on a dental image.

16. List the classifications of occlusal caries on a dental image.

17. Describe the appearance of root caries on a dental image.

18. Describe the appearance of recurrent caries on a dental image.

19. Describe the appearance of rampant caries on a dental image.

20. Discuss the factors that may influence the interpretation of dental caries.

chapter 34

Interpretation of Periodontal Disease

OUTLINE

DESCRIPTION OF THE PERIODONTIUM
DESCRIPTION OF PERIODONTAL DISEASE
DETECTION OF PERIODONTAL DISEASE
    Clinical Examination
    Dental Image Examination

INTERPRETATION OF PERIODONTAL DISEASE ON
    DENTAL IMAGES
    Bone Loss
    Classification of Periodontal Disease
    Predisposing Factors

LEARNING OBJECTIVES

After completion of this chapter, the student will be able to do the following:

- Define the key terms associated with interpreting periodontal disease
- Describe the healthy periodontium
- Briefly describe periodontal disease
- Discuss the importance of the clinical examination and interpretation of dental images in the diagnosis of periodontal disease
- Describe the limitations of dental images in the detection of periodontal disease
- Describe the type of dental images that should be used to document periodontal disease and the preferred exposure technique
- State the difference between horizontal bone loss and vertical bone loss

- State the difference between localized bone loss and generalized bone loss
- State the differences among mild, moderate, and severe bone loss
- List each of the four American Dental Association (ADA) case types and describe the corresponding appearance on dental images
- Recognize each of the four ADA case types on dental images
- List two predisposing factors for periodontal disease
- Recognize and describe the appearance of calculus on dental images

KEY TERMS

Alveolar crest	Calculus	Periodontal
Bone loss, generalized	Clinical attachment loss	Periodontal disease
Bone loss, horizontal	Furcation area	Periodontal ligament space
Bone loss, localized	Lamina dura	Periodontium
Bone loss, vertical		

Dental images play an integral role in the assessment of periodontal disease. An examination of dental images is essential for diagnostic purposes because it enables the dental professional to obtain vital information about supporting bone, as this information cannot be obtained clinically. Detailed information about periodontal disease is beyond the scope of this text. The purpose of this chapter is to introduce the dental radiographer to the description and detection of periodontal disease. The interpretation of periodontal disease,

with an emphasis on a description of bone loss, ADA case types, and identification of predisposing factors, is also presented.

DESCRIPTION OF THE PERIODONTIUM

The term **periodontium** refers to tissues that invest and support teeth, such as the gingiva and alveolar bone. As

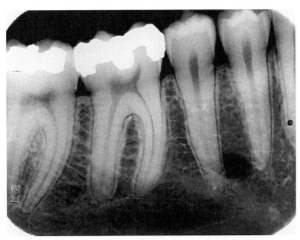

FIGURE 34-1 Healthy alveolar crest, normal lamina dura, and periodontal ligament space on a periapical image. (From Haring JI, Lind LJ: *Radiographic interpretation for the dental hygienist*, Philadelphia, 1993, Saunders.)

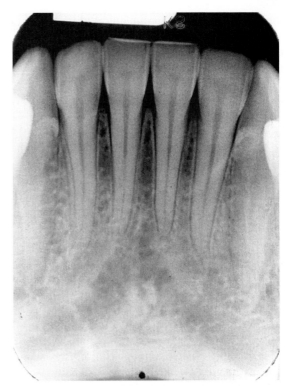

FIGURE 34-2 Healthy alveolar crest in the anterior region that appears pointed and highly radiopaque. (From Haring JI, Lind LJ: *Radiographic interpretation for the dental hygienist*, Philadelphia, 1993, Saunders.)

described in Chapter 27, the normal anatomic landmarks of alveolar bone include the lamina dura, alveolar crest, and periodontal ligament space. The appearance of healthy alveolar bone on a dental image can be described as follows:

Lamina dura: In health, the lamina dura of teeth appears as a dense radiopaque line around the roots (Figure 34-1).

Alveolar crest: The normal healthy alveolar crest is located approximately 1.5 to 2.0 mm apical to the cemento-enamel junctions (CEJs) of adjacent teeth (see Figure 34-1). The shape and density of the alveolar crest vary between the anterior and posterior regions of the mouth. In the anterior regions, the alveolar crest appears pointed and sharp and is normally very radiopaque (Figure 34-2). In the posterior regions, the alveolar crest appears flat, smooth, and parallel to a line between adjacent CEJs (Figure 34-3). The alveolar crest in the posterior regions appears slightly less radiopaque than that in the anterior regions.

Periodontal ligament space: The normal periodontal ligament space appears as a thin radiolucent line between the root of the tooth and the lamina dura. In health, the periodontal ligament space is continuous around the root structure and is of uniform thickness (see Figure 34-1).

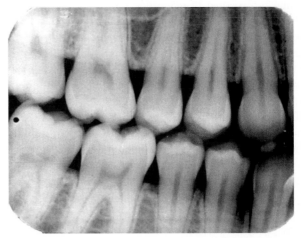

FIGURE 34-3 Healthy alveolar crest in the posterior region that appears flat, smooth, and radiopaque. (From Haring JI, Lind LJ: *Radiographic interpretation for the dental hygienist*, Philadelphia, 1993, Saunders.)

DESCRIPTION OF PERIODONTAL DISEASE

The term **periodontal** literally means "around a tooth." **Periodontal disease** refers to a group of diseases that affect the tissues around teeth. Periodontal disease may range from a superficial inflammation of the gingiva to the destruction of supporting bone and the periodontal ligament. With periodontal disease, the gingiva exhibits varying degrees of inflammation. Gingival tissues affected by periodontal disease may not appear stippled, pink, and firm. Instead, the gingiva may appear swollen, red, and bleeding, and formation of soft tissue pockets is seen.

On a dental image, the appearance of alveolar bone affected by periodontal disease differs from that of healthy alveolar bone. With periodontal disease, the alveolar crest is no longer located 1.5 to 2.0 mm apical to the CEJs and no longer appears radiopaque. Instead, the alveolar crest appears indistinct, and bone loss is seen. Periodontal disease may result in severe destruction of bone and loss of teeth.

DETECTION OF PERIODONTAL DISEASE

To detect periodontal disease, both clinical examinations and interpretation of dental images are necessary. Dental images *must* be used in conjunction with a clinical examination. In general, what is seen clinically cannot be evaluated on dental images, and what is viewed on dental images cannot be evaluated clinically. Clinical examination provides information about soft tissues, while dental images permit evaluation of bone.

Clinical Examination

Clinical examination must be performed by the dentist and dental hygienist and should include an evaluation of soft tissues (gingiva) for signs of inflammation (e.g., redness, bleeding, swelling, pus). A thorough clinical assessment must include periodontal probing. Whenever clinical evidence of periodontal disease is present, images must be obtained in order to get maximum diagnostic information.

Dental Image Examination

Dental images, along with clinical examination, enable the dental professional to determine the extent of periodontal disease. Dental images provide an overview of the amount of bone present and indicate the pattern, distribution, and severity of bone loss resulting from periodontal disease. In addition, dental images enable the dental professional to document periodontal disease at specific points in time.

The *periapical image* is recommended for the evaluation of periodontal disease. The *paralleling technique* is the preferred periapical exposure method for the demonstration of the anatomic features of periodontal disease. With the paralleling technique, the height of crestal bone is accurately recorded in relation to the tooth root. If the bisecting technique is used to expose periapical images, a dimensional distortion of bone results due to vertical angulation. Therefore, periapical images using the bisecting technique may show more or less bone loss than actually present (Figures 34-4 and 34-5).

The horizontal bite-wing image alone should not be used to document moderate to severe periodontal disease. This image has limited use in the detection of periodontal disease; severe interproximal bone loss cannot be adequately visualized on horizontal bite-wing images.

The vertical bite-wing image can be used to examine bone levels and is best used for post-treatment and follow-up purposes. The panoramic image has little diagnostic value in the identification of periodontal disease and is not recommended to demonstrate the anatomic features of this condition.

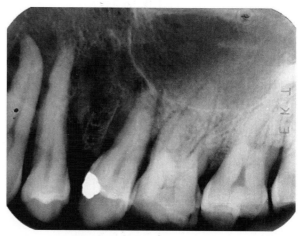

FIGURE 34-4 Bisecting technique distorting the level of bone present seen on an image because of the vertical angulation used. (From Haring JI, Lind LJ: *Radiographic interpretation for the dental hygienist*, Philadelphia, 1993, Saunders.)

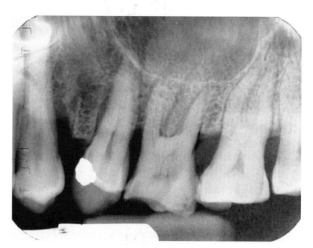

FIGURE 34-5 Paralleling technique used to examine the same area seen in Figure 34-4. Note the difference in bone level. With the paralleling technique, the height of crestal bone is accurately recorded in relation to the tooth root. (From Haring JI, Lind LJ: *Radiographic interpretation for the dental hygienist*, Philadelphia, 1993, Saunders.)

Dental images alone cannot be used to diagnose periodontal disease because of limitations in detecting and diagnosing the condition; images must be used in conjunction with a thorough clinical examination. For example, dental images do not provide information about the condition of soft tissues or the early bony changes seen in periodontal disease. Because dental images record two-dimensional images of three-dimensional structures, certain areas of teeth and bone are difficult, if not impossible, to examine in this manner. Buccal and lingual areas are particularly difficult to evaluate. For example, bone loss in the **furcation area**—the area between the roots of multirooted teeth—may not be detected on a dental image because of the superimposition of buccal and lingual bone.

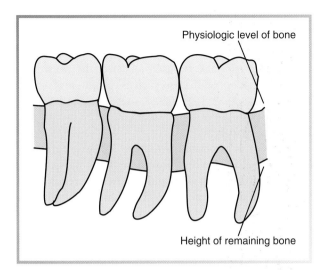

FIGURE 34-6 Bone loss estimated as the difference between the physiologic level of bone and the height of the remaining bone. (From Haring JI, Lind LJ: *Radiographic interpretation for the dental hygienist*, Philadelphia, 1993, Saunders.)

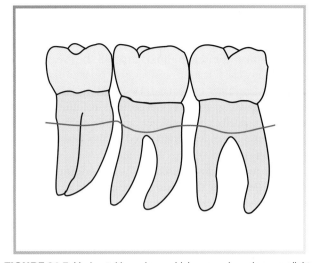

FIGURE 34-7 Horizontal bone loss, which occurs in a plane parallel to the cemento-enamel junctions (CEJs) of adjacent teeth. (From Haring JI, Lind LJ: *Radiographic interpretation for the dental hygienist*, Philadelphia, 1993, Saunders.)

INTERPRETATION OF PERIODONTAL DISEASE ON DENTAL IMAGES

The dental radiographer must be familiar with the appearance of periodontal disease. All images should be evaluated for bone loss and examined for other predisposing factors that may contribute to periodontal disease.

Bone Loss

A dental image allows the dental professional to view the amount of bone remaining rather than the amount of bone lost. However, in documenting bone levels, the amount of bone loss that has occurred is recorded rather than the amount of bone that remains. The amount of bone loss can be estimated as the difference between the physiologic bone level and the height of remaining bone (Figure 34-6). Bone loss can be described in terms of the pattern, distribution, and severity of loss.

Pattern

The pattern of bone loss viewed on a dental image can be described as horizontal or vertical. The CEJs of adjacent teeth can be used as a plane of reference in determining the pattern of bone loss present. With **horizontal bone loss**, the bone loss occurs in a plane parallel to the CEJs of adjacent teeth (Figures 34-7 and 34-8). With **vertical bone loss** (also known as *angular bone loss*), the bone loss does not occur in a plane parallel to the CEJs of adjacent teeth (Figures 34-9 and 34-10).

Distribution

The distribution of bone loss seen on a dental image can be described as localized or generalized, depending on the areas involved. **Localized** bone loss occurs in isolated areas, with

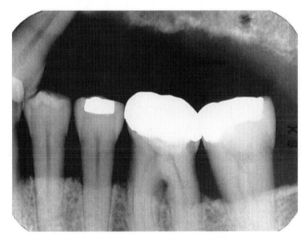

FIGURE 34-8 Horizontal bone loss. (From Haring JI, Lind LJ: *Radiographic interpretation for the dental hygienist*, Philadelphia, 1993, Saunders.)

less than 30% of the sites involved (Figure 34-11). **Generalized** bone loss occurs evenly throughout the dental arches, with more than 30% of the sites involved (Figure 34-12).

Severity

Bone loss viewed on a dental image can be classified as slight, moderate, or severe. The severity of bone loss is measured by the **clinical attachment loss** (CAL). The CAL is a measurement of the distance in millimeters from the CEJ to the base of the sulcus or periodontal pocket; CAL is measured by the calibrated periodontal probe. (*Note*: Clinical conditions, such as recession or gingival overgrowth, must be considered when determining CAL.) The severity of bone loss can be defined as follows:

- *Slight* bone loss: 1 to 2 mm
- *Moderate* bone loss: 3 to 4 mm
- *Severe* bone loss: 5 mm or greater

Classification of Periodontal Disease

Classification systems are routinely used to provide a framework to study clinical findings and for the treatment of disease. The classification system for periodontal disease was revised in 1999 (Armitage, 1999). More clinical information regarding disease categories, including gingival disease, age-related terminology, and the pathogenesis of periodontal disease, was highlighted in this latest classification system.

Dental images can be used in the classification of periodontal disease. On the basis of the amount of bone loss, periodontal disease can be classified as follows: the American Dental Association (ADA) Case Type I (*gingivitis)*, ADA Case Type II (*mild or slight periodontitis*), ADA Case Type III (*moderate periodontitis*), or ADA Case Type IV (*advanced or severe periodontitis*). Each disease type has a specific appearance. Dental images can also be used to detect the contributing factors for periodontal disease, such as calculus and defective restorations.

ADA Case Type I

No bone loss is associated with type I disease (gingivitis); therefore, no change in bone is seen on the dental image. The crestal lamina dura is present, and the alveolar crest is approximately 1 to 2 mm apical to the CEJ. Clinically, bleeding may or may not be present. Only the gingival tissues are affected by the inflammatory process in ADA Case Type I.

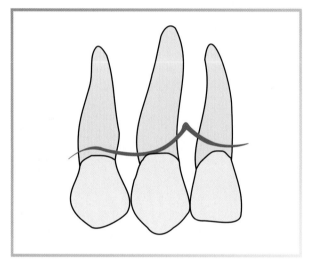

FIGURE 34-9 Vertical bone loss, which occurs in a plane that is not parallel to the cemento-enamel junctions (CEJs) of adjacent teeth. (From Haring JI, Lind LJ: *Radiographic interpretation for the dental hygienist*, Philadelphia, 1993, Saunders.)

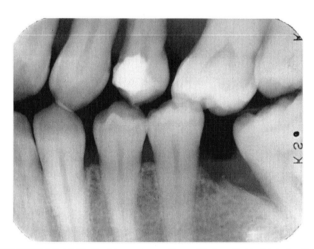

FIGURE 34-10 Vertical bone loss. (From Haring JI, Lind LJ: *Radiographic interpretation for the dental hygienist*, Philadelphia, 1993, Saunders.)

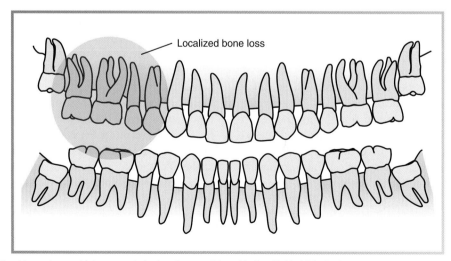

FIGURE 34-11 Localized bone loss, which occurs in isolated areas. (From Haring JI, Lind LJ: *Radiographic interpretation for the dental hygienist*, Philadelphia, 1993, Saunders.)

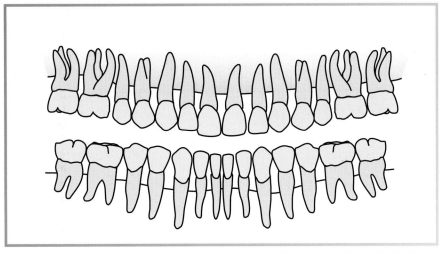

FIGURE 34-12 Generalized bone loss, which occurs throughout the dental arches. (From Haring JI, Lind LJ: *Radiographic interpretation for the dental hygienist*, Philadelphia, 1993, Saunders.)

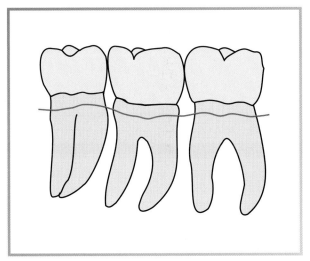

FIGURE 34-13 Mild bone loss. (From Haring JI, Lind LJ: *Radiographic interpretation for the dental hygienist*, Philadelphia, 1993, Saunders.)

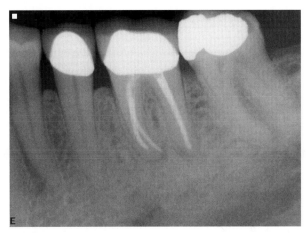

FIGURE 34-15 ADA Case Type II. (Courtesy Timothy W. Godsey and Liliana Gandini, Chapel Hill, NC.)

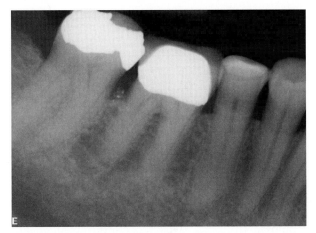

FIGURE 34-14 Horizontal bone loss and mild crestal changes seen in ADA Case Type II. (Courtesy Timothy W. Godsey, DDS, MS, and Liliana Gandini, DMD, Chapel Hill, NC.)

ADA Case Type II

The bone loss associated with type II disease (mild or slight periodontitis) is mild crestal changes (Figures 34-13 to 34-15). The lamina dura becomes unclear and fuzzy and no longer appears to be a continuous radiopaque line. Horizontal bone loss is seen more often in type II disease, with the alveolar bone level approximately 3 to 4 mm apical to the CEJ. Clinically, bleeding may occur on probing, pocket depths resulting from attachment loss as well as localized areas of recession may be evident.

ADA Case Type III

Horizontal or vertical bone loss may be present in type III disease; the distribution of the bone loss may be localized or generalized (Figures 34-16 to 34-19). The alveolar bone level is approximately 4 to 6 mm apical to the CEJs of adjacent

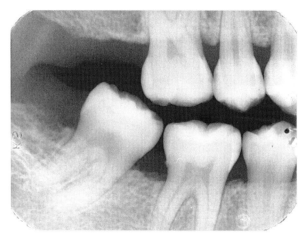

FIGURE 34-16 ADA Case Type III. (From Haring JI, Lind LJ: *Radiographic interpretation for the dental hygienist*, Philadelphia, 1993, Saunders.)

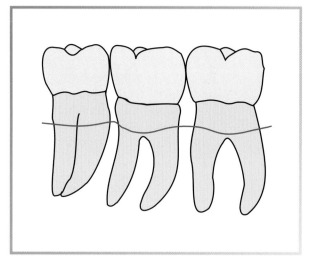

FIGURE 34-17 Moderate bone loss. (From Haring JI, Lind LJ: *Radiographic interpretation for the dental hygienist*, Philadelphia, 1993, Saunders.)

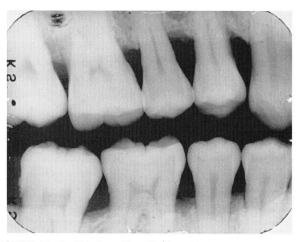

FIGURE 34-18 ADA Case Type III. (From Haring JI, Lind LJ: *Radiographic interpretation for the dental hygienist*, Philadelphia, 1993, Saunders.)

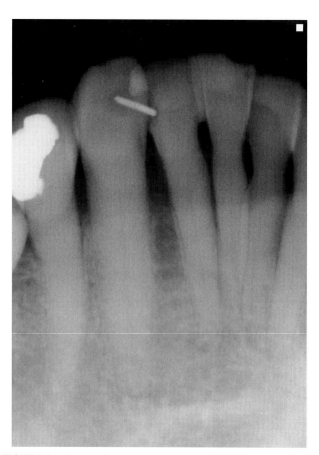

FIGURE 34-19 ADA Case Type III demonstrating generalized horizontal bone loss. (Courtesy Timothy W. Godsey, DDS, MS, and Liliana Gandini, DMD, Chapel Hill, NC.)

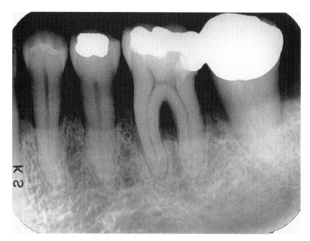

FIGURE 34-20 Furcation area of the mandibular first molar that appears radiolucent. (From Haring JI, Lind LJ: *Radiographic interpretation for the dental hygienist*, Philadelphia, 1993, Saunders.)

teeth. Furcation involvement, or the extension of periodontal disease between the roots of multirooted teeth, may also be seen in type III disease. When bone in the furcation area is destroyed, a radiolucent area is evident on the dental image (Figure 34-20). Clinically, pocket depths and attachment loss

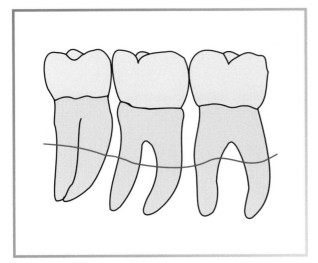

FIGURE 34-21 Severe bone loss. (From Haring JI, Lind LJ: *Radiographic interpretation for the dental hygienist*, Philadelphia, 1993, Saunders.)

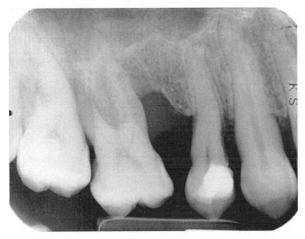

FIGURE 34-22 ADA Case Type IV. (From Haring JI, Lind LJ: *Radiographic interpretation for the dental hygienist*, Philadelphia, 1993, Saunders.)

up to 6 mm are evident. Recession, furcation involvement areas, and slight mobility may also be present.

ADA Case Type IV

The bone loss associated with type IV disease (advanced or severe periodontitis) indicates further progression of the disease and is considered severe (Figures 34-21 to 34-23). The pattern of bone loss may be horizontal or vertical, and the alveolar bone level is 6 mm or greater from the CEJ. Furcation involvement is readily viewed on posterior images. Clinically, pocket depths and attachment loss are greater than 6 mm, and furcation involvement and mobility are more severe.

Predisposing Factors

The effects of certain medications, tobacco use, and various medical conditions are all considered risk factors for periodontal disease. A number of other factors may predispose the patient or contribute to periodontal disease. The

identification, detection, and elimination of local irritants are important in the management and treatment of periodontal disease. Dental images play a major role in the detection of local irritants such as calculus and defective restorations.

Calculus

Calculus is a stonelike concretion that forms on the crowns and roots of teeth due to the calcification of bacterial plaque. Calculus acts as a contributing or predisposing factor to periodontal disease. Calculus appears radiopaque (white or light) on a dental image (Figure 34-24). Although calculus may have a variety of appearances on dental images, it most often appears as pointed or irregular radiopaque projections extending from proximal root surfaces (Figure 34-25). Calculus may also appear as a ringlike radiopacity encircling the cervical portion of a tooth (Figure 34-26), a nodular radiopaque projection (Figure 34-27), or a smooth radiopacity on a root surface (Figure 34-28).

Defective Restorations

Faulty dental restorations act as potential food traps and lead to the accumulation of food debris and bacterial deposits. Defective restorations act as contributing factors to periodontal disease and can be detected both clinically and on dental images. Dental images allow the dental professional to identify restorations with open or loose contacts, poor contours uneven marginal ridges, overhangs, and inadequate margins, all of which may contribute to periodontal disease (Figures 34-29 to 34-35).

SUMMARY

- The term *periodontal disease* refers to a group of diseases that affect the tissues around teeth.
- Thorough clinical and dental image examinations are necessary to detect, diagnose, and evaluate periodontal disease. Clinical examination provides information about soft tissues, and the dental image examination provides information about supporting bone.
- Dental images can be used to document periodontal disease and determine the success or failure of periodontal therapy.
- Interpretation of periodontal disease on dental images should include an evaluation of alveolar bone; bony changes can be described in terms of pattern (horizontal or vertical), distribution (localized or generalized), and severity (slight, moderate, or severe).
- Dental images can be used in the classification of periodontal disease. On the basis of the amount of bone loss, periodontal disease can be classified as ADA Case Type I (gingivitis), Case Type II (mild/slight periodontitis), Case Type III (moderate periodontitis), and Case Type IV (advanced/severe periodontitis).
- Dental images can also be used to detect local irritants, including calculus and defective restorations, that contribute to periodontal disease.

Text continued on p. 424

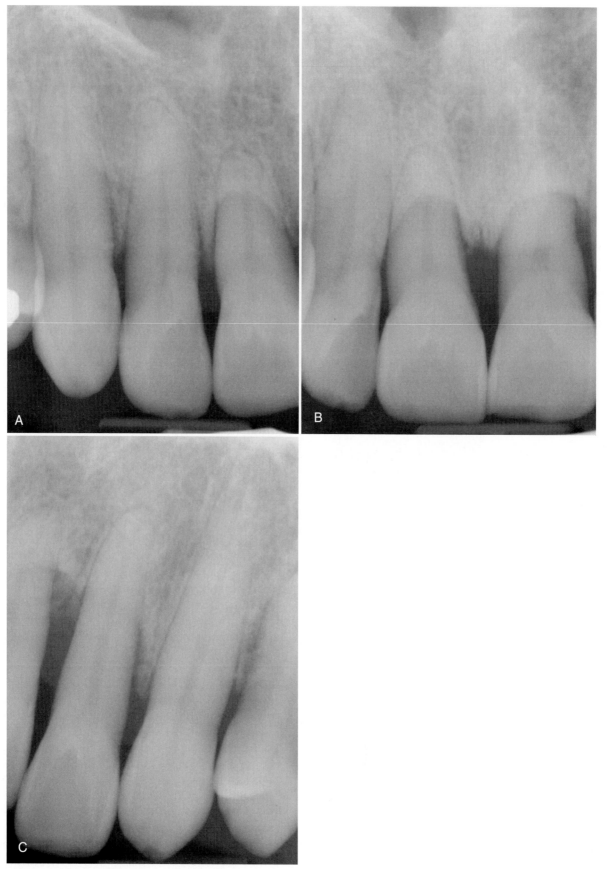

FIGURE 34-23 A–C, Advanced periodontitis seen on images of the maxillary anterior teeth. (Courtesy of Timothy W. Godsey, DDS, MS, and Liliana Gandini, DMD, Chapel Hill, NC.)

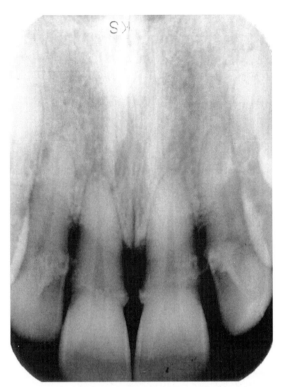

FIGURE 34-24 Subgingival calculus that appears as irregular radiopaque projections in the maxillary anterior region. (From Haring JI, Lind LJ: *Radiographic interpretation for the dental hygienist*, Philadelphia, 1993, Saunders.)

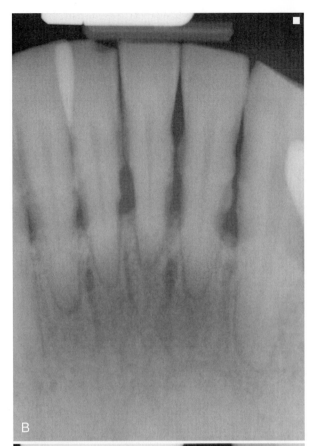

B

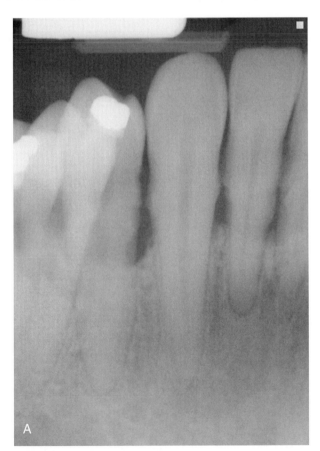

A

FIGURE 34-25 A–C, Calculus that appears as sharp, pointed radiopacities along the surfaces of mandibular anterior teeth. (Courtesy Timothy W. Godsey, DDS, MS, and Liliana Gandini, DMD, Chapel Hill, NC.)

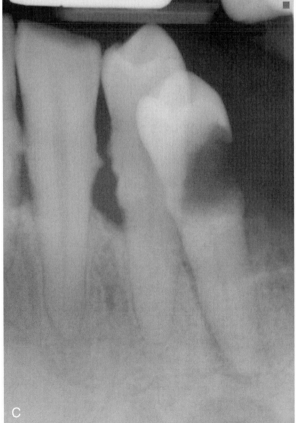

C

FIGURE 34-25, cont'd

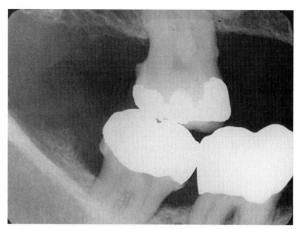

FIGURE 34-26 Calculus appearing as a ring-like radiopacity around the cervical region of a tooth. (From Haring JI, Lind LJ: *Radiographic interpretation for the dental hygienist*, Philadelphia, 1993, Saunders.)

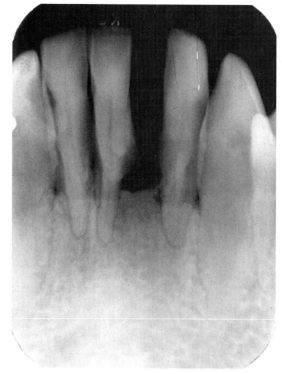

FIGURE 34-27 Calculus appearing nodular, as seen here between two mandibular incisors. (From Haring JI, Lind LJ: *Radiographic interpretation for the dental hygienist*, Philadelphia, 1993, Saunders.)

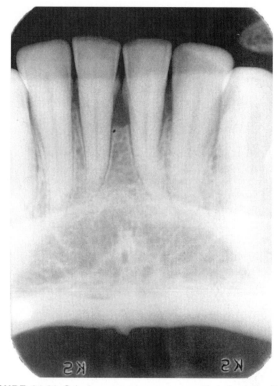

FIGURE 34-28 Calculus appearing as a smooth radiopacity. (From Haring JI, Lind LJ: *Radiographic interpretation for the dental hygienist*, Philadelphia, 1993, Saunders.)

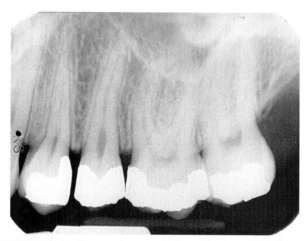

FIGURE 34-29 Open contact between maxillary premolars. (From Haring JI, Lind LJ: *Radiographic interpretation for the dental hygienist*, Philadelphia, 1993, Saunders.)

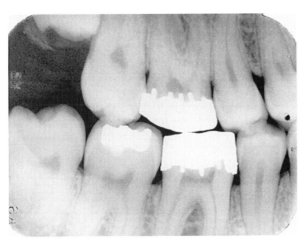

FIGURE 34-30 Poorly contoured crowns on maxillary and mandibular first molars. (From Haring JI, Lind LJ: *Radiographic interpretation for the dental hygienist*, Philadelphia, 1993, Saunders.)

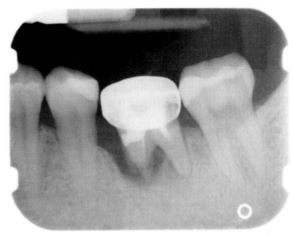

FIGURE 34-31 A poorly contoured stainless steel crown causing bone loss on a mandibular first molar.

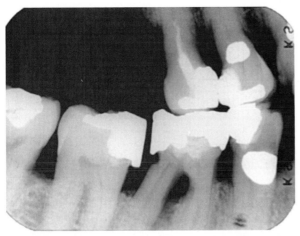

FIGURE 34-32 Uneven marginal ridges, open contacts, overhangs, and poorly contoured restorations on a bite-wing image. (From Haring JI, Lind LJ: *Radiographic interpretation for the dental hygienist*, Philadelphia, 1993, Saunders.)

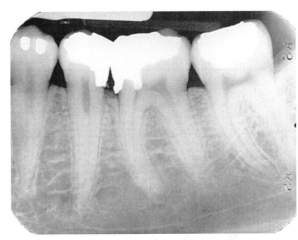

FIGURE 34-33 Amalgam overhang on the mesial surface of the mandibular first molar. (From Haring JI, Lind LJ: *Radiographic interpretation for the dental hygienist*, Philadelphia, 1993, Saunders.)

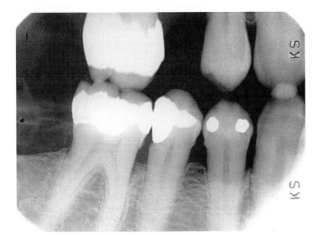

FIGURE 34-34 Inadequate margin on the distal surface of a mandibular second premolar. (From Haring JI, Lind LJ: *Radiographic interpretation for the dental hygienist*, Philadelphia, 1993, Saunders.)

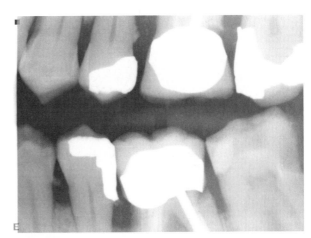

FIGURE 34-35 Ill-fitting restorations and open contacts between teeth contributing to the periodontal condition of this patient. (Courtesy of Timothy W. Godsey, DDS, MS, and Liliana Gandini, DMD, Chapel Hill, NC.)

BIBLIOGRAPHY

American Academy of Periodontology: Treatment of plaque-induced gingivitis, chronic periodontitis and other clinical conditions. *J Periodontol* 72:1790–1800, 2001.

Armitage GC: Development of a classification system for periodontal diseases and conditions. *Ann Periodontol* 4:1–6, 1999.

Frommer HH, Savage-Stabulas JJ: Caries and periodontal disease. In *Radiology for the dental professional*, ed 9, St. Louis, 2011, Mosby.

Haring JI, Lind LJ: Periodontal disease. In *Radiographic interpretation for the dental hygienist*, Philadelphia, 1993, Saunders.

Miles DA, Van Dis ML, Jensen CW, Williamson GF: Basics of interpretation: normal versus abnormal and common radiographic presentation of lesions. In *Radiographic imaging for the dental team*, ed 4, Philadelphia, 2009, Saunders.

Newman MG, Takei H, Carranza FA: Classification of diseases and conditions affecting the periodontium. In *Carranza's clinical periodontology*, ed 10, Philadelphia, 2006, Saunders.

White SC, Pharoah MJ: Periodontal diseases. In *Oral radiology: principles of interpretation*, ed 6, St. Louis, 2009, Mosby.

QUIZ QUESTIONS

IDENTIFICATION

For questions 1 to 5, identify the pattern of bone loss, severity of bone loss, and ADA Case Type (I to IV) represented by each dental image in Figures 34-36 to 34-40.

1. _____

2. _____

3. _____

4. _____

5. _____

MATCHING

For questions 6 to 9, match each of the ADA case types with the appropriate dental image description.

a. Mild crestal changes
b. Bone loss is more than 6 mm apical to the cemento-enamel junction (CEJ)
c. No bone change seen
d. Bone loss is 4 to 6 mm apical to the CEJ

___ 6. ADA Case Type I
___ 7. ADA Case Type II
___ 8. ADA Case Type III
___ 9. ADA Case Type IV

FILL IN THE BLANK

10. A term that refers to tissues that invest and support teeth.

_____

11. A term that means "around a tooth."

_____

12. A term that refers to the area between the roots of multirooted teeth.

_____

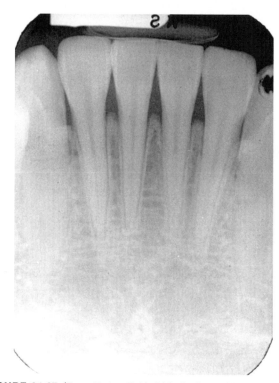

FIGURE 34-37 (From Haring JI, Lind LJ: *Radiographic interpretation for the dental hygienist*, Philadelphia, 1993, Saunders.)

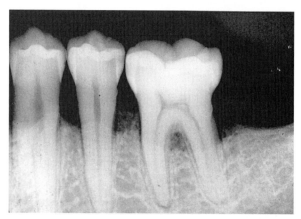

FIGURE 34-36 (From Haring JI, Lind LJ: *Radiographic interpretation for the dental hygienist*, Philadelphia, 1993, Saunders.)

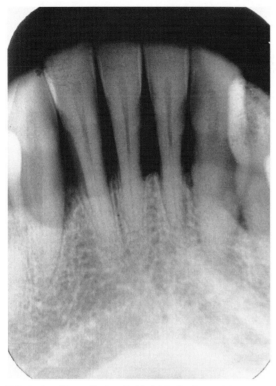

FIGURE 34-38 (From Haring JI, Lind LJ: *Radiographic interpretation for the dental hygienist*, Philadelphia, 1993, Saunders.)

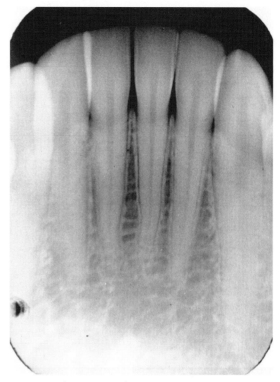

FIGURE 34-40 (From Haring JI, Lind LJ: *Radiographic interpretation for the dental hygienist*, Philadelphia, 1993, Saunders.)

15. The term that describes bone loss that occurs in a plane parallel to the CEJs of adjacent teeth.

___

16. The term that describes bone loss that does not occur in a plane parallel to the CEJs of adjacent teeth.

___

17. The term that describes a group of diseases that affect the tissues found around teeth.

___

18. The term that describes bone loss that occurs in isolated areas.

___

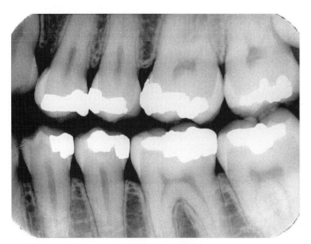

FIGURE 34-39 (From Haring JI, Lind LJ: *Radiographic interpretation for the dental hygienist*, Philadelphia, 1993, Saunders.)

13. The image of choice for the evaluation of periodontal disease.

___

14. The preferred method of exposure for receptors documenting periodontal disease.

___

19. The term that describes bone loss that occurs evenly throughout the arches.

___

20. The term that describes a stonelike concretion that forms on the crowns and roots of teeth as a result of the calcification of plaque.

chapter 35

Interpretation of Trauma, and Pulpal and Periapical Lesions

OUTLINE

TRAUMA VIEWED ON DENTAL IMAGES
    Fractures
    Injuries
RESORPTION VIEWED ON DENTAL IMAGES
    External Resorption
    Internal Resorption

PULPAL LESIONS VIEWED ON DENTAL IMAGES
    Pulpal Sclerosis
    Pulpal Obliteration
    Pulp Stones
PERIAPICAL LESIONS VIEWED ON DENTAL IMAGES
    Periapical Radiolucencies
    Periapical Radiopacities

LEARNING OBJECTIVES

After completion of this chapter, the student will be able to do the following:

- Define the key terms associated with the interpretation of trauma, pulpal lesions, and periapical lesions as viewed on a dental image
- Describe and identify the appearance of crown, root, and jaw fractures as viewed on a dental image
- Describe and identify the appearance of an avulsion as viewed on a dental image
- Describe and identify the appearance of internal and external resorption as viewed on a dental image

- Describe and identify the appearance of pulpal sclerosis, pulpal obliteration, and pulp stones as viewed on a dental image
- Describe and identify the appearance of periapical granuloma, cyst, and abscess as viewed on a dental image
- Describe and identify the appearance of condensing osteitis, sclerotic bone, and hypercementosis as viewed on a dental image

KEY TERMS

Avulsion	Periapical abscess	Pulpal sclerosis
Condensing osteitis	Periapical cyst	Resorption, external
Extrusion	Periapical granuloma	Resorption, internal
Fracture	Periapical lesion	Resorption, pathologic
Hypercementosis	Periodontal abscess	Resorption, physiologic
Intrusion	Pulp stones	Sclerotic bone
Luxation	Pulpal obliteration	Trauma

In many cases, the dental image shows changes and thus acts as a detector. Changes associated with trauma, resorption, and pulpal and periapical lesions can all be viewed on dental images. Dental images allow the dental professional to evaluate areas that cannot be examined clinically, such as the roots, pulp chambers, and periapical regions of teeth. Detailed information about trauma, pulpal lesions, and periapical lesions is beyond the scope of this text. For more complete information on these topics, the dental radiographer should consult a text on interpretation.

The purpose of this chapter is to provide a brief overview of the common features of trauma, pulpal lesions, and periapical lesions as viewed on dental images.

TRAUMA VIEWED ON DENTAL IMAGES

Trauma can be defined as an injury produced by an external force. Trauma may affect the crowns and roots of teeth as well as alveolar bone. Trauma may result in fractures of teeth and

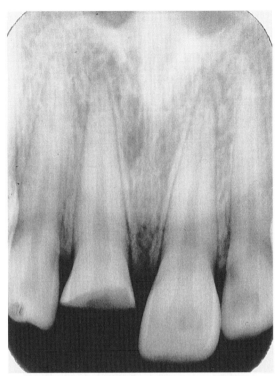

FIGURE 35-1 A fractured central incisor. (From Haring JI, Lind LJ: *Radiographic interpretation for the dental hygienist*, Philadelphia, 1993, Saunders.)

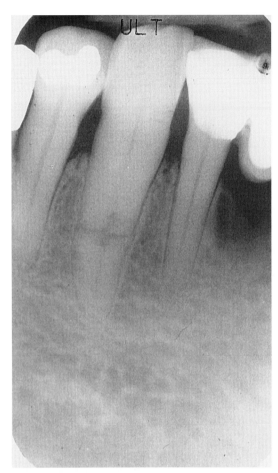

FIGURE 35-2 A root fracture on a mandibular canine. (From Haring JI, Lind LJ: *Radiographic interpretation for the dental hygienist*, Philadelphia, 1993, Saunders.)

bone and injuries such as intrusion, extrusion, and avulsion.

Fractures

A **fracture** can be defined as the breaking of a part. Fractures may affect the crowns and roots of teeth or the bones of the maxilla and the mandible. Whenever a fracture is evident or suspected, dental imaging of the injured area is necessary.

Crown Fractures

Fractures that affect tooth crowns most often involve anterior teeth. Most crown fractures result from a fall or a motor vehicle accident. Crown fractures may involve enamel only; enamel and dentin; or enamel, dentin, and pulp. The missing part of a crown caused by a fracture is evident on a dental image (Figure 35-1). The image allows the dental professional to evaluate the proximity of the pulp chamber to the fracture and to examine the root for any additional fractures.

Root Fractures

Root fractures are less common than crown fractures and also result from an accident or a traumatic blow. Root fractures occur most often in the maxillary central incisor region. Tooth roots may be fractured at any level along the root and may involve more than one root of a multirooted tooth. If the x-ray beam is parallel with the plane of the fracture, the root fracture appears as a sharp radiolucent line on a periapical image (Figure 35-2). If the x-ray beam is not parallel with

the fracture, adjacent areas of the tooth structure obscure the fracture site; as a result, the fracture cannot be seen on the dental image. With time, root fractures have a tendency to enlarge because of displacement of root fragments, hemorrhage, or edema. A root fracture that was initially overlooked may be identified on a later dental image.

Jaw Fractures

Fractures of the mandible occur more often than do fractures of any other bone of the face and frequently as a result of assaults, accidents, and sports injuries. The panoramic image is recommended for the evaluation of mandibular fractures. On a panoramic image, a mandibular fracture appears as a radiolucent line at the site where the bone has separated (Figure 35-3). Fractures of the maxilla occur less frequently than do mandibular fractures and most often involve anterior alveolar bone and teeth. Maxillary fractures are typically difficult to detect on a dental image.

Injuries

In addition to fractures, trauma may result in the displacement of teeth. Dental images enable the dental professional to evaluate structures after tooth displacement. Tooth

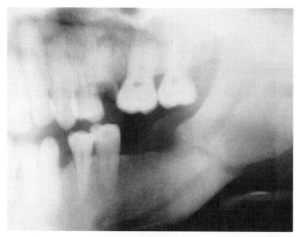

FIGURE 35-3 A fractured mandible. (From Haring JI, Lind LJ: *Radiographic interpretation for the dental hygienist*, Philadelphia, 1993, Saunders.)

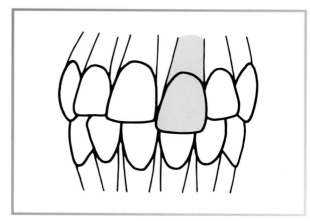

FIGURE 35-5 An extruded crown. (From Haring JI, Lind LJ: *Radiographic interpretation for the dental hygienist*, Philadelphia, 1993, Saunders.)

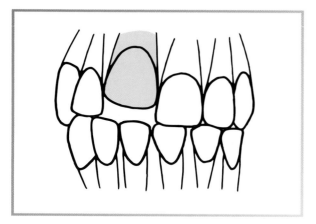

FIGURE 35-4 An intruded crown. (From Haring JI, Lind LJ: *Radiographic interpretation for the dental hygienist*, Philadelphia, 1993, Saunders.)

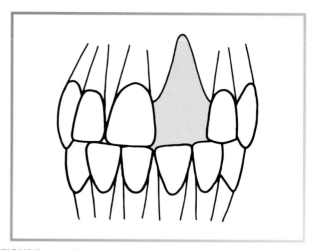

FIGURE 35-6 Empty tooth socket, with avulsion, seen on a dental radiograph. (From Haring JI, Lind LJ: *Radiographic interpretation for the dental hygienist*, Philadelphia, 1993, Saunders.)

displacement includes luxation (intrusion or extrusion) and avulsion.

Luxation

Luxation, the abnormal displacement of teeth, can be categorized as either intrusion or extrusion. **Intrusion** refers to the abnormal displacement of teeth *into* bone (Figure 35-4). **Extrusion** refers to the abnormal displacement of teeth *out of* bone (Figure 35-5). Teeth that have been luxated should be evaluated using a periapical image and examined for root and adjacent alveolar bone fractures, damage to the periodontal ligament, and pulpal problems.

Avulsion

Avulsion is the complete displacement of a tooth from alveolar bone. Most avulsions result from trauma associated with assault or accidental fall. An avulsed tooth is not actually seen on a dental image; instead, a periapical image shows a tooth socket without a tooth (Figure 35-6). Dental images are important in the evaluation of the socket area and should be used to examine the region for splintered bone.

RESORPTION VIEWED ON DENTAL IMAGES

Two types of resorption are associated with teeth: physiologic and pathologic.

Physiologic resorption is a process that is seen with the normal shedding of primary teeth. The roots of a primary tooth are resorbed as the permanent successor moves in an occlusal direction; the primary tooth is shed when resorption of the roots is complete (Figure 35-7).

Pathologic resorption is a regressive alteration of tooth structure that is observed when a tooth is subjected to abnormal stimuli.

Resorption of teeth can be described as external or internal, depending on the location of the resorption process.

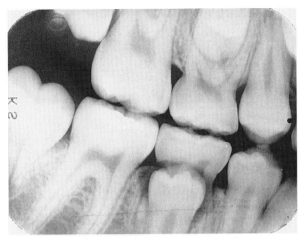

FIGURE 35-7 Physiologic resorption of a mandibular deciduous second molar. (From Haring JI, Lind LJ: *Radiographic interpretation for the dental hygienist*, Philadelphia, 1993, Saunders.)

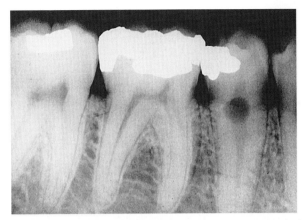

FIGURE 35-9 Internal resorption seen as a round radiolucency in the cervical region of a mandibular second premolar. (From Haring JI, Lind LJ: *Radiographic interpretation for the dental hygienist*, Philadelphia, 1993, Saunders.)

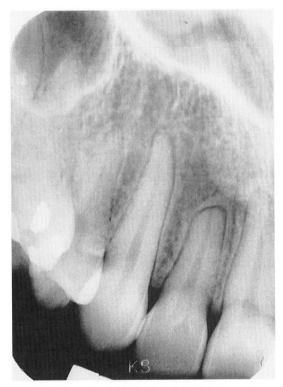

FIGURE 35-8 External resorption of the apical region of a maxillary lateral incisor. (From Haring JI, Lind LJ: *Radiographic interpretation for the dental hygienist*, Philadelphia, 1993, Saunders.)

External Resorption

External resorption is seen along the periphery of the root surface and is often associated with reimplanted teeth, abnormal mechanical forces, trauma, chronic inflammation, tumors and cysts, impacted teeth, or idiopathic causes. External resorption most often affects the apices of teeth; the apical region appears blunted, and the length of the root appears shorter than normal (Figure 35-8). Both the lamina dura and the bone around the blunted apex appear normal.

External resorption is not associated with any signs or symptoms and is not detected clinically. Teeth that undergo external resorption do not exhibit mobility. Currently, no effective treatment is available for external resorption.

Internal Resorption

Internal resorption occurs within the crown or root of a tooth and involves the pulp chamber, pulp canals, and surrounding dentin. Precipitating factors such as trauma, pulp capping, and pulp polyps are believed to stimulate the internal resorption process. Internal resorption appears as a round-to-ovoid radiolucency in the midcrown or midroot portion of a tooth (Figures 35-9 and 35-10).

Internal resorption is generally asymptomatic. Treatment is variable; endodontic therapy may be used if the resorptive process has not physically weakened the tooth. If the tooth is weakened by the resorptive process, extraction is recommended.

PULPAL LESIONS VIEWED ON DENTAL IMAGES

Many dental procedures require information about the size and location of the pulp cavity before treatment begins. Without dental images, examination of pulp chambers and canals is impossible. Pulpal sclerosis, pulpal obliteration, and pulp stones are common conditions of the pulp cavity that can be seen on dental images.

Pulpal Sclerosis

Pulpal sclerosis, a diffuse calcification of the pulp chamber and pulp canals of teeth, results in a pulp cavity of decreased size (Figure 35-11). For unknown reasons, pulpal sclerosis is associated with aging. No clinical features are associated with pulpal sclerosis; it is generally considered an incidental finding that is of little clinical significance unless endodontic therapy is indicated.

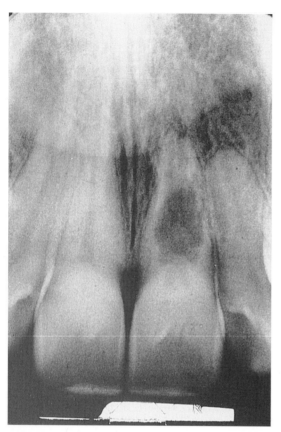

FIGURE 35-10 Internal resorption seen as a radiolucency in the root of a maxillary central incisor. (From Haring JI, Lind LJ: *Radiographic interpretation for the dental hygienist*, Philadelphia, 1993, Saunders.)

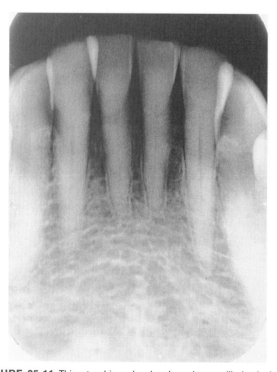

FIGURE 35-11 Thin atrophic pulp chambers in mandibular incisors. (From Haring JI, Lind LJ: *Radiographic interpretation for the dental hygienist*, Philadelphia, 1993, Saunders.)

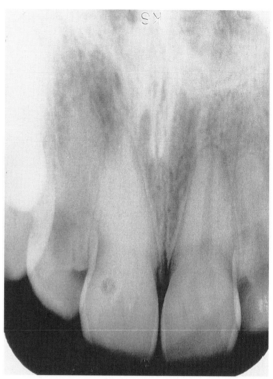

FIGURE 35-12 Pulpal obliteration in a maxillary central incisor. (From Haring JI, Lind LJ: *Radiographic interpretation for the dental hygienist*, Philadelphia, 1993, Saunders.)

Pulpal Obliteration

Some conditions (e.g., attrition, abrasion, caries, dental restorations, trauma, abnormal mechanical forces) may act as irritants to the pulp and stimulate the production of secondary dentin, which results in obliteration of the pulp cavity. On a dental image, a tooth with **pulpal obliteration** does not appear to have a pulp chamber or pulp canals (Figure 35-12). Teeth that exhibit pulpal obliteration are nonvital and therefore do not require treatment.

Pulp Stones

Pulp stones are calcifications that are found in the pulp chamber or pulp canals of teeth. The cause of pulp stones is unknown. On a dental image, pulp stones appear as round, ovoid, or cylindrical radiopacities; some pulp stones may conform to the shape of the pulp chamber or canal (Figures 35-13 and 35-14). Pulp stones may vary in shape, size, and number. Pulp stones do not cause any problems and therefore do not require treatment.

PERIAPICAL LESIONS VIEWED ON DENTAL IMAGES

A **periapical lesion** is a lesion that is located around the apex (tip of the root) of a tooth. The use of dental imaging is particularly important in the identification of periapical problems. Periapical lesions cannot be evaluated on a clinical

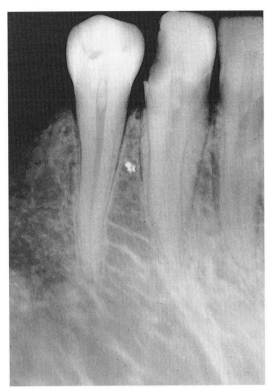

FIGURE 35-13 Cylindrical pulp stones in the mandibular canine and premolar. (From Haring JI, Lind LJ: *Radiographic interpretation for the dental hygienist*, Philadelphia, 1993, Saunders.)

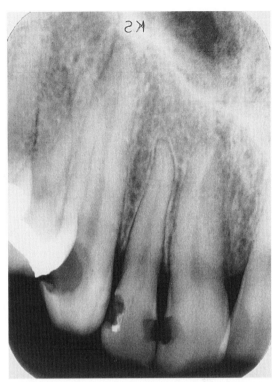

FIGURE 35-15 A widened periodontal ligament space at the apex of a maxillary lateral incisor. (From Haring JI, Lind LJ: *Radiographic interpretation for the dental hygienist*, Philadelphia, 1993, Saunders.)

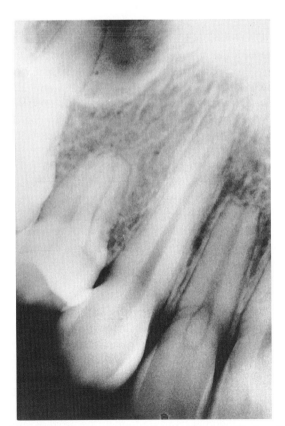

FIGURE 35-14 An ovoid pulp stone in a maxillary lateral incisor. (From Haring JI, Lind LJ: *Radiographic interpretation for the dental hygienist*, Philadelphia, 1993, Saunders.)

basis alone. On dental images, periapical lesions may appear either *radiolucent* (dark or black) or *radiopaque* (light or white).

Periapical Radiolucencies

Periapical granulomas, cysts, and abscesses are common periapical radiolucencies that can be seen on dental images. These lesions cannot be diagnosed by their appearances alone; instead, diagnosis is based on clinical features, dental imaging, and microscopic appearances. Because it is impossible to distinguish these three periapical lesions based on their dental image features, the dental radiographer should refer to these lesions simply as "periapical radiolucencies."

Periapical Granuloma

A **periapical granuloma** is a localized mass of chronically inflamed granulation tissue at the apex of a nonvital tooth. It results from pulpal death and necrosis and is the most common sequela of *pulpitis* (inflammation of the pulp). A periapical granuloma may give rise to a periapical cyst or periapical abscess. A tooth with a periapical granuloma is typically asymptomatic but has a previous history of prolonged sensitivity to heat or cold. Treatment for a periapical granuloma may include endodontic therapy or removal of the tooth with curettage of the apical region.

On a dental image, a periapical granuloma is initially seen as a widened periodontal ligament space at the root apex (Figure 35-15). With time, the widened periodontal ligament

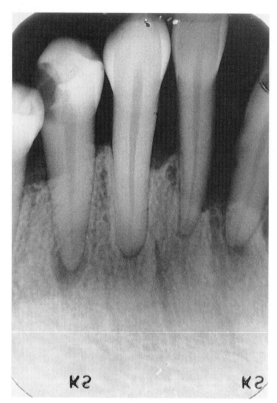

FIGURE 35-16 A periapical radiolucency associated with a mandibular premolar. (Note that the lamina dura is not visible.) (From Haring JI, Lind LJ: *Radiographic interpretation for the dental hygienist*, Philadelphia, 1993, Saunders.)

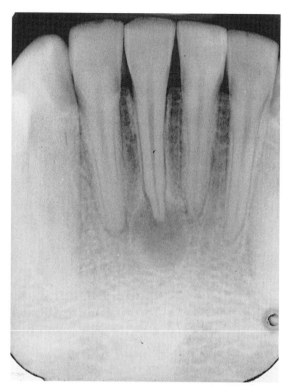

FIGURE 35-17 A well-defined round radiolucency seen at the apex of a mandibular central incisor. (From Haring JI, Lind LJ: *Radiographic interpretation for the dental hygienist*, Philadelphia, 1993, Saunders.)

space enlarges and appears as a round or ovoid radiolucency (Figure 35-16). The lamina dura is not visible between the root apex and the apical lesion.

Periapical Cyst

A **periapical cyst** (also known as a *radicular cyst*) is a lesion that develops over a prolonged period; cystic degeneration takes place within a periapical granuloma and results in a periapical cyst. The periapical cyst results from pulpal death and necrosis. Periapical cysts are the most common of all tooth-related cysts and comprise 50% to 70% of all cysts in the oral region. Periapical cysts are typically asymptomatic. Treatment may include endodontic therapy or extraction of the tooth as well as curettage of the apical region. On a dental image, the typical periapical cyst appears as a round or ovoid radiolucency (Figure 35-17).

Periapical Abscess

A **periapical abscess** is a localized collection of pus in the periapical region of a tooth that results from pulpal death. Periapical abscesses may be acute or chronic. An *acute* periapical abscess has features of an acute pus-producing process and inflammation. An acute abscess may result from an acute inflammation of the pulp or an area of chronic infection, such as a periapical granuloma. A *chronic* periapical abscess has features of a long-standing, low-grade, pus-producing

process. A chronic abscess may develop from an acute abscess or a periapical granuloma.

An acute periapical abscess is painful; the pain may be intense, throbbing, and constant. The tooth is nonvital and is sensitive to pressure, percussion, and heat. Chronic periapical abscesses are usually asymptomatic because the pus drains through bone or the periodontal ligament space. Clinically, a *gum boil* (parulis) may be seen in the apical region of the tooth at the site of drainage. Treatment of the periapical abscess includes drainage and endodontic therapy or extraction.

With an acute periapical abscess, no change may be evident on a dental image. Early changes viewed on dental images include increased widening of the periodontal ligament space (Figure 35-18). A chronic periapical abscess appears as a round or ovoid apical radiolucency with poorly defined margins (Figure 35-19). The lamina dura cannot be seen between the root apex and the radiolucent lesion.

It is important to differentiate between a periapical abscess and a periodontal abscess. A **periodontal abscess** results from bacterial infection within the walls of periodontal tissues and typically results from a pre-existing periodontal condition. The most common symptom of a periodontal abscess is pain. Therapy includes deep scaling and débridement of periodontal tissues, although the prognosis for the tooth's periodontal health depends on the amount of bone loss and mobility.

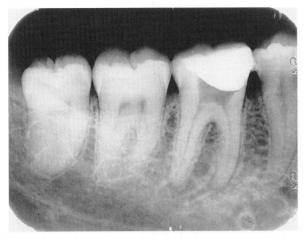

FIGURE 35-18 An increased widening of the periodontal ligament space seen in the periapical region of the mandibular first molar. (From Haring JI, Lind LJ: *Radiographic interpretation for the dental hygienist*, Philadelphia, 1993, Saunders.)

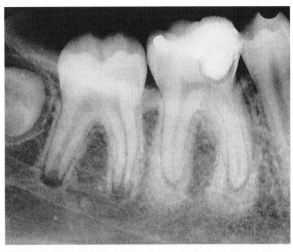

FIGURE 35-20 A diffuse radiopacity seen along the roots of a mandibular first molar. (From Haring JI, Lind LJ: *Radiographic interpretation for the dental hygienist*, Philadelphia, 1993, Saunders.)

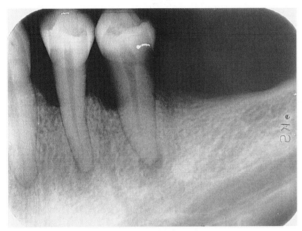

FIGURE 35-19 Periapical radiolucencies associated with mandibular premolars. (From Haring JI, Lind LJ: *Radiographic interpretation for the dental hygienist*, Philadelphia, 1993, Saunders.)

To summarize, the term *periapical abscess* refers to an infection in the pulp of a tooth; *periodontal abscess* refers to a purulent inflammation within periodontal tissues.

Periapical Radiopacities

Condensing osteitis, sclerotic bone, and hypercementosis are some common periapical radiopacities seen on dental images. Unlike periapical radiolucencies, periapical radiopacities can be diagnosed on the basis of dental images, clinical information, and patient history.

Condensing Osteitis

Condensing osteitis (also known as *chronic focal sclerosing osteomyelitis*) is a well-defined radiopacity that is seen below the apex of a nonvital tooth with a history of long-standing pulpitis (Figure 35-20). The opacity represents a proliferation of periapical bone that is a result of low-grade inflammation or mild irritation. The inflammation that

stimulates condensing osteitis occurs in response to pulpal necrosis. Condensing osteitis may vary in size and shape and does not appear to be attached to the tooth root.

Condensing osteitis is the most common periapical radiopacity observed in adults. The tooth most frequently involved is the mandibular first molar. Teeth associated with condensing osteitis are nonvital and typically have a large carious lesion or a large restoration. Because condensing osteitis is believed to represent only a physiologic reaction of bone to inflammation, no treatment is necessary.

Sclerotic Bone

Sclerotic bone (also known as *osteosclerosis* or *idiopathic periapical osteosclerosis*) is a well-defined radiopacity that is seen below the apices of vital, noncarious teeth (Figure 35-21). The cause of sclerotic bone is unknown; however, it is not believed to be associated with inflammation. The lesion is not attached to a tooth and varies in size and shape. The margins may appear smooth or irregular and diffuse. The borders are continuous with adjacent normal bone, and no radiolucent outline is seen. Sclerotic bone is asymptomatic and is usually discovered during routine dental imaging.

Hypercementosis

Hypercementosis is the excessive deposition of cementum on root surfaces. Hypercementosis results from supra-eruption, inflammation, or trauma; sometimes there is no obvious cause. On dental images, hypercementosis is visible as an excessive amount of cementum along all or part of a root surface (Figure 35-22). The apical area is most often affected and appears enlarged and bulbous. Root areas affected by hypercementosis are separated from periapical bone by a normal-appearing periodontal ligament space; the surrounding lamina dura appears normal as well.

No signs or symptoms are associated with hypercementosis; most cases are discovered during routine dental imaging.

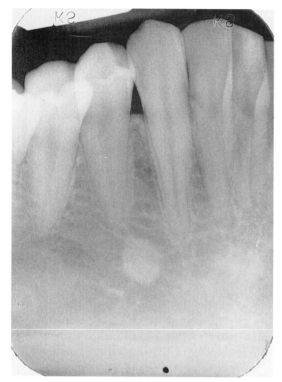

FIGURE 35-21 A well-defined radiopacity below the apex of a mandibular premolar. (From Haring JI, Lind LJ: *Radiographic interpretation for the dental hygienist*, Philadelphia, 1993, Saunders.)

Teeth affected by hypercementosis are vital and do not require treatment.

SUMMARY

- Changes associated with trauma, resorption, and pulpal and periapical lesions can be viewed on dental images.
- Dental imaging allows the dental professional to evaluate the roots, pulp cavities, and periapical regions of teeth, all of which are areas that cannot be examined clinically.
- Dental imaging is important in the evaluation of trauma and injury and can be used for diagnostic, treatment, and post-treatment purposes.
- Dental imaging is useful in the evaluation of tooth and jaw fractures and of tooth injuries, including intrusion, extrusion, and avulsion.
- Dental imaging is useful in identifying regressive alterations of teeth, such as external and internal resorption. These alterations are usually asymptomatic and discovered only through dental imaging.
- Dental imaging is also useful in examining and in obtaining information about the pulp cavity. Pulpal sclerosis, obliteration of the pulp cavity, and pulp stones are common conditions that can be viewed on dental images.
- Periapical lesions cannot be examined without the aid of dental images. Examples include periapical granulomas, periapical cysts, periapical abscesses, condensing osteitis, sclerotic bone, and hypercementosis.

BIBLIOGRAPHY

Frommer HH, Savage-Stabulas JJ: Pulpal and periapical lesions. In *Radiology for the dental professional*, ed 9, St. Louis, 2011, Mosby.

Haring JI, Lind LJ: Trauma, pulpal and periapical lesions. In *Radiographic interpretation for the dental hygienist*, Philadelphia, 1993, Saunders.

Herrera D, Roldán S, Sanz M: The periodontal abscess: A review, *J Clin Periodontol* 27(6):377–386, 2000.

Johnson ON, McNally MA, Essay CE: Preliminary interpretation of the radiographs. In *Essentials of dental radiography for dental assistants and hygienists*, ed 8, Upper Saddle River, NJ, 2007, Pearson Education, Inc.

Manson-Hing LR: Interpretation and value of radiographs. In *Fundamentals of dental radiography*, ed 3, Philadelphia, 1990, Lea & Febiger.

Miles DA, Van Dis ML, Jensen CW, Williamson GF: Basics of interpretation: normal versus abnormal and common radiographic presentation. In *Radiographic imaging for the dental team*, ed 4, Philadelphia, 2009, Saunders.

White SC, Pharoah MJ: Inflammatory lesions of the jaws. In *Oral radiology: principles of interpretation*, ed 6, St. Louis, 2009, Mosby.

White SC, Pharoah MJ: Trauma to teeth and facial structures. In *Oral radiology: principles of interpretation*, ed 6, St. Louis, 2009, Mosby.

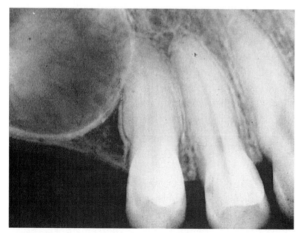

FIGURE 35-22 Hypercementosis of a maxillary premolar. (From Haring JI, Lind LJ: *Radiographic interpretation for the dental hygienist*, Philadelphia, 1993, Saunders.)

QUIZ QUESTIONS

MATCHING

For questions 1 to 6, match the terms with the appropriate definition.

a. Abnormal displacement of teeth
b. An injury produced by an external force
c. Complete displacement of a tooth from alveolar bone
d. Abnormal displacement of teeth out of bone
e. The breaking of a part
f. Abnormal displacement of teeth into bone

____ **1.** Trauma
____ **2.** Fracture
____ **3.** Luxation
____ **4.** Intrusion
____ **5.** Extrusion
____ **6.** Avulsion

IDENTIFICATION

For questions 7 to 12, refer to Figures 35-23 to 35-28. Identify or describe the periapical and pulpal lesions shown in each figure.

7. _____

8. _____

9. _____

10. _____

11. _____

12. _____

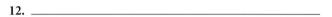

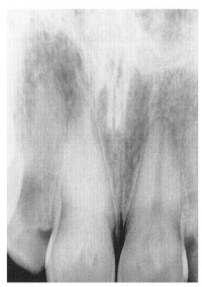

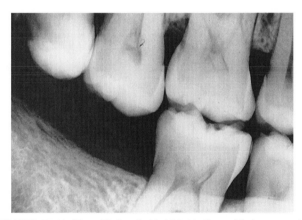

FIGURE 35-23 (From Haring JI, Lind LJ: *Radiographic interpretation for the dental hygienist*, Philadelphia, 1993, Saunders.)

FIGURE 35-25 (From Haring JI, Lind LJ: *Radiographic interpretation for the dental hygienist*, Philadelphia, 1993, Saunders.)

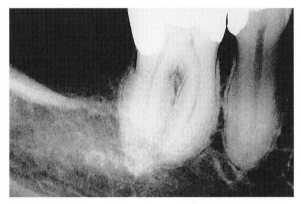

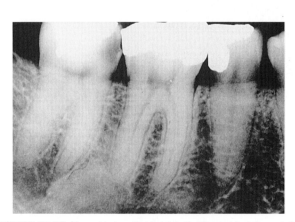

FIGURE 35-24 (From Haring JI, Lind LJ: *Radiographic interpretation for the dental hygienist*, Philadelphia, 1993, Saunders.)

FIGURE 35-26 (From Haring JI, Lind LJ: *Radiographic interpretation for the dental hygienist*, Philadelphia, 1993, Saunders.)

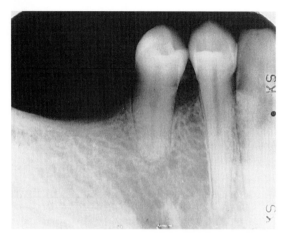

FIGURE 35-27 (From Haring JI, Lind LJ: *Radiographic interpretation for the dental hygienist*, Philadelphia, 1993, Saunders.)

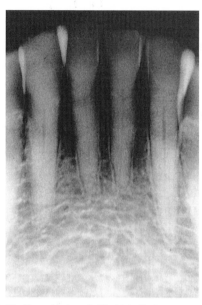

FIGURE 35-28 (From Haring JI, Lind LJ: *Radiographic interpretation for the dental hygienist*, Philadelphia, 1993, Saunders.)

Glossary

Absorption The total transfer of energy from the x-ray photon to the atoms of matter through which the x-ray beam passes. Absorption depends on the energy of the x-ray beam and the composition of the absorbing matter or tissues.

Accelerator One of the basic ingredients of the developer solution; sodium carbonate activates and provides an alkaline environment for the developing agents and softens the film emulsion.

Acetic acid See **Acidifier**.

Acidifier One of the basic ingredients of the fixer solution (e.g., acetic acid or sulfuric acid); the acidifier neutralizes the alkaline developer and stops further action of the developer.

ADA Case Types The American Dental Association categorization of periodontal disease used by the American Academy of Periodontology; four categories are described: ADA Case Types I, II, III, and IV.

Adhesive layer A thin layer of adhesive material that covers both sides of the receptor base and attaches the emulsion to the base.

Air bubbles A film handling error; white spots appear on a film as a result of trapped air that remains on the film surface after the film has been placed in the processing solution.

ALARA concept A concept of radiation protection that states that all exposure to radiation must be kept to a minimum, or "as low as reasonably achievable."

Alignment, object-receptor One of the influencing factors for image distortion that refers to the alignment of the tooth and receptor; less image distortion results when the tooth and receptor are parallel to each other.

Alpha particles A type of particulate radiation emitted from the nuclei of heavy metals; alpha particles contain two protons and two neutrons and are positively charged.

Aluminum discs Discs or sheets of aluminum, usually 0.5 mm thick, that are placed in the path of the x-ray beam; filter out the nonpenetrating, longer-wavelength x-rays.

Alveolar bone Bone of the maxilla and the mandible that supports and encases the roots of teeth; appears radiopaque.

Alveolar bone loss A loss of bone that surrounds and supports teeth in the maxilla or the mandible.

Alveolar crest The most coronal portion of alveolar bone found between teeth; composed of dense cortical bone and appears radiopaque (also known as *crestal bone*).

Alveolar process Portion of the mandible that encases and supports teeth.

Amalgam Most common restorative material used in dentistry.

Ammonium thiosulfate A chemical found in the fixing agent that clears the unexposed, undeveloped silver halide crystals from the film emulsion.

Amperage The number of electrons that pass through a conductor; the strength of an electrical current.

Ampere (A) The unit of measure used to describe the number of electrons passing through a conductor (electrical current strength); the intensity of an electric current produced by 1 volt acting through a resistance of 1 ohm.

Analog image A radiographic image produced by conventional film.

Anatomic order The order in which teeth are arranged within the dental arches.

Angle In geometry, a figure formed by two lines diverging from a common point.

Angle, right In geometry, an angle of 90 degrees formed by two lines perpendicular to each other.

Angle of mandible Area of the mandible where the body meets the ramus.

Angulation The alignment of the central x-ray beam in the horizontal and vertical planes.

Angulation, horizontal The positioning of the position-indicating device (PID) and direction of the central ray in a horizontal, or side-to-side, plane.

Angulation, negative vertical The positioning of the position-indicating device (PID) below the occlusal plane that directs the central ray upward.

Angulation, positive vertical The positioning of the position-indicating device (PID) above the occlusal plane that directs the central ray downward.

Angulation, vertical Positioning of the position-indicating device (PID) in a vertical, or up and down, plane.

Anode The positive electrode in the x-ray tube; consists of a wafer-thin tungsten plate embedded in a solid copper rod; converts electrons into x-ray photons.

Anterior nasal spine A sharp projection of the maxilla located at the anteroinferior portion of the nasal cavity; appears radiopaque.

Antiseptic A substance that inhibits the growth of bacteria.

Articular eminence A rounded projection of the temporal bone located anterior to the glenoid fossa.

Asepsis The absence of pathogens or disease-causing microorganisms.

Atom A tiny, invisible particle that is the fundamental unit of matter; the smallest part of an element that has the properties of that element.

Atom, neutral An atom that contains an equal number of protons (positive charges) and electrons (negative charges).

Atomic number The total number of protons in the nucleus, which is also equal to the number of electrons outside of the nucleus.

Atomic weight The total number of protons and neutrons in the nucleus of an atom (also known as *mass number*).

Autotransformer A voltage compensator that corrects for minor fluctuations in the current flowing through the x-ray machine.

Avulsion The complete displacement of a tooth from alveolar bone.

Barrier envelope A plastic shield that protects an intraoral receptor from saliva and is used to minimize contamination.

Beam alignment device A device used to align the position-indicating device (PID) in relation to tooth and receptor; positions the intraoral receptor in the mouth and retains the receptor in position during exposure; helps stabilize the receptor in the mouth and reduces the chances of movement, thus reducing the patient's exposure to x-radiation.

Beta particles Fast-moving electrons emitted from the nucleus of radioactive atoms.

Binding energy The attraction between the positive nucleus and the negative electrons that maintains electrons in their orbits; determined by the distance between the nucleus and electrons (also known as *electrostatic force* or *binding force*).

Bisect To divide into two equal parts.

Bisecting technique An intraoral radiographic technique used to expose periapical receptors: the receptor is placed along lingual surface of the tooth; the central ray of x-ray beam is directed perpendicular to the imaginary bisector formed by the receptor and the long axis of the tooth; and receptor holder or the patient's finger is used to stabilize the receptor.

Bisector, imaginary An imaginary plane that divides in half the angle formed by the receptor and the long axis of the tooth; creates two equal angles and provides a common side for the two imaginary equal triangles.

Bit-depth image The number of possible gray-scale combinations for each pixel.

Bite-wing, horizontal The bite-wing receptor is placed in the mouth with the long portion of the receptor in a horizontal direction.

Bite-wing, vertical The bite-wing receptor is placed in the mouth with the long portion of the receptor in a vertical direction.

Bite-wing tab A heavy paperboard tab or loop fitted around an intraoral receptor and used to stabilize the receptor during the exposure (also known as *bite loop* or *bite tab*).

Bite-wing technique An intraoral radiographic technique in which the interproximal surfaces of teeth are examined; also known as *interproximal technique*.

Bloodborne pathogens Microorganisms present in blood that cause disease in humans.

Body of mandible The body of the mandible is the horizontal, U-shaped portion that extends from ramus to ramus.

Bone loss, angular See **Bone loss, vertical**.

Bone loss, generalized Bone loss occurring evenly throughout the dental arches.

Bone loss, horizontal Bone loss that occurs in a plane parallel to the cemento-enamel junctions of adjacent teeth.

Bone loss, localized Bone loss occurring in isolated areas.

Bone loss, mild Bone loss appearing as crestal changes.

Bone loss, moderate Bone loss of 10% to 33%, measured on a dental radiograph.

Bone loss, severe Bone loss of 33% or more, measured on a dental radiograph.

Bone loss, vertical Bone loss that does not occur in a plane parallel to the cemento-enamel junctions of adjacent teeth (also known as *angular bone loss*).

Bremsstrahlung See **Radiation, general**.

Buccal object rule Governs the orientation of structures portrayed in two images exposed at different angulations; used to determine the buccal–lingual relationship of an object.

Calculus A stonelike concretion that forms on the crowns and roots of teeth as a result of the calcification of bacterial plaque; appears radiopaque.

Canal A tubelike passageway through bone that houses nerves and blood vessels; appears radiolucent.

Cancellous Refers to a latticelike structure; the soft, spongy bone located between two layers of dense cortical bone; appears radiolucent.

Caries Tooth decay caused by microorganisms; appears radiolucent.

Caries, buccal Caries found on the buccal tooth surface.

Caries, interproximal Caries found between two adjacent teeth.

Caries, interproximal advanced Caries found between two teeth that extends to the dentino-enamel junction (DEJ) or through the DEJ and into dentin but does not extend through the dentin more than half the distance toward the pulp.

Caries, interproximal incipient Caries found between two teeth that extends less than halfway through the thickness of enamel.

Caries, interproximal moderate Caries found between two teeth that extends more than halfway through the thickness of enamel but does not involve the dentino-enamel junction (DEJ).

Caries, interproximal severe Caries found between two teeth that extends through enamel, through dentin, and more than half the distance toward the pulp.

Caries, lingual Caries found on the lingual tooth surface.

Caries, occlusal Caries found on the chewing surface of posterior teeth.

Caries, occlusal incipient Caries found on the chewing surface of posterior teeth; cannot be seen on a dental radiograph.

Caries, occlusal moderate Caries found on the chewing surface of posterior teeth that extends into dentin; appears as a thin radiolucent line.

Caries, occlusal severe Caries found on the chewing surface of posterior teeth that extends into dentin; appears as a large radiolucency.

Caries, rampant Caries that affects numerous teeth in the dentition.

Caries, recurrent Caries found adjacent to a pre-existing restoration (also known as *secondary caries*).

Caries, root surface Caries found on the roots of teeth.

Cassette A light-tight device used in extraoral radiography to hold the film and intensifying screens.

Cathode The negative electrode in the x-ray tube; consists of a tungsten wire filament in a molybdenum cup; supplies the electrons necessary to generate x-rays.

Cathode ray A stream of high-speed electrons that originates from the cathode in an x-ray tube.

Cavitation A hole or cavity in a tooth that results from the caries process; appears radiolucent.

Cavity See **Cavitation**.

Cell The basic structural unit of living organisms.

Cell differentiation Individual characteristics of a cell that determine the response of the cell to radiation exposure (e.g., cells that are immature [not highly specialized] are more sensitive to radiation).

Cell metabolism The physical and chemical processes of a cell that determine the response of the cell to radiation exposure (e.g., cells with a high metabolic rate are more sensitive to radiation).

Central ray The central portion of the primary beam of x-radiation.

Cephalostat In extraoral radiography, a device that includes a receptor holder and head positioner that allow the dental radiographer to position both receptor and patient easily.

Chairside manner The manner in which a dental professional conducts himself or herself at the chairside of a patient.

Charge-coupled device (CCD) A solid-state detector used in many devices (e.g., fax machine, home video camera); in digital radiography, a CCD is an image receptor found in the intraoral sensor.

Circuit A path of electrical current.

Circuit, filament The circuit that regulates the flow of electrical current to the filament of the x-ray tube; controlled by the milliampere settings (also known as *low-voltage circuit*).

Circuit, high-voltage The circuit that provides the high voltage required to accelerate electrons and to generate x-rays in the x-ray tube; controlled by the kilovoltage settings.

Circuit, low-voltage See **Circuit, filament**.

Clinical attachment loss (CAL) The measurement in millimeters of the distance between the cemento-enamel junction (CEJ) and the base of the sulcus or periodontal pocket; measurement of bone loss.

Coherent scatter One of the interactions of x-radiation with matter in which the path of an low-energy x-ray photon interacts with an outer-shell electron. No change in the atom occurs, and an x-ray photon of scattered radiation is produced (also known as *unmodified scatter*).

Collimating device See **Collimator**.

Collimation The restriction of the size and shape of the x-ray beam in order to reduce patient exposure.

Collimator A diaphragm, usually made of lead, used to restrict the size and shape of the x-ray beam.

Communication The process by which information is exchanged between two or more persons.

Compartment, developer A component part of the automatic processor that holds the developer solution.

Compartment, fixer A component part of the automatic processor that holds the fixer solution.

Compartment, water A component part of the automatic processor that holds circulating water.

Complementary metal oxide semiconductor/active pixel sensor (CMOS/APS) Silicon-based dectector used in digital imaging; differs from the charge-coupled device (CCD) detector in the way that the pixels are read.

Complete mouth radiographic series (CMRS) An intraoral series of dental radiographs that show all the tooth-bearing areas of the upper and lower jaws (also known as *full mouth series or complete series*).

Compton electron An outer-shell electron that is ejected from its orbit during Compton scatter; this electron carries a negative charge.

Compton scatter One of the interactions of x-radiation with matter in which the x-ray photon collides with a loosely bound, outer-shell electron and gives up part of its energy to eject the electron from its orbit. The x-ray photon loses energy and continues in a different direction at a lower energy level.

Condensing osteitis A well-defined radiopacity seen below the apex of a nonvital tooth that has a history of long-standing pulpitis (also known as *chronic focal sclerosing osteomyelitis*); appears radiopaque.

Cone beam computer tomography (CBCT) Computer-assisted digital imaging in dentistry; this imaging technique uses a cone-shaped x-ray beam to acquire information and present it in three dimensions.

Cone-beam technology A three-dimensional imaging technique that uses a cone-shaped radiation beam to acquire a digital image.

Cone beam volume tomography (CBVT) Computer-assisted digital imaging in dentistry; used interchangeably with cone beam volume imaging (CBVI); terms used to differentiate this procedure from medical computer tomography.

Cone-cut A clear, unexposed area on a dental radiograph that occurs when the position-indicating device (PID) is misaligned and the x-ray beam is not centered over the film.

Confidential Private; in dental radiography, information contained in the dental record is confidential.

Contact areas The area where adjacent tooth surfaces contact each other.

Contacts, open On a dental radiograph, open contacts appear as a thin radiolucent line between adjacent tooth surfaces.

Contacts, overlapped On a dental image, the area where the contact area of one tooth is superimposed over the contact area of an adjacent tooth.

Contrast How sharply dark and light areas are differentiated or separated on an image; the difference in the degrees of blackness (densities) between adjacent areas on a dental radiograph.

Contrast, high A term describing an image with many very dark areas and very light areas and few shades of gray.

Contrast, long-scale A term describing an image with many densities, or many shades of gray; long-scale contrast results from the use of a higher kilovoltage range.

Contrast, low A term describing an image with many shades of gray and few areas of black and white.

Contrast, receptor The characteristics of the receptor that influence radiographic contrast; includes the inherent qualities of the receptor and receptor processing and the qualities of the sensor.

Contrast, scale of The range of useful densities seen on a dental image.

Contrast, short-scale A term describing an image with only two densities, areas of black and white; short-scale contrast results from the use of a lower kilovoltage range.

Contrast, subject The characteristics of the subject that influence radiographic contrast; characteristics include thickness, density, and composition of the subject.

Control devices The components of the control panel of the x-ray machine that regulate the x-ray beam; includes the timer, kilovoltage, and milliamperage selectors.

Control panel A part of the dental x-ray machine that contains an on-off switch and an indicator light, an exposure button and indicator light, and control devices to regulate the x-ray beam.

Copper stem A portion of the anode that dissipates heat away from the tungsten target.

Coronoid notch A scooped-out concavity of bone located distal to the coronoid process on the ramus of the mandible.

Coronoid process A marked prominence of bone located on the anterior ramus of the mandible; appears radiopaque.

Cortical The dense outer layer of bone; appears radiopaque. Also known as *compact bone*.

Coulomb (C) A unit of electrical charge; the quantity of electrical charge transferred by 1 ampere in 1 second.

Coulombs per kilogram (C/kg) The unit of measurement used to describe the number of electrical charges, or the number of ion pairs, in 1 kilogram of air.

Crestal bone See **Alveolar crest**.

Critical organ An organ that, if damaged, diminishes the quality of an individual's life (e.g., skin, thyroid gland, lens of the eye, bone marrow).

Cumulative effects The additive effects of repeated radiation exposure.

Current, alternating (AC) A current in which electrons flow in opposite directions.

Current, direct (DC) A current in which electrons flow in one direction.

Darkroom A completely darkened room where x-ray film is handled and processed.

Darkroom plumbing Plumbing in the darkroom that includes hot and cold water and mixing valves to adjust water temperature.

Darkroom storage space An area in the darkroom used to store chemical processing solutions, film cassettes, and other miscellaneous supplies.

Darkroom work space A clean counter area where films can be unwrapped before processing.

Daylight loader A light-shielded compartment on an automatic film processor; films can be unwrapped in a daylight loader in a room with white light.

Density The overall darkness or blackness of an image.

Dentin The tooth layer found beneath the enamel and surrounding the pulp cavity; appears radiopaque.

Dentino-enamel junction (DEJ) The junction between the dentin and enamel of a tooth.

Dentulous With teeth; areas that exhibit teeth.

Developer cutoff A film-handling error; a straight white border appears on a film as a result of using too low a level of developer solution during processing; represents an undeveloped portion of the film.

Developer solution A chemical solution used in film processing that distinguishes between the exposed and unexposed silver halide crystals and makes the latent image visible.

Developer spots A chemical contamination error; dark spots appear on the film because the developer solution has come in contact with the film before processing.

Developing agent One of the four basic ingredients of the developer solution; contains two chemicals, hydroquinone and elon, which reduce halides in the film emulsion to black metallic silver.

Development The first step in film processing; the developer solution reduces the halides in the film emulsion to black metallic silver and softens the film emulsion.

Diagnosis Identification of a disease by examination or analysis.

Diatorics Metal retention pins that are included in anterior porcelain denture teeth.

DICOM Data The universal format for handling, storing and transmitting three-dimensional images; the acronym refers to Digital Imaging and Communications in Medicine.

Digital image An image composed of pixels.

Digital Imaging, Three-Dimensional An image that demonstrates structures in three dimensions.

Digital imaging A filmless imaging system; a method of capturing a radiographic image using a sensor, breaking it into electronic pieces, and presenting and storing the image using a computer.

Digital subtraction One of the features of digital radiography; a method of reversing the gray scale as an image is viewed; radiolucent images (normally black) appear white and radiopaque images (normally white) appear black.

Digitize In digital radiography, to convert an image into digital form that, in turn, can be processed by a computer.

Direct digital imaging A method of obtaining a digital image in which an intraoral sensor is exposed to x-radiation to capture a radiographic image that can be viewed on a computer monitor.

Direct theory A theory that suggests that cell damage results when ionizing radiation hits critical areas directly within the cell.

Disability A physical or mental impairment that substantially limits one or more of an individual's major life activities.

Disability, developmental A substantial impairment of mental or physical functioning that occurs before age 22 and is of indefinite duration.

Disability, physical A physical impairment involving vision, hearing, or mobility.

Disclosure In dental radiography, the process of informing a patient about the particulars of exposing dental radiographs.

Disinfect To inhibit or destroy disease-causing microorganisms through use of a chemical or physical procedure.

Disinfectant, high-level Chemicals classified by the U.S. Environmental Protection Agency (EPA) as "sterilants–disinfectants"; used to disinfect heat-sensitive, semicritical dental instruments.

Disinfectant, intermediate-level U.S. Environmental Protection Agency (EPA)-registered chemical germicides labeled as both "hospital disinfectants" and "tuberculocidals"; recommended for all surfaces that have been contaminated.

Disinfectant, low-level U.S. Environmental Protection Agency (EPA)-registered chemical germicides labeled only as "hospital disinfectants"; recommended for general housekeeping purposes.

Disinfection The act of disinfecting; see **Disinfect**.

Distance, object-receptor One of the influencing factors of image magnification; refers to the distance between the object being radiographed (e.g., tooth) and the receptor; less image magnification results when the tooth and the receptor are as close as possible.

Distance, target-receptor One of the influencing factors of image magnification; refers to the distance between the source of x-rays and the receptor; less image magnification results when a longer position-indicating device (PID) is used.

Distortion A geometric characteristic that refers to a variation in the true size and shape of the object being radiographed; radiographic distortion is influenced by object-receptor alignment and x-ray beam angulation.

Dose The amount of energy absorbed by a tissue.

Dose, total The quantity of radiation received, or the total amount of radiation energy absorbed.

Dose equivalent A measurement used to compare the biologic effects of different types of radiation.

Dose rate Rate at which exposure to radiation occurs and absorption takes place (dose rate = dose/time).

Dose–response curve A curve that can be used to correlate the "response," or damage, of tissues with the "dose," or amount, of radiation received.

Drying chamber A component part of the automatic processor in which heated air is used to dry the wet films.

Ear The organ of hearing.

Edentulous Without teeth; areas where teeth are no longer present.

Edentulous patient A patient without teeth.

Edentulous zone Areas where teeth are no longer present.

Electrical current The flow of electrons through a conductor; an electrical current is used to produce x-rays.

Electricity Electrical current used as a source of power; the energy used to make x-rays.

Electromagnetic radiation Propagation of wavelike energy (without mass) through space or matter.

Electromagnetic spectrum Energies of electromagnetic radiation arranged in diagrammatic form on a chart.

Electron A tiny negatively charged particle found outside of the nucleus in the atom.

Electron volt The unit of measurement for the binding energies of orbital electrons.

Electrostatic force The attraction between the positive nucleus and the negative electrons that maintains electrons in their orbits; determined by the distance between the nucleus and electrons (also known as *binding energy* or *binding force*).

Element Substances made up of only one type of atom.

Elon A chemical found in the developing agent that generates the many shades of gray of the radiographic image.

Elongated images On a dental radiograph, images of the teeth that appear long and distorted; see **Elongation**.

Elongation A term used in radiography to describe the images of teeth that appear longer than the actual teeth; elongation is the result of insufficient vertical angulation.

Enamel The densest structure found in the human body; the outermost radiopaque layer of the crown of a tooth.

Endodontia Within a tooth.

Endodontic patient A patient who has undergone root canal therapy.

Endodontics A branch of dentistry dealing with the diagnosis and treatment of diseases of the dental pulp.

Energy What occurs when matter is altered.

Erg A unit of energy equivalent to 1.0×10^{-7} joules or 2.4×10^{-8} calories.

Expansile Capable of expansion.

Exposure A measure of ionization produced in air by x-radiation or gamma radiation.

Exposure, occupational Contact with blood or other infectious materials involving the skin, eye, or mucous membranes that results from procedures performed by the dental professional.

Exposure, parenteral Contact with blood or other infectious materials that results from piercing or puncturing the skin barrier.

Exposure button A component of the dental x-ray machine control panel; activates the dental x-ray machine to produce x-rays.

Exposure factors Factors that influence the density of a radiograph (e.g., milliamperage, kilovoltage, exposure time).

Exposure incident A specific incident involving contact with blood or other potentially infectious materials that results from procedures performed by the dental professional.

Exposure light A component of the dental x-ray machine control panel; provides a visible signal when x-rays are produced.

Exposure sequence A definite order for periapical receptor placement and exposure that must be followed in the placement and exposure of intraoral films.

Exposure time The interval during which x-rays are produced.

Extension arm A part of the dental x-ray machine; suspends the x-ray tubehead and houses electrical wires that extend from the control panel to the tubehead.

External auditory meatus A hole or opening in the temporal bone located superior and anterior to the mastoid process.

External oblique ridge A linear prominence of bone located on the external surface of the body of the mandible; appears radiopaque.

Extraoral Outside the mouth.

Extraoral imaging A radiographic inspection of large areas of the skull or jaws; requires the use of extraoral imaging receptors.

Extraoral radiography See **Radiographic examination, extraoral**.

Extrusion The abnormal displacement of teeth out of bone.

Facilitation skills Interpersonal skills used to ease communication and to develop a trusting relationship between the dental professional and the patient.

Field of view The area that can be captured when performing imaging procedures.

Filament circuit Uses 3 to 5 volts; regulates the flow of electrical current to the filament of the x-ray tube, and is controlled by the milliampere settings.

Receptor, bite-wing An intraoral receptor used to examine the crowns of both maxillary and mandibular teeth on one image.

Film, blue-sensitive An extraoral film that requires the use of a screen for exposure and is sensitive to blue fluorescent light; this film must be paired with screens that produce blue light.

film, cephalometric see lateral cephalometric projection.

Film, cleaning An extraoral-size film used to clean the rollers of the automatic processor.

Film, D-speed The slowest intraoral film; used before E-speed film; the letter D identifies the film speed.

Film, duplicating A special type of photographic film used to make an identical copy (duplicate) of an intraoral or extraoral radiograph; this film is not exposed to x-radiation.

Film, E-speed The fastest intraoral film before the introduction of F-speed film; the letter E identifies the film speed.

Film, F-speed The fastest intraoral film available; the letter F identifies the film speed; also called *InSight*.

Film, fast A type of dental x-ray film that requires less radiation for exposure (e.g., D-speed film, E-speed film).

Film, fogged A processing error; fogged film appears gray and lacks detail and contrast; results from improper safelighting or light leaks in the darkroom.

Film, green-sensitive An extraoral film that requires the use of a screen for exposure and is sensitive to green fluorescent light; this film must be paired with screens that produce green light.

Receptor, intraoral A receptor placed inside the mouth during x-ray exposure; intraoral receptors are used to examine teeth and supporting structures.

Film, nonscreen An extraoral film that does not require the use of a screen for exposure.

Receptor, occlusal A receptor used to examine large areas of the maxilla or the mandible; the patient "occludes" or bites on the entire receptor.

Film, overdeveloped A processing error; an overdeveloped film appears dark; results from excessive development time, inaccurate timer, hot developer solution, inaccurate thermometer, or concentrated developer solution.

Film, overlapped A film handling error; white or dark areas appear on films where overlap has occurred , results from two films come into contact with each other during processing .

Receptor, periapical An intraoral receptor used to examine the entire tooth (crown and root) and supporting bone.

Film, scratched A film handling error; white lines appear on films; results from the emulsion having been removed from the film base by a sharp object (e.g., a film clip or hanger).

Film, screen An extraoral film that requires the use of a screen for exposure; this film is sensitive to the light emitted from intensifying screens.

Film, underdeveloped A processing error; an underdeveloped film appears light; results from inadequate development time, inaccurate timer, cool developer temperature, inaccurate thermometer, or depleted or contaminated developer solution.

Film, underexposed An exposure error that results in a light film; results from inadequate exposure time, kilovoltage, or milliamperage or a combination of these factors.

Film, x-ray An image receptor that consists of a film base, adhesive layer, film emulsion, and protective layer; three types of x-ray film may be used in dental radiography: (1) intraoral film, (2) extraoral film, and (3) duplicating film .

Film, yellow-brown A processing error; this film appears yellow-brown; results from exhausted developer or fixer, insufficient fixation time, or insufficient rinsing.

Film badge A device used to measure and monitor radiation exposure; worn by persons frequently exposed to radiation.

Film base A flexible piece of plastic that is constructed to withstand heat, moisture, and chemical exposure and provides strength and stable support for the film emulsion.

Film composition The formulation of the film emulsion; depends on the size of the crystals in the film emulsion (the smaller the crystals, the sharper the radiographic image).

Film duplicator A light source used to expose duplicating film.

Film emulsion A coating attached to both sides of the film base by the adhesive layer to give the film greater sensitivity to x-radiation; homogenous mixture of gelatin and silver halide crystals .

Film feed slot An opening on the outside of the automatic processor housing; used to insert unwrapped films into the automatic processor.

Film hangers A stainless steel device equipped with clips; used to hold films during manual processing.

Film holder See **Beam alignment device**.

Film holder, EEZEE-Grip A type of film-holding device used to stabilize film (formerly known as *Snap-A-Ray*).

Film holder, hemostat A small surgical clamp inserted through a rubber bite-block and used to stabilize the film.

Film holder, precision A type of film-holding device that includes a metal collimating shield and film-holding devices that restrict the size of the x-ray beam to the size of the film.

Film holder, Stabe A disposable film holder designed for one-time use only.

Film-holding device See beam alignment device.

Film mount A cardboard, plastic, or vinyl holder used to support and arrange dental radiographs in anatomic order.

Film mounting The placement of radiographs in a supporting structure or holder.

Film placement The specific area where a film is positioned before exposure.

Film recovery slot An opening on the outside of the automatic processor housing where dry, processed radiographs emerge.

Film speed The amount of radiation required to produce a radiograph of standard density .

Film viewing In dental radiography, the examining of dental radiographs on a light source.

Filtration The use of absorbing materials (e.g., aluminum) for removing the low-energy x-rays from the primary beam.

Filtration, added Aluminum discs inserted in the dental x-ray machine between the x-ray tubehead seal and collimator; absorb low-energy x-rays.

Filtration, inherent Occurs when the primary beam passes through the glass window of the x-ray tube, the insulating oil, and the tubehead seal.

Filtration, total The combination of the inherent filtration and added filtration in an x-ray machine.

Finger-holding method A method of exposing receptors in which the patient's finger or thumb stabilizes the receptor from behind the teeth.

Fingernail artifact A film handling error; a fingernail artifact exhibits black, crescent-shaped marks where the film has been damaged by the operator's fingernail during rough handling of the film.

Fingerprint artifact A film handling error; a black fingerprint appears on a film where the film has been touched by fingers contaminated with fluoride or developer.

Fixation A step in film processing; the fixer solution removes the unexposed, undeveloped silver halide crystals from the film emulsion and hardens the film emulsion.

Fixer cutoff A film handling error; a straight black border appears on a film as a result of using too low a level of fixer solution during processing; represents an unfixed portion of the film.

Fixer solution A chemical solution used in film processing; removes the unexposed silver halide crystals and creates white or clear areas on the film.

Fixer spots A chemical contamination error; white spots appear on a film as a result of fixer solution contacting the film before processing.

Fixing One of the five steps in film processing; A chemical solution known as the fixer removes the unexposed, unenergized silver halide crystals from the film emulsion.

Fixing agent One of the four basic ingredients of the fixer solution; contains hypo (sodium thiosulfate or ammonium thiosulfate), which removes or clears all unexposed and undeveloped silver halide crystals from the film emulsion (also known as *clearing agent*).

Floor of nasal cavity A bony plate formed by the palatal processes of the maxilla and the horizontal processes of the palatine bones; appears radiopaque.

Fluoresce To emit visible light in the blue or green spectrum.

Fluorescence The emission of a glowing light by certain substances when struck by a particular wavelength (e.g., calcium tungstate screens have phosphors that emit blue light, or fluoresce, when exposed to x-rays).

Focal opacity A term used to describe a well-defined, localized radiopaque lesion.

Focal spot The tungsten target of the anode; converts bombarding electrons into x-ray photons, concentrating the electrons and creating an enormous amount of heat.

Focal spot size The size of the tungsten target of the anode; ranges from 0.6 mm^2 to 1.0 mm^2 and is determined by the manufacturer of the x-ray machine.

Focal trough A three-dimensional curved zone in which structures are clearly demonstrated on a panoramic image; in panoramic radiography, a patient must be positioned so that the dental arches are located within the focal trough area; (also called *image layer*).

Foramen An opening or hole in bone that permits the passage of nerves and blood vessels; appears radiolucent.

Foreshortened images Images of teeth that appear short with blunted roots; see **Foreshortening**.

Foreshortening A term describing images of teeth that appear too short; foreshortening is the result of excessive vertical angulation.

Fossa A broad, shallow, scooped-out or depressed area of bone; appears radiolucent.

Fracture The breaking of a part; appears as a thin radiolucent line.

Frankfort plane The imaginary plane that intersects the orbital rim of the eye and the opening of the ear.

Free radical An atom, molecule or ion that carries a negative, positive or zero charge; it exists with a single, unpaired electron in its outermost shell.

Frequency The number of wavelengths that pass a given point in a certain amount of time; frequency indicates the energy of a radiation (e.g., high-frequency radiations have more energy than do low-frequency radiations).

Full mouth series (FMS or FMX) See **Complete mouth radiographic series (CMRS)**.

Furcation area The area between the roots of multi-rooted teeth.

Gag reflex Retching that is elicited by stimulation of the sensitive tissues of the soft palate region (also known as *pharyngeal reflex*).

Gagging The strong involuntary effort to vomit (also known as *retching*).

Gelatin A component of the film emulsion that suspends and disperses silver halide crystals over the film base.

Genetic cells Cells that contain genes; reproductive cells (e.g., ova, sperm).

Genetic effects Effects of radiation that are not seen in the person irradiated but are passed on to future generations through genetic cells.

Genial tubercles Tiny bumps of bone located on the lingual aspect of the mandible in the anterior region of the mandible; serve as attachment sites for the genioglossus and geniohyoid muscles; appear radiopaque.

Ghost image An artifact on a dental radiograph produced when a radiodense object (e.g., earring) is penetrated twice by the x-ray beam; appears radiopaque.

Glenoid fossa A concave, depressed area of the temporal bone on which the mandibular condyle rests.

Glossopharyngeal air space Refers to the portion of the pharynx (*pharyngeal*) located posterior to the tongue (*glosso*) and oral cavity; on a panoramic image, the glossopharyngeal air space appears as a vertical *radiolucent* band superimposed over the ramus of the mandible.

Gray (Gy) A unit for measuring absorbed dose; the SI unit equivalent to the rad; 1 gray = 100 rad.

Grid In extraoral imaging, a device used to prevent scatter radiation from reaching the film during exposure.

Ground glass A term used to describe a radiopacity; refers to a granular, pebbled, or pulverized-glass appearance of bone that resembles pulverized glass; also referred to as an *orange-peel appearance*.

Gutta percha Claylike material used in endodontic therapy to fill the canals of the pulp.

Half-value layer (HVL) The thickness of material that, when placed in the path of the x-ray beam, reduces the exposure rate by one-half.

Halide A chemical compound that is sensitive to radiation or light; in dental radiography, a halide, such as silver bromide, is suspended in the gelatin of the emulsion.

Hamulus A small, hooklike projection of bone that extends from the medial pterygoid plate of the sphenoid bone; appears radiopaque.

Hardening agent One of the four basic ingredients of the fixer solution; contains the chemical potassium alum, which hardens and shrinks the gelatin in the film emulsion.

Head positioner One of the component parts of a panoramic unit consisting of a chin rest, notched bite-block, forehead rest, and lateral head supports.

Hemostat A small surgical clamp.

Herringbone pattern An image on a dental radiograph that has been placed in the mouth backward and exposed (also known as *tire-track pattern*).

High-voltage circuit Uses 65,000 to 100,000 volts; provides the high voltage required to accelerate electrons and to generate x-rays in the x-ray tube, and is controlled by the kilovoltage settings.

Humidity level The amount of moisture in the air.

Hydroquinone A chemical found in the developing agent that generates the black tones and sharp contrast of the radiographic image.

Hypercementosis The excess deposition of cementum on the root surfaces of teeth; appears radiopaque.

Hypo Sodium thiosulfate or ammonium thiosulfate; a common name for these chemicals found in the fixing agent.

Hypotenuse In geometry, the side of a right triangle opposite the right angle.

Identification dot A small raised bump that appears in one corner of an intraoral film; used to determine film orientation.

Image A picture or likeness of an object.

Image, extraoral An image that results when a receptor is placed outside the mouth and exposed to x-rays; extraoral receptors are used to examine large areas of the skull or jaws.

Image, overexposed An exposure error that results in a dark image; results from excessive exposure time, kilovoltage, or milliamperage or a combination of these factors.

Image receptor A recording medium; examples include x-ray film or digital sensors.

Image, underexposed An exposure error that results in a light image; results from inadequate exposure time, kilovoltage, or milliamperage or a combination of these factors.

Impulse In dental radiography, a measure of exposure time; 60 impulses occur in 1 second.

Incipient Small; beginning to exist or appear.

Incisive canal A passageway through bone that extends from the superior foramina of the incisive canal to the incisive foramen.

Incisive foramen An opening or hole in bone located at the midline of the anterior portion of the hard palate directly posterior to the maxillary central incisors; appears radiolucent.

Indicator light A component of the dental x-ray machine control panel; when illuminated, indicates that the dental x-ray machine is turned on.

Indirect digital imaging A method of obtaining a digital image in which an existing radiograph is scanned and converted into digital form using a charge-coupled device (CCD) camera.

Indirect theory A theory suggesting that cell damage results indirectly; x-ray photons are absorbed with the cell, causing the formation of toxins; toxins, in turn, damage the cell.

Infectious waste Waste that consists of blood, blood products, contaminated sharps, or other microbiologic products.

Inferior border of mandible A linear prominence of cortical bone that defines the lower border of the mandible.

Inferior nasal conchae Wafer-thin, curved plates of bone that extend from the lateral walls of the nasal cavity and appear radiopaque.

Informed consent Consent given by a patient following complete disclosure about the particulars of a procedure.

Infraorbital foramen A hole or opening in bone found inferior to the border of the orbit.

Instrument, critical Instruments that are used to penetrate soft tissue or bone; must be sterilized after each use.

Instrument, noncritical Instruments that do not come in contact with mucous membranes.

Instrument, Rinn XCP A type of beam alignment devices that are used with the paralleling technique; these include plastic bite-blocks, plastic aiming rings, and metal indicator arms (X = extension, C = cone, P = paralleling).

Instrument, semicritical Instruments that contact but do not penetrate soft tissue or bone; must be sterilized after each use.

Insulating oil Oil that surrounds the x-ray tube and transformers inside the tubehead.

Intensity The total energy of the x-ray beam; the product of the quantity (number of x-ray photons) and quality (energy of each photon) per unit of area per time of exposure.

Internal oblique ridge A linear prominence of bone located on the internal surface of the mandible that extends downward and forward from the ramus; appears radiopaque.

Interpersonal skills Skills that promote good relationships between individuals.

Interpret To offer an explanation.

Interpretation An explanation.

Interpretation, image An explanation of what is viewed on a dental radiograph; the ability to read what is revealed by a dental radiograph.

Interproximal Between two adjacent surfaces.

Interproximal examination A radiographic inspection used to examine the crowns of both maxillary and mandibular teeth on a single image.

Inter-radicular Between the roots of adjacent teeth.

Intersecting Cutting across or through.

Intraoral Inside the mouth.

Intraoral radiographic examination A radiographic inspection of teeth and intraoral adjacent structures.

Intraoral radiography See **Intraoral radiographic examination**.

Intrusion The abnormal displacement of teeth into bone.

Inverse square law A rule that states that "the intensity of radiation is inversely proportional to the square of the distance from the source of radiation"; as distance is increased, radiation intensity at the object is decreased, and vice versa.

Inverted Y A radiographic landmark that represents the intersection of the maxillary sinus and the nasal cavity; appears radiopaque.

Ion An electrically unbalanced particle; an atom that gains or loses an electron.

Ion pair A pair of ions, one positive and one negative, that results when an electron is removed from an atom in the ionization process. The atom becomes the positive ion, and the ejected electron becomes the negative ion.

Ionization The production of ions; the process of converting an atom into an ion, resulting in the formation of a positive atom and a dislodged negative electron.

Ionizing radiation Radiation that is capable of producing ions by removing or adding an electron to an atom. It can be classified into two groups: (1) particulate radiation and (2) electromagnetic radiation.

Irregular, radiopacities Terms used to describe a radiopacity that has irregular borders and is not well defined.

Isometry Equality of measurement.

Isometry, rule of A geometric principle that states that "two triangles are equal if they have two equal angles and share a common side."

Joule (J) The SI unit of measurement equivalent to the work done by the force of 1 newton acting over the distance of 1 meter.

Kilo electron volt (keV) 1000 electron volts; the unit of measurement for the binding energies of orbital electrons.

Kilogram (kg) 1000 grams; a unit equivalent to 2.205 pounds.

Kilovolt (kV) 1000 volts; unit of measure for voltage.

Kilovoltage In radiography, the x-ray tube peak voltage used during an exposure; measured in kilovolts.

Kilovoltage peak (kVp) The maximum or peak voltage that is used during an x-ray exposure.

Kinetic energy Energy of motion.

Label side The outer side of the x-ray film packet that is color-coded and contains printed information; the label side of the film faces the tongue.

Labial mounting A film mounting method in which radiographs are placed in the film mount with the raised side of the identification dot facing the viewer; the dental radiographer then views the radiographs from the labial aspect.

Lamina dura The wall of the tooth socket that surrounds the root of a tooth; appears radiopaque.

Latent image The pattern of stored energy on the exposed film; the invisible image produced when the film is exposed to x-rays and that remains invisible until the film is processed.

Latent image centers Aggregates of neutral silver atoms on exposed crystals that collectively become the latent image on the emulsion of the film.

Latent period The amount of time that elapses between exposure to ionizing radiation and the appearance of observable clinical signs.

Lateral cephalometric projection An extraoral image that is used to determine facial growth and development, trauma, disease, and developmental abnormalities.

Lateral fossa A smooth, depressed area of the maxilla located just inferior and medial to the infraorbital foramen between the maxillary canine and lateral incisors; appears radiolucent.

Lateral jaw projection–body of mandible An extraoral radiographic projection used to image the posterior body of the mandible; used to evaluate impacted teeth, fractures, and lesions located in the body of the mandible.

Lateral jaw projection–ramus of mandible An extraoral radiographic projection used to image the ramus of the mandible; used to evaluate impacted third molars, large lesions, and fractures that extend into the ramus of the mandible.

Lateral pterygoid plate A wing-shaped bony projection of the sphenoid bone located distal to the maxillary tuberosity region.

Lead apron A flexible lead shield used to protect the patient's reproductive and blood-forming tissues from scatter radiation.

Lead collimator A lead diaphragm or tubular device used to restrict the size and shape of the x-ray beam.

Lead foil sheet One of the four components of the dental x-ray film packet; a single piece of embossed lead foil placed behind the film to shield the film from scattered radiation.

Leaded-glass housing Leaded-glass vacuum tube that prevents x-rays from escaping in all directions.

Liability Legal accountability.

Liable Accountable; legally obligated.

Light leak (1) Any white light that is seen when all the lights are turned off and the door is closed; (2) an exposure error; a black area appearing on a film as a result of exposure of the film to white light.

Light-tight A term used to describe the darkroom, a room that is completely dark and excludes all white light.

Line pairs/millimeter (lp/mm) A measurement used to evaluate the ability of the computer to capture the resolution (or detail) of a radiographic image.

Lingula A small, tongue-shaped projection of bone seen adjacent to the mandibular foramen.

Lingual foramen An opening or hole in bone located on the internal surface of the mandible near the midline; it is surrounded by the genial tubercles and appears radiolucent.

Lingual mounting A film mounting method in which radiographs are placed in the film mount with the depressed side of the identification dot facing the viewer; the dental radiographer then views the radiographs from the lingual aspect.

Lipline An artifact seen on panoramic radiographs formed by the positioning of the patient's lips.

Localization techniques Method used to locate the position of a tooth or object in the jaws.

Long axis (of tooth) An imaginary line that divides a tooth longitudinally into two equal halves.

Long-term effects Effects of radiation that appear years, decades, or generations after exposure; associated with small amounts of radiation absorbed repeatedly over a long period.

Luxation The abnormal displacement of teeth.

Magnification A geometric characteristic; refers to a radiographic image that appears larger than the actual size of the object it represents; influenced by target-film distance and object–receptor distance.

Malpractice Improper or negligent conduct or treatment.

Mandibular canal A tubelike passageway through bone that travels the length of the mandible; appears radiolucent.

Mandibular condyle A rounded projection of bone extending from the posterosuperior border of the ramus of the mandible.

Mandibular foramen A round or ovoid hole in bone on the lingual aspect of the ramus of the mandible.

Mass Weight; the physical volume or bulk of a solid body.

Mass number See **Atomic weight**.

Mastoid process A marked prominence of bone located posteroinferior to the temporomandibular joint.

Matter Anything that occupies space and has mass.

Maxillary sinuses Paired cavities or compartments of bone located within the maxilla and located superior to the maxillary posterior teeth; appear radiolucent.

Maxillary tuberosity A rounded prominence of bone that extends posterior to the third molar region; appears radiopaque.

Maximum accumulated dose (MAD) The maximum accumulated lifetime radiation dose that may be received by persons who are occupationally exposed to radiation.

Maximum permissible dose (MPD) Maximum dose equivalent that a body is permitted to receive in a specific period. MPD is the dose of radiation that the body can endure with little or no injury.

Median palatal suture The immovable joint between the two palatine processes of the maxilla; appears radiolucent.

Mental foramen An opening or hole in bone located on the external surface of the mandible in the region of the mandibular premolars; appears radiolucent.

Mental fossa A scooped-out, depressed area of bone located on the external surface of the anterior mandible; appears radiolucent.

Mental ridge A linear prominence of cortical bone located on the external surface of the anterior portion of the mandible; appears radiopaque.

Metal housing The metal body of the dental x-ray tubehead that surrounds the x-ray tube and transformers.

Metallic restoration Restorations that completely absorb x-rays; as a result, little to no radiation contacts the receptor, and the radiographic appearance is totally radiopaque (e.g., amalgam, gold).

Midsagittal plane An imaginary line or plane passing through the center of the body that divides it into right and left halves.

Milliamperage In radiography, the quantity, or number, of x-rays emitted from the tubehead; measured in milliamperes.

Milliampere (mA) 1/1000 of an ampere; a unit of measurement used to describe the intensity of an electrical current.

Milliampere-second (mAs) A unit of radiographic exposure equal to the product of milliamperage and exposure time.

Mitotic activity Process of cell division; determines the response of a cell to radiation exposure (cells that divide frequently are more sensitive to radiation).

Mixed lucent–opaque A term used to describe a lesion that exhibits both radiolucent and radiopaque components.

Molecule Two or more atoms joined together by chemical bonds, or the smallest amount of a substance that possesses its characteristic properties. Molecules are formed in one of two ways: (1) by the transfer of electrons or (2) by the sharing of electrons between the outermost shells of atoms.

Molybdenum cup A portion of the cathode in the x-ray tube; focuses the electrons into a narrow beam and directs the beam across the tube toward the tungsten target in the anode.

Mount To place in an appropriate setting, as for display or study.

Movement Movement or motion of the receptor or patient during radiographic exposure; movement results in a radiographic image with less sharpness.

Multifocal confluent A term used to describe multiple radiopacities that appear to overlap or flow together.

Multilocular A term used to describe a radiolucent lesion that exhibits multiple compartments.

Multiplanar reconstruction (MPR) The reconstruction of raw data into images when imported into viewing software to create three anatomic planes of the body.

Mylohyoid ridge A linear prominence of bone located on the internal surface of the mandible that extends from the molar region downward and forward toward the lower border of the mandibular symphysis; appears radiopaque.

Nanometer A measurement used for wavelength; 1 nanometer equals one-billionth (10^{-9}) of a meter.

Nasal cavity A pear-shaped compartment of bone located superior to the maxilla; appears radiolucent.

Nasal septum A vertical bony wall or partition that divides the nasal cavity into the right and left nasal fossae; appears radiopaque.

Nasopharyngeal air space Refers to the portion of the pharynx (*pharyngeal*) located posterior to the nasal cavity (*naso*); on a panoramic image, the nasopharyngeal air space appears as a diagonal *radiolucency* located superior to the radiopaque shadow of the soft palate and uvula.

Negligence Omission or failure to provide reasonable precaution, care, or action; occurs when the diagnosis made or the dental treatment delivered falls below the standard of care.

Neutral atom An atom that contains an equal number of protons (positive charges) and electrons (negative charges).

Neutron An electrically neutral or uncharged particle.

Nonmetallic restoration Restorations that do not completely absorb x-rays; these restorations vary in radiographic appearance from slightly radiopaque to radiolucent, depending on the density of the material (e.g., porcelain, composite, acrylic).

Nonstochastic effects Somatic effects that have a threshold and increase in severity with increasing absorbed dose.

Normalizing device A commercially available device used to monitor developer strength and film density.

Nucleon Part of an atomic nucleus (e.g., protons, neutrons).

Nucleus The central, positively charged core of an atom; composed of *protons* and *neutrons*.

Nutrient canal(s) A tiny tubelike passageway through bone, which contains blood vessels and nerves that supply maxillary teeth and interdental areas ; appears radiolucent.

Occlusal examination A type of intraoral radiographic examination used to inspect large areas of the maxilla or the mandible on one image.

Occlusal projection, mandibular cross-sectional A type of occlusal projection used to examine the buccal and lingual aspects of the mandible and locate foreign bodies (e.g., salivary stones) in the floor of the mouth.

Occlusal projection, mandibular pediatric A type of occlusal projection used to examine the anterior teeth of the mandible; recommended for children aged 5 years or younger.

Occlusal projection, mandibular topographic A type of occlusal projection used to examine the anterior teeth of the mandible.

Occlusal projection, maxillary lateral A type of occlusal projection used to examine the palatal roots of molar teeth and locate foreign bodies or lesions in the posterior maxilla.

Occlusal projection, maxillary pediatric A type of occlusal projection used to examine the anterior teeth of the maxilla; recommended for children aged 5 years or younger.

Occlusal projection, maxillary topographic A type of occlusal projection used to examine the palate and anterior teeth of the maxilla.

Occlusal surfaces The chewing surfaces of posterior teeth.

Occlusal technique The method used to expose a receptor in occlusal examination.

On-off switch A component of the control panel on the dental x-ray machine; turns the dental x-ray machine on or off.

Operating kilovoltage See **Kilovoltage**.

Operating kilovoltage peak See **Kilovoltage peak.**

Orbit (1) The well-defined path of an electron around the nucleus of an atom (also known as *shell*); (2) The bony cavity that contains the eyeball.

Outer package wrapping One of the four components of the dental x-ray film packet; a soft vinyl or paper wrapper that serves to protect the film from exposure to light and saliva. It has two sides: the tube side and the label side.

Oxidation A chemical reaction that occurs when processing solutions are exposed to air; the chemicals break down, resulting in a decreased concentration of solution strength.

Packet, film The intraoral film and its surrounding packaging.

Packet, one-film A film packet containing one film.

Packet, two-film A film packet containing two films.

Palate Roof of the mouth.

Palate, hard The bony plate that separates the nasal cavity from the oral cavity; the anterior portion of the roof of the mouth.

Palate, soft The posterior portion of the roof of the mouth separating the mouth and pharynx.

Palatoglossal air space Refers to the space found between the palate (*palato*) and tongue (*glossal*); on a panoramic image, the palatoglossal air space appears as a horizontal *radiolucent* band located superior to the apices of maxillary teeth.

Panoramic view A wide view.

Panoramic imaging An extraoral technique used to examine the upper and lower jaws on a single projection (also known as *rotational panoramic radiography*).

Paper film wrapper One of the four components of the dental x-ray film packet; a black paper protective sheet covers the film and shields it from light.

Parallel Moving or lying in the same plane; always separated by the same distance and not intersecting.

Paralleling technique An intraoral radiographic technique used to expose periapical receptors: the receptor is placed parallel to the long axis of the tooth; the central ray is directed perpendicular to the receptor and the long axis of tooth; a beam alignment device must be used to keep the receptor parallel to the long axis of the tooth. Also known as *extension cone paralleling [XCP] technique*, *right-angle technique*, and *long-cone technique*.

Particulate radiations Tiny particles of matter that possess mass and travel in straight lines and at high speeds. Particulate radiations transmit kinetic energy by means of their extremely fast-moving small masses. Four types of particulate radiation are recognized.

Pathogen A microorganism capable of causing disease.

Patient relations The relationship between the patient and the dental professional.

Pediatric A term derived from the Greek word *pedia*, meaning child.

Pediatric patient A child patient.

Pediatrics, dental A branch of dentistry dealing with the diagnosis and treatment of dental diseases in children.

Penumbra The fuzzy, unclear area that surrounds a radiographic image.

Periapical Around the apex of a tooth.

Periapical abscess A lesion characterized by a localized collection of pus around the apex of a nonvital tooth that results from pulpal death; appears radiolucent.

Periapical cyst A lesion characterized by an epithelial-lined cavity or sac located around the apex of a nonvital tooth that results from pulpal death; appears radiolucent.

Periapical examination A radiographic inspection used to examine the entire tooth (crown and root) and supporting bone.

Periapical granuloma A lesion characterized by a localized mass of granulation tissue around the apex of a nonvital tooth; appears radiolucent.

Periapical lesion A lesion located around the apex of a tooth.

Pericoronal Around the crown of a tooth.

Periodic table of the elements A chart that arranges elements in increasing atomic number.

Period of injury Occurs after the latent period following exposure to radiation; can include a variety of cellular injuries.

Periodontal Around a tooth.

Periodontal abscess A lesion that originates in a soft tissue pocket and is characterized by the accumulation of pus and destruction of bone; is often painful; appears radiolucent.

Periodontal disease A group of diseases that affects the tissues around teeth.

Periodontal ligament space (PDL) A space that exists between the root of a tooth and the lamina dura; contains connective tissue fibers, blood vessels, and lymphatics; appears radiolucent.

Periodontium Tissues that invest and support teeth, such as the gingiva and alveolar bone.

Perpendicular Intersecting at or forming right angles.

Personal protective equipment (PPE) Equipment worn by dental professionals to protect themselves from hazards; includes protective attire, gloves, mask, and eyewear.

Phalangioma An error on a dental radiograph; refers to the distal phalanx of the finger seen in the radiograph. This error occurs when the finger-holding method is used with the bisecting technique.

Phosphors Minute fluorescent crystals that cover intensifying screens and fluoresce, or emit visible light, when exposed to x-rays.

Photoelectric effect One of the interactions of x-radiation with matter; the x-ray photon collides with a tightly bound, inner-shell electron and gives up all its energy to eject the electron from its orbit. All the energy of the photon is absorbed by the displaced electron in the form of kinetic energy.

Photon A bundle of energy with no mass or weight that travels as a wave at the speed of light and moves through space in a straight line.

Pixel A discrete unit of information; in digital electronic images, digital information is contained in, and presented as, discrete units of information (also known as *picture element*).

Plane, axial A horizontal plane that divides the body into superior and inferior parts; runs parallel to the ground.

Plane, coronal A vertical plane that divides the body into anterior and posterior sides; runs perpendicular to the ground.

Plane, sagittal A vertical plane that divides the body into right and left sides; runs perpendicular to the ground. A midsagittal plane describes a plane that runs through the midline of the body.

Polychromatic x-ray beam An x-ray beam containing many different wavelengths of varying intensities.

Position-indicating device (PID) An open-ended, lead-lined cylinder extending from the opening of the metal housing of the tubehead; aims and shapes the x-ray beam (also called the *cone*).

Posteroanterior projection An extraoral radiographic projection of the skull used to evaluate facial growth, trauma, diseases, and developmental abnormalities.

Potassium alum See **Hardening agent**.

Potassium bromide See **Restrainer**.

Preservative (1) One of the four basic ingredients of the developer solution; sodium sulfite prevents the developer solution from oxidizing in the presence of air; (2) one of the four basic ingredients of the fixer solution; sodium sulfite prevents the chemical deterioration of the fixing agent.

Primary beam See **Radiation, primary**.

Process A marked prominence or projection of bone; appears radiopaque.

Processing, automatic A method used to process films in which all film processing steps are automated.

Processing, film A series of steps that collectively produce a visible, permanent image on a dental radiograph.

Processing, manual A method used to process films in which all film processing steps are performed manually (also known as *hand processing or tank processing*).

Processor, automatic A machine that automates all film processing steps.

Processor housing The housing, or protective covering, of the automatic film processor; encases all the component parts of the automatic processor.

Protective barrier A barrier of radiation-absorbing material used to protect the operator from primary and scatter radiation (e.g., a wall).

Protective layer One of the four basic components of x-ray film; a thin, protective coating on top of the emulsion that protects the film from manipulation and mechanical and processing damage.

Proton A positively charged particle with a mass of one.

Pterygomaxillary fissure A narrow space or cleft that separates the lateral pterygoid plate and the maxilla; appears radiolucent.

Pulp cavity A cavity within a tooth that includes both the pulp chamber and the pulp canals; contains blood vessels, nerves, and lymphatics; appears radiolucent.

Pulp stones Calcifications found in the pulp chamber or pulp canals of teeth; appear radiopaque.

Pulpal obliteration Total calcification of the pulp cavity; appears radiopaque.

Pulpal sclerosis A diffuse calcification of the pulp chamber and pulp canals of teeth that results in a pulp cavity of decreased size; appears radiopaque.

Quality (of x-ray beam) The mean energy or penetrating ability of the x-ray beam; the quality of the x-ray beam is controlled by kilovoltage.

Quality administration The management of the quality assurance plan in the dental office.

Quality assurance Special procedures used to ensure the production of high-quality, diagnostic radiographs.

Quality control tests Specific tests designed to maintain and monitor dental x-ray equipment, supplies, and film processing.

Quality factor (QF) A factor used for radiation protection purposes that accounts for the exposure effects of different types of radiation; for x-rays, QF = 1.

Quanta See **Photon**.

Quantity (of x-ray beam) The number of x-rays produced in the dental x-ray unit ; the quantity of x-rays produced is controlled by milliamperage.

Radiation A form of energy carried by waves or a stream of particles.

Radiation, background A form of ionizing radiation that is ubiquitous in the environment; includes cosmic and terrestrial radiation.

Radiation, braking See **Radiation, general**.

Radiation, characteristic A form of radiation that occurs when a high-speed electron dislodges an inner-shell electron from an atom, causing excitation, or ionization, of the atom.

Radiation, electromagnetic The propagation of wavelike energy through space or matter; the propagated energy is accompanied by electric and magnetic fields, thus the term *electromagnetic*; examples include cosmic rays, gamma rays, x-rays, ultraviolet rays, visible light, infrared light, radar waves, microwaves, and radio waves.

Radiation, general A form of radiation that occurs when speeding electrons slow down because of their interactions with the tungsten target in the anode (also known as *bremsstrahlung* or *braking radiation*).

Radiation, ionizing Radiation capable of producing ions; includes particulate or electromagnetic radiation.

Radiation, leakage Any radiation, with the exception of the primary beam, that is emitted from the dental tubehead.

Radiation, particulate Tiny particles of matter that possess mass, travel in straight lines, and travel at high speeds (e.g., electrons, β-particles, α-particles, protons, and neutrons).

Radiation, primary The penetrating x-ray beam produced at the target of the anode and that exits the tubehead (also known as the *primary beam* or *useful beam*).

Radiation, scatter A form of secondary radiation; results from an x-ray beam that has been deflected from its path by the interaction with matter.

Radiation, secondary Radiation created when the primary beam interacts with matter; secondary radiation is less penetrating than primary radiation.

Radiation absorbed dose (rad) A unit for measuring absorbed dose; the traditional unit of dose equivalent to the gray (Gy); 100 erg of energy per gram of tissue; 100 rad = 1 Gy.

Radiation biology The study of the effects of ionizing radiation on living tissues.

Radioactivity The process by which certain unstable atoms or elements undergo spontaneous disintegration, or decay, in an effort to attain a more balanced nuclear state.

Radiograph A two-dimensional representation of a three-dimensional object. In practice, often called an "x-ray"; this is not correct. X-ray (also *x-ray*) is a term that refers to a beam of energy.

Radiograph, dental Two-dimensional representation of a three-dimensional object produced on an image receptor by the passage of x-rays through teeth and related supporting structures.

Radiograph, diagnostic A radiograph that provides much information with images that have proper density and contrast, have sharp outlines, and are of the same shape and size as the object being radiographed.

Radiograph, duplicate An identical copy of a radiograph that is made through the process of film duplication.

Radiograph, extraoral See **Receptor, extraoral**.

Radiograph, intraoral See **Receptor intraoral**.

Radiograph, reference A radiograph processed under ideal conditions and then used to compare the film densities of radiographs that are processed daily.

Radiographer, dental Any person who positions, exposes, and processes dental x-ray image receptors.

Radiography The art and science of making radiographs by the exposure of film to x-rays.

Radiography, dental The production of radiographs of teeth and adjacent structures by the exposure of an image receptor to x-rays.

Radiology The science or study of radiation as used in medicine; a branch of medical science that deals with the use of x-rays, radioactive substances, and other forms of radiant energy in the diagnosis and treatment of disease.

Radiolucent The portion of an image that is dark or black; a radiolucent structure readily permits the passage of the x-ray beam and allows more x-rays to reach the receptor.

Radiopaque The portion of an image that is light or white; a radiopaque structure is one that resists the passage of the x-ray beam and limits the amount of x-rays that reach the receptor.

Radioresistant cell A cell that is resistant to radiation (e.g., bone, muscle, and nerve cells).

Radiosensitive cell A cell that is sensitive to radiation (e.g., small lymphocytes; blood, immature reproductive, young bone, and epithelial cells).

Rampant Growing or spreading unchecked.

Ramus Vertical portion of the mandible that is found posterior to the third molar. The mandible has two rami, one on each side.

Receptor Something that responds to a stimulus; a recording medium (examples: x-ray film or digital sensors).

Receptor, bite-wing Receptor used in the interproximal examination.

Receptor, extraoral Receptor placed outside the mouth to examine large areas of the skull or jaws.

Receptor, intraoral Receptor placed inside the mouth to examine the teeth and supporting structures.

Receptor, occlusal Receptor used in occlusal examination.

Receptor, panoramic Receptor used in panoramic examination, shows a wide view of the maxilla and the mandible.

Receptor, periapical Receptor used in periapical examination.

Receptor placement The specific area where the receptor must be positioned before exposure.

Recoil electron See **Compton electron**.

Recovery period The period during which cellular damage caused by radiation is followed by repair.

Rectification The conversion of alternating current to direct current.

Reduction A chemical reaction during film processing in which the halide portion of the exposed energized silver halide crystal is removed.

Reduction, selective A chemical reaction during film processing in which the energized exposed silver halide crystals are changed into black metallic silver, while the unenergized unexposed silver halide crystals are removed from the film.

Replenisher A superconcentrated solution added to a processing solution to compensate for the loss of volume and strength that results from oxidation.

Replenisher pump A component part of the automatic film processor; automatically maintains proper concentrations and levels of solutions.

Replenisher solutions See **Replenisher**.

Resolution, contrast The number of gray scale colors available to be chosen for each pixel in the image.

Resolution, spatial A measurement of pixel size in multiplanar reconstruction.

Resorption, external A regressive alteration of tooth structure that occurs along the periphery of the root surface.

Resorption, internal A regressive alteration of tooth structure that occurs within the crown or root of a tooth; appears as a radiolucency.

Resorption, pathologic Resorption of a tooth *not* associated with the normal shedding of deciduous teeth.

Resorption, physiologic Resorption of the teeth associated with the normal shedding of deciduous teeth.

Restrainer One of the four basic ingredients of the developer solution; potassium bromide is used to prevent the development of unexposed silver halide crystals; also prevents film fogging.

Reticulation of emulsion A temperature error; a film has a cracked appearance as a result of being subjected to sudden temperature changes between the developer solution and the water bath.

Reverse Towne projection An extraoral radiographic projection used to identify fractures of the condylar neck and ramus area.

Ridge A linear prominence or projection of bone; appears radiopaque.

Right-angle technique A localization technique in which the orientation of structures can be seen in two radiographs (one periapical and one occlusal).

Rinsing One of the five steps in film processing; a water bath is used to rinse the developer from the film and stop the development process.

Risk The likelihood of adverse effects or death resulting from exposure to a hazard.

Risk management The policies and procedures that the dental professional should follow to reduce the chance that a patient will take legal action against the dental professional or the supervising dentist.

Roentgen (R) The traditional unit of exposure for x-rays; the quantity of x-radiation or gamma radiation that produces an electrical charge of 2.58×10^{-4} coulombs in 1 kilogram of air at standard pressure and temperature conditions.

Roentgen equivalent (in) man (rem) The traditional unit of the dose equivalent; the product of absorbed dose (rad) and a quality factor (QF) specific for the type of radiation; 100 rems = 1 sievert (Sv).

Roller film transporter A component part of the automatic film processor; a system of rollers is used to move the film rapidly through the developer, fixer, water, and the drying compartments.

Room lighting One of the two essential types of lighting in a darkroom; room lighting provides adequate illumination for the size of the room to perform tasks such as cleaning, stocking of materials, and mixing of chemicals.

Rotation center In panoramic radiography, the axis or pivotal point on which the receptor and x-ray tubehead rotate around the patient.

Safelight filter A filter placed over the safelight that is designed to remove the short wavelengths in the blue-green portion of the visible light spectrum that are responsible for exposing and damaging x-ray film.

Safelighting One of the two essential types of lighting in a darkroom; a low-intensity light composed of long wavelengths in the red-orange portion of the visible light spectrum; safelighting provides sufficient illumination in the darkroom to carry out processing activities without exposing or damaging the film.

Sclerotic bone A well-defined radiopacity seen below the apices of vital, noncarious teeth (also known as *osteosclerosis* or *idiopathic periapical osteosclerosis*).

Screen, calcium tungstate A type of intensifying screen used in extraoral radiography; contains phosphors that emit blue light.

Screen, intensifying A device used in extraoral radiography that converts x-ray energy into visible light; the light, in turn, exposes the screen film.

Screen, rare earth A type of intensifying screen used in extraoral radiography; contains phosphors not usually found in the earth that emit green light.

Self-determination The legal rights of an individual to make choices about the care he or she receives, including the opportunity to consent to or refuse treatment.

Sensitivity speck An irregularity within the lattice structure of the exposed silver halide crystals that attracts the silver atoms.

Sensor In digital radiography, a small detector that is placed intraorally to capture a radiographic image.

Septum Bony wall or partition that divides a cavity into separate areas; appears radiopaque (plural: septa).

Sharp Any object that can penetrate skin, including, but not limited to, needles and scalpels.

Sharpness Refers to the capability of the receptor to reproduce the distinct outlines of an object; influenced by focal spot size, film composition, and movement.

Shell See **Orbit**.

Short-term effects Effects of radiation that appear within minutes, days, or weeks; associated with large amounts of radiation absorbed in a short time.

Sievert (Sv) A unit of measurement for dose equivalent; the SI unit of measurement equivalent to the rem; 1 Sv = 100 rems.

Silver halide crystals Crystals that are suspended in the emulsion of the dental x-ray film (e.g., silver bromide, silver iodide); function to absorb radiation during x-ray exposure and store energy from the radiation.

Sinus A hollow space, cavity, or recess in bone; appears radiolucent.

Sodium carbonate See **Accelerator**.

Sodium sulfite See **Preservative**.

Sodium thiosulfate See **Fixing agent**.

Soft tissue opacity A well-defined radiopacity located in soft tissue and viewed on a radiograph.

Somatic cells All the cells in the body, with the exception of the reproductive cells.

Somatic effects Radiation injuries that produce changes in somatic cells and produce poor health in the irradiated individual (e.g., the induction of cancer, leukemia, or cataracts).

Spine A sharp, thornlike projection of bone; appears radiopaque.

Standard of care In dentistry, the quality of care that is provided by dental practitioners in a similar locality under the same or similar conditions.

Standard precautions Measures that integrate and expand the elements of universal precautions into a standard of care designed to protect health care personnel and patients from pathogens that can be spread by blood or any other body fluid, excretion, or secretion.

Static electricity A film handling error; thin, black, branching lines on a film that result from opening a film packet too quickly.

Statute of limitations A period during which a patient may bring a malpractice action against a dentist or an auxiliary.

Stepwedge A device constructed of uniform-layered thicknesses of an x-ray absorbing material, usually aluminum; different steps absorb varying amounts of x-rays and are used to demonstrate film densities and contrast scales.

Sterilization The act of sterilizing; see **Sterilize**.

Sterilize The use of a physical or chemical procedure to destroy all pathogens, including highly resistant bacterial and fungal spores.

Stimuli, psychogenic Stimuli originating in the mind.

Stimuli, tactile Stimuli originating from touch.

Stirring paddle A device used in manual processing; agitates the developer and fixer solutions and equalizes the temperature of the solutions before processing.

Stirring rod See **Stirring paddle**.

Stochastic effects Biologic effects from radiation that occur as a direct function of dose; the probability of occurrence increases with increasing absorbed dose; however, the severity of effects does not depend on the magnitude of the absorbed dose.

Storage phosphor imaging A method of obtaining a digital image in which the image is recorded on phosphor-coated plates and then placed into an electronic processor, where a laser scans the plate and produces an image on a computer screen.

Styloid process A long, pointed, and sharp projection of bone that extends downward from the inferior surface of the temporal bone; located anterior to the mastoid process.

Subject thickness The thickness of soft tissue and bone in a patient.

Submandibular fossa A depressed area of bone located on the internal surface of the mandible inferior to the mylohyoid ridge; appears radiolucent.

Submentovertex projection An extraoral radiographic projection used to identify the position of the condyles, demonstrate the base of the skull, and evaluate fractures of the zygomatic arch.

Sulfuric acid See **Acidifier**.

Superior foramina of the incisive canal Two tiny openings or holes in bone that are located on the floor of the nasal cavity; appear radiolucent.

Suture An immovable joint that represents a line of union between adjoining bones of the skull; appears radiolucent.

Tank, insert In manual processing, a component part of the processing tank; two removable insert tanks are placed in the master tank and hold the developer and fixer solutions.

Tank, master In manual processing, a component part of the processing tank; the master tank is filled with circulating water that surrounds and suspends the two insert tanks.

Tank, processing A tank used in manual processing; divided into compartments for the developer solution, water bath, and fixer solution; a processing tank has two insert tanks and one master tank.

Target lesion A well-defined, localized radiopacity surrounded by a uniform radiolucent halo.

Teeth, anterior Incisors and canines.

Teeth, posterior Premolars and molars.

Temporomandibular joint (TMJ) The jaw joint ; includes the temporal bone (glenoid fossa and articular eminence) and the mandible (condyle) and the articular disc between the two bones.

Temporomandibular joint tomography An extraoral radiographic technique used to examine the temporomandibular joint (TMJ).

Thermionic emission The release of electrons from the tungsten filament when the electrical current passes through it and heats the filament.

Thermometer A device used to measure temperature.

Three-dimensional volume rendering A three-dimensional shape that is created from two-dimensional images.

Thyroid collar A flexible lead shield used to protect the thyroid gland from scatter radiation.

Timer A mechanical device used to measure time intervals.

Tomogram An extraoral radiograph used to examine the bony components of the temporomandibular joint (TMJ).

Tomography Radiography technique that allows the imaging of one layer or section of the body while blurring images from structures in other planes.

Tongue A movable muscular organ attached to the floor of the mouth.

Tooth-bearing areas Regions of the maxilla and mandible in which the 32 teeth of the human dentition are normally located.

Torus A bony growth in the oral cavity (plural, *tori*).

Torus, mandibular A bony growth seen along the lingual aspect of the mandible (also known as *torus mandibularis*).

Torus, maxillary A nodular mass of bone along the midline of the hard palate (also known as *torus palatinus*).

Total dose Quantity of radiation received, or the total amount of radiation energy absorbed.

Transcranial projection An extraoral radiographic projection used to evaluate the superior surface of the condyle and the articular eminence; this view can also be used to evaluate the movement of the condyle when the mouth is opened (also called *Lindblom technique*).

Transformer A device used to increase or decrease the voltage of incoming electricity.

Transformer, step-down In dental radiography, a device used to decrease the incoming voltage from 110 or 220 volts to the low voltage required, usually 3 to 5 volts.

Transformer, step-up In dental radiography, a device used to increase the incoming line voltage from 110 or 220 volts to the high voltage required, usually 65,000 to 100,000 volts.

Trauma Injury produced by an external force.

Triangle In geometry, a figure formed by connecting three points not in a straight line by three straight-line segments; the figure has three angles.

Triangle, equilateral In geometry, a triangle with three equal sides.

Triangle, right In geometry, a triangle with one 90-degree angle (right angle).

Triangles, congruent In geometry, triangles that are identical and correspond exactly when superimposed.

Tube side The outer side of the x-ray film packet that is solid white and exhibits a raised bump in one corner; the tube side of the film faces the teeth and tubehead.

Tubehead The tightly sealed heavy metal housing that contains the dental x-ray tube; includes the metal housing, insulating oil, tubehead seal, x-ray tube, transformers, aluminum discs, lead collimator, and position-indicating device (PID); contains a filament used to produce electrons and a target used to produce x-rays.

Tubehead seal The aluminum or leaded-glass covering of the tubehead that permits the exit of x-rays from the tubehead; seals the oil in the tubehead and filters the x-ray beam.

Tubercle A small bump or nodule of bone; appears radiopaque.

Tuberosity A rounded prominence of bone; appears radiopaque.

Tungsten filament A portion of the cathode in the x-ray tube; a coiled wire of tungsten that produces electrons when heated.

Tungsten target A portion of the anode in the x-ray tube; serves as a focal spot and converts bombarding electrons into x-ray photons.

Unilocular corticated A term used to describe a radiolucent lesion that exhibits one compartment with a well-defined outer border.

Unilocular noncorticated A term used to describe a radiolucent lesion that exhibits one compartment without a well-defined outer border.

Useful beam See **Radiation, primary**.

Uvula A small, muscular structure located on the free edge of the soft palate.

Vacuum tube A sealed glass tube from which most of the air has been evacuated.

Valve, mixing In manual processing, a device that mixes the incoming hot and cold water to produce a water bath of optimum temperature (68°F).

Velocity Speed; in dental radiography, the speed of a wave.

Viewbox A light source used to view dental radiographs (also called the *illuminator*).

Viewing Examining or inspecting; see **Film viewing**.

Volt (V) Unit of measure for voltage.

Voltage In dental radiography, measurement of force that refers to the potential difference between two electrical charges.

Voxel The smallest element of a three-dimensional image; also referred to as *volume element* or *three-dimensional pixel*.

Washing A step in film processing; water is used to wash a film after fixation; removes excess chemicals from the emulsion.

Waters projection An extraoral radiographic projection used to evaluate the maxillary sinus area.

Wavelength The distance between the crest of one wave to the crest of the next wave; determines the energy and penetrating power of the radiation (the shorter the wavelength, the higher is the energy).

X-radiation A high-energy radiation produced by the collision of a beam of electrons with a metal target in an x-ray tube; see **X-ray(s)**.

X-ray(s) A beam of energy that has the power to penetrate substances and record image shadows on photographic film or digital sensors.

X-ray beam angulation One of the influencing factors for image distortion; refers to the direction of the x-ray beam; less image distortion results when the x-ray beam is directed perpendicular to the tooth and receptor.

X-ray tube A component part of the x-ray tubehead that generates x-rays; includes a leaded-glass vacuum tube, cathode, and anode.

Zygoma The cheekbone; articulates with the zygomatic process of the maxilla and appears as a diffuse radiopaque band posterior to the zygomatic process of the maxilla (also call *zygomatic bone* or *malar bone*).

Zygomatic process of maxilla A bony projection of the maxilla that articulates with the zygoma; appears as a J-shaped or U-shaped radiopacity on a maxillary molar periapical image.

Index

A

AAOMR. *See* American Academy of Oral and Maxillofacial Radiology (AAOMR).
Abscess
  periapical, 432–433, 433f
  periodontal, 432
Absorbed dose, patient exposure and, 42, 42t
Absorption
  definition of, 35
  of energy, 20
  radiation injury and, 35
AC (alternating current), 16–17
Accelerator, in developer solution, 89t, 90
Acetic acid, in fixing solution, 90, 90t
Acidifier, in fixing solution, 90
Acrylic restorations, identification of, 390
Activator, in developer solution, 90
ADA. *See* American Dental Association (ADA).
Added filtration, in radiation protection, 46, 46f
Adhesive layer, of film, 64, 64f
Age, radiation injury and, 37
Air bubbles on film, 101t, 105, 105f
Air spaces on panoramic images, 363, 365f
Airway analysis, three-dimensional digital imaging for, 317
ALARA concept, in radiation protection, 53
Alignment
  object-film, image distortion and, 81t, 83, 83f
  x-ray beam. *See* X-ray beam alignment.
Alpha particles, 12
Alternating current (AC), 16–17
Aluminum disks in x-ray tubehead, 14–15, 15f
  in radiation protection, 46, 46f, 48f
Alveolar bone, 340–341, 341f
  anatomy of, 341, 341f
  definition of, 211, 211f
  loss of, location of, 376–377, 377f
  shape and density of, 341–342, 342f
Alveolar crest, 341, 342f
  appearance of, on dental image, 413, 413f
Alveolar process, anatomy of, 335, 336f
Amalgam fragments, identification of, 385, 385f–386f
Amalgam overhangs, identification of, 384, 385f
Amalgam restorations, identification of, 384–385, 384f–385f
American Academy of Oral and Maxillofacial Radiology (AAOMR)
  on collimator selection, 157
  F-speed film recommended by, 68
American Dental Association (ADA)
  on collimator selection, 157
  F-speed film recommended by, 68
  guidelines of, for prescribing dental radiographs, 46, 47t
  periodontal disease classification by, 416–419, 417f–420f
Ammonium thiosulfate, as fixing agent, 90, 90t
Amperage, 17
  x-ray beam quantity and, 29–30
Ampere (A), 17
  definition of, 29, 39t

Analog image, 302
  definition of, 302
Analog-to-digital converter (ADC), 302–303
Anatomic landmarks, 328–339
  mandibular, 335–339, 360–363
    angle of mandible as, 362f, 363, 364f
    coronoid notch as, 360, 362f–363f
    coronoid process as, 327f, 339, 340f, 360–361, 362f–363f
    external oblique ridge as, 339, 339f, 362f, 363, 364f
    genial tubercles as, 327f, 335–336, 336f, 362, 362f–363f
    interior border of mandible as, 362, 362f, 364f
    internal oblique ridge as, 327f, 338–339, 339f, 362f, 363, 364f
    lingual foramen as, 327f, 336, 336f, 362, 362f
    lingula as, 361, 362f
    mandibular canal as, 338, 338f, 361–362, 362f, 364f
    mandibular condyle as, 360, 362f–363f
    mandibular foramen as, 361, 362f–363f
    mental foramen as, 327f, 337, 338f, 362, 362f–363f
    mental fossa as, 327f, 337, 338f, 362, 362f
    mental ridge as, 327f, 337, 337f, 362, 362f
    mylohyoid ridge as, 327f, 337–338, 338f, 362, 362f
    nutrient canals as, 336–337, 337f
    for periapical images, 348t
    submandibular fossa as, 327f, 339, 339f
  maxillary, 328–335
    anterior nasal spine as, 328f, 332, 332f, 358f, 359
    articular eminence as, 358f, 359
    external auditory meatus as, 358, 358f
    floor of nasal cavity as, 327f, 332, 332f
    glenoid fossa as, 358–359, 358f
    hamulus as, 328f, 334, 335f, 358f, 360
    hard palate as, 358f, 359
    incisive canal as, 358f, 359
    incisive foramen as, 329, 329f–330f, 358f, 359
    inferior nasal conchae as, 327f, 332, 333f
    infraorbital foramen as, 358f, 359
    inverted Y as, 334, 334f
    lateral fossa as, 327f, 330–331, 331f
    lateral pterygoid plate as, 358f, 359
    mastoid process as, 358, 358f
    maxillary sinus and floor of maxillary sinus as, 358f, 359–360
    maxillary sinus as, 328f, 332, 333f
    maxillary tuberosity as, 328f, 334, 334f, 358f, 359
    median palatal suture as, 329f–330f, 330
    nasal cavity as, 327f, 331, 331f, 358f, 359
    nasal septum as, 327f, 331, 331f, 358f, 359
    nutrient canals within maxillary sinus as, 334, 334f
    orbit as, 358f, 359
    for periapical images, 348t
    pterygomaxillary fissure as, 358f, 359
    septa within maxillary sinus as, 332, 333f
    styloid process as, 358, 358f

Anatomic landmarks *(Continued)*
    superior foramina of incisive canal as, 327f, 329–330, 330f
    zygoma as, 335, 335f–336f, 358f, 360
    zygomatic process of maxilla as, 334–335, 335f, 358f, 360, 360f
Anatomic order
  for dental radiographs, 346–347
  for digital images, 348
Anatomy
  of alveolar bone, 341, 341f
  film mounting and, 348, 348t
  on intraoral images, 325–343
    of bone, 326
     cancellous, 326, 326f–327f
     cortical, 326, 326f
     prominences of, 326–327, 327f–328f
     spaces and depressions in, 327f–328f, 328
  on panoramic images, 257f, 357–367
    air spaces in, 363, 365f
    mandibular landmarks as, 360–363. *See also* Anatomic landmarks, mandibular.
    maxillary landmarks as, 358–360. *See also* Anatomic landmarks, maxillary.
    soft tissues in, 363–365, 366f
  on three-dimensional digital images, 317, 318f
    accuracy of, 321
    beyond maxilla and mandible, lack of training on, 321–322
  of tooth, 340–342
Anesthetic, topical, for gag reflex, 292
Angle
  definition of, 181, 181f
  of mandible, 362f, 363, 364f
Angulation
  in bisecting technique, 183–185
    horizontal, 183, 184f
     problems with, 206
    vertical, 183–185, 184f–185f, 185t
  in bite-wing technique, 213–214
    horizontal, 214
     incorrect, 231–232, 232f
    vertical, 214, 215f–216f
     incorrect, 232, 232f
  definition of, 183–184
  horizontal. *See* Horizontal angulation.
  in paralleling technique, 156f, 158–159, 159f
    with shallow palate, 173
  vertical. *See* Vertical angulation.
Anode, x-ray tube, 16, 16f
Anterior nasal spine
  on intraoral image, 328f, 332, 332f
  on panoramic image, 358f, 359, 360f
Antiseptic, definition of, 141
Apron, lead
  artifact from, in panoramic imaging, 262, 265f
  infection control and, 143, 145
  for pediatric patient, 293
  in radiation protection, 50, 50f
  removal of, 146
Articular eminence, 358f, 359, 361f
Artifact(s)
  fingernail, 101t, 105, 105f
  fingerprint, 101t, 105, 105f

Artifact(s) *(Continued)*
  lead apron, in panoramic imaging, 262, 265f
  motion, in three-dimensional digital imaging, 321
  static electricity, 101t, 105–106, 105f
Asepsis, definition of, 141
Atom
  atomic number of, 9
  definition of, 9
  neutral, 11
  structure of, 9–11, 9f
Atomic number, 9
Atomic weight, 9
Attitude, patient relations and, 128
Auditory meatus, external, 358, 358f, 360f
Automatic processor
  care and maintenance of, 97
  components of, 96–97, 96f
  quality control tests for, 114
Autotransformer, 17, 17f
Avulsion, 428, 428f
Axial plane
  definition of, 313–314, 314f
  image through, 315f

B
Background radiation, 40, 41t
BAI beam alignment devices, 61
Barrier envelopes, for intraoral films, 143–145
Base materials, identification of, 390, 390f
Beam. *See* X-ray beam.
Beam alignment devices, 59
  in bisecting technique, 182–183, 183f
  in bite-wing technique, 212, 213f
  infection control for
    during exposure, 146
    postexposure, 146
    preexposure, 145–146
  in paralleling technique, 157–158
  in radiation protection, 50, 51f
  types of, 60–61
Beta particles, 12
Binding energy, of electrons, 10
Biology, radiation, 34–44
Bisect, definition of, 181, 181f
Bisecting angle instruments (BAIs), 182–183, 183f
Bisecting technique, 180–209
  advantages of, 189
  angulation in, problems with, 206
  angulation of position-indicating device for, 183–185
    horizontal, 183, 184f
    vertical, 183–185, 184f–186f, 185t
  charting of full-mouth series with, 206t
  disadvantages of, 189–206
  equipment preparation for, 186, 187b
  exposure sequence in, 187–188
    anterior, 187, 187t
    posterior, 187–188, 187t
  helpful hints for, 206
  history of, 6
  patient preparation for, 186, 186b
  in periodontal disease evaluation, 414, 414f
  principles of, 181–182, 181f–182f
  procedures for, 185–189
  receptor for, 183
  receptor placement in
    guidelines for, 189b
    for mandibular canine exposure, 188, 194b, 194f–195f
    for mandibular incisor exposure, 188, 196b, 196f–197f

Bisecting technique *(Continued)*
    for mandibular molar exposure, 189, 204b, 204f–205f
    for mandibular premolar exposure, 189, 202b, 202f–203f
    for maxillary canine exposure, 188, 190b, 190f–191f
    for maxillary incisor exposure, 188, 192b, 192f–193f
    for maxillary molar exposure, 189, 200b–206b, 200f–201f
    for maxillary premolar exposure, 189, 198b, 198f–199f
  rules of, 185
  terminology for, 181
Bisector, imaginary, 182
Bit-depth image, 305
  definition of, 302
Bite-block, 59–60, 60f
Bite-wing
  horizontal, definition of, 211
  vertical, 222, 222f–223f
    definition of, 212
Bite-wing film, 67–68, 67f
  sizes of, 68, 69f–70f
Bite-wing receptor, definition of, 211
Bite-wing tab, 213, 214f
Bite-wing technique, 210–225
  absorbed doses from, 42t
  angulation of position-indicating device in, 213–214
    horizontal, 214
    vertical, 214, 215f–216f
  beam alignment device for, 212, 213f
  bite-wing tab in, 213, 214f
  charting exposures with, 222t
  equipment preparation for, 215, 216b
  errors in, 230–233
    angulation problems as, 231–232
    receptor placement problems as, 230–231
  exposure sequence in, 215–216, 216f
  helpful hints for, 223–224
  history of, 6
  modifications of, 222–224
    for bony growths, 223
    for edentulous spaces, 222–223
  patient preparation for, 215, 216b
  for pediatric patient, 295f
  principles of, 212, 212f
  procedures for, 214–217
  receptor placement in, 216–217
    guidelines for, 217b
    for molar exposure, 217, 220b–222b, 220f–222f
      correct, 231, 231f
      incorrect, 231, 232f
    for premolar exposure, 217, 217b–218b, 217f–219f
      correct, 231, 231f
      incorrect, 231, 232f
  receptors for, 213
  rules of, 214
  terminology for, 211–212
Blind patients, modifications for, 292
Bloodborne pathogens, definition of, 141
Body, mandibular, anatomy of, 335, 336f
Body movement, in nonverbal communication, 126
Bone
  alveolar, 340–341, 341f
    anatomy of, 341, 341f
    definition of, 211
  cancellous, 326, 326f–327f
  cortical, 326, 326f

Bone *(Continued)*
  crestal, definition of, 211
  loss of. *See also* Periodontal disease.
    horizontal, 415, 415f
    vertical, 415, 416f
  prominences of, 326–327, 327f–328f
  sclerotic, 433, 434f
  spaces and depressions in, 327f–328f, 328
Bone marrow, dental radiation risks to, 41
Bony landmarks
  mandibular, 335–339. *See also* Anatomic landmarks, mandibular.
  maxillary, 328–335. *See also* Anatomic landmarks, maxillary.
Braking radiation, 18
Bremsstrahlung, 18
Bridge, gold, 386, 387f
Buccal caries, 407, 407f–408f
Buccal object rule, 242, 248b–250b, 248f–250f, 252f

C
Calcium tungstate intensifying screens, 71
Calculus, periodontal disease and, 419, 421f–422f
Canal
  definition of, 328
  incisive
    on panoramic image, 358f, 359
    superior foramina of, 327f, 329–330, 330f
  mandibular, 328f
    on intraoral images, 338, 338f
    on panoramic image, 361–362, 362f, 364f
Cancellous bone, 326, 326f–327f
Canine exposure
  mandibular
    in bisecting technique, 188, 194b, 194f–195f
    in paralleling technique, 163, 167b, 167f
  maxillary
    in bisecting technique, 188, 190b, 190f–191f
    in paralleling technique, 163, 165b, 165f
Caries. *See* Dental caries.
Cassette(s)
  for extraoral imaging, 276
  for panoramic film, 72, 72f, 261, 261f–262f
  quality control tests for, 112–113
  for screen films, 71–72, 71f–72f
Cathode, x-ray tube, 16, 16f
Cathode rays, 12
  early studies of, 4
CBCT. *See* Cone beam computed tomography (CBCT).
CBVT (cone beam volume tomography), definition of, 313
Cell(s)
  definition of, 38
  genetic, 37
  radiation effects on, 38
  radioresistant, 38, 38t
  radiosensitive, 38, 38t
  radiosensitivity of, radiation injury and, 37
  somatic, 37
Cell differentiation, radiosensitivity and, 38
Cell metabolism, radiosensitivity and, 38
Centers for Disease Control and Prevention (CDC), guidelines of, for infection control practices, 141
Central ray, definition of, 156, 181
Cephalometric film, 68
  image on, 71f
Cephalostat, for extraoral imaging, 275, 275f

Chair, dental
  adjustment of, 145
  infection control and, 143
Chairside manner, patient relations and, 127–128
Characteristic radiation, 19, 19f
Charge-coupled device (CCD), 304
  definition of, 302
Chemicals, contamination errors in film processing from, 101t, 103, 103f
Chrome crowns, identification, 386–387
Chronic focal sclerosing osteomyelitis, 433
Circuits, 17
Circular collimator, 46–48, 49f
Cleaning
  of dental unit and environmental surfaces, 143
  of processing tank, 94, 95b
Cleaning film, 97
Clear film mounts, 346–347, 346f
Clinical attachment loss (CAL), in periodontal disease, 415
Coherent scatter, 20, 21f
Coin test for safelighting, 114, 114f
Collar, thyroid, in radiation protection, 48–50, 50f
Collimation
  patient exposure and, 41
  in radiation protection, 46–48
Collimator
  lead, in x-ray tubehead, 15, 15f
  of panoramic x-ray machine, 259, 260f
  in radiation protection, 46, 48f–49f
  XCP Universal, 61, 61f
Communication skills, in patient relations, 125–126
Complementary metal oxide semiconductor/ active pixel sensor (CMOS/APS), 304–305
Complete mouth radiographic series (CMRS), 153
Composite restorations, identification of, 389, 390f
Compton electron, 20
Compton scatter, 20, 21f
Computed tomography, cone beam, 312. *See also* Cone beam computed tomography (CBCT).
Conchae, nasal, inferior, 327f, 332, 333f
Condensing osteitis, 433, 433f
Condyle, mandibular, 360, 362f–363f
Cone. *See* Position-indicating device (PID).
Cone beam computed tomography (CBCT). *See also* Three-dimensional digital imaging.
  cone-shaped beam in, 313, 313f
  definition of, 313
  development of, 312
Cone beam computed tomography (CBCT) machine, 315, 316f–317f
Cone beam volume tomography (CBVT), definition of, 313
Cone cuts, in periapical technique, problems with, 229–230, 230f–231f
Confidentiality, 137
Congruent triangles, definition of, 181, 181f
Conical position-indicating device, 48, 49f
Consent, informed, 136–137
Consumer-Patient Radiation Health and Safety Act (1981), 52–53
  on safe use of dental x-ray equipment, 135–136
Contact areas, definition of, 211, 211f
Contacts
  opened, definition of, 211, 212f
  overlapped, definition of, 212, 212f

Contrast
  high, 78
  kilovoltage peak and, 28, 28t, 29f, 78t, 79, 79f, 80t
  long-scale, 79, 80t
  low, 78
  of radiographic image, 78–80, 79f–80f, 80t
    factors influencing, 79
    receptor, 78–79
    scales of, 79–80, 80f, 80t
    subject, 79
  short-scale, 79, 80t
  stepwedge, 79–80, 80f
Contrast resolution
  definition of, 313
  in three-dimensional digital imaging, 315
Control devices, 59
Control panel, 14, 14f, 58–59, 59f
Coolidge, William D., x-ray tube developed by, 5
Copper stem, in anode, 16, 16f
Coronal plane
  definition of, 313–314, 314f
  image through, 315f
Coronoid notch, 360, 362f–363f
Coronoid process
  on intraoral images, 327f, 337, 340f
  on panoramic image, 360–361, 362f–363f
Cortical bone, 326, 326f
Cosmic radiation, 40, 41t
Cotton rolls, in paralleling technique with shallow palate, 173, 173f
Coulomb (C), definition of, 39t, 40
Coulombs/kilogram (C/kg), 39, 39t
  in exposure measurement, 40
Craniostat, for extraoral imaging, 275
Crestal bone, definition of, 211, 211f
Critical instruments, sterilization and disinfection of, 143
Critical organ(s), 38
  dental radiation risks to, 41
Crookes, William, in early study of cathode rays, 4
Crowns
  chrome, identification of, 386–387
  fractured, 427, 427f
  gold, 386, 386f
  porcelain, identification of, 388–389, 388f–389f
  porcelain-fused-to-metal, identification of, 389, 389f–390f
  stainless steel, identification of, 386–387, 387f–388f
Cumulative effects of radiation exposure, 37
Cyst, periapical, 432, 432f

D
D-speed film, 50, 68
Darkroom
  disinfection of, for processing, 146
  function of, 97
  lighting for, 98, 98f
    quality control tests for, 113–114
  location and size of, 97–98
  plumbing for, 99
  requirements for, 97
  storage space in, 99
  supplies for, infection control and, 146
  temperature and humidity controls in, 99
  waste management in, 99
  work space in, 98–99

Data
  DICOM, definition of, 313
  raw, in three-dimensional digital imaging, 314
Daylight loaders, 86, 95f
  infection control procedures for, 146–147
DC (direct current), 16–17
Deaf patients, modifications for, 292
Deep breathing, for gag reflex, 292
Density
  exposure time and, 78, 78t
  kilovoltage peak and, 27–28, 28f, 28t, 78, 78t
  milliamperage and, 30, 30t, 78, 78t
  of radiographic image, 77–78, 77f
    factors influencing, 77–78, 78t
  subject thickness and, 78
Dental caries
  classification of, 404–408
    buccal and lingual, 407, 407f–408f
    interproximal, 404–406, 404f–405f
    occlusal, 406, 407f
    rampant, 408, 409f
    recurrent, 408, 408f
    root surface, 407–408, 408f
  description of, 403, 403f
  detection of, 403
  examination of
    clinical, 403, 403f
    dental image in, 403
  interpretation of, 402–411
  interproximal, bite-wing images in detection of, 211
  radiolucency of, 373, 373f
Dental chair
  adjustment of, 145
  infection control and, 143
Dental radiograph(s)
  benefits of, 122
  in caries evaluation, 403–404
  definition of, 3, 121
  diagnostic, 77
  duplicate, 72
  importance of, 3, 121
  information found on, 122
  interpretation of, 369–371. *See also* Image interpretation.
  mounting of, 345–352. *See also* Film mounting.
  ownership and retention of, 137–138
  patient refusal of, legal significance of, 138
  prescribing, 154
    for pediatric patients, 293
    radiation protection and, 46, 47t
  risk versus benefit of, 42
  uses of, 3b, 122
  x-ray versus, 373
Dental radiographer, 122–123
  attitude of, gag reflex in patient and, 291
  competence of, 123
    in quality assurance, 117
  definition of, 3
  dental radiographs and, 121–124
  description of, 122
  duties of, 122–123
  efficiency of, 123
  in infection control, 140–150
  infection control for, 145–146
  interpersonal skills of, 125–127
  knowledge requirements for, 122
  legal issues and, 135–139
  in patient education, 123, 130–134. *See also* Education, patient.
  in patient protection, 123

Dental radiographer *(Continued)*
  patient relations and, 125–129. *See also* Patient relations.
  in production of quality radiographs, 123
  professional goals of, 123
  protection of, 123
  quality care and, 123
  radiation protection for, 51–52, 123
    guidelines for, 51–52
    radiation monitoring in, 52
  responsibilities of, 122–123
  skill requirements for, 122
Dental radiographic techniques. *See also* Bisecting technique; Bite-wing technique; Panoramic radiography; Paralleling technique.
  history of, 6
Dental radiography
  definition of, 3
  federal and state regulations on, 135–136
  history of, 3–6, 6t
  infection control in, 143–147
    checklist for, 144b
  legal issues and, 135–136
  licensure requirements for, 136
  measurements used in, 40
Dental x-radiation, pioneers in, 4–5
Dental x-ray equipment, history of, 5
Dental x-ray film. *See* Film.
Dental x-ray image, 76–85. *See also* Image(s).
Dental x-rays, production of, 17–18, 18f
Dentin, 340, 340f
Dentino-enamel junction (DEJ), 340, 340f
  caries at, 404–405, 404f–405f
Dentistry, x-radiation and, 2–3
Dentures
  complete, identification of, 391–392, 392f
  removable partial, identification of, 392, 393f
Descriptive terminology, 372–382
  definition of, 372
  diagnosis versus, 373
  reasons to use, 373
Developer compartment, of automatic processor, 96, 96f
Developer cutoff, 101t, 103–104, 104f
Developer solution, 87, 89–90., 89t
  care and maintenance of, 94
  disposal of, 99
  strength of, quality control tests for, 114–116
Developer spots, 101t, 103, 103f
Developing agent, 89–90, 89t
Development, in film processing, 87
  manual, 88–89
Developmental disabilities, 292–293
Diagnosis
  definition of, 369
  descriptive terminology versus, 373
  interpretation versus, 370
Diagnostic image, enhancement of, with digital imaging, 309
Diagnostic radiograph, 77, 153
Diaphragm collimator, 48f
Diatorics, identification of, 391–392, 392f
DICOM data, definition of, 313
DICOM images, in three-dimensional digital imaging, 314
Digital image(s), 302, 303f
  definition of, 302, 373
  mounts for, 348, 348f
  patient questions about, 133
  quality assurance procedures for, 116–117
  quality of, 309
  retrieval of, for radiation protection, 51

Digital imaging, 301–311
  advantages of, 307–309
  background of, 301
  computer for, 305, 305f
  definition of, 302
  direct, 306
  disadvantages of, 309–310
  efficiency of, 308–309, 308f
  equipment for, 303–305
  fundamentals of, 302–303
  indirect, 306–307
  intraoral sensor for, 304–305
  legal issues and, 309–310
  patient questions about, 133
  procedures for, 307
  purpose and use of, 302
  quality assurance procedures for, 116–117
  radiation exposure in, 303, 308
  sensor placement in, 307, 308f
  sensor preparation for, 307, 307f
  terminology for, 302
  three-dimensional, 312–323
  types of, 305–307
  x-radiation source for, 303
Digital radiography, 301–311. *See also* Digital imaging.
Digital subtraction
  definition of, 302
  in enhancement of diagnostic image, 309, 309f
Digitize, 302–303
  definition of, 302
Direct current (DC), 16–17
Direct digital imaging, 306
  definition of, 302
Direct theory of radiation injury, 36
Disability, definition of, 292
Disabled patients, 292–293
Disinfect, definition of, 141
Disinfectants
  intermediate-level, 143
  low-level, 143
Disinfection
  definition of, 141
  of dental unit and environmental surfaces, 143
  of instruments, in infection control, 142–143
  surface, postexposure, 146
Distance
  image magnification and, 81t, 82–83, 82f–83f
  radiation protection for operator and, 51
Distortion, image, 83
  in bisecting technique, 189–206
  definition of, 83
  factors influencing, 81t, 83, 83f
Distraction, for gag reflex, 292
Documentation, in patient record, 137
Dose
  absorbed, patient exposure and, 42, 42t
  of background radiation exposure, 54
  definition of, 54
  low, with three-dimensional digital imaging, 319–321
  maximum accumulated, 53
  maximum permissible, 53
  measurement of, 40
  radiation injury and, 37
Dose equivalent measurement, 41
Dose-response curve for radiation exposure, 36, 36f
Drying, in film processing, manual, 89
Drying chamber, of automatic processor, 96, 96f
Duplicate radiograph, 72
Duplicating film, 72

Duplication, film, 99
  equipment for, 99, 99f
  procedure for, 99, 100b, 100f
Duplicator, film, 99, 99f

E
E-speed film, 50
  discontinuation of, 68
Ear, on panoramic image, 365, 366f
Earrings, identification of, 395, 396f–397f
Edentulous, definition of, 296, 376–377
Edentulous patients, 296–298
Edentulous space, bite-wing technique modifications for, 222–223
Edentulous zone
  radiolucent lesions in, 376–377, 377f
  radiopaque lesions in, 380, 380f
Education, patient
  dental radiographer in, 123, 130–134
  digital images in, 309
  image interpretation and, 370
  importance of, 130–131
  methods of, 131
  questions and answers in, 131–133
    about digital imaging, 133
    about exposure, 132
    about necessity, 131–132
    about safety, 133
    miscellaneous, 133
  radiation protection and, 53
EEZEE-Grip film holder, 59–60, 60f
  in bisecting technique, 182–183, 183f
  in paralleling technique, 157, 158f
Efficiency, of digital imaging, 308–309, 308f
Ektaspeed film, 50
Electrical currents, for generating x-rays, 16–17
Electricity
  for generating x-rays, 16–17
  static, as artifact, 101t, 105–106, 105f
Electromagnetic radiation, 12–13
  properties of, 13b
Electromagnetic spectrum, 12, 13f
Electron(s), 9–11
  binding energy of, 10
  Compton, 20
Electron volts (eV), 10
Electrostatic force, 10
Elements
  definition of, 9
  periodic table of, 9, 10f
Elon, in developing agent, 89–90, 89t
Elongated image
  in bisecting technique, 185, 186f
  in periapical technique, 229, 230f
Emulsion, film, 64, 64f
  reticulation of, 101t, 102, 103f
Enamel, 340, 340f
Endodontic assessment, three-dimensional digital imaging for, 317, 318f
Endodontic patients, 295–296
Endodontics
  definition of, 295–296
  materials used in, identification of, 391
EndoRay film holder, 59–60, 60f
Energy
  absorption of, 20
  definition of, 9
  kinetic, in production of dental x-rays, 18
Environmental Protection Agency (EPA), sterilant and disinfectant classifications of, 143
EPA (Environmental Protection Agency), sterilant and disinfectant classifications of, 143

Equilateral triangle, definition of, 181, 181f
Equipment and supplies, 57–62
    beam alignment devices as, 59–61
        in radiation protection, 50, 51f
    for digital imaging, 303–305
        lower cost of, 308
    film holding, 59–61. *See also* Film holders.
    for film processing
        automatic, 96–97, 96f
            quality control tests for, 114
        manual, 90–91, 91f–92f
            quality control tests for, 114
    for film viewing, 352
    history of, 5
    infection control and, 143–145
    for panoramic imaging, 259–261
    personal protective, definition of, 141
    preparation of
        for bisecting technique, 186, 187b
        for bite-wing technique, 215, 216b
        for extraoral imaging, 276, 276b
        gag reflex and, 291
        for localization techniques, 248
        for panoramic imaging, 261, 262b
        for paralleling technique, 159, 160b,
            160f–161f
        for pediatric patient, 293
    quality control tests for, 112–113
    radiation monitoring for, 52
    in radiation protection
        leakage monitoring in, 52
        proper use of, 46–48
    for three-dimensional digital imaging,
        314–317
        cost of, 321
Erg (erg), definition of, 39t
Examination, radiographic, 152–154. *See also*
        Radiographic examination.
Exposure
    in bisecting technique
        of mandibular canine, 188, 194b,
            194f–195f
        of mandibular incisor, 188, 196b,
            196f–197f
        of mandibular molar, 189, 204b, 204f–205f
        of mandibular premolar, 189, 202b,
            202f–203f
        of maxillary canine, 188, 190b, 190f–191f
        of maxillary incisor, 188, 192b, 192f–193f
        of maxillary molar, 189, 200b–206b,
            200f–201f
        of maxillary premolar, 189, 198b,
            198f–199f
    in bite-wing technique
        of molars, 217, 220b–222b, 220f–222f
        of premolars, 217, 217b–218b, 217f–219f
    infectious. *See also* Infection control.
        occupational, definition of, 141
        parenteral, definition of, 141
    in paralleling technique
        of mandibular canines, 163, 167b, 167f
        of mandibular incisors, 163, 168b, 168f
        of mandibular molar, 164, 172b–173b,
            172f
        of mandibular premolar, 164, 171b, 171f
            modifications for, 174–176, 176f
        of maxillary canines, 163, 165b, 165f
        of maxillary incisors, 163, 166b, 166f
        of maxillary molar, 164, 170b, 170f
        of maxillary premolar, 164, 169b, 169f
    radiation
        cumulative effects of, 37
        in digital imaging, 308
        excess

Exposure *(Continued)*
        operator protection from, 51–52
        patient protection from
            before, 46–48
            during, 48–51
            after, 51
        factors affecting, 41–42
        guidelines for, 52–53
        measurement of, 39–40
        patient questions about, 132
        sources of, 40–41, 41t
    sequencing of, gag reflex and, 291
Exposure button, 59
Exposure errors, 227–228
Exposure factors
    in extraoral imaging, for lateral jaw
            projections, 277
    for panoramic x-ray machine, 259, 261f
    for pediatric patients, 293
    selection of, in radiation protection, 51
    x-ray beam intensity and, 48–50
    x-ray beam quality and, 27–29
    x-ray beam quantity and, 29–30
Exposure incident, 141
Exposure light, 59
Exposure time
    density and, 78, 78t
    kilovoltage peak and, 29
    milliamperage and, 30, 30t
    in three-dimensional digital imaging, 321
Extension arm, 14, 14f, 58
Extension cone paralleling technique, 156. *See
        also* Paralleling technique.
External auditory meatus, 358, 358f, 360f
External oblique ridge
    on intraoral images, 339, 339f
    on panoramic image, 362f, 363, 364f
External resorption, 429, 429f
Extraoral film, 68–72, 153
    cephalometric, 68, 71f
    equipment for use of, 69–72
    nonscreen, 69
    packaging of, 68–69, 71f
    panoramic, 68. *See also* Panoramic film.
    screen, 69, 71f
    types of, 69
    x-ray machines used for, 58, 58f
Extraoral image, definition of, 274–275
Extraoral imaging, 274–289
    cassette for, 276
    definition of, 274–275
    digital, 303
    equipment for, 275–276
    equipment preparation for, 276, 276b
    film for, 275–276
    grid for, 276, 276f
    intensifying screens for, 276
    panoramic, 256–272. *See also* Panoramic
            imaging.
    patient positioning for, 277
    patient preparation for, 276, 277b
    procedures for, 276–277
    projection techniques in, 277–287
        lateral jaw, 277, 278t, 279f–280f
        skull, 277–282
        for temporomandibular joint, 282–287,
            287f–288f
    purpose and use of, 275
Extraoral radiographic examination, 153
Extraoral receptors, 153
Extrusion, definition of, 428, 428f
Eye contact, in nonverbal communication, 126
Eyeglasses, identification of, 397, 398f
Eyes, dental radiation risks to, 41

Eyewear
    in infection control, 146
    protective, in infection control, 142

F
F-speed film, 68
    in radiation protection, 50
Facilitation, definition of, 126
Facilitation skills, in patient relations, 126–127
Fast film, in radiation protection, 50
Federal regulations, on dental radiography,
        135–136
Field of view
    in cone beam computed tomography, 313,
        314f
    definition of, 313
    in three-dimensional digital imaging, 315, 321
Filament circuit, 17
Film, 63–75. *See also* Receptor(s).
    air bubbles on, 101t, 105, 105f
    artifacts of. *See* Artifacts.
    blue-sensitive, 71
    cleaning, 97
    composition of, 64, 64f
        sharpness of image and, 81, 81t
    disposal of, 99
    duplicating, 72
    expiration date for, 73, 73f
    extraoral, 68–72. *See also* Extraoral film.
    for extraoral imaging, 275–276
    fast, in radiation protection, 50
    fogged, 102t, 106, 106f
    green-sensitive, 71
    handling of
        film processing problems associated with,
            101t, 103–106, 104f–106f
        postexposure, infection control and, 144b,
            146, 147f–148f
        during processing, infection control and,
            144b
        for radiation protection, 51
    history of, 5–6
    as image receptor, 64
    infection control and, 143–145
    intraoral, 65–68. *See also* Intraoral film.
    latent image formation on, 64–65, 65f
    nonscreen, 69
        for extraoral imaging, 275–276
    overdeveloped, 101t, 102, 102f
    overlapped, 101t, 104–105, 104f
    panoramic, 68. *See also* Panoramic film.
    for panoramic imaging, 260–261
    processing of. *See* Film processing.
    quality control tests for, 112
    scratched, 101t, 106, 106f
    screen, 64–65, 71f. *See also* Screen film(s).
    storage and protection of, 72–73
    transport of, infection control during,
        146–147
    types of, 65–72
    underdeveloped, 100–102, 101t, 102f
Film base, 64, 64f
Film duplicator, 99, 99f
Film emulsion, 64, 64f–65f
Film feed slot, 96, 96f
Film hangers, for film processing, 91, 92f
Film holders, 59–61
    in bisecting technique, 182–183, 183f
    definition of, 59
    in paralleling technique, 157–158, 158f
    types of, 59–60
Film mounting, 345–352
    basic concepts of, 346–348
    helpful hints for, 352

Film mounting (Continued)
labial, 349, 349f
lingual, 349, 349f
normal anatomy and, 348, 348t
procedure for, 349, 350b, 350f–351f
qualified personnel for, 347
timing and location for, 347
Film mounts, 346–347, 346f–347f
clear versus opaque, 346–347, 346f
information placed on, 347–348
reasons for use of, 347
sizes of, 347, 347f
Film packaging
duplicating, 72
extraoral, 68–69, 71f
intraoral, 65–67, 65f–66f
Film packet, 65
Kodak, color codes for, 67t
label side of, 67, 67f
labeled, 66f
one-film versus two-film, 65
tube side of, 67
Film placement. See also Receptor placement.
for paralleling technique, 158. See also
Paralleling technique, film placement in.
Film processing, 86–110
automatic, 95–97, 95f
advantages of, 95–96
care and maintenance in, 97
equipment for, 96–97, 96f
quality control tests for, 114
procedure for, 97, 97b
steps in, 95–96
darkroom for, 97–99. See also Darkroom.
development in, 87
duplication in, 99
equipment for, 99, 99f
procedure for, 99, 100b, 100f
film handling during, infection control and,
144b
fixing in, 88
fundamentals of, 87–88
infection control during, 146–147
manual, 88–95
care and maintenance in, 94–95
equipment for, 90–91, 91f–92f
quality control tests for, 114
procedure for, 92, 92b–93b, 93f
solutions for, 89–90
steps in, 88–89
temperatures and times for, 94t
problems with, 99–106
air bubbles as, 101t, 105, 105f
from chemical contamination, 101t, 103,
103f
developer cutoff as, 101t, 103–104, 104f
developer spots as, 101t, 103, 103f
from film handling, 101t, 103–106,
104f–106f
fingernail artifacts as, 101t, 105, 105f
fingerprint artifact as, 101t, 105, 105f
fixer cutoff as, 101t, 104, 104f
fixer spots as, 101t, 103, 103f
from lighting, 102t, 106, 106f
overdeveloped film as, 101t, 102, 102f
overlapped films as, 101t, 104–105, 104f
reasons for, 100
reticulation of emulsion as, 101t, 102, 103f
scratched film as, 101t, 106, 106f
static electricity as, 101t, 105–106, 105f
from time and temperature, 100–102, 101t,
102f–103f
underdeveloped film as, 100–102, 101t, 102f
yellow-brown stains as, 101t, 103, 103f

Film processing (Continued)
quality control tests for, 113–116, 115t
for radiation protection, 51
rinsing in, 87
solutions used in, 89–90
care and maintenance of, 94, 97
quality control tests for, 114–116
Film receptor exposure, in paralleling
technique, 159, 159f
Film recovery slot, of automatic processor, 96f,
97
Film speed
definition of, 68
intraoral, 68
patient exposure and, 41
radiation protection and, 50
Film-to-screen contact tests, 112–113, 113f
Film viewing, 352–355
equipment for, 352
helpful hints for, 354–355
procedure for, 352–353, 354b, 354f
qualified personnel for, 352
timing and location for, 352
Filtration, in radiation protection, 46
Fingernail artifacts, on film, 101t, 105, 105f
Fingerprint artifact, on film, 101t, 105, 105f
First impressions, patient relations and, 127,
127b
Fissure, pterygomaxillary, 358f, 359, 360f
Fixer compartment, of automatic processor, 96,
96f
Fixer cutoff, 101t, 104, 104f
Fixer solution, 88, 90, 90t
care and maintenance of, 94
disposal of, 99
strength of, quality control tests for, 116
Fixer spots, 101t, 103, 103f
Fixing, in film processing, 88
manual, 89
Fixing agent, 90, 90t
Fluoresce, 71
Fluorescence
early study of, 4
of phosphors, in intensifying screens, 71, 71f
Focal opacities, 377–378, 378f
Focal spot, 80
Focal spot size, sharpness of image and, 80–81,
81f, 81t
Focal trough in panoramic imaging, 259, 259f
positioning of teeth anterior to, 266,
267f–268f
positioning of teeth posterior to, 266,
268f–269f
Fogged film, 102t, 106, 106f
Food and Drug Administration (FDA),
guidelines of, for prescribing dental
radiographs, 46, 47t
Foramen(ina)
definition of, 328
incisive, on intraoral image, 329,
329f–330f
infraorbital, 358f, 359, 360f
lingual
on intraoral images, 327f, 336, 336f
on panoramic image, 362, 362f
mandibular, 361, 362f–363f
mental, 327f, 328
on intraoral images, 327f, 337, 338f
on panoramic image, 362, 362f–363f
superior, of incisive canal, 327f, 329–330,
330f
Foreshortened images
in bisecting technique, 184, 185f
in periapical technique, 229, 230f

Fossa
definition of, 328
glenoid, 358–359, 358f, 361f
lateral, 327f, 330–331, 331f
mental
on intraoral images, 327f, 337, 338f
on panoramic image, 362, 362f
submandibular, 327f, 339, 339f, 364f
Fractures, image interpretation of, 427,
427f–428f
Frankfort plane positioning, in panoramic
imaging, 265–266, 266f–267f
Free radical formation, radiation injury from,
35, 35f
Frequency of electromagnetic radiation, 13
Fresh film test, 112
Full mouth series (FMS/FMX), 153
Full-mouth survey, absorbed doses from, 42t
Furcation area
bone loss in, detection of, 414
definition of, 414

G
Gag reflex
definition of, 291
hypersensitive, managing, 291
Gagging, definition of, 291
Geissler, Heinrich, vacuum tube first made
by, 4
Gelatin, in film emulsion, 64
General radiation, 18–19
Generalized bone loss, 415, 417f
Genetic cells, 37
Genetic effects of radiation, 34, 37–38, 38f
Genial tubercles
on intraoral images, 327f, 335–336, 336f
on panoramic image, 362, 362f–363f
Germicides, Environmental Protection
Agency-registered, 143
Ghost images
from jewelry, identification of, 395, 396f–397f
in panoramic imaging, 262, 264f
Glenoid fossa, 358–359, 358f, 361f
Glossopharyngeal air space, 363, 365f
Gloves, in infection control, 142, 146
Gold restorations, identification of, 385–386,
386f–387f
Granuloma, periapical, 431–432, 431f–432f
Gray (Gy), 39, 39t
in dose measurement, 40
Gray-scale resolution, in digital imaging,
307–309, 308f
Grid, for extraoral imaging, 276, 276f
Ground glass opacities, 378–379, 379f
Guidelines for Infection Control in Dental Health
Care Settings (CDC), 141
Guidelines for Prescribing Dental Radiographs,
154
on prescribing for pediatric patients, 293
Gutta percha, identification of, 391, 391f

H
Half-value layer (HVL), 32
Halide crystals, in film emulsion, 64
Hamulus, 328f
on intraoral image, 328f, 334, 335f
on panoramic image, 358f, 360
Hand hygiene, in infection control, 142
Hand processing, 88. See also Film processing,
manual.
Hands, care of, in infection control, 142
Handwashing, in infection control, 146
Hard palate, 358f, 359
Hardening agent, in fixing solution, 90, 90t

Head positioner, of panoramic x-ray machine, 259, 260f
Head positioning, in extraoral imaging
  for lateral cephalometric projection, 278, 278t
  for lateral jaw imaging, 277, 278t
  for posteroanterior projection, 278t, 282
  for reverse Towne projection, 278t, 282
  for skull imaging, 278, 278t
  for submentovertex projection, 278t, 282
  for transcranial projection, 278t, 287
  for Waters projection, 278t, 282
Headrest adjustment, 145
Hearing impairment, 292
Heliodent intraoral x-ray machine, 58f
Hemostat film holder, in paralleling technique, 157, 158f
Herringbone pattern, 235, 235f
High-voltage circuit, 17
Hittorf, Johann Wilhelm, in early study of fluorescence, 4
Hittorf-Brookes tube, 4, 5f
Horizontal angulation
  in bisecting technique, 183, 184f, 185
  in bite-wing technique, 214
    incorrect, 231–232, 232f
  definition of, 183, 228–229
  in localization techniques, 242
  in paralleling technique, 159, 159f
  in periapical technique, incorrect, 229, 229f
Horizontal bite-wing, definition of, 211
Horizontal bone loss, 415, 415f
Humidity control, in darkroom, 99
Hydroxyquinone, in developing agent, 89–90, 89t
Hygiene, hand, in infection control, 142
Hyoid, 364f
Hypercementosis, 433–434, 434f
Hypo, as fixing agent, 90
Hypotenuse, definition of, 181, 181f

I
Identification dot, on intraoral film, 65–66, 66f, 348–349
  in film mounting, 349
Idiopathic periapical osteosclerosis, 433
Illuminator, 352
  quality control tests for, 113, 113f
Image(s)
  analog, 302
  bit-depth, 305
    definition of, 302
  bite-wing, in caries evaluation, 403
  characteristics of, 76–85
    geometric, 80–83
      distortion as, 81t, 83, 83f
      magnification as, 81–83, 81t, 82f–83f
      sharpness as, 80–81
    radiolucent, 77, 77f
    radiopaque, 77, 77f
    visual, 77–80
      contrast as, 78–80, 79f–80f, 80t
      density as, 77–78
  definition of, 64
  DICOM, in three-dimensional digital imaging, 314
  digital, 302, 303f. See also Digital image(s); Digital imaging.
  distortion of, 83. See also Distortion, image.
  ease of saving and transport of, with three-dimensional digital imaging, 321
  extraoral, definition of, 274–275
  latent
    formation of, 64–65, 65f
    to visible image, 87–88

Image(s) (Continued)
  multiplanar reconstructed, in three-dimensional digital imaging, 314
  panoramic, 256–272. See also Panoramic imaging.
  periapical, in caries evaluation, 403
  visible, 88
    from latent image to, 87–88
Image interpretation, 369–371
  basic concepts of, 369–370
  definition of, 369
  of dental caries, 402–411. See also Dental caries.
    factors influencing, 404
    tips on, 404
  descriptive terminology in, 372–382. See also Descriptive terminology.
  diagnosis versus, 370
  eyeglasses and napkin chain identification in, 397, 398f
  guidelines for, 370
  in identification of materials
    used in dentistry, 390–393
    used in endodontics, 391
    used in oral surgery, 393, 395f–396f
    used in orthodontics, 393, 393f–394f
    used in prosthodontics, 391–392
    used in restorative dentistry, 390–391
  importance of, 369–370
  jewelry identification in, 396f–398f
  metal plate with screw identification in, 396f
  patient education and, 370
  of periapical lesions, 430–434, 431f–434f
  of periodontal disease, 412–425
  of pulpal lesions, 429–430, 430f–431f
  qualified personnel for, 370
  of resorption, 428–429, 429f–430f
  restoration identification in, 384–390. See also Restorations, identification.
  terminology for, 369
  time and place for, 370
  of trauma, 426–428, 427f–428f
Image receptor, film as, 64
Imaginary bisector, 182
Impacted teeth, three-dimensional digital imaging for, 317, 318f
Implant placement, three-dimensional digital imaging for, 317, 317f
Impulse, exposure time and, 29
Incipient interproximal caries, 405, 405f
Incisive canal
  on panoramic image, 358f, 359
  superior foramina of, 327f, 329–330, 330f
Incisive foramen, on intraoral image, 329, 329f–330f
Incisor exposure
  mandibular
    in bisecting technique, 188, 196b, 196f–197f
    in paralleling technique, 163, 168b, 168f
  maxillary
    in bisecting technique, 188, 192b, 192f–193f
    in paralleling technique, 163, 166b, 166f
Indicator light, 59
Indirect digital imaging, 306–307
  definition of, 302
Indirect theory of radiation injury, 36
Infection control
  dental radiographer and, 140–150
  in dental radiography, 143–147
    checklist for, 144b
    during exposure, 146
    during film processing, 146–147

Infection control (Continued)
  guidelines for, 141–143, 142b
  intraoral sensor in digital imaging and, 145, 145f, 307, 307f, 309
  postexposure, 146
  preexposure, 143–146
  rationale for, 141
  terminology for, 141
Infectious waste, definition of, 141
Inferior nasal conchae, 327f, 332, 333f
Informed consent, 136–137
Infraorbital foramen, 358f, 359, 360f
Inherent filtration, in radiation protection, 46
Injury
  image interpretation of, 427–428, 428f
  radiation, 35–37
    determining factors for, 37
    dose-response curve and, 36, 36f
    free radical formation causing, 35, 35f
    ionization causing, 35, 35f
    mechanisms of, 35
    period of, 37
    sequence of, 37
    theories of, 35–36
Insert tanks, 90, 91f
  care and maintenance of, 94, 95b
InSight film, in radiation protection, 50
Instruments, sterilization and disinfection of, in infection control, 142–143
Insulating oil of x-ray tubehead, 14
Intensifying screens, 69–71, 71f
  calcium tungstate, 71
  for extraoral imaging, 276
  for panoramic imaging, 261
  quality control tests for, 112–113
  rare earth, 71
  for screen films, 69–71, 71f
Intensity, of x-ray beam, 30–32
Inter-radicular lesions
  radiolucent, 376, 376f
  radiopaque, location of, 380, 380f
Intermediate-level disinfectants, 143
Internal oblique ridge
  on intraoral images, 327f, 338–339, 339f
  on panoramic image, 362f, 363, 364f
Internal resorption, 429, 429f–430f
International System of Units (SI system), 39, 39t
Interpersonal skills
  definition of, 125
  in patient relations, 125–127
Interpret, definition of, 369
Interpretation
  definition of, 369
  diagnosis versus, 370
  image, 369–371. See also Image interpretation.
  importance of, 369–370
Interproximal, definition of, 211
Interproximal caries, 404–406, 404f–405f
  advanced, 405–406, 406f
  incipient, 405, 405f
  moderate, 405, 405f
  severe, 406, 406f
Interproximal examination, 153
  definition of, 211
Interproximal tooth surfaces, bite-wing film for, 67–68
Intersecting, definition of, 156, 156f
Intraoral film
  barrier envelopes for, 143–145
  bite-wing, 67–68, 67f
  identification dot on, 65–66, 66f, 348–349
    in film mounting, 349

Intraoral film (Continued)
  occlusal, 68, 68f
  packaging of, 65–67, 65f–66f
  periapical, 67, 67f
  sizes of, 68, 69f–70f
    for bite-wing technique, 68, 69f–70f
  speed of, 68
  types of, 67–68
Intraoral radiographic examination, 152–153
  definition of, 152
Intraoral radiographs, diagnostic criteria for, 153, 153b
Intraoral receptors, 152
Intraoral sensor, in digital imaging, 60, 60f, 304–305
  charge-coupled device as, 304
  complementary metal oxide semiconductor/active pixel sensor as, 304–305
  infection control and, 145, 145f, 307, 307f, 309
  placement of, 307, 308f
  preparation of, 307, 307f
  size and thickness of, 309, 310f
Intrusion, definition of, 428, 428f
Inverse square law, 31–32, 31b, 31f
Inverted Y, 334, 334f
Ion pair, 11, 11f
Ionization, 11
  definition of, 11
  radiation injury from, 35, 35f
Ionizing radiation, 12–13
Irregular ill-defined radiopacity, 378–379, 379f
Isometry
  definition of, 181
  rule of, 181–182

J
Jaw(s). See Mandible; Maxilla.
  fractures of, 427, 428f
  lateral imaging of, 277, 278t, 279f–280f
  radiolucent lesions of, 375b
Jewelry, identification of, 395–397, 396f–398f
Joule (J), definition of, 39t

K
Kells, C. Edmund
  dental radiograph use and, 5
  paralleling technique introduced by, 6
Kilo electron volts (keV), 10
Kilogram (kg), definition of, 39t
Kilovoltage, x-ray beam quality and, 27
Kilovoltage peak (kVp)
  contrast and, 28, 28t, 29f, 78t, 79, 79f, 80t
  definition of, 27
  density and, 27–28, 28f, 28t, 78, 78t
  exposure time and, 29
  patient exposure and, 42
  rule for, 29b
  x-ray beam quality and, 27, 27f–28f
Kilovoltage peak (kVp) controls, 27f
Kilovolts (kV), 17, 27
Kinetic energy, in production of dental x-rays, 18

L
Label side of film packet, 67, 67f
Labial mounting, 349, 349f
Lamina dura, 341, 341f
  appearance of, on dental image, 413, 413f
Latent image
  formation of, 64–65, 65f
  to visible image, 87–88
Latent image centers, in latent image formation, 65, 65f

Latent period, in radiation injury, 37
Lateral cephalometric projection, in extraoral imaging, 278–282, 278t, 281f
Lateral fossa, 327f, 330–331, 331f
Lateral jaw imaging, 277, 278t, 279f–280f
Lateral pterygoid plate, 358f, 359, 361f
Lead, in undeveloped film packets, disposal of, 99
Lead apron
  artifact from, in panoramic imaging, 262, 265f
  infection control and, 143, 145
  for pediatric patient, 293
  in radiation protection, 50, 50f
  removal of, 146
Lead collimator in x-ray tubehead, 15, 15f
Lead foil sheet, in film packet, 66, 66f
Leaded-glass housing for x-ray tube, 16, 16f
Leakage radiation, monitoring for, 52
Legal issues
  dental patient and, 136–138
  dental radiography and, 135–136
  digital imaging and, 309–310
  websites on, 138t
Legislation, radiation safety, 52–53
Lenard, Philip, in early study of cathode rays, 4
Lenard tube, 4
Liability, 137
Licensure requirements, 136
Light
  exposure, 59
  indicator, 58–59
  source of, for film viewing, 352
Light leak
  in darkroom, 98
    testing for, 113–114
  film processing problems from, 102t, 106, 106f
Light-tight, for darkroom, 98
  testing for, 113–114
Lighting
  for darkroom, 98, 98f
    quality control tests for, 113–114
  film processing problems associated with, 102t, 106, 106f
Lindblom technique, in temporomandibular joint imaging, 282–287, 287f
Line pairs/millimeter (lp/mm), definition of, 302
Linear curve, 36f
Linear nonthreshold curve, 36, 36f
Lines pairs/millimeter (lp/mm), in digital imaging, 307–308
Lingual caries, 407, 407f
Lingual foramen
  on intraoral images, 327f, 336, 336f
  on panoramic image, 362, 362f
Lingual mounting, 349, 349f
Lingula, 361, 362f
Lip positioning, in panoramic imaging, 265, 265f
Lipline, on panoramic image, 364, 366f
Listening skills, in patient relations, 126
Localization techniques
  buccal object rule and, 242, 248b–250b, 248f–250f, 252f
  equipment preparation for, 248
  helpful hints for, 250
  patient preparation for, 248
  procedures for, 248–250
  purpose and use of, 242
  receptor placements and image comparisons in, 248–250, 248b

Localization techniques (Continued)
  right-angle, 248, 249b–250b, 249f, 251f–252f
  types of, 242–248
Localizations techniques, 242–250
Localized bone loss, 415, 416f
Long axis of tooth, 156, 156f, 181, 181f
Long-cone technique, 156. See also Paralleling technique.
Long-scale contrast, 79, 80t
Long-term effects of radiation, 37
Low-level disinfectants, 143
Low palatal vault, paralleling technique modifications for, 173
Luxation, definition of, 428

M
Magnification
  for film viewing, 352, 353f
  image, 81–83, 82f
    definition of, 81
    factors influencing, 81t, 82–83, 82f–83f
Malar bone, 360
Malpractice issues, 137
Mandible
  angle of, 362f, 363, 364f
  body of, anatomy of, 335, 336f
  bony landmarks of, 335–339. See also Anatomic landmarks, mandibular.
  inferior border of, 362, 362f, 364f
  lateral jaw imaging of, 277, 279f–280f
Mandibular canal, 328, 328f
  on intraoral images, 338, 338f
  on panoramic image, 361–362, 362f, 364f
Mandibular canine exposure
  in bisecting technique, 188, 194b, 194f–195f
  in paralleling technique, 163, 167b, 167f
Mandibular condyle, 360, 362f–363f
Mandibular foramen, 361, 362f–363f
Mandibular fossa, 339, 358
Mandibular incisor exposure
  in bisecting technique, 188, 196b, 196f–197f
  in paralleling technique, 163, 168b, 168f
Mandibular molar exposure
  in bisecting technique, 189, 204b, 204f–205f
  in paralleling technique, 164, 172b–173b, 172f
Mandibular occlusal projections, 242
  cross-sectional, 242, 246b, 246f
  pediatric, 242, 247b, 247f
  topographic, 242, 245b, 245f
Mandibular premolar exposure
  in bisecting technique, 189, 202b, 202f–203f
  in paralleling technique, 164, 171b, 171f
  modifications for, 174–176, 176f
Mandibular torus
  bite-wing technique modifications for, 223
  paralleling technique modifications for, 173–174, 174f–175f
Masks, in infection control, 142, 146
Mass number, 9
Master tank, 90, 91f
  care and maintenance of, 94, 95b
Mastoid process, 358, 358f
Matter, definition of, 9
Maxilla
  bony landmarks of, 328–335. See also Anatomic landmarks, maxillary.
  zygomatic process of, on intraoral image, 334–335, 335f
Maxillary canine exposure
  in bisecting technique, 188, 190b, 190f–191f
  in paralleling technique, 163, 165b, 165f
Maxillary incisor exposure
  in bisecting technique, 188, 192b, 192f–193f
  in paralleling technique, 163, 166b, 166f

Maxillary molar exposure
  in bisecting technique, 189, 200b–206b, 200f–201f
  in paralleling technique, 164, 170b, 170f
Maxillary occlusal projections, 240–242
  lateral, 240–242, 243b, 243f
  pediatric, 242, 244f
  topographic, 240, 241b, 241f
Maxillary premolar exposure
  in bisecting technique, 189, 198b, 198f–199f
  in paralleling technique, 164, 169b, 169f
Maxillary sinus
  floor of, on panoramic image, 358f, 359–360
  on intraoral image, 328, 328f, 332, 333f
    nutrient canals within, 333f, 334
    septa within, 332, 333f
  on panoramic image, 358f, 359–360, 361f
Maxillary torus, paralleling technique modifications for, 173–174, 174f
Maxillary tuberosity
  on intraoral image, 328f, 334, 334f
  on panoramic image, 358f, 359, 361f
Maximum accumulated dose, in radiation protection, 53
Maximum permissible dose, in radiation protection, 53
McCormack, Franklin W., paralleling technique and, 6
Median palatal suture, 328, 329f–330f, 330
Medical radiation, 40–41, 41t
Mental foramen, 327f, 328
  on intraoral images, 327f, 337, 338f
  on panoramic image, 362, 362f–363f
Mental fossa
  on intraoral images, 327f, 337, 338f
  on panoramic image, 362, 362f
Mental ridge
  on intraoral images, 327f, 337, 337f
  on panoramic image, 362, 362f
Metal housing of x-ray tubehead, 14
Metallic pins, identification of, 391, 391f
Metallic restorations, radiopacity of, 373, 374f
Midsagittal plane positioning, in panoramic imaging, 266–267, 269f–270f
Milliamperage
  density and, 30, 30t, 78, 78t
  exposure time and, 30, 30t
  x-ray beam quantity and, 29–30
Milliamperage (mA) controls, 27f
Milliampere (mA), 17
  definition of, 29
Milliampere-seconds (mAs), x-ray beam quantity and, 29–30
Mitotic activity of cells, radiosensitivity and, 38
Mixed lucent-opaque lesions, 378–379, 379f
Mobility impairment, 292
Molar exposure
  in bite-wing technique, 217, 220b–222b, 220f–222f
    receptor placement for, 231, 231f
  mandibular
    in bisecting technique, 189, 204b, 204f–205f
    in paralleling technique, 164, 172b–173b, 172f
  maxillary
    in bisecting technique, 189, 200b–206b, 200f–201f
    in paralleling technique, 164, 170b, 170f
Molecule
  formation of, 11
  structure of, 11
Molybdenum cup, in cathode, 16, 16f
Monitoring, radiation, in operator protection, 52

Morton, W.J., first dental radiograph made in U. S. by, 4–5
Moth-eaten radiolucencies, 375
Mount(s)
  digital, 348, 348f
  film, 346–347, 346f–347f. *See also* Film mount(s).
Mounting, film, 345–352. *See also* Film mounting.
Movement
  patient, artifacts from, in three-dimensional digital imaging, 321
  sharpness of image and, 81, 81t, 82f
  technique errors from, 234, 235f
Multifocal confluent radiopacity, 378, 378f
Multifocal radiolucencies, 375
Multifocal radiopacities, 380
Multilocular radiolucent lesions, 374–375, 375f
Multiplanar reconstructed images (MPR images), in three-dimensional digital imaging, 314
Multiplanar reconstruction (MPR), definition of, 313
Mylohyoid ridge
  on intraoral images, 327f, 337–338, 338f
  on panoramic image, 362, 362f

N
Nanometers, 12–13
Napkin chain, identification of, 397
Nasal cavity
  floor of, 327f, 332, 332f
  on intraoral image, 327f, 331, 331f
  on panoramic image, 358f, 359
Nasal conchae, inferior, 327f, 332, 333f
Nasal septum
  on intraoral image, 327f, 331, 331f
  on panoramic image, 358f, 359, 360f
Nasal spine, anterior
  on intraoral image, 328f, 332, 332f
  on panoramic image, 358f, 359, 360f
Nasopalatine canal, 359
Nasopalatine foramen, 359
Nasopharyngeal air space, 363, 365f
Necklace, identification of, 397, 397f
Negative vertical angulation, 214, 215f
Negligence, 137
Neutral atom, 11
Neutrons, 9, 9f, 12
Newton (N), definition of, 39t
Noncritical instruments, sterilization and disinfection of, 143
Nonscreen film, 69
  for extraoral imaging, 275–276
Nonstochastic effects of radiation, 36–37
Nonverbal communication skills, in patient relations, 126
Normalizing device, in quality control, 116
Nose jewelry, identification of, 397, 398f
Nucleons, 9
Nucleus, of atom, 9, 9f
Numata, Hisatugu, panoramic radiography introduced by, 6
Nutrient canals
  mandibular, 336–337, 337f
  in maxillary sinus, 333f, 334

O
Object-film alignment, image distortion and, 81t, 83, 83f
Object-receptor distance
  image magnification and, 81t, 82–83, 83f
  in paralleling technique, 157, 157f
Obliteration, pulpal, 430, 430f

Occlusal caries, 406
  moderate, 406, 407f
  severe, 406, 407f
Occlusal examination, 153
  definition of, 240
Occlusal film/receptor, 68, 68f
  definition of, 240
  for extraoral imaging, 275–276
  sizes of, 68, 69f–70f
Occlusal-periapical examination, of edentulous patient, 297–298, 297f
Occlusal surfaces, definition of, 240
Occlusal technique, 239–242
  definition of, 240
  equipment preparation for, 240, 240b
  mandibular occlusal projections in, 242
    cross-sectional, 242, 246b, 246f
    pediatric, 242, 247b, 247f
    topographic, 242, 245b, 245f
  maxillary occlusal projections in, 240–242
    lateral, 240–242, 243b, 243f
    pediatric, 242, 244f
    topographic, 240, 241b, 241f
  patient preparation for, 240, 240b
  principles of, 240
  procedures for, 240–242
  purpose and use of, 240
  terminology for, 239–240
  vertical angulations for, 242, 242t
Occupational exposure, definition of, 141
Occupational Exposure to Bloodborne Pathogens (OSHA), 141–142
Occupational Safety and Health Administration (OSHA), infection control practices recommended by, 141–142
Oil, insulating, of x-ray tubehead, 14
On-off switch, 59
Opaque film mounts, 346–347, 346f
Opened contacts, definition of, 211, 212f
Operating kilovoltage peak
  image contrast and, 78t, 79, 79f
  image density and, 78, 78t
Operator. *See* Dental radiographer.
Oral surgery, materials used in, identification of, 393, 395f–396f
Orbit, 358f, 359, 360f
  electron, 9–10, 10f–11f
Organs
  critical, 38
    dental radiation risks to, 41
  radiation effects on, 38
Orthodontic evaluation, three-dimensional digital imaging for, 317, 320f
Orthodontics, materials used in, identification of, 393, 393f–394f
Orthophos XG 5 extraoral x-ray machine, 260f–261f, 275f
Orthophos XGPlus extraoral x-ray machine, 58f, 259, 260f
Orthoralix 8500 extraoral x-ray machine, 259, 260f
Osteitis, condensing, 433, 433f
Osteomas, three-dimensional digital imaging for evaluation of, 317, 320f
Osteomyelitis, sclerosing, chronic focal, 433
Osteosclerosis, 433
Outer package wrapping, of film packet, 66–67, 66f
Overexposed receptor, 227–228, 227f
Overlapped contacts, definition of, 212, 212f
Overlapped films, 101t, 104–105, 104f
Oxidation
  definition of, 94
  of fixer and developer solutions, 94

P

Paatero, Yrjo, panoramic radiography and, 6
Palatal suture, median, 328, 329f–330f, 330
Palate
 hard, 358f, 359
 shallow, paralleling technique modifications for, 173, 173f
 soft, 364, 366f
Palatoglossal air space, 363, 365f
Pancreatic images, anatomy on. *See also* Anatomy, on panoramic images.
Panoramic film, 68
 cassette for, 72, 72f
 image on, 70f
Panoramic images, anatomy on, 357–367
Panoramic imaging, 256–272
 advantages of, 267–268
 anatomy with, 257f
 basic concepts of, 256–261
 cassette for, 261, 261f–262f
 definition of, 256–257
 digital, 303, 303f
 disadvantages of, 268
 of edentulous patient, 296, 296f
 equipment for, 259–261
  preparation of, 261, 262b
 film for, 260–261
 focal trough in, 259, 259f
 fundamentals of, 257–259
 helpful hints for, 268
 history of, 6
 intensifying screens for, 261
 patient positioning for, 261–262, 263b–264b, 263f–264f
  errors in
   with aligning teeth to focal trough, 266, 267f–269f
   with Frankfort plane, 265–266, 266f–267f
   with lips and tongue, 265, 265f
   with midsagittal plane alignment, 266–267, 269f–270f
   with spinal alignment, 267, 270f
 patient preparation for, 261, 263b, 263f
  errors in, 262
   ghost images from, 262, 264f
   lead apron artifact from, 262, 265f
 for pediatric patient, 295f
 procedures for, 261–262
 purpose and use of, 257
 rotation center in, 258–259, 258f
 tomography and, 257–258
Paper film wrapper, 66, 66f
Parallel, definition of, 156, 156f
Paralleling technique, 155–179
 advantages of, 176
 beam alignment devices in, 157–158
 charting of full-mouth series with, 173t
 for digital imaging, 307
 disadvantages of, 176
 equipment preparation for, 159, 160b, 160f–161f
 exposure sequence in, 159–163
  anterior, 159–162, 162f, 162t
  posterior, 162–163, 163t
 helpful hints for, 176–177
 history of, 6
 modifications of, 164–176
  for bony growths, 173–174, 174f–175f
  for mandibular premolar region, 174–176, 176f
  for shallow palate, 173, 173f
 patient preparation for, 159, 159b
 in periodontal disease evaluation, 414, 414f

Paralleling technique *(Continued)*
 principles of, 156–157
 procedures for, 159–164
 receptor placement in, 163–164
  anterior, 163, 165b–168b, 165f–168f
   disadvantages of, 176
   for mandibular canine exposure, 163, 167b, 167f
   for mandibular incisor exposure, 163, 168b, 168f
   for mandibular molar exposure, 164, 172b–173b, 172f
   for mandibular premolar exposure, 164, 171b, 171f
    modifications of, 174–176, 176f
   for maxillary canine exposure, 163, 165b, 165f
   for maxillary incisor exposure, 163, 166b, 166f
   for maxillary molar exposure, 164, 170b, 170f
   for maxillary premolar exposure, 164, 169b, 169f
   posterior, 163–164, 169b–173b, 169f–172f
  rules for, 158–159
  terminology for, 156, 156f
Parenteral exposure, definition of, 141
Particle concept, 12
Particulate radiation, 12
Pathogen
 bloodborne, definition of, 141
 definition of, 141
Pathologic resorption, 428
Pathology, three-dimensional digital imaging for evaluation of, 317, 320f
Patient
 education of. *See* Education, patient.
 legal issues and, 136–138
  confidentiality as, 137
  documentation as, 137
  informed consent as, 136–137
  liability as, 137
  malpractice issues as, 137
  ownership and retention of dental radiographs as, 137–138
  patient records as, 137–138
  patient refusal of dental radiographs as, 138
  risk management as, 136–137
 movement of, artifacts from, in three-dimensional digital imaging, 321
 radiation protection for, 46–51. *See also* Radiation protection, for patient.
 with special needs, 290–299. *See also* Special needs patients.
Patient positioning
 for extraoral imaging, 277
 for panoramic imaging, 261–262, 263b–264b, 263f–264f
  errors in, 262–267. *See also* Panoramic imaging, patient positioning for, errors in.
 for three-dimensional digital imaging, 319, 320f
Patient preparation
 for bisecting technique, 186, 186b
 for bite-wing technique, 215, 216b
 for extraoral imaging, 276, 277b
 gag reflex and, 291
 infection control and, 145
 for localization techniques, 248
 for panoramic imaging, 261, 263b, 263f
  errors in, 262

Patient preparation *(Continued)*
  ghost images from, 262, 264f
  lead apron artifact from, 262, 265f
 for paralleling technique, 159, 159b
 for pediatric patient, 293
 for three-dimensional digital imaging, 319
Patient records, 137–138
 dental radiographs in, 122
Patient relations
 attitude and, 128
 chairside manner and, 127–128
 dental radiographer and, 125–129
 first impressions and, 127, 127b
 interpersonal skills for, 125–127
Pediatric patient, occlusal projections in
 mandibular, 242, 247b, 247f
 maxillary, 242, 244f
Penumbra, definition of, 80
Periapical abscess, 432–433, 433f
Periapical cyst, 432, 432f
Periapical examination, 153
 of edentulous patient, 296–297, 297f
Periapical film, 67, 67f
 sizes of, 68, 69f–70f
 technique errors with, 228–230
  angulation problems as, 228–230, 229f–230f
  PID alignment problems as, 229–230, 230f–231f
  receptor placement problems as, 228, 228f–229f, 236f
Periapical granuloma, 431–432, 431f–432f
Periapical image, in periodontal disease evaluation, 414
Periapical lesions
 image interpretation of, 430–434, 431f–434f
 radiolucent
  image interpretation of, 431–433, 431f–433f
  location of, 375–376, 376f
 radiopaque
  image interpretation of, 433–434, 433f–434f
  location of, 380, 380f
Pericoronal lesions
 radiolucent, location of, 376–377, 377f
 radiopaque, 380, 380f
Period of injury, in radiation injury, 37
Periodic table of elements, 9, 10f
Periodontal, definition of, 413
Periodontal abscess, 432
Periodontal disease
 definition of, 413
 description of, 413–414
 detection of, 414
  clinical examination in, 414
  dental image examination in, 414, 414f
 image interpretation of, for bone loss, 415
  distribution of, 415, 416f–417f
  pattern of, 415, 415f–416f
  predisposing factors for, 419, 421f–423f
  severity of, classification of, 415, 417f–420f
 interpretation of, 412–425
Periodontal ligament space, 341, 342f
 appearance of, on dental image, 413, 413f
 widened, 375
Periodontium
 definition of, 412–413
 description of, 412–413
Perpendicular, definition of, 156, 156f
Personal protective equipment (PPE)
 definition of, 141
 in infection control, 142

Phalangioma, 234, 234f
Phosphors, in intensifying screens, 71, 71f
Photo-stimulable phosphor imaging (PSP), 306, 306f
Photoelectric effect, 20, 20f
Photoelectron, 20
Photons
    definition of, 12
    x-ray, absorption of, 20
Physical disability, 292
Physics, radiation, 8–25
Physiologic resorption, 428, 429f
Picture elements, 302
PID. *See* Position-indicating device (PID).
Pit amalgams, identification of, 384, 384f
Pixel, definition of, 302
Plane
    axial
        definition of, 313–314, 314f
        image through, 315f
    coronal
        definition of, 313–314, 314f
        image through, 315f
    sagittal
        definition of, 313–314, 314f
        image through, 315f
Plumbing, for darkroom, 99
Polychromatic x-ray beam, 27
Porcelain restorations, identification of, 388–389, 388f–390f
Position-indicating device (PID), 15, 16f
    alignment problems with, 229–230, 230f–231f
    angulation of
        for bisecting technique, 183–185
        for bite-wing technique, 213–214
    in radiation protection, 48, 49f–50f
Positioning, operator, in radiation protection, 51–52, 52f
Positive vertical angulation, 214, 215f
Post and core restorations, 387–388, 388f
Posteroanterior projection, in extraoral imaging, 278t, 282, 283f
Posture, in nonverbal communication, 126
Potassium alum, in fixing solution, 90, 90t
Potassium bromide, in developer solution, 89t, 90
PPE. *See* Personal protective equipment (PPE).
Precision film holders, 60, 61f
    in paralleling technique, 157–158, 158f
Premolar exposure
    in bite-wing technique, 217, 217b–218b, 217f–219f
        receptor placement for, 231, 231f
    mandibular
        in bisecting technique, 189, 202b, 202f–203f
        in paralleling technique, 164, 171b, 171f
            modifications for, 174–176, 176f
    maxillary
        in bisecting technique, 189, 198b, 198f–199f
        in paralleling technique, 164, 169b, 169f
Prescribing of dental radiographs, 154
    for pediatric patients, 293
    radiation protection and, 46, 47t
Preservative
    in developer solution, 89t, 90
    in fixing solution, 90, 90t
Price, Weston, bisecting technique introduced by, 6
Primary beam, 19
Primary radiation, definition of, 19

Process(es)
    coronoid, 327f
        on intraoral images, 327f, 337, 340f
    definition of, 326
    hamular, 360
    mastoid, 358, 358f
    styloid, 358, 358f
Processing tank
    care and maintenance of, 94, 95b
    manual, 90–91, 91f
Processor housing, 96, 96f
Prosthodontics, materials used in, identification of, 391–392
Protection
    film, 72–73
    radiation, 45–55. *See also* Radiation protection.
Protective barriers, for operators, 52
Protective clothing, in infection control, 142
Protective layer, of film, 64, 64f
Protons, 9, 9f, 12
PSP system (storage phosphor imaging), 306–307, 306f
    definition of, 302
    receptors for, wear and tear on, 309
Psychogenic stimuli, initiating gag reflex, 291
Pterygoid plate, lateral, 358f, 359, 361f
Pterygomaxillary fissure, 358f, 359, 360f
Pulp cavity, 340, 340f
Pulp stones, 430, 431f
Pulpal lesions, 429–430, 430f–431f
Pulpal obliteration, 430, 430f
Pulpal sclerosis, 429, 430f

Q

Quality, of x-ray beam, 27–29
Quality administration, 117
Quality assurance, 111–119
    for darkroom lighting, 113–114, 114f
    definition of, 111
    for digital imaging, 116–117
    for film processing, 113–116, 115t
    monitoring schedule in, 118t
    operator competence in, 117
    for processing equipment, 114
    for processing solutions, 114–116, 116f
    for screens and cassettes, 112–113, 113f
    for viewing equipment, 113, 113f
    for x-ray film, 112
    for x-ray machines, 112, 112b
Quality assurance plan, 111, 112b
Quality care, dental radiographer in, 123
Quality control tests, 111–117
Quality Control Tests for Dental Radiography, 117
Quality factor (Qf), for exposure effects, 40
Quanta, 12
Quantity, of x-ray beam, 29–30

R

Rad (radiation absorbed dose), 39, 39t
    in dose measurement, 40
Radiation, 12
    background, 40, 41t
    biologic effects of, 34–44
        on cells, 38
        cumulative, 37
        genetic, 34, 37–38, 38f
        long-term, 37
        nonstochastic, 36–37
        on organs, 38, 38t
        short-term, 37
        somatic, 37–38, 38f
        stochastic, 36
        on tissues, 37–38, 37t–38t

Radiation (*Continued*)
    braking, 18
    characteristic, 19, 19f
    characteristics of, 26–33
    cosmic, 40, 41t
    definition of, 2
    dentistry and, 2–3
    dose of. *See* Dose.
    electromagnetic, 12–13
        properties of, 13b
    exposure to. *See* Exposure, radiation.
    general, 18–19
    history of, 2–7
    injury from, 35–37. *See also* Injury, radiation.
    ionizing, 12–13
    leakage, monitoring for, 52
    measurements of, 39–40
        units of, 39, 39t
        used in dental radiography, 40
    medical, 40–41, 41t
    monitoring of, in operator protection, 52
    particulate, 12
    physics of, 8–25
    primary, definition of, 19
    risks of, 40–42
    scatter, definition of, 19
    secondary, definition of, 19
    terrestrial, 40, 41t
Radiation absorbed dose (rad), 39, 39t
    in dose measurement, 40
Radiation Control for Health and Safety Act (1968), 52–53
Radiation monitoring badge, 52, 52f
Radiation protection, 45–55
    ALARA concept in, 53
    maximum accumulated dose in, 53
    maximum permissible dose in, 53
    for operator, 51–52
    for patient, 46–51
        dental radiographer in, 123
        during exposure, 48–51
        patient education in, 53
        post-exposure, 51
        pre-exposure, 46–48
    safety legislation and, 52–53
Radioactivity, definition of, 12
Radiograph(s)
    definition of, 3, 373
    dental. *See* Dental radiograph(s).
    diagnostic, 77, 153, 153b
    image of patient's finger on, 234, 234f
    mounting of, 345–352. *See also* Film mounting.
    reference, in quality control, 115, 115t
    stepwedge, in quality control, 115–116, 115t, 116f
    traditional, digital scanning of, 306
    x-ray versus, 373
Radiographer. *See* Dental radiographer.
Radiographic examination, 152–154
    complete mouth/full-mouth, 153
    extraoral, 153
    intraoral, 152–153
    for pediatric patient, 293–294, 294t, 295f
Radiographic interpretation, 369–371. *See also* Image interpretation.
Radiographic techniques
    patient exposure and, 41
    radiation protection and, 51
Radiography
    definition of, 3
    dental, definition of, 3
    digital, 301–311. *See also* Digital imaging.

Radiography (Continued)
  panoramic, 256–272. See also Panoramic
    imaging.
Radiology, definition of, 3
Radiolucent
  definition of, 373
  dental caries as, 373, 373f
  radiopaque versus, 373
Radiolucent lesions
  descriptive terminology for, 374–377
    for appearance, 374–375
    for location, 375–377
    for size, 377, 377f
  of jaws, 375b
Radiolucent structures, 77, 77f, 88
Radiopaque
  definition of, 373
  radiolucent versus, 373
Radiopaque lesions, descriptive terminology for,
    377–381
    for appearance, 377–379
    for location, 379–380, 380b
    for size, 381
Radiopaque structures, 77, 77f, 88
Radioresistant cells, 38, 38t
Radiosensitive cells, 38, 38t
Rampant caries, 408, 409f
Ramus, mandibular
  anatomy of, 335, 336f
  lateral jaw projection of, 275f, 277, 280f
Raper, Howard Riley
  first college course in dental radiography by,
    5
  intraoral radiographic techniques and, 6
Rare earth intensifying screens, 71
Raw data, in three-dimensional digital imaging,
    314
Reassurance
  for gag reflex, 292
  for pediatric patient, 294
Receptor(s). See also Film.
  bending of, 233–234, 233f
  for bisecting technique, 183
  bite-wing, 213
    definition of, 211
  ceasing of, 234, 234f
  definition of, 64
  double exposure of, 234, 234f
  exposed, handling of, infection control and,
    146
  exposed to light, 227, 227f
  extraoral, 153
  intraoral, 152
  occlusal, definition of, 240
  overexposed, 227–228, 227f
  for paralleling technique, 158
  reversed, 235, 235f
  size of, for pediatric patients, 293
  underexposed, 227–228, 228f
  unexposed, 227, 227f
Receptor contrast, 78–79
Receptor exposure
  in bisecting technique, 185
  in bite-wing technique, 214
Receptor exposure errors, 227–228
Receptor placement
  in bisecting technique, 185
  in bite-wing technique, 214, 216–217, 217b
    errors in, 230–231
    guidelines for, 217b
  for endodontic patient, 296
  in extraoral imaging
    for lateral cephalometric projection, 278,
      278t

Receptor placement (Continued)
    for lateral jaw projections, 277, 278t
    for posteroanterior projection, 278t, 282
    for reverse Towne projection, 278t, 282
    for skull projections, 278, 278t
    for submentovertex projection, 278t, 282
    for transcranial projection, 278t, 287
    for Waters projection, 278t, 282
  gag reflex and, 291
  in paralleling technique, 158
  in periapical technique
    correct, 228, 228f
    incorrect, 228, 229f
Receptor position
  in bisecting technique, 185, 186f
  in bite-wing technique, 214
  in paralleling technique, 156f, 158
Recoil electron, 20
Recovery period, in radiation period, 37
Rectangular collimator, 46–48, 48f–49f
Rectangular position-indicating device, 48, 50f
Rectification, 16–17
Recurrent caries, 408, 408f
Reduction in film processing, 87
  selective, 87–88
Reference radiograph, in quality control, 115,
    115t
Rem (roentgen equivalent (in) man), 39–40,
    39t
  definition of, 40
Replenisher, definition of, 94
Replenisher pump, of automatic processor, 96,
    96f
Replenisher solution(s)
  for automatic processor, 96, 96f
  care and maintenance of, 94
Resolution
  contrast
    definition of, 313
    in three-dimensional digital imaging, 315
  spatial
    definition of, 313
    in three-dimensional digital imaging,
      315
Resorption, image interpretation of, 428–429,
    429f–430f
Restoration(s)
  defective, periodontal disease and, 419,
    422f–423f
  identification of, 384–390
    acrylic, 390
    amalgam, 384–385, 384f–386f
    composite, 389, 390f
    gold, 385–386, 386f–387f
    metallic, 384, 384f
    nonmetallic, 384
    porcelain, 388–389, 388f–390f
    post and core, 387–388, 388f
    stainless steel and chrome crowns,
      386–387, 387f–388f
  metallic, radiopacity of, 373, 374f
Restorative dentistry, materials used in,
    identification of, 390–391
Restrainer, in developer solution, 89t, 90
Reverse Towne projection, in extraoral imaging,
    278t, 282, 286f
Ridge
  definition of, 327
  external oblique
    on intraoral images, 339, 339f
    on panoramic image, 362f, 363, 364f
  internal oblique
    on intraoral images, 327f, 338–339, 339f
    on panoramic image, 362f, 363, 364f

Ridge (Continued)
  mental
    on intraoral images, 327f, 337, 337f
    on panoramic image, 362, 362f
  mylohyoid
    on intraoral images, 327f, 337–338, 338f
    on panoramic image, 362, 362f
Right angle, definition of, 156, 156f
Right-angle technique, 156. See also Paralleling
    technique.
  for localization, 248, 249b–250b, 249f,
    251f–252f
Right triangle, definition of, 181, 181f
Rinn BAI instruments, 182–183, 183f
Rinn XCP instruments
  in bite-wing technique, 212, 213f
  in paralleling technique, 157–158, 158f
Rinsing, in film processing, 87
  manual, 89
Risk(s)
  definition of, 41
  of dental radiography, benefit versus, 42
  radiation, 40–42
Risk management, 136–137
Roentgen, Wilhelm Conrad, 3f
  x-ray discovery by, 3–4
Roentgen equivalent (in) man (rem), 39–40, 39t
  definition of, 40
Roentgen (R), 39, 39t
  in exposure measurement, 39–40
Roller film transporter, 96, 96f
Rollins, William H, radiation experimentation
    by, 5
Room lighting, for darkroom, 98
Root fractures, 427, 427f
Root surface caries, 407–408, 408f
Rotational panoramic imaging, 256–257. See
    also Panoramic imaging.
Round collimator, 46–48, 49f
Round position-indicating device, 48, 50f

S
Safelight filter, 98, 98f
Safelighting, for darkroom, 95, 98f
  testing of, 114, 114f
Safety. See also Radiation protection.
  patient questions about, 133
Sagittal plane
  definition of, 313–314, 314f
  image through, 315f
Scatter
  coherent, 20, 21f
  Compton, 20, 21f
  unmodified, 20
Scatter radiation, definition of, 19
Sclerosis, pulpal, 429, 430f
Sclerotic bone, 433, 434f
Scratched film, 101t, 106, 106f
Screen film(s), 69, 71f
  cassettes for, 71–72, 71f–72f
  for extraoral imaging, 275
  intensifying screens for, 69–71, 71f. See also
    Intensifying screens.
  for panoramic imaging, 260–261
Screens
  intensifying. See Intensifying screens.
  quality control tests for, 112–113
Seal, tubehead, 14
Secondary radiation, definition of, 19
Selective reduction in film processing, 87–88
Semicritical instruments, sterilization and
    disinfection of, 143
Sensitivity specks, in latent image formation, 65,
    65f

Sensor
  definition of, 302
  handling of, for radiation protection, 51
  intraoral, in digital imaging, 60, 60f, 304–305.
    See also Intraoral sensor, in digital
    imaging.
Septum(a)
  definition of, 328
  within maxillary sinus, 332, 333f
  nasal, 327f
    on intraoral image, 327f, 331, 331f
Sharpness of image, 80–81
  definition of, 80
  factors influencing, 80–81, 81f–82f, 81t
Sharps, definition of, 141
Shells, electron, 9–10, 10f–11f
Shielding
  for operators, 52
  for patients, 48–50, 50f
Short-scale contrast, 79, 80t
Short-term effects of radiation, 37
Show and tell approach, for pediatric patient,
  294
SI system of radiation measurement, 39, 39t
Sialolity, 379
Sievert (Sv), 39–40, 39t
Silver
  in fixer solutions, disposal of, 99
  in undeveloped film packets, disposal of, 99
Silver bromide, in film emulsion, 64, 64f–65f
Silver halide crystals, in film emulsion, 64
Silver iodide, in film emulsion, 64
Silver points, identification of, 391, 391f
Sinus(es)
  assessment of, three-dimensional digital
    imaging for, 317, 319f
  definition of, 328
  maxillary. *See* Maxillary sinus.
    floor of, on panoramic image, 358f,
      359–360
    on panoramic image, 358f, 359–360, 361f
Size
  of bite-wing film, 68, 69f–70f
  focal spot, sharpness of image and, 80–81,
    81f, 81t
  of intraoral films, 68, 69f–70f
  of occlusal film, 68, 69f–70f
  of periapical film, 68, 69f–70f
Skin, dental radiation risks to, 41
Skull, extraoral imaging of
  lateral cephalometric projection in, 278–282,
    278t, 281f
  posteroanterior projection in, 278t, 282, 283f
  reverse Towne projection in, 278t, 282, 286f
  submentovertex projection in, 278t, 282, 285f
  Waters projection in, 278t, 282, 284f
SLOB mnemonic, 242
Snap-A-Ray film holder, 59–60, 60f. *See also*
  EEZEE-Grip film holder.
Sodium carbonate, in developer solution, 89t, 90
Sodium sulfite
  in developer solution, 89t, 90
  in fixing solution, 90, 90t
Sodium thiosulfate, as fixing agent, 90, 90t
Soft palate, 364, 366f
Soft tissue opacity, 378–379, 379f
Soft tissues on panoramic images, 363–365,
  366f
Software, viewing, for three-dimensional digital
  imaging, 315–317, 317f
Solution(s), processing
  care and maintenance of, 94–95, 97
  developer, 87, 89–90, 89t
  fixer, 88

Solution(s), processing *(Continued)*
  fixing, 90, 90t
  quality control tests for, 114–116
Somatic cells, 37
Somatic effects of radiation, 37–38, 38f
Spatial resolution
  definition of, 313
  in three-dimensional digital imaging, 315
Special needs patients, 290–299
  with disabilities, 292–293
  edentulous, 296–298
  endodontic, 295–296
  with hypersensitive gag reflex, 291
  pediatric, 293–294
Spectrum, electromagnetic, 12, 13f
Spine
  alignment of, in panoramic imaging, 267, 270f
  anterior nasal, 327f
  definition of, 327
  nasal, anterior
    on intraoral image, 328f, 332, 332f
    on panoramic image, 358f, 359, 360f
Stabe Bite-Block, 59–60, 60f
  in bisecting technique, 182–183, 183f
  in paralleling technique, 157, 158f
Stainless steel crowns, identification of,
  386–387, 387f–388f
Standard of care, 137
Standard precautions, definition of, 141
State regulations, on dental radiography,
  135–136
Static electricity artifact, 101t, 105–106, 105f
Statute of limitations, 137
Step-down transformer, 17, 17f
Step-up transformer, 17, 17f
Stepwedge contrast, 79–80, 80f
Stepwedge radiographs, in quality control,
  115–116, 115t, 116f
Sterilization
  definition of, 141
  of instruments, in infection control, 142–143
Sterilize, definition of, 141
Stirring paddle, for film processing, 92
Stirring rod, for film processing, 92
Stochastic effects of radiation, 36
Stones, pulp, 430, 431f
Storage, film, 72–73
Storage phosphor imaging, 306–307, 306f
  definition of, 302
  receptors for, wear and tear on, 309
Storage space, in darkroom, 99
Styloid process, 358, 358f
Styrofoam bite-block, 59–60, 60f
Subject contrast, 79
Subject thickness, density and, 78
Submandibular fossa, 327f, 339, 339f, 364f
Submaxillary fossa, 339
Submentovertex projection, in extraoral
  imaging, 278t, 282, 285f
Sulfuric acid, in fixing solution, 90, 90t
Superior foramina, of incisive canal, 327f,
  329–330, 330f
Surgery, oral, materials used in, identification
  of, 393, 395f–396f
Suture
  definition of, 328
  median palatal, 328, 329f–330f, 330
Système International de'Unités (International
  System of Units, SI system), 39, 39t

T
Tactile stimuli
  initiating gag reflex, 291
  reduction of, for gag reflex, 292

Tank processing, 88. *See also* Film processing,
  manual.
Target lesion, 378, 378f
Target-object distance, 30, 31f
Target-receptor distance, 30, 31f
  image magnification and, 81t, 82, 82f
  in paralleling technique, 157
Target-surface distance, 30, 31f
Teeth. *See* Tooth (teeth).
Temperature
  control of, in darkroom, 99
  film processing problems associated with,
    101t, 102f–103f, 103
Temporomandibular joint (TMJ)
  definition of, 282
  three-dimensional digital imaging in
    evaluation of, 317, 319f
Temporomandibular joint (TMJ) imaging
  tomography in, 287, 288f
  transcranial projection in, 282–287, 287f
Terminology
  for bisecting technique, 181
  for bite-wing technique, 211–212
  descriptive, 372–382. *See also* Descriptive
    terminology.
  for digital imaging, 302
  for infection control, 141
  for occlusal technique, 239–240
  for paralleling technique, 156, 156f
Terrestrial radiation, 40, 41t
Thermionic emission, 17–18
Thermometer for film processing, 91, 91f, 94t
Thickness, subject, density and, 78
Three-dimensional digital imaging, 312–323.
    See also Cone beam computed tomography
    (CBCT).
  advantages of, 319–321
  background of, 312
  computer for, 315
  cone beam computed tomography machine
    for, 315, 316f–317f
  definition of, 313
  disadvantages of, 321–322
  equipment for, 314–317
  fundamentals of, 313–314
  patient positioning for, 319, 320f
  patient preparation for, 319
  procedures for, 319
  terminology for, 313
  uses of, 317–319
  viewing software for, 315–317
Three-dimensional volume rendering, definition
  of, 313
Threshold curve, 36f
Thyroid collar, in radiation protection, 48–50,
  50f
Thyroid gland, dental radiation risks to, 41
Time, film processing problems associated with,
  101t, 102f–103f, 103
Timer, for film processing, 91, 94t
Tire-track pattern, 235, 235f
Tissue(s)
  radiation effects on, 37–38, 37t–38t
  soft, on panoramic images, 363–365, 366f
TMJ. *See* Temporomandibular joint (TMJ).
Tomogram, 287
Tomography
  definition of, 287
  in panoramic imaging, 257–258
  transmandibular joint, 287
Tongue
  on panoramic image, 364, 366f
  positioning of, in panoramic imaging, 265,
    270f

Tooth-bearing areas, definition of, 153
Tooth (teeth)
  anatomy of, 340–342
  anterior, exposure sequence for
    in bisecting technique, 187, 187t
    in paralleling technique, 159–162, 162f, 162t
  dentin of, 340, 340f
  dentino-enamel junction of, 340, 340f
  enamel of, 340, 340f
  impacted, three-dimensional digital imaging for, 317, 318f
  long axis of, 156, 156f, 181, 181f
  positioning of, in panoramic imaging, 266, 267f–269f
  posterior, exposure sequence for
    in bisecting technique, 187–188, 187t
    in paralleling technique, 162–163, 163t
  pulp cavity of, 340, 340f
  structure of, 340, 340f
  supporting structures of, 340–342, 341f
Topical anesthetic, for gag reflex, 292
Torus
  bite-wing technique modifications for, 223
  paralleling technique modifications for, 173–174, 174f–175f
Total filtration, in radiation protection, 46
Traditional system of radiation measurement, 39, 39t
Transcranial projection, in temporomandibular joint imaging, 282–287, 287f
Transformer, 14, 17, 17f
Trauma, image interpretation of, 426–428, 427f–428f
Treatment area, infection control for, 143, 144b
Triangle
  congruent, definition of, 181, 181f
  definition of, 181, 181f
  equilateral, definition of, 181, 181f
  right, definition of, 181, 181f
Tube side of film packet, 67
Tubehead, 14–15, 14f–15f, 58, 59f
  of panoramic x-ray machine, 259, 260f
Tubehead seal, 14
Tubercle(s)
  articular, 359
  definition of, 327
  genial, 327f
    on intraoral images, 327f, 335–336, 336f
    on panoramic image, 362, 362f–363f
Tuberosity
  definition of, 327
  maxillary, 328f
    on intraoral image, 328f, 334, 334f
    on panoramic image, 358f, 359, 361f
Tungsten filament in cathode, 16
Tungsten target, in anode, 16, 16f

U
Ultra-Speed film, 50
Underexposed receptor, 227–228, 228f
Unexposed receptor, 227, 227f
Uni-bite film holder, 59–60, 60f
Unilocular corticated lesion, 374, 374f
Unilocular noncorticated lesion, 374, 375f
Unilocular radiolucent lesions, 374–375
Unmodified scatter, 20
Uvula, on panoramic image, 364, 366f

V
Van Woert, Frank, intraoral film use and, 5
Velocity of electromagnetic radiation, 12

Verbal communication skills, in patient relations, 125–126
Vertical angulation
  in bisecting technique, 183–185, 184f–186f, 185t
    problems with, 184–185, 185f–186f
  in bite-wing technique, 212f, 214, 215f–216f
    incorrect, 232, 232f
  definition of, 228–229
  in localization techniques, 242
  negative, 214, 215f
  for occlusal projections, 242, 242t
  in periapical technique, incorrect, 229, 230f
  positive, 214, 215f
Vertical bite-wing, 222, 222f–223f
  definition of, 212
Vertical bone loss, 415, 416f
Victor CDX shockproof tube housing, 5, 5f
Viewbox, 352, 353f
  quality control tests for, 113, 113f
Viewing
  of dental radiographs, 352–355
  of digital images, speed of, 308
Viewing software, for three-dimensional digital imaging, 315–317, 317f
Visible image, 88
  from latent image to, 87–88
Vision impairment, 292
Voltage, 17
  x-ray beam quality and, 27
Volts (V), 17
Voxels
  definition of, 313
  spatial resolution and, 315

W
Walkhoff, Otto, first dental radiograph made by, 4–5
Warmth, in patient relations, 126–127
Washing, in film processing, manual, 89
Waste, infectious, definition of, 141
Waste management, in darkroom, 99
Water compartment, of automatic processor, 96, 96f
Waters projection, in extraoral imaging, 278t, 282, 284f
Wave concept, 12–13
Wavelength, 12–13, 13f
Wired intraoral sensor, 304, 304f
Wireless intraoral sensor, 304
Work area
  in darkroom, 98–99
  infection control and, 143

X
X-radiation, 13–14. See also Radiation.
  definition of, 2
  definitions of, 19
  discovery of, 3–4
  interactions of, 19–20, 19f
  production of, 17–19, 18f
X-ray(s)
  definition of, 3, 373
  discovery of, 3–4
  properties of, 14, 14b
  radiograph/dental image versus, 373
  types of, 18–19
X-ray beam
  alignment of. See X-ray beam alignment.
  amperage and, 29
  cone-shaped, in cone beam computed tomography, 313, 313f

X-ray beam (Continued)
  distance and, 30–31
  exposure time and, 30
  half-value layer and, 32
  intensity of, 30–32
  inverse square law and, 31–32, 31b, 31f
  kilovoltage and, 27
  kilovoltage peak and, 27
    contrast and, 28, 28t, 29f
    density and, 27–28, 28f, 28t
    exposure time and, 29, 29b
    intensity and, 30
  milliamperage and, 29
    density and, 30, 30t
    exposure time and, 30, 30t
    intensity and, 30
  milliampere-seconds and, 29–30
  polychromatic, 27
  quality of, 27–29
  quantity of, 29–30
  voltage and, 27
X-ray beam alignment
  devices for. See Beam alignment devices.
  in extraoral imaging
    for lateral cephalometric projection, 282
    for lateral jaw projections, 277
    for posteroanterior projection, 282
    for reverse Towne projection, 282
    for submentovertex projection, 282
    for transcranial projection, 287
    for Waters projection, 282
X-ray beam angulation, image distortion and, 81t, 83, 83f
X-ray equipment. See Equipment and supplies; X-ray machine(s).
X-ray film. See Film.
X-ray generating apparatus, 16–17
X-ray image, 76–85. See also Image(s).
X-ray machine(s), 14–17, 57–59
  component parts of, 14–15, 14f, 57–59, 59f
  control devices of, 59
  control panel of, 58–59
  for digital imaging, 303, 304f
  exposure button of, 59
  extension arm of, 58
  extraoral, 58, 58f, 275, 275f
  infection control and, 143
  intraoral, 58, 58f
  on-off switch of, 59
  panoramic, 258–259, 258f, 260f–261f
  performance standards for, 57
  quality control tests for, 112, 112b
  tubehead of, 58, 59f
  types of, 58
X-ray tube, 14–16, 15f–16f
XCP beam alignment devices, 61, 61f
XCP Bite-Block, 59–60, 60f
XCP Universal Collimator, 61, 61f

Y
Yellow-brown stains on film, 101t, 103, 103f

Z
Zygoma
  on intraoral image, 335, 335f–336f
  on panoramic image, 358f, 360, 361f
Zygomatic process of maxilla
  on intraoral image, 334–335, 335f
  on panoramic image, 358f, 360, 360f